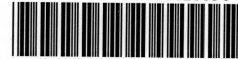

The
Inconstant Gene

The Evolution and Functioning of the Genetic Mechanism

LAWRENCE S. DILLON

The Genetic Mechanism and the Origin of Life
Ultrastructure, Macromolecules, and Evolution
The Inconstant Gene

The
Inconstant Gene

LAWRENCE S. DILLON

Texas A & M University
College Station, Texas

PLENUM PRESS · NEW YORK AND LONDON

Library of Congress Cataloging in Publication Data

Dillon, Lawrence S.
  The inconstant gene.

  Bibliography: p.
  Includes index.
  1. Gene expression. 2. Genetic regulation. I. Title. [DNLM: 1. Gene expression
regulation. QH 450 D579i]
QH450.D54 1982   574.87′322   82-20414
ISBN 0-306-41084-2

© 1983 Plenum Press, New York
A Division of Plenum Publishing Corporation
233 Spring Street, New York, N.Y. 10013

Printed in the United States of America

Preface

Why should the gene be suggested to be inconstant when the contrary view, that gene structure is invariant except through mutagenic processes induced by potent external factors, has long been a universal doctrine of genetics? Indeed, during the early part of the present century before mutation was recognized as being of general occurrence, the seeming unvarying nature of the gene led to skepticism regarding the validity of the evolutionary theory; only later could the origins of the morphological differences between individuals and species be attributed to a combination of mutation and evolution, involving natural forces selecting between favorable and unfavorable genetic changes. But during the past several decades, as knowledge of the macromolecular constitution of organisms has increased to the point where even the primary structures of the genes themselves are being revealed on a routine basis, it has become increasingly difficult to ascribe all the resulting observations to ordinary mutagenesis and natural selection. Some more profound mechanism often seems to be present that influences both the constancy and inconstancy of the genes, an apparatus whose existence this study hopes to reveal.

In seeking to demonstrate the universality of this mechanism, data are sought through the numerous activities of organisms of many types wherever gene action changes are manifest. Since the ontogenies of multicellular organisms, and to a lesser extent, even unicellular ones, are replete with such alterations in gene expression, the search for facts commences at the very start of the reproductive processes by examining the formative steps of ova and sperm and continues through fertilization into the development and differentiation of the individual into the adult form. But as the changes do not cease at birth or hatching but carry on through the full life cycle, the nature of senescence likewise receives attention.

In contrast to the often long-term changes wrought during ontogeny, organisms experience rhythmic fluctuations in gene actions of a diversity of types. At the multicellular level of organization at least, the diurnal modulations are of both qualitative and quantitative nature, and are frequently so extensive that is has been stated that an organism is completely different at midnight than it is at noon. Regrettably, the fields of circadian and circannual rhythms are found fuller of promise for the future than valuable at the present, insofar as the nature of the involved gene changes is concerned, for the necessary explorations at the macromolecular level are still too insufficient in quantity to be convincing.

However, the final topic to be searched for supportive data, gene changes during immune reactions, more than compensates for this lack. As a consequence of researches conducted in literally hundreds of laboratories scattered over the face of the earth, the immunoglobulins and their coding regions in the genome have become the most thoroughly investigated macromolecules of today. The results of these studies, combined with others, make amply clear both the invariable and inconstant nature of the gene. But the facts supplied by the two previous studies in this trilogy, as well as all those contained in this one, are essential to a full appreciation of the mechanism that is involved in governing the behavior of the usual DNA–RNA protein system.

Like the two preceding components, the present one is not to be considered merely a review of the literature but rather an analysis of the existing state of knowledge. Because of the in-depth approach into a number of biological disciplines concerned in diverse ways with changes in gene expression, many novel points of view are presented. As in the other studies, areas requiring more intensive investigation are brought to light, and weaknesses in interpreting results of experimental researches have had to be pointed out. Far too frequently in the literature, broad generalizations are advanced, based on very limited data, and these superficial hypotheses do not withstand thorough scrutiny.

The assistance of a large number of scientists has been required for the completion of this book, most of whom happily can be acknowledged individually in association with the light or electron micrographs they have generously supplied. But the author hopes that the others who have contributed in diverse ways will know that their contribution is also deeply appreciated, although they cannot be named individually here. Conversations with a number of colleagues here at Texas A&M University and elsewhere have aided in clarifying the author's views, those with Drs. Sydney W. Fox, of Miami University, Dennis Opheim, of Quinnepiac College, and Donald Killebrew, of the University of Texas at Tyler, being especially profitable. Special thanks are also extended to Galen Jennings for suggesting the title for this work. Finally as always, my wife has been the most indispensable aid of all in collaborating with me throughout the long search of the literature, tedious preparation of the manuscript and illustrations, and interpretation of the data.

LAWRENCE S. DILLON

Contents

1

Gene Action Changes in Gametogenesis

Probably nowhere else are gene action changes so rampant as they are during those earliest stages in the developmental histories of organisms represented by the preparation of the gametes. In the formation of the egg and sperm, generalized cells become converted to types highly specialized for their respective functions. While the specializations of the spermatozoon are obvious features, those of the ovum, although not evident on the surface, are no less marked internally, as becomes even more apparent in the next two chapters. For only during and following fertilization into early development does the remarkable internal organization that exists in the egg cell become revealed. Then, too, the best indicators of gene expression changes, alterations in protein profiles, are manifested. Here then in the present discussion, one must largely be content with changes in the fine structural characteristics and similar topics that merely imply, rather than clearly demonstrate, the activation of new genes and the abandonment of former ones.

Since this is thus the first of several chapters concerned with the nature of gene expression during development from the gametes to adulthood and senescence, the method of employing certain broad terms needs to be made clear. This is especially necessitated by the wide spectrum of organisms that are viewed, including fungi to green plants and metazoans, and even bacteria on a few occasions where they are appropriate. Inevitably, in the literature a certain few of the terms have been loosely applied or given different senses in the several taxa. Development, for example, is a nonspecific word, equally applicable to the changes found in the embryo, fetus, neonatal, or adult. Thus, development of the individual, or ontogeny, is considered to consist of the following stages:

1. Gametogenesis, the development of specific gametes from unspecialized germ plasm or other cells.
2. Fertilization, the union of gametes of opposite types.
3. Embryogenesis, the events following fertilization to the point where the anlagen of the organs have been established.
4. Differentiation, the development of diverse tissues from the relatively unspecialized cells of the embryo.

The latter, perhaps, is the most inclusive stage of ontogeny, for it embraces fetal and neonatal changes in most vertebrates, the larval periods and the metamorphoses in metazoans as a whole, and metagenesis and pregermination events in the metaphytans. Regeneration, too, is perceived as representing a special facet of this topic, during which lost appendages or other body parts are re-formed. The latter aspect is to be distinguished from aggregation, in which groups of free individual cells congregate and differentiate to produce organs or whole organisms, as in fungi and sponges, respectively. Likewise, sporulation involves differentiation of specialized cells from others of a contrasting nature. Finally, age-associated differentiation, or maturation and senescence, follows birth, metamorphosis, germination, or hatching and continues until the death of the organism, gerontology being a subdivision that deals with those modifications associated with advanced years.

1.1. GAMETOGENESIS IN GENERAL

The very first step in the development of the individual is the preparation of the reproductive cells, or gametes, typically ova and spermatozoa. One important cytological event appears to be a universal feature, that of reducing the chromosome number from the diploid condition, in which pairs of homologous chromosomes are present, to the haploid, in which each chromosomal type is represented only once. Meiosis, then, the processes of which carry out the reduction steps, is one of the few activities common to the preparation of eggs and sperm alike; however, this event may occur in widely disparate times of the life cycle in the several taxa, and thus is not always a particular aspect of gametogenesis.

1.1.1. Meiosis

As a whole, the processes of meiotic division of the nucleus in metazoans and metaphytans are not greatly different from those of ordinary mitosis, one of the most apparent distinctions being the occurrence of two complete division cycles in close sequence, with little or no interphase intervening. The second division is identical to mitosis in fact, except for minor details of chromosomal behavior, but the first one contains a number of unusual features. Of these, the most prominent and important occur at the onset of division, so that prophase consists of a series of substages. Typically five such subdivisions are distinguishable, with a sixth one added at the very beginning in a few special cases.

Prophase I. In the usual first substage of prophase I, referred to as the leptotene (Figure 1.1B), the chromosomes are scarcely condensed, so that they appear long and threadlike and are devoid of coils. Although replication of the DNA they contain has already occurred in the preceding S phase, they appear to be unpaired. Towards the latter portion of this substage, the chromosomes are in the form of loose loops and are attached at each end to one region of the nuclear envelope, usually adjacent to the centriolar region. This attachment probably is a continuation of an interphase condition, for all chromosomes appear to be permanently associated at their termini with the envelope, except during division in metaphytans, metazoans, and others, when the latter breaks down.

The second subdivision, zygotene, is characterized by the homologous pairs of chromosomes being brought together and corresponding regions aligned point-by-point (Figure 1.1C). Viewed in its essentials, this synapsis formation often appears to begin at the ends attached to the nuclear envelope, but it may seem to commence at the kinetochore or other region, from where it proceeds in zipperlike fashion throughout the length of the structure. When isolated in this substage, the chromosomes, still threadlike and elongate, have been found to be poorly condensed, with strands of chromatin forming loose mats around them (Wolfe and John, 1965).

Pachytene, the third substage, is more readily observed than the two preceding, for at this point the chromosomes are more fully condensed and appear as the characteristic rods, although more elongate than in later stages (Figure 1.1D, E). Frequently the members of each homologous pair are coiled around one another, so that their dual nature is not readily perceived.

This close association is relaxed at the next substage, diplotene, so that the individual chromatids comprising each pair are more plainly visible, the tetrads becoming apparent accordingly (Figure 1.1F). The dual chromosomes, or bivalents, are held together at points where one of the chromatids crosses over the other, as many as 12 such chiasmata being present occasionally. Although typically a chiasma forms between only one chromatid of each homologous pair, only nonsister elements thus being involved, chiasmata do occur between sister chromatids (Alves and Jonasson, 1978; Conner *et al.*, 1979; Kanda and Kato, 1979; Kato, 1979; Jonasson *et al.*, 1980; Lin, 1980). Between pachytene and diplotene, there frequently is a diffuse phase, in which the bivalents elongate and loosen, so that they appear fuzzy (Moens, 1968). During diplotene, or perhaps earlier, breakage and rejoining occurs at each chiasma, permitting recombination of genetic information to take place. Some evidence exists which indicates that an enzyme, DNA synaptase, mediates the fusing of DNA molecules at regions of homology, at least in bacteria (Potter and Dressler, 1980). While homologs seemingly are often held together as tetrads

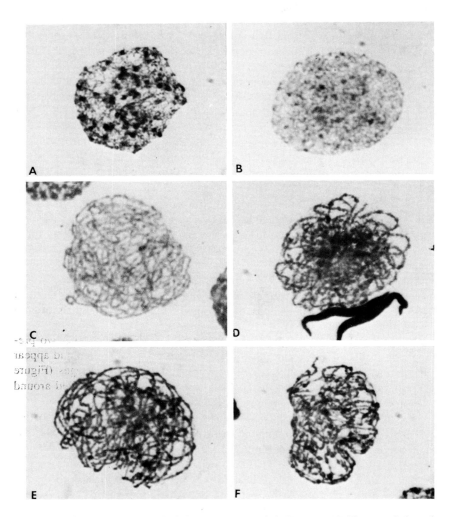

Figure 1.1. Major stages in meiosis during spermatogenesis in *Xenopus*. (A) The premeiotic nucleus exhibits numerous heterochromatic clumps. (B) In the early leptotene stage the chromatin is thin and fine, with a few remnant heterochromatic clumps. (C) Late zygotene nucleus with the chromosomes in synapsis. (D) Thickened loops of chromatin characterize the pachytene nucleus. The dark bodies are sperm heads. (E) At late pachytene the nucleus displays the characteristic bouquet configuration. (F) During diplotene the sets of chromosomes begin to separate. All squash preparations; 1800×. (Courtesy of Kalt, 1976.)

by these chiasmata, they can unite and remain as pairs even in the absence of such structures, as in male *Drosophila* and certain other metazoans (Brown and Bertke, 1974). As becomes apparent shortly, the adherence is not due so much to the chiasmata proper but to the presence of special organelles described in a following paragraph.

In diakinesis, the last special subdivision, the chromatids shorten and assume their definitive form, while the nucleolus detaches from the chromosomes and disappears, at least in many metazoans. Among metaphytans its disappearance does not occur until just before metaphase I. During this stage, a process called terminalization may often be noted, in which the location of chiasmata migrates outwards on each arm of the chromatids away from the kinetochore.

The Synaptonemal Complex. In metazoans in which chiasmata and subsequent crossing over occur, a striking apparatus, referred to as the synaptonemal complex, is present at least from zygotene to diplotene, but often through much of the division processes in altered form. Each such structure is a narrow ribbon, bordered on the sides by a thin, electron-opaque plate, and contains an actinlike substance called protein C (Hofstein *et al.*, 1980). At one end, the complex is attached to the nuclear envelope, where a small, dense plate occurs, and between the members of a tetrad at the other (Kalt, 1973). Some variation is found among various taxa, as in the spermatids of certain insects (Schin, 1965; Sotelo and Wettstein, 1966), green plants (Stack, 1973), and fungi (Lu 1967; Garber and Aist, 1979). However, the complexes appear to be universally present among eukaryotes, for they have been reported even from yeasts, the chromatin of which does not condense into chromosomes (Byers and Goetsch, 1975; Horesh *et al.*, 1979).

As becomes apparent later in the present discussion, the synaptonemal complex seems to be of great importance in such genetic events as crossing over, recombination, and sister chromatid cohesiveness (Maguire, 1979); consequently, currently it forms the focus of an extremely active field of research (Figure 1.2). The results of the ensuing rapid progress naturally are sometimes conflicting, or at best, subject to differing interpretations that time alone can sort out and make firm. At least in *Drosophila*, the complex was shown not to be of uniform construction throughout its length, but within a given chromosome the heterochromatic (central) portions differed structurally from the euchromatic (distal) (Carpenter, 1975a). In the latter sector its central element was comprised of two fine bars that were interconnected by a close-set series of cross-bars. At a short distance on each side was a somewhat thicker, more electron-opaque plate, much less regular in configuration than the central structure. Contrastingly, in the heterochromatic region, the synaptonemal complex was less well defined, especially the central element, which seemed to be more amorphous; the lateral plates, however, were thicker and more diffuse and each was connected to the central part by irregular transverse filaments. The latter varied both in thickness and in orientation, being squarely transverse in some

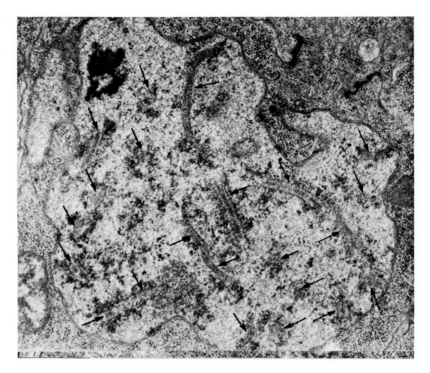

Figure 1.2. Synaptonemal complexes in *Drosophila melanogaster*. In this section of an early pachytene nucleus, the arrows indicate synaptonemal complexes in various planes of section. 18,000×. (Courtesy of Carpenter, 1975a.)

instances and strongly oblique in others. As a given complex was associated with only a single major arm of a chromosome in *D. melanogaster,* there was a total of five—one each for the right and left arms of both chromosomes 2 and 3 and one for the single arm of the X, but none for the minute chromosome 4. The complexes attained their maximum lengths at early pachytene, diminishing gradually thence until at diplotene they were only half as long. In contrast, in the crane fly *Pales ferruginea*, a form which lacks leptotene and zygotene stages, these structures were much longer in diplotene than in pachytene (Figure 1.3A, C; Fuge, 1979). As the chromosomes began to undergo desynapsis later in this stage, the synaptonemal complex broke down, and the resulting subunits crystallized into so-called polycomplexes. Quite similar behavior of these organelles has been reported also in Chinese hamster spermatocytes (Pathak *et al.*, 1979; Dresser and Moses, 1980). The polycomplexes remained associated with sister chromatids in metaphase I of certain insects, dissociating from them only at anaphase I (Moens and Church, 1979).

Although the dual nature of the central element is not always apparent, depending upon the plane of the section, that condition has been noted in the aquatic fungi, *Allomyces macrogynus* and *Catenaria allomycis* (Borkhardt and Olson, 1979; Sykes and Porter, 1981). In these forms the dual long plates of the central element were interconnected by a few widely spaced bars, and a

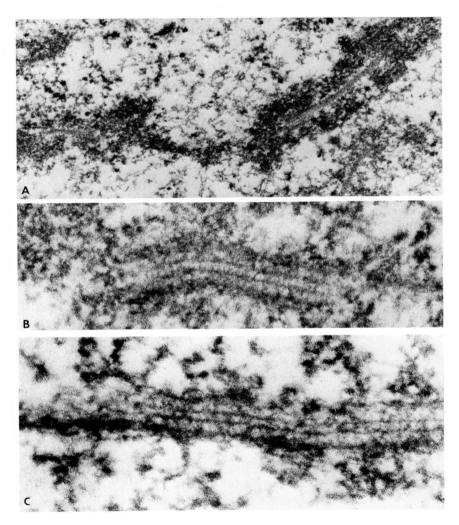

Figure 1.3. Synaptonemal complexes in the crane fly *Pales ferruginea*. (A) Two synaptic regions in a single bivalent during early prophase. 40,000×. (B) Structure of the synaptonemal complex in early prophase. 150,000×. (C) Same as (B), but in diplotene. 150,000×. (All courtesy of Fuge, 1979.)

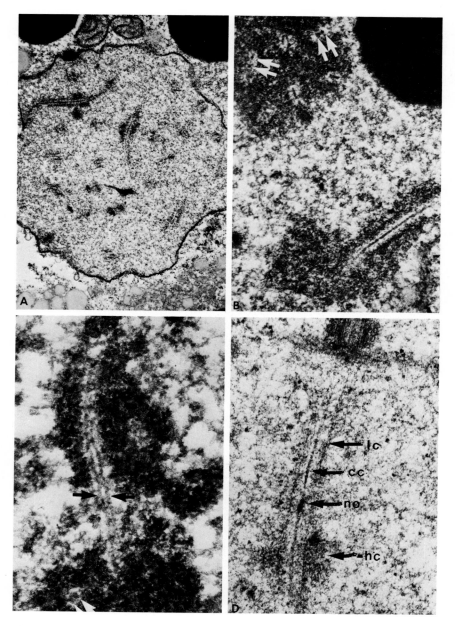

Figure 1.4. Synaptonemal complex structure in *Allomyces macrogynus*. (A) Appearance of the synaptonemal complex at midpachytene. 13,000×. (B) Higher magnification view of the complex at early pachytene. White arrows indicate cross sections of these structures showing two central

similar paucity of interconnections was evident between them and the lateral bars (Figure 1.4A–D). The latter were even more irregular in outline than those of *Drosophila* and also thicker and more variable in density.

Another feature of synaptonemal complexes that has been reported from diverse species is provided by the recombination nodules that are spaced along the central elements (Carpenter, 1975b; Moses *et al.*, 1979). Two types of these bodies have now been described in *Drosophila*, spherical and ellipsoidal; the latter has its long axis lying along that of the central element, whose width this type scarcely exceeds (Carpenter, 1979a). The spherical form varies widely in diameter, but it correlates closely numerically both with the number of reciprocal exchange events per nucleus, and with the presence and magnitude of chiasma interference. Hence, this class of nodules appears to mark sites of exchange of segments between chromosomes. This involvement in crossing over and related phenomena has been further confirmed through use of recombination-defective *Drosophila* mutant forms (Carpenter, 1979b). These mutations also exhibited similar effects during mitosis of somatic cells in both sexes, suggesting that the complexes or comparable structures were active there also (Baker *et al.*, 1978) as has been clearly demonstrated in mouse cerebral cortical cells (Bird, 1980). Moreover, they have been shown to be present at meiotic interphase in mouse spermatocytes (Grell *et al.*, 1980). Since the recombination nodules differ in shape from taxon to taxon, however, it is difficult at this time to infer the respective functions of the two types from their shape on a comparative basis; for example, in *Neurospora* the size of both types varied so greatly that considerable overlap in length occurred (Gillies, 1979), and a similar condition appeared to prevail in *Chlamydomonas* (Storms and Hastings, 1977).

The Remaining Events. The remainder of the meiotic steps show few noteworthy differences from those of mitosis (Dillon, 1981, pp. 525–550). During prometaphase, the nuclear membrane breaks down, the spindle develops, and the chromosomes are moved about, finally becoming aligned on the metaphase plate. In addition, in plants the nucleolus disappears at this point. One difference from ordinary nuclear division which occurs in animal cells at meiosis is that the kinetochores of homologs are separate, permitting the opposite members of each bivalent to move apart somewhat, so that each projects off the plane of the equatorial plate. Complete separation, however, is prevented by persistent chiasmata or synaptonemal complexes. Moreover, the chromatids appear to be single in spite of their dual composition, a condition

---

components. 32,000×. (C) Longitudinal section through a complex at the same stage as (B), in which two central components are visible (black arrows). 50,000×. (D) In this longitudinal section of a complex at pachytene, two poorly defined lateral components (1c) are visible, along with a tripartite central region containing an electron-opaque central component (cc) bordered by a transparent band on each side. In addition, recombination nodes (no), a heterochromatic knob (hc), and a centriole are discernible. 45,000×. (All courtesy of Borkhardt and Olson, 1979.)

that prevails into early anaphase I. In the latter phase, the chromosomal homologs are pulled towards opposite poles, often notwithstanding the chiasmata resisting such separation and consequently greatly elongating some of the chromosomal arms.

Telophase I may involve the relaxation of the chromosomes or not, depending on the species, so that anaphase I may lead almost directly into prophase II or even prometaphase II. Beyond the latter point, nothing of pertinence is to be noted.

Premeiotic Mitosis. Evidence has accumulated from metaphytan and fungal sources that indicates the occurrence of some of the events characteristic of meiosis during the last mitotic division preceding those processes. In seed plants, pairing of homologs appears to commence in prometaphase of the premeiotic division cycle and then to continue through the ensuing anaphase (Smith, 1942; Brown and Stack, 1968; Grell *et al.*, 1980). Moreover, the pairs remain associated during the succeeding interphase, at least in *Plantago* (Stack and Brown, 1969). Similar premeiotic pairing has been reported also in a number of fungi, including members of the genera *Neurospora* (Singleton, 1953), *Neottiella* (Rossen and Westergaard, 1966), and *Preussia* (Kowalski, 1965, 1966), in which it takes place during the interphase preceding meiosis, rather than during mitosis. Thus, no possible phylogenetic relationships are indicated by these two comparable, but unidentical, processes. Similar pairing of homologous chromosomes is not an uncommon event even in somatic tissues, having been reported from newt and other animal tissues (Boss, 1954, 1955). Whether synapsis follows the formation of pairs in the premeiotic division has not been firmly established, but it seems to do so in some fungi (Rossen and Westergaard, 1966). However, in the fruiting bodies of *Coprinus,* union of the gametic nuclei (karyogamy) leads immediately to synapsis and the rest of the meiotic steps (Lu and Raju, 1970).

1.1.2. Early Gametogenesis

As in meiosis, the precise sequence of events varies to some degree from one taxon to another, although the basic processes are remarkably uniform (Hardisty, 1978). Since the details have been worked out most extensively in higher vertebrates, they serve as the primary models, descriptions from a comparative standpoint being provided later to indicate some of the more important deviations from the standard pattern.

Primordial Germ Cells. Variations are rampant, too, in the formation of the primordial germ cells that eventually give rise to either eggs or sperm. As a general rule in the vertebrates, they can be identified at an early stage by their large size and their low nucleus-to-cytoplasm ratio (Jordon, 1917) and by their frequent location in the midgut or hindgut. From there they migrate through the gut mesentery to a site on the genital ridge between the parietal peritoneum and the developing mesonephric kidney. The region surrounding the primordial germ cells then undergoes differentiation, at first into a simple gonad or ovotestis, containing both ovarian and testicular structures. Later in females, the outer portion, or cortex, gives rise to an ovary, whereas in males, the central, medullary portion differentiates into a testis, the other parts in each case undergoing degeneration to a greater or lesser extent.

Although at first primordial germ cells range from 10 to 25 μm, they gradually become reduced in size, both through division and loss of yolk. To cite a specific case, the cells of the 7-day embryo of *Xenopus*, then still in the genital ridge, average 25 μm in diameter but become reduced to about 20 μm at day 12, possibly due to loss of yolk (Ijiri and Egami, 1975). By 53 days, this dimension has been reduced to 15 μm, chiefly through cleavage. These cells in anuran amphibians have an additional distinctive characteristic in the form of so-called germinal plasm that has enabled their origin in the zygote to be traced. This trait is provided by granular islets of yolk-free cytoplasm that possesses characteristic staining properties and is closely associated with aggregates of mitochondria (Bournoure, 1939; Blackler, 1970). In addition, electron microscopic studies have demonstrated the existence of electron-dense cylinders, mostly about 30 to 40 nm in diameter, that are referred to as nuage (Czolowska, 1972; Ikenishi *et al.*, 1974). These were closely associated with mitochondrial clusters and appeared to consist of short fibrils and densely placed granules.

Formation of Primordial Germ Cells. In the fertilized egg from which the embryo had developed, the islets described in the preceding paragraph were scattered through the subcortical layer of the lower portion of the vegetal pole, but with the commencement of cleavage, they gradually coalesced as they moved upwards along the forming furrows. At the second cleavage, all blastomeres contained some germinal plasm, but after the first horizontal division, those of the animal pole were found to no longer possess any. As cleavage progressed further, the granular islets eventually became confined to a small number of cells derived from four blastomeres that had been located between the blastocoel and vegetal pole. This number then remained constant, for, although 11 or 12 mitoses followed, division was carried out in such a fashion that only one of each pair of daughter cells received the germinal plasm (Whitington and Dixon, 1975). However, between the gastrula and neurula stages, the number of these primordial germ cells was increased by ordinary mitosis from about 5 to 14 (Dziadek and Dixon, 1975).

Although the topic is not especially pertinent to the present account, it should be noted that the origin of these cells in the anurans is by no means consistent throughout the vertebrates. In sharks and rays, they seemed to arise in the extraembryonic endoderm (Woods, 1902), as they may also in certain teleost and holostean fishes (Allen, 1911; Richards and Thompson, 1921), but in other teleosts, such as *Gambusia,* they formed around the dorsal lip of the blastopore (Pala, 1970). Among avian species, as represented by the chicken, they were localized in endoderm anterior and lateral to the embryo proper in a region near the junction of the area pellucida and vitelline wall (Benoit, 1930; Simon, 1960); however, much variation has been shown to exist from species to species (Fargeix, 1966; Bruel, 1973). The mammalian site of origin proved equally variable with the species, but these cells often first appeared in the yolk sac endoderm as already mentioned or in the splanchnic mesoderm around the base of the allantois (Vanneman, 1917; Ozdzenski, 1967; Spiegelman and Bennett, 1973).

More Mature Primordial Germ Cells. As they undergo further development, the primordial germ cells of mammals change from their smooth, spheroidal or ovate conformation in the yolk sac to an amoeboid type with blunt pseudopodia as they enter the mesenchyme. Once within the germinal epithelium, however, the smooth spheroidal form is reassumed. Few ultrastructural features are especially distinctive, aside from the germinal plasm. Endoreticulum is sparse (Spiegelman and Bennett, 1973), and dictyosomes are only moderately abundant. In contrast to the aggregates found in anuran primordial germ cells, mitochondria are not numerous in those of mammals, but the nuage is present, as in the germinal plasm of frogs. The mitochondria frequently are subovate, often to the point of being spheroidal, and contain cristae that are irregular in form and few in number.

1.2. OOGENESIS

The production of female gametes (Figure 1.5), oogenesis, is at once a simpler and more complex process than its counterpart, the production of sperm. It is simpler in that the resulting ova undergo less marked changes in form than spermatozoa, but far more complicated in development of its genome and macromolecular content. For although the egg is an undifferentiated cell in that it eventually gives rise to all parts of the resulting organism, it is highly specialized for its function of development.

1.2.1. The Cell Generations

The Oogonia. Following their migration to the developing ovary, the primary germ cells of vertebrates are at first associated with the surface (coelomic) epithelium. At this time the female gonad is a diffusely cellular organ comprised of a mixture of the tissue just mentioned and mesenchymal elements, along with the primitive sex cells. As the ovarian tissues become more organized, the primordial germ cells move into the cortex, accompanied by supporting epithelial cells, in the form of "cords" (Gondos, 1978). Once within the interior, the minute cells, now referred to as oogonia, undergo proliferation

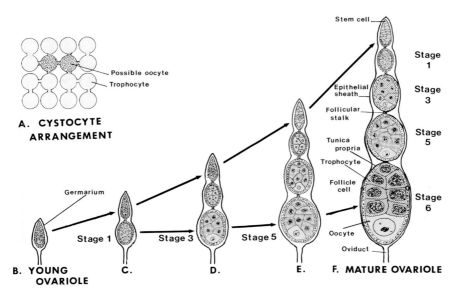

Figure 1.5. Development of the oocyte and ovariole in *Drosophila*.

by ordinary mitosis, the cords elongating accordingly. This close association between oogonia and the epithelium is continued throughout the later maturation of the ova in the form of the oocyte–granulosa cell relationship described in a subsequent section (p. 36).

In ultrastructural details, oogonia scarcely differ from the primary germ cells, except that now they lack the pseudopodia noted earlier. Mitochondria appear to be slightly less abundant but still retain their primitive spheroidal form; however, the cristae often appear to be of the microvillose rather than the flattened-sac type (Gondos, 1978), and they are more uniformly distributed throughout the cytoplasm, packets being absent. Another distinctive feature is provided by the intercellular bridges between adjacent oogonia that result from not-quite-complete separation of daughter cells during mitotic division. These and other provisions for intercellular communication (Figure 1.6), which do not exist in the primordial germ cells, are believed to function in synchronizing groups of the oogonia during the steps of oogenesis (Gondos and Zamboni, 1969; Moens and Go, 1972), because all members of each such group have been found to be in identical stages of development (Gondos, 1970).

One activity that appears to be synchronized by intercellular communication is division, for groups of the cells divide in unison, clusters of mitotic figures often being observed as proliferation proceeds. The period of duration of oogonial multiplication varies considerably, even among the higher mam-

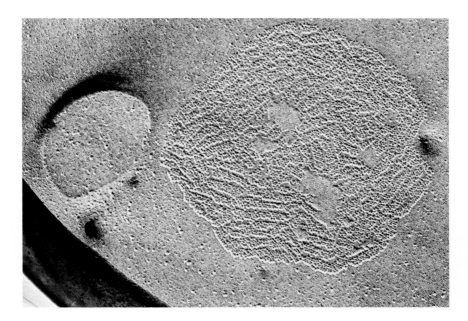

Figure 1.6. Gap junctions of rat granulosa cells. While intercellular bridges unite adjacent oogonia, the associated granulosa cells communicate with one another by way of such connectives as these gap junctions. 75,000×. (Unpublished electron micrograph, courtesy of Robert C. Burghardt.)

mals. In such forms in which oogonia persist postnatally as the rabbit, all germ cells of female neonatals are oogonia, but all become transformed into the succeeding cell type (oocytes) by the 10th day (Peters *et al.*, 1965). In the mouse, in which proliferation has ceased by the end of term, at 13 days postpartum 95% of the ovarian germ cells are oogonia (Figure 1.7), at day 14 only 43%, and by day 17 none remain (Peters *et al.*, 1962). A similar condition prevails in human beings; consequently, many of these cells are several decades old before they undergo maturation and ovulation. What controls the commencement and termination of proliferation remains undetermined, but gonadotropic hormones do not seem to be involved (Baker and Neal, 1973, 1974; Challoner, 1975). The results of this period of cell reproduction are best illustrated by the human being; while only 1700 primordial germ cells migrate to the pair of ovaries, by the eighth week of gestation these have increased to 600,000, and by the fifth month have reached 7,000,000, at which point mitosis of these cells ceases (Baker and O, 1976). Many of these, however, undergo degeneration as described in a later section.

The Primary Oocytes. The primary oocytes that mature from the oogonia differ from the latter in several traits, the most outstanding of which is

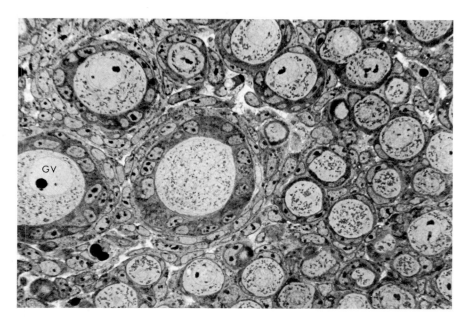

Figure 1.7. Mouse ovary at birth. This section reveals the numerous stages of development of the female gametes at birth. GV, germinal vesicle. 535×. (Unpublished micrograph, courtesy of Robert C. Burghardt.)

the nucleus. This structure becomes greatly enlarged and is given the name germinal vesicle because of its resemblance to a vacuole; its envelope contains rather numerous pores, and perinuclear spaces between the two membranous components are frequent. Mitochondria, rounded as in earlier stages, are conspicuously plentiful, the relatively few cristae in each being of the flattened-sac type (Figure 1.8A, B). Only a single dictyosome is present orginally, but as the oocyte matures this undergoes frequent divisions to become quite abundant (Baca and Zamboni, 1967). Endoreticulum is entirely of the rough vesicular type in the early period; after diplotene, however, the multilayered cisternal kind becomes evident, as do multivesicular bodies, the remnants of lysosomes (Dillon, 1981, pp. 285–290).

Undoubtedly the most important distinctive feature of the primary oocyte is the occurrence of meiotic division. In many mammalian species the usual first stage of these processes is preceded by a preleptotene stage in which the chromosomes first undergo condensation and then relaxation (often called decondensation), a trait that occurs also in cells which do not progress to meiosis (Mauléon, 1975; Mauléon et al., 1976). As a rule in mammals, meiosis begins in the midterm fetus, progressing through the several stages of prophase I to

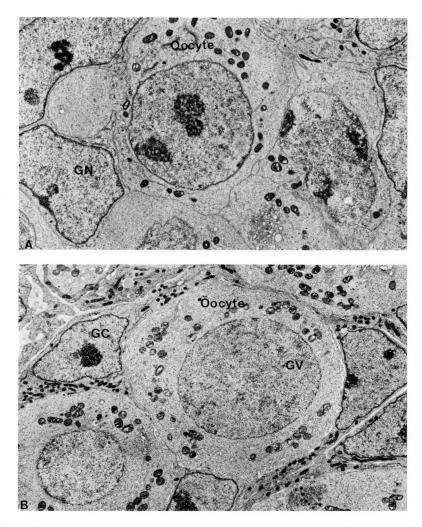

Figure 1.8. Stages in the development of the follicle. (A) In the early stages of follicle formation the granulosa cells (GC) are separately placed here and there about the oocyte. GN, granulosa cell nucleus. 4500×. (B) As the follicle develops, the granulosa cells gradually form a continuous layer around the gamete. GV, germinal vesicle. 4650×. (Both micrographs unpublished, courtesy of Robert C. Burghardt.)

diplotene, in which condition they remain until shortly after birth. This "first meiotic arrest" persists until shortly before ovulation, being maintained by a substance called oocyte-maturation inhibitor, secreted by follicle cells (Tsafriri and Channing, 1975a,b; Channing, 1979). This is a small peptide, with a molecular weight of around 2000, whose inhibitory action can be overcome by a gonadotropin. Thus, the surge of gonadotropins that precedes ovulation initiates resumption of meiosis in the oocyte (Tsafriri, 1978). The latter events then proceed to metaphase II during a period known as meiotic maturation, at which point a second meiotic arrest occurs, to be broken only after fertilization or parthenogenetic stimulation.

The oocyte in first meiotic arrest is commonly considered as being in the "dictyate" stage. Although nuclear division is interrupted, often for such very long periods as up to 40 or more years in human beings, growth and synthesis of various macromolecules take place actively during this period. Among the features of oocyte structure that develop during this span of time is the zona pellucida (Figure 1.9A). This acellular covering over the germ cell first appears as fibrillar material located in intercellular spaces between the oocyte and the adjacent granulosa cells (Wartenberg, 1962; Baker, 1970). As these scattered areas enlarge, they coalesce until a continuous layer several micrometers thick is formed about the oocyte. Sometimes the zona seems to consist of two layers, the one adjacent to the oocyte being homogeneous and consisting largely of neutral mucopolysaccharides, whereas the outer layer is flocculent and consists of acid mucopolysaccharides in which are electron-dense particles. In contrast, high-resolution, two-dimensional electrophoresis disclosed only three species of proteins in the zona pellucida of the mouse oocyte (Bleil and Wassarman, 1980). These three, having molecular weights of 200,000, 120,000, and 83,000, respectively, comprised in the same order 36, 47, and 17% of the total protein; only the heaviest appeared to be oligomeric. The functions of this layer appear to be chiefly in fertilization and early embryonic development, in which discussions it receives appropriate attention accordingly. Many other proteins are synthesized in the oocytes at this time, including a species of 28,000 daltons that becomes concentrated largely in the germinal vesicle (Wassarman et al., 1979).

Later in maturation in mammals, when the follicle acquires the large chamber known as the antrum, a number of follicle cells remain around the zona pellucida. This cluster, known as the cumulus oophorus (Figure 1.9B), gains intimate connections to the oocyte by way of numerous cytoplasmic bridges which penetrate through the zona pellucida (Moor et al., 1980a,b). These projections terminate on the oocyte plasmalemma, where gap junctions exist at the points of contact, permitting the passage of substances such as phosphocholine and lecithin into the maturing egg cell. Just before the occurrence of ovulation the cumulus is shed. Another distinctive feature of the mammalian ovum develops during this period, provided by the presence of numerous, fine, electron-dense particles lying around the periphery just beneath the plasmalemma. These spherical and membrane-enclosed cortical granules appear to be primary lysosomes of an unusual nature, but their precise identification in terms of cell organelles remains uncertain (Gulyas, 1980). Depending on the species of organism, the time of their formation varies from very early primary oocyte before the cell commences to grow, as in rats and mice (Szöllösi, 1967; Kang,

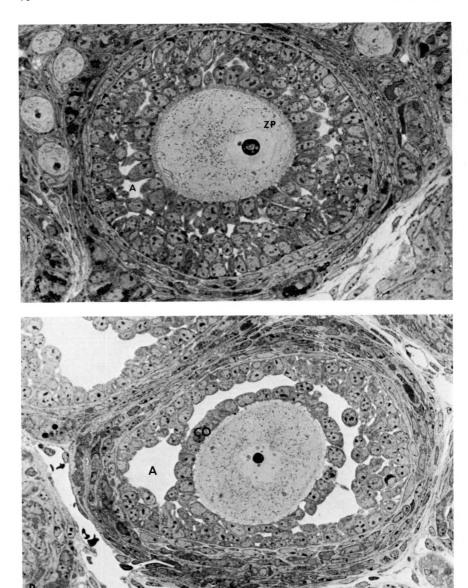

Figure 1.9. Late stages in follicle formation. (A) The zona pellucida (ZP) has now formed around the oocyte as the first hint of the cavity called the antrum (A) can be noted in the layers of numerous granulosa cells. 585×. (B) As the antrum becomes more marked, a layer of granulosa cells called the cumulus oophorus (CO) remains attached to the growing gamete. 540×. (Both micrographs unpublished, courtesy of Robert C. Burghardt.)

1974), to its fully grown condition, as in the human being and rabbit (Zamboni, 1974; Selman and Anderson, 1975). In all cases, the granules appear to be a product of the dictyosomes and play an obscure role in fertilization.

The Secondary Oocytes. Between the first and second arrest periods, nuclear division is accompanied by a characteristic type of cell division. This cytokinesis is highly asymmetrical, the products being a minute polar body and a secondary oocyte that is virtually as large as the primary cell. However, the nucleus now is small and no longer vesicular. This division, as well as the next, may not take place until fertilization, depending on the species. For instance, in starfish the eggs can be fertilized any time after ovulation, in mammals only the secondary oocyte can receive sperm, and in sea urchins only the very end product of oogenesis is fertilizable. The next division is equally as asymmetrical as its predecessor and results in the ootid and a second polar body; usually this division is accompanied by symmetrical cytokinesis of the first polar body. Since the term ovum is applied to any stage of oogenesis that can receive sperm, subsequent cell types, including the secondary oocytes and ootids of mammals, are not customarily distinguished by the latter terms.

An interesting development has come to light through the employment of nucleate and anucleate fragments of the mouse oocyte (Schultz *et al.*, 1978a). Before the fragments were isolated, the intact fully grown dictyate oocytes were treated with cytochalasin B, which disrupts microtubule formation. The nucleated portions were found to resume meiosis *in vitro*, progressing to metaphase II and exhibiting all the changes in proteins of normal meiotic maturation. Moreover, despite the absence of nuclear progression, the anucleated fragments likewise underwent a number of the same changes of protein synthesis. Consequently, it was proposed that the ability to undergo meiotic maturation during early oocyte development ensued from changes in the quality of the cytoplasm, not just the increase in quantity, and that the reprogramming of protein synthesis during meiotic maturation resulted from mRNA molecules already present in the cytoplasm.

During meiotic maturation, the chromosomes of mouse oocytes have been shown to undergo a sequence of changes in protein content (Rodman and Barth, 1979). The evidence for the alterations was derived from two sets of observations, one from alterations in resistance of the chromosomes to degradation by trypsin, the other from patterns of incorporation of labeled amino acids. During the dictyate stage, the chromosomes were found to be moderately resistant to trypsin treatment, a resistance that was greatly enhanced following activation from first meiotic arrest as the chromosomes became still more condensed. This condition persisted until telophase I, when they were revealed to be greatly sensitive to the protease while in the characteristic chromatin mass. Later, after separation from the mass, the chromosomes decompacted into relaxed coils and regained their original moderate degree of resistance. In the autoradiographic studies, which employed tritium-labeled arginine and tryptophan, both amino acids were found to be incorporated into the cytoplasm, but only the former one was combined into chromosomal proteins. Incorporation into the latter structures occurred as two distinct events, the first in late diplotene and the other after telophase I. Moreover, the products of the first utilization of arginine were transitory in nature and were not retained on metaphase II chromosomes.

In amphibians the newly formed primary oocyte is about 50 nm in diameter, as are the oogonia; during maturation in *Rana*, its volume increases about 100,000 times and about 25,000 times in *Xenopus*, in the former case achieving a diameter of 1.5 mm. This growth is accompanied by the first meiotic division, the whole development being a very protracted process. In *Xenopus* the premeiotic S phase requires 1 to 2 weeks, leptotene from 3 to 7 days, zygotene 5 to 9 days, and pachytene about 20 days (occurring about the time of metamorphosis), while diplotene may extend over a year or two (Wischnitzer, 1966). In amphibians as a whole, the maturing oocyte is surrounded by two layers of cells, the inner one comprised of a single layer of granulosa cells, the outer one thickened to form a theca containing several cell types. When the oocyte is undergoing meiosis as it matures, it is under control of pituitary secretions, but the specific path of action of these hormones has been deciphered only recently. When exposed to pituitary homogenates *in vitro,* the oocytes of intact follicles underwent normal maturation, whereas those deprived of the granulosa layer did not (Heilbrunn *et al.*, 1939; Masui, 1967; Schatz and Ziegler, 1979). However, they did respond to progesterone or to pituitary homogenates if granulosa cells were added. More recently, use of radiolabeled compounds has demonstrated that the granulosa cells converted the Δ^5-pregnenolone of the homogenates to progesterone and that the oocyte alone could further reduce the progesterone.

In the maturing oocytes of *X. laevis*, a spherical aggregate consisting mainly of mitochondria has been shown to lie close to the nucleus during the early stages (Dumont, 1972). Although various names have been applied to the formation, mitochondrial mass is currently in vogue. In oocytes from young toads, the mass increases in size during maturation but not so rapidly as the oocyte; consequently, the relative size decreases with the age of the cell (Callen *et al.*, 1980). The DNA in very small oocytes undergoes multiple rounds of replication in close succession, then at a greatly diminished pace after the oocytes have attained a diameter of 120 μm, achieving about 12 rounds in the interval. As the toads mature and become senescent, the mitochondrial mass is in a state of arrest and does not replicate.

1.2.2. Lampbrush Chromosomes

The chromosomes during the first meiotic arrest are in the lampbrush state (Figure 1.10A, B), a condition that occurs in many other metazoans, both vertebrate (including man) and invertebrate. The prevailing interpretation of lamp-

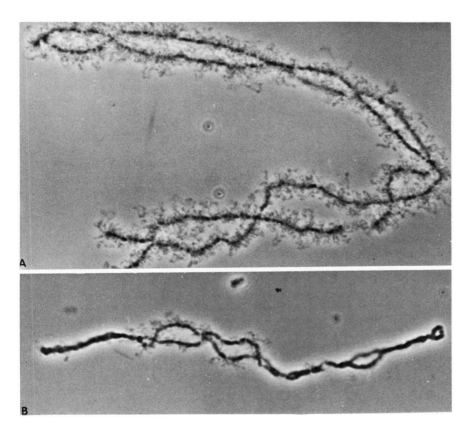

Figure 1.10. Lampbrush chromosomes from a salamander. (A) Chromosome from the oocyte of *Pleurodeles*, showing the normal appearance. (B) Same but from an oocyte that had been injected with anti-H2B serum, suggesting the role this histone plays in the formation of the loops. Both 730×. (Courtesy of Scheer *et al.*, 1979b.)

brush chromosomal structure is that one pair of loops arises from each of numerous common points along the length of the closely paired chromatids that form the backbone of the structure. Each loop is believed to consist of one double-stranded molecule of DNA and protein, quite like each half of the chromosomal backbone. At the base of the loops is a swelling called a chromomere, which is interpreted as being a folded segment of the backbone.

Transcriptional Organization. In this state, the loops are actively transcribed to form the various RNAs needed for the high level of protein synthesis that provides the basis for oocyte growth. At one time it was believed that the entire genome was transcribed during the long period of the diplotene (Gall and

Callan, 1962; Callan, 1967), but hybridization studies between the RNA and DNA have shown that only around 1.2% of the nonrepeated genes in *Xenopus* is actually transcribed. This seemingly small proportion, however, is sufficient to encode perhaps 30,000 average-sized polypeptide chains (Berrill and Karp, 1976). Analyses of the arrays resulting from transcription of lampbrush chromosomes of amphibians have demonstrated that most loops bear one or more transcriptional products (or units), usually of a large size (Figure 1.11A, B; Angelier and Lacroix, 1975; Hill, 1979; Scheer, 1981). When multiple units occur on a given loop, they often are dissimilar in length and polarities (Scheer *et al.*, 1976, 1979b) and hence have been interpreted to signify that they do not represent repeats of a single basic sequence. However, by means of hybridization studies with nascent RNA, both moderately- and highly-repetitive sequences of many loops have been revealed to undergo transcription (Macgregor and Andrews, 1977; Varley *et al.*, 1980), including genes coding for 5 S rRNA, tRNAs, and histones (Brown *et al.*, 1971; Brown and Sugimoto, 1973; Clarkson *et al.*, 1973; Sommerville, 1979). In addition a new family of tandemly arranged transcriptional units of homogeneous size has currently been described, which differs from all the foregoing but whose nature remains unknown (Scheer, 1981).

Recent studies at the ultrastructural level to a large extent have clarified the molecular organization of these chromosomes and have demonstrated the existence within them of two kinds of chromatin (Hill, 1979). One type, found primarily in the arms, consisted of deoxyribonucleoproteins (DNP) having high levels of transcriptive activity, plus spacer sequences, showing little or no transcription. In addition there were large aggregates of loosely packed DNPs, also inactive in transcription, which formed the chromomeres (Figure 1.11C). As a whole, the transcriptive units were closely covered with polymerase, there being 13 to 20 of these enzymes per micrometer. When freed of these enzymes, regular beads were disclosed along the nucleoprotein axis of both types, that were distinctly larger (17–20 nm) than the usual nucleosomes (10 nm). The ribonuclear products transcribed from the active sectors were bushlike in appearance, the molecules being complexly folded into circles and branches and carrying beads. More recent studies on earlier stages of oocyte development have cast light on the formation of this type of chromosomal structure (Hill and Macgregor, 1980). It was proposed that the basic structure was provided by unwinding the DNA molecule at multiple points to form the individual loops, possibly by unraveling the 20- to 30-nm fiber (Finch and Klug, 1976; Olins, 1977) into a less supercoiled form. RNA polymerase molecules then attached at specific initiation sites, each reading through an entire transcription unit. With the passage of time, an increasing number of polymerase molecules engaged in transcription, so that RNP transcripts became spaced along the active loops. Thus, at first in small oocytes, perhaps beginning in early pachytene, the loops have only scattered RNP particles on them (Figure 1.12A; Hill and

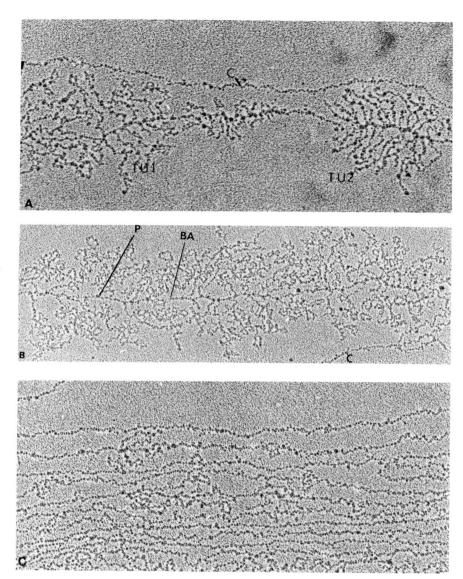

Figure 1.11. The nature of *Xenopus* lampbrush chromatin. (A) Two types of RNP transcriptional units (TU), TU1 showing a gradation in length of the RNP transcripts that is not evident in TU2. C marks an unraveled DNP chromomere. 31,300×. (B) Transcriptional units often have a bushlike appearance as a result of the folding of their axes. Here the polymerases (P) are well spaced, leaving much of the beaded axis (BA) exposed. 24,300×. (C) An aggregate of chromomeric DNP fibers, whose inactive nature contrasts strongly with the several transcriptional units intermixed with them. 31,000×. (All courtesy of Hill, 1979.)

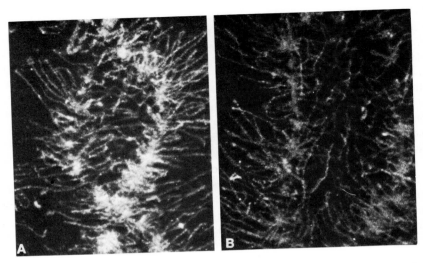

Figure 1.13. Involvement of histone H2B in lampbrush formation. Immunofluorescent preparations of *Pleurodeles* lampbrush chromosomes. (A) With antibodies against calf thymus H2B, the histones are seen to be localized along the chromomeric axes, whereas with antibodies to the protein of RNP particles (B), the staining is largely confined to the lateral loops. Both 1300×. (Courtesy of Scheer *et al.*, 1979b.)

much more DNA present in a *Triturus* loop than in one of *Xenopus*, but why this should be so is not evident, if each loop contains corresponding genes as just indicated. Furthermore, the number of loops is very much greater in the lampbrush chromosomes of *Triturus* than in those of the toad, but this can scarcely imply that there is a corresponding discrepancy in the number of genes present in the two amphibians. Repetitive genes have been ruled out by Rosbach and co-workers (1974) in a series of investigations that indicated most of the structural genes which are active during oogenesis are represented by single-copy sequences. However, it has now been more positively demonstrated that short repetitive sequences do occur in the DNA of *Plethodon* and *Triturus*, but these are interspersed among single-copy genes in members of both genera (Macgregor *et al.*, 1976; Sommerville and Malcolm, 1976).

The specialized nature of the respective loop pairs has been indicated also by results of researches into the organization of RNP particles. Ultrastructural investigations have disclosed that these were constructed from 20-nm subparticles that became assembled in different ways from one loop to another (Malcolm and Sommerville, 1974), suggesting that each may bear distinctive species of nonhistone chromosomal proteins. This proposal has been confirmed to some extent in lampbrush chromosomes of *Triturus* through employment of immunofluorescent procedures, which disclosed that certain fractions of the antibodies reacted with as few as 10 loops (Scott and Sommerville, 1974). One explanation that has been offered for the observed limited distribution of the antigens is that the 20-nm subparticles represent areas of recent transcripts of the DNA molecule to which peptides have been added (Malcolm and Sommerville, 1974), as has already been indicated. Thus, the different RNPs were conceived to be mRNAs that bore proteins as they typically do. When this line of reasoning is carried still further, however, in view of the differing immunological reactions that were actually observed, it clearly implies that the proteins of each mRNA differ from one another. Thus, the problem of specialization is removed from the central structure, only to become an equally difficult aspect of the morphology of messengers transcribed from it.

Molecular investigations into lampbrush chromosome activities have disclosed a number of interesting aspects of these structures, particularly regarding the size of the products and rates of transcription in oocytes. Frequently, as pointed out earlier, each loop is transcribed along its entire length, but occasional ones in salamanders show transcriptional activity in two regions separated by an inactive sector (Figure 1.14; Gall and Callan, 1962; Angelier and Lacroix, 1975). Nevertheless, in either case the transcript is quite lengthy, conservative estimates yielding values from 50,000 to as much as 100,000 nucleotides long. Calculations based on number of loop estimates and observed transcript length yield values for rate of transcription at about 15 nucleotides/polymerase per sec (Davidson, 1976) or a total rate of RNA synthesis of 6×10^8 nucleotides/sec or 20 pg/min per oocyte for *Triturus*, whereas it is only about 3 pg/min per oocyte for *Xenopus*. These figures compare with 0.01 to 0.02 pg/min per cell in postgastrular *Xenopus* embryos. Although these figures are only approximations, it is nevertheless quite evident that oocytes are far more active in RNA synthesis than are the cells of embryos.

A recent investigation has demonstrated that extreme caution must be exercised in interpreting the results of *in situ* hybridization experiments with these chromosomes (Callan and Old, 1980). Denatured tritium-labeled DNA molecules containing *Xenopus* or human globin sequences hybridized with complementary DNA segments on a single pair of lateral loops on lampbrush chromosome IX of the crested newt and to no others. But they did so as a result of the plasmids bearing the DNA having been constructed with G·C homopolymer tails, because simple poly[d(C·G)] hybridized solely with the DNA of the same pair of loops (Figure 1.15A, B). Thus, the first reaction had nothing to do with the globin sequences.

Transcription in nucleoli, which has recently been followed in amphibian oocytes by means of high-resolution autoradiography, proved to be quite comparable to that of lampbrush chromosomes (Figure 1.16A, B; Angelier *et al.*, 1979). Tritium-labeled RNP particles were found to be scattered throughout the transcriptional units, indicating that polymerization continued from one end to the other in each instance, as hypothesized in the beginning of this discussion

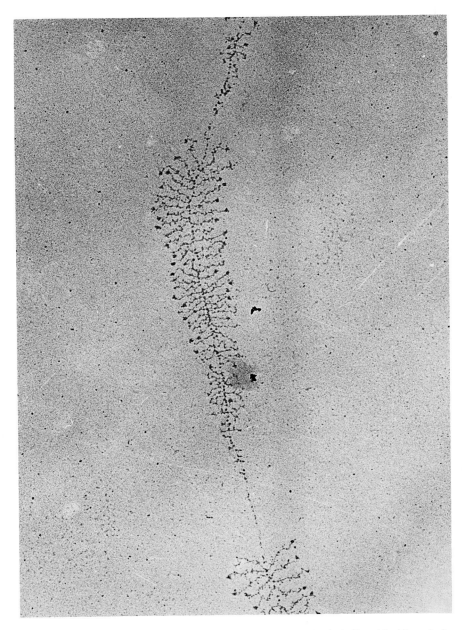

Figure 1.14. Spaced transcriptional units. The several transcriptional units indicated in this nucleolar preparation from *Pleurodeles* probably represent copies from multiple genes for ribosomal RNA. 34,500×. (Courtesy of N. Angelier and J. C. Lacroix, unpublished.)

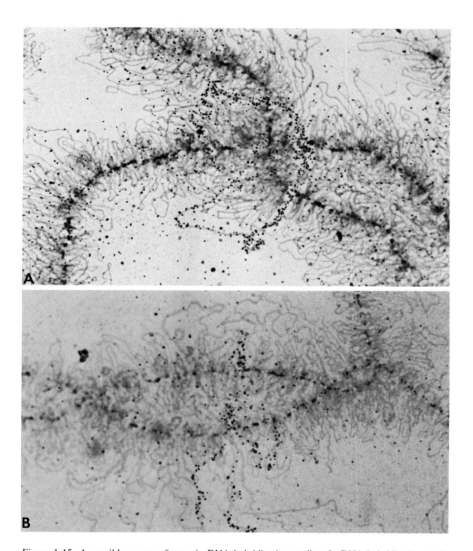

Figure 1.15. A possible source of error in DNA hybridization studies. In DNA hybridization studies of lampbrush structure or function, the use of poly[d(G·C)] homopolymers could prove to be a source of error. (A) Bivalent IX of a *Triturus cristatus* oocyte hybridized with tritiated complementary DNA, a single pair of loops being distinctly labeled. (B) A similar bivalent treated with tritiated poly[d(G·C)] showed radioactivity over the corresponding pair of loops. Both 35,000×. (Courtesy of Callan and Old, 1980.)

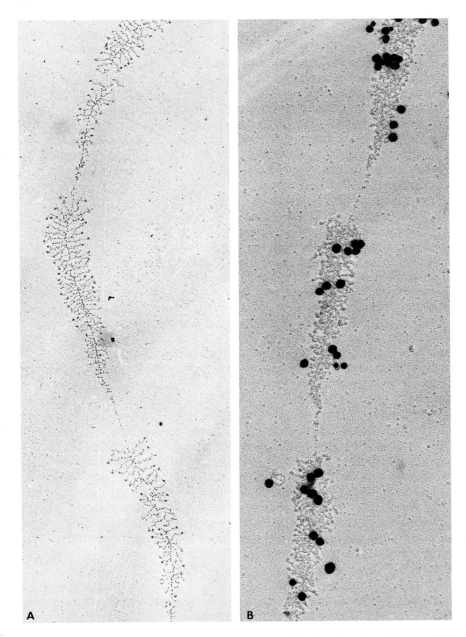

Figure 1.16. Activity in repeated ribosomal RNA genes. (A) A series of repetitious or RNA transcriptional units from nucleolar DNA of an oocyte of *Pleurodeles waltlii*. (B) Similar transcriptional units labeled by means of tritiated precursors revealed a surprising lack of uniformity in activity. 26,500×. (Courtesy of Angelier *et al.*, 1979.)

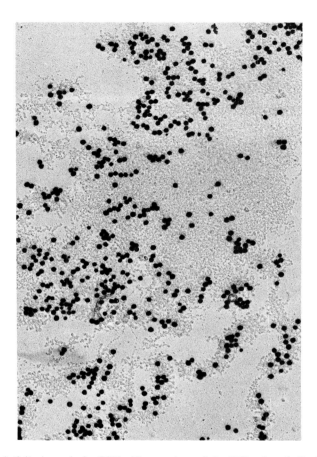

Figure 1.17. Activity in nucleolar DNA. Many regions of the DNA of nucleoli of salamander oocytes show no transcriptional activity, as indicated by this nucleolar spread treated with tritiated ribonucleotides. 13,500×. (Courtesy of Angelier *et al.*, 1979.)

(Figure 1.17). However, as in the chromosomes, transcription did not occur equally throughout the chromatin, some areas as well as individual fibers being entirely devoid of silver deposition. Moreover, there were multiple transcriptional units per individual fiber, with short inactive regions in between; thus, the occurrence of highly repetitive genes, probably of rRNAs, separated by untranscribed spacers was strongly supported.

1.2.3. Vitellogenesis

Vitellogenesis in Birds. Further differentiation of the oocyte takes place during maturation through the acquisition of proteins, and usually also lipids, from outside sources to form its major storage material.* Regardless of its precise biochemical composition, which varies from taxon to taxon, this material is referred to as yolk, and the accumulative processes are given the term vitellogenesis. In vertebrates as a whole, most of the yolk biochemicals are secreted by the liver into the bloodstream, from which they are taken in by pinocytotic vesicles forming between the microvilli of the oocyte. Once inside the cell, the yolk may either be stored temporarily just below the plasmalemma as cortical granules or immediately transported to the dictyosomes and rough and smooth endoreticula.

The processes, not surprisingly, first received close attention in the chicken egg. For instance, Klemperer (1893) reported that when hens were immunized with specific antigens, the yolk of their eggs demonstrated antibodylike activity. More recently, blood serum proteins of various sorts have been found in this portion of the egg (Jukes and Kay, 1932; Abe et al., 1958; McCulley et al., 1959; Williams, 1962), and the major proteins of yolk have been purified and characterized (Cook, 1961). One of these, the phosphoprotein phosvitin, has been isolated from blood serum of laying hens and those treated with estrogen (Mok et al., 1961; Heald and McLachlan, 1963) and was subsequently demonstrated to be formed in the liver and released by that organ into the bloodstream (Heald and McLachlan, 1965; Wallace, 1978). Actually the constitution of yolk has been revealed to be far more complex. In the first place vitellogenin has been resolved by gel electrophoresis into two species, VTG1 and VTG2, which differed markedly in amino acid composition and proteolytic mapping (Wang and Williams, 1980). After arrival at the egg, these proteins underwent enzymatic cleavage into α- and β-lipovitellins and at least two species of phosvitins (Bergink et al., 1974; Christmann et al., 1977), not just one as reported earlier.

Some progress has been made concerning the processes of taking in the yolk constituents and transporting them to their final destinations. When yolk was subjected to centrifugation, two major fractions were separated: the first, accounting for 66% of total yolk solids, consisted of a low-density lipoprotein (lipovitellenin), and the second, making up 16%, differed in being high density (lipovitellin; Cook, 1968). These lipids were deposited in the final phase of rapid growth, commencing about 7 days before ovulation, and involved growth of the follicle from 0.15 g to 17 g (Gilbert, 1971). Both classes of lipids were taken into the cell from the bloodstream by micropinocytosis. In laying hens, the very-low-density lipoprotein occurred at a higher level in the plasma than it did in immature chickens or cockerels, as a result of hormonal stimulation of its synthesis in the liver (Tarlow et al., 1977). This material has been re-

---

*Although Waddington (1962) defines yolk in this loose fashion, a more precise definition is given by Szöllösi (1970) to the effect that yolk consists of proteins and lipids chemically combined, for even heavily yolked eggs contain other stored foodstuffs.

ported to occur in the basal lamina of the granulosa layer and in the granulosa cells, as well as in the space around the vitelline membrane and on the plasmalemma of the oocyte (Perry and Gilbert, 1979). Within the peripheral region of the oocytes, yolk spheres have been noted to contain particles similar in size and substance to those of the plasmalemma. From these observations, it was deduced that the particles of very-low-density lipoprotein were first transferred to the oocyte plasmalemma by way of channels between the granulosa cells, taken into the egg cell by adsorptive endocytosis, and transferred directly to yolk spheres with little alteration.

Vitellogenesis in Amphibians. Among amphibians, the product of the liver is vitellogenin, a lipophosphoprotein that is broken down enzymatically in the oocyte endoreticulum and Golgi bodies to form two substances, each of 200,000 molecular weight. One of these, phosphovitin, is a highly phosphorylated protein, while the second, lipovitellin, is a lipoprotein with a rich lipid content (Wallace, 1978); together these become organized along with various enzymes into the inactive autosomes (lysosomes) known as yolk platelets (Dillon, 1981, pp. 285–288), through the activity of Golgi complexes (Kessel and Ganion, 1980a,b). Deposition of the yolk platelets commences near the surface and progresses centripetally and continues until the formative processes approach the germinal vesicle. The particles are deposited more abundantly on the side of the oocyte away from the attachment to the ovarian wall, which thus becomes the vegetal pole and the attached end, the animal pole. Here, then, is an instance where the physical location of a cell region may influence its immediate and subsequent differentiation, but it could equally be that the polarity of the cell has been established before the deposition of the yolk, which takes place in harmony with that arrangement.

The control of vitellogenesis has received particular attention in *Xenopus.* Chorionic gonadotropin injected into female clawed toads stimulated the synthesis of vitellogenin, but, as it had no effect on males, it has been presumed to act by stimulating ovarian secretion of estrogens. This hypothesis has been corroborated by experimental injection of estradiol into males and females, in both of which massive amounts of vitellogenin were noted in the blood (Follett and Redshaw, 1968; Wallace and Jared, 1968). The ability to react in this fashion was absent in the larva until just prior to metamorphosis (Follett and Redshaw, 1974), at which time synthesis of the protein becomes induced under the influence of thyroxine (May and Knowland, 1980). Since many hormones react with their specific target tissues by means of receptors on the surface of the latter's cells, the induction of vitellogenin production by the liver of males has aroused the interest of many laboratories (for a review see Tata, 1976). Other hormones, including testosterone, progesterone, and cortisol, exercised no effect in either sex (Redshaw *et al.*, 1969). In the liver the vitellogenin is translated from precursorial mRNAs containing a number of introns separated by several exons (Ryffel *et al.*, 1980). Moreover, as in the chicken, vitellogenin was a composite of more than one species of that protein, four actually being present in these amphibians (Felber *et al.*, 1980; Jaggi *et al.*, 1980); these were synthesized from precursorial mRNAs transcribed from about 4 genes out of a complement of nearly 16, most of which were not expressible (Tata *et al.*, 1980; Wahli *et al.*, 1980).

In female *Xenopus*, the vitellogenin of the blood serum was not taken into the oocyte specifically, other blood proteins being taken in concurrently. However, the yolk-forming substance was phagocytosed about 50 times more rapidly than the others (Wallace and Jared, 1969). From the capillaries of the ovarian wall, the vitellogenin and other serum constituents seep around the developing oocyte within the interstices between the follicle cells that cover the latter. Then, as stated earlier, the substances are taken into the oocyte by micropinocytotic activities that occur largely at the bases of the microvilli covering the surface (Brummett and Dumont, 1977). Quite a different picture of vitellogenesis is developing at the current time, for in *Rana pipiens* the primary yolk precursor has been clearly shown to be produced in the Golgi complexes and multivesicular bodies of the oocyte itself (Ward, 1978; Kessel and Ganion, 1980a). Perhaps neither account of the processes is complete, for Opresko *et al.* (1980) have demonstrated that the yolk proteins taken into the oocyte by endocytosis are compartmentalized within the cell into vesicles, whereas others, such as albumin, are not.

Vitellogenesis in Mammals. The question of the occurrence of vitellogenesis in eutherian mammals can be answered in several ways, depending upon the definition of the term yolk. If defined in the loose sense of Waddington (1962) as given earlier, then vitellogenesis does take place in these mammals, for fat droplets and glycogen deposits definitely are present in advanced mammalian oocytes, the former, for example, being more predominant in carnivore eggs than the latter substance (Szabo, 1967; Szöllösi, 1970). Furthermore, in a number of rodent secondary oocytes, a series of fibrous sheets has been described, whose behavior and association with ribosomes suggest the fibers to be proteinaceous (Hadek, 1966; Zamboni, 1970). In rabbit oocytes a better case can be made for yolk in a stricter sense, for membrane-enclosed vesicles containing flocculent material are fairly abundant (Zamboni and Mastroianni, 1966; Gulyas, 1971); however, these contents have not been clearly identified as lipoprotein. Hence, if yolk in the sense of abundant stored lipoprotein is meant, then vitellogenesis has not as yet been confirmed in oogenesis of the placental mammals.

Vitellogenesis in Insects. The yolk-depositing events among insects frequently parallel those of vertebrates. However, here the fat body, not the liver, secretes the principal yolk protein, referred to as vitellogenin, and deposits it in the hemolymph for transport (Telfer, 1965; Wyatt and Pan, 1978; Chen, 1980; Sams *et al.*, 1980). Both this synthesis and the eventual uptake of this protein are controlled by juvenile hormone in many insects (Brookes, 1969;

Koeppe and Ofengand, 1976). In a locust, production of this substance involves the translation of the transcripts of two structural genes, both of which then undergo cleavage into several subunits; dimerization then occurs as additions of carbohydrate and lipid are made before leaving the fat body (Chen *et al.*, 1978, 1979; Couble *et al.*, 1979; Chen, 1980; Applebaum *et al.*, 1981). The two translation products had molecular weights of 235,000 and 225,000, respectively, while the subunits following processing ranged from 52,000 to 126,000 (Chen, 1980).

In the moth *Hyalophora cecropia*, the secretory organelles of the oocytes form the yolk from proteins provided by a variety of sources. At least one of these, the major yolk protein called vitellogenin as elsewhere, is secreted by the fat body and reaches the ovary by way of the hemolymph as in the locust (Pan *et al.*, 1969; Pan, 1971; Hagedorn and Judson, 1972). There, along with other blood proteins, it permeates the intercellular spaces of the follicular epithelium, to which mixture the latter tissue itself adds another constituent (Telfer, 1961; Anderson and Telfer, 1969; Bast and Telfer, 1976). From this assortment of macromolecules, the oocyte selectively takes in by micropinocytosis a specific combination of proteinaceous yolk precursors (Telfer, 1954, 1960; Stay, 1965). As metamorphosis of the insect approaches completion, one by one the follicles of each ovariole cease their pinocytotic intake of the blood proteins (Anderson, 1969), even though the latter's composition remains unchanged. The question therefore has arisen as to what induces the termination of vitellogenesis. At least part of the answer seems to have been provided by an ultrastructural investigation, which indicated the follicular epithelium to form occlusion zones (tight junctions) that late in the processes barricaded the entrance of blood proteins to the oocyte surface (Rubenstein, 1979). Further, it was suggested that the follicular epithelial secretion continued to be taken into the oocyte beyond vitellogenesis, where it may have provided the macromolecular basis for formation of the membrane-bounded particles occupying the cortex of mature silkworm eggs. Perhaps the development of the tight junctions was in turn induced by juvenile hormone, which substance has been disclosed as being active in the control of vitellogenesis in certain orthopterans (Chen *et al.*, 1976) and in the cockroach *Periplaneta americana* (Bell, 1969; Bell and Barth, 1971).

Three major yolk proteins were recently isolated from *D. melanogaster* yolk spheres, whose respective molecular weights were 44,000, 45,000, and 46,000 according to SDS-polyacrylamide electrophoresis. Although thus quite similar to one another in molecular weight, they had distinctly different isoelectric points; moreover, limited proteolysis yielded distinctive digestion products as shown by peptide mapping. The latter type of analysis, as well as immunoelectrophoretic studies, showed that two of the trio were related chemically, whereas the third was obviously unique (Warren and Mahowald, 1979).

1.2.4. Associated Cells

Follicle Cells. The primary oocytes of vertebrates and a number of other major taxa are accompanied by one or more layers of accessory cells called follicle cells, derived from the germinal epithelium of the ovary. As a rule they do not have direct cytoplasmic connections with the developing oocyte as do the nurse cells (trophocytes) described below. Apparently their main function is assisting in the collection of yolk or other nutrients from the ovarian sac or follicle, for all are equipped with microvilli on their exposed surfaces, often interdigitating with those of the oocyte. Once the antrum (Figure 1.9B) has been formed in *Xenopus,* the follicle cells, together with the enclosed oocyte, secrete a number of proteins into the environs. But the presence of the former has been demonstrated not to be essential to the egg cell in regard to this function (Mohun *et al.,* 1981), because if the follicle layers were removed, the oocyte continued to synthesize and export secretory products. Moreover, it was found that the secreted proteins were sequestered into vesicles after their synthesis, whereas nonsecretory ones were not. Both in the oocytes and follicle cells, secretion was by means of exocytosis. In part the distinctions between secreted and retained proteins depended upon the precursor's gaining access to the endoreticulum (Colman *et al.,* 1981); however, the precise length of time of processing and retention in the vesicles appeared to depend upon the particular protein (Lane *et al.,* 1981).

Similarly in mammals, eggs *in vitro* have been demonstrated to mature whether or not the cumulus oophorus cells were present (Magnusson, 1980). Nevertheless, the respiratory rate of oocytes with the cumulus intact showed an increase of 40% after 4–8 hr in culture, whereas that of denuded cells remained at a constant level, but even this difference in behavior could not be found to have material effect on nuclear maturation.

The functional distinctions between follicle and nurse cells are not always readily drawn, a point made especially clear by studies of oogenesis in the squid *Loligo pealei* (Selman and Arnold, 1978; Ramirez and Guajardo, 1980). Very early primary oocytes, less than 25 μm in diameter, are covered by a single follicle cell; as the forming egg cell increases in diameter to about 100 μm, the covering cell undergoes proliferation by mitosis to form squamous-shaped cells, which as the oocyte grows to around 200 μm become increasingly cuboidal and numerous. As additional mitotic divisions occur, they penetrate the enlarging oocyte, forming deep folds. By the time the oocyte has attained a diameter of 700 μm or more, these folds constitute up to 80% of the latter's bulk. No further increase in size or extent of folds occurs beyond this point, as the follicle cells become columnar in shape and fuse into a syncytium. Yolk granules form within this syncytium along with RNA, both of which substances are passed into oocyte cytoplasm; however, the oocyte itself may also synthesize part of the yolk. As the egg cell increases in diameter up to 1.5 mm, the folds are gradually lost, as chorionic material is deposited around the plasma-lemma. Finally, when the chorion is completed, the follicle cells are sloughed off.

Trophocytes or Nurse Cells. The trophocytes just mentioned differ from those of the follicle in several important aspects. First, they are derivatives of primary oogonia; second, their cytoplasm has direct communication both with one another and the oocyte (Figure 1.5A). However, they resemble the follicle cells in being secretory, but differ in not being involved in transport. To cite an especially thoroughly documented example, *D. melanogaster* oogonia divide mitotically four times. One of the resulting 16 cells becomes the primary oocyte and lies at one end of an ovarian follicle (Figure 1.5B–F), surrounded by a layer of follicle cells, except for one region. The other 15 cells become trophocytes having extremely large nuclei and occupying the follicle opposite the oocyte (King, 1970).

Yolk and other foodstuffs, as well as great quantities of RNA, are passed through the cytoplasmic interconnections into the oocyte. In the polychaete *Diopatra cuprea*, loops of cells that project from the ovarian wall eventually break free and float in the coelomic fluid, where further development occurs. One of these oogonia located near the center of the string becomes the oocyte; as it enlarges, the remaining oogonia develop into chains of nurse cells that migrate to one end of the developing gamete, which side matures into the vegetal pole. As in *Drosophila*, the nurse cells have large nuclei and are equipped with numerous microvilli, features which have provided the basis for the assumption that they serve in supplying the oocyte with large quantities of RNA as well as yolk and other nutrients (Allen, 1961; Anderson and Huebner, 1968; Huebner and Anderson, 1976). Similar interconnected chains of cells are produced in other polychaetes, such as *Enchytraeus*, the oligochaete *Eisenia*, and the archiannelid *Dinophilus* (Dumont, 1969; Chapron and Relexans, 1971; Grün, 1972), but in each of these cases all the oogonia develop into oocytes, although presumably they also engage in exchange of RNA, ribosomes, and perhaps other organelles.

1.2.5. Macromolecular Aspects of Oogenesis

As the oocyte undergoes maturation and subsequently ovulation, a number of changes can be observed in its patterns of synthesis and utilization of nucleic acids and proteins. One of the most prominent set of alterations that have been observed is in RNA content, which accordingly receives the greater share of attention in the discussion that follows. However, some interesting results have also been obtained with protein aspects, as well as with DNA synthesis and transcription.

Gene Amplification in Oogenesis. One of the more striking facets of oocyte development was the discovery that certain genes became amplified in number during those processes, the most thoroughly documented of which are the genes for ribosomal RNAs in *Xenopus*. In most metazoans these have been demonstrated to be localized within the nuceolus at the so-called organizer center, where in somatic cells between 200 and 250 tandemly repeated copies of the precursors of 18 S and 28 S rRNAs have been reported in *Drosophila* and about 400 copies of each in *Xenopus* (Brown and Weber, 1968; Brown and Dawid, 1968; Dillon, 1978, p. 191). Contrasting to the somatic cell values, the germinal vesicles of the clawed toad's oocyte contain about 1000 nucleoli, often called micronucleoli because of their relatively small size. These multiple bodies first appear at diplotene of meiosis, when transcription begins, as just discussed. Although the actual length of ribosomal-coding DNA (rDNA) varies from one micronucleolus to another, the total present suggests that about 2500 times as many rRNA genes exist in an oocyte as in a somatic cell (Brown and Dawid, 1968; Kalt and Gall, 1974). Oocytes of echiurid worms like *Urechis* and a surf clam (*Spicula*), while not showing multiple nucleoli in the germinal vesicle, nevertheless exhibited about 5 times as much rDNA as the somatic cells of the same species. Similar enrichment of the genome of oocytes has been detected for 5 S rRNA, amounting to 20,000 copies in *Xenopus*, but this amplification persists in the somatic cells of the adult; however, no similar amplification could be detected in a shark, although 5 S rRNA accumulated in excess amounts in the oocytes (Wegnez *et al.*, 1978).

Light and electron microscopic studies have more recently established that multiple micronucleoli exist in the germinal vesicles of mammals (Luciani and Stahl, 1971; Chouinard, 1973), 40 being reported for the human oocyte in addition to the main nucleolus (Stahl *et al.*, 1975; Wolgemuth *et al.*, 1979). However, the latter study found only a twofold enhancement of rDNA in early oocytes and a fourfold increase in late pachytene and diplotene cells. Thus, amplification of specific sectors of chromosomes appears to be a general phenomenon among metazoans at least, but how the supernumerary copies of the genes are engendered has not been ascertained.

A somewhat more detailed account of the developmental history of rDNA amplification in *X. laevis* has been presented by Kalt and Gall (1974). The primordial germ cells were reported to remain in an extended interphase condition from day 4 of development when they first reached the genital ridge until day 22; during this time span, they did not synthesize DNA, as shown by their failing to incorporate tritiated thymidine. Moreover, they contained only the somatic cell level of rDNA in their one or two nucleoli. Then between day 22 and 24, rDNA amplification and sexual differentiation began, accompanied by the onset of mitotic cell division and the appearance of additional nucleoli. The amplification of the rRNA genes continued as long as mitosis occurred, which period varied with the individual germ cell. Some seemed to divide in this fashion only four times before entering meiotic prophase, but the mean number apparently was closer to nine times, each division requiring about 4 days at

21°C. During the entire set of processes, segments of DNA about 200 pairs of nucleotides long were associated with the nucleosomes, regardless of the rate of rRNA synthesis (Reeves, 1978).

RNA Synthesis in Oocytes. The actual synthesis of RNA varies with the stage of development. In small quiescent follicles, transcription was observed to proceed at a very low rate, but as the oocyte grew, it gradually increased to peak in the fully grown oocyte (Ford, 1972), and then ceased entirely when the follicle matured (Oakberg, 1968; Bachvarova, 1974; Tsafriri, 1978). DNA-dependent RNA polymerase activity also apparently ceased in mature oocytes, although it was demonstrated to be present in both the nucleoplasm and nucleolus of growing ones (Moore and Lintern-Moore, 1974). Quite to the contrary, investigations employing a labeled precursor injected into the ovarian bursa or mature follicles made it clear that those observations were in error, for RNA synthesis was found to occur in mature oocytes (Rodman and Bachvarova, 1976; Wassarman and Letourneau, 1976). This synthesis continued past ovulation until the breakdown of the germinal vesicle, after which synthesis of RNA by mitochondria alone remained (Webb *et al.*, 1975).

That the changes in synthesis of RNA involve a complex series of events has been clearly indicated by microinjection of nucleic acids or nuclei into oocytes or postovulated eggs (Diberardino, 1980). Nuclei of somatic cells continued to synthesize RNA, but not DNA, when introduced into oocytes (Gurdon, 1968); on the other hand, when the same type of nuclei were injected into ovulated eggs, they did quite the opposite, producing DNA but not RNA (Graham *et al.*, 1966; Gurdon, 1967). Corresponding reactions have been secured by microinjections of DNA, for only in eggs was newly synthesized DNA demonstrated (Laskey and Gurdon, 1973; Ford and Woodland, 1975; Davidson, 1976). When synthetic DNAs of known constituency were employed, such as poly[d(A-T) · d(A-T)], production of RNA was stimulated in eggs as well as oocytes, being about 10 times greater in the former than in the latter (Colman, 1975). However, when a series of other synthetic DNAs was used, only poly-[d(I-C) · d(I-C)] proved to be transcribed as efficiently as the first type cited. Native DNA from calf thymus also was effective, but not denatured DNA from the same source, nor were the native genomes of various DNA-viruses.

The RNA synthesized by oocytes represents a broad spectrum of types. In addition to the several rRNAs already discussed, an extensive variety of tRNAs is present, being especially abundant in amphibian and teleost oocytes (Denis *et al.*, 1980), but mRNAs make up the great bulk of the total. In mature eggs of the sea urchin *Strongylocentrotus purpuratus*, the complexity has been reported to be 37×10^6 nucleotides, with about 1600 copies of each mRNA sequence (Hough-Evans *et al.*, 1977). A subsequent study revealed that less than half of the complexity of the mature egg had been accumulated before vitellogenesis began, leaving the rest to be acquired during the last several weeks of oocyte development (Hough-Evans *et al.*, 1979).

The oocytes of *Drosophila* have been shown to contain an equal complexity of mRNA sequences. About 14,500 different sequences bearing poly(A) have been demonstrated, which averaged 2017 nucleotides in length and represented about 2% of the total RNA population (Lovett and Goldstein, 1977); 102 of these were abundant, 2877 were of moderate frequency, and 11,500 were rare (Arthur *et al.*, 1979). Two classes have been described, one bearing short poly(A) sequences accumulated from early vitellogenesis to the mature oocyte stage, while the other had longer poly(A) sections and was synthesized only to the initiation of vitellogenesis (Sagata *et al.*, 1980). Forty percent of the poly(A)-bearing mRNAs were found on polysomes, the remainder as free RNP particles (Lovett and Goldstein, 1977; Goldstein and Arthur, 1979). When polysomal and nonpolysomal sequences from mature oocytes of these flies were separated in a sucrose gradient, 60% of the poly(A)-bearing RNAs were found in the nonpolysomal region, along with 75% of the ribosome population. This sequestered group of mRNAs, deduced to be of the same types as those in polysomes, thus probably represented excess copies (Goldstein, 1978). The distribution of mRNAs between polysomes and RNP particles does not appear to be random, however, for in these insects three DNA-binding proteins were confined to the RNP fraction in mature oocytes that occurred only on polysomes after fertilization (Mermod *et al.*, 1980). Such selectivity in translation is further indicated by the nature of the diversity of mRNA species just discussed. In *Xenopus*, as a case in point, it has been found that only a few of the species present in the oocyte were translated into products used only during development of the egg, most being for substances shared by the late embryo or larva or even the adult (Perlman and Rosbash, 1978). For example, mRNAs for the tadpole and mature toad hemoglobins have been reported to be present, albeit in small quantities (Perlman *et al.*, 1977; Jacob, 1980).

All 5 S rRNA molecules and most of the tRNAs have been found in *Xenopus* oocytes to be stored as two types of RNP particles, one sedimenting at 42 S, the other at 7 S (Denis and Wegnez, 1977; Picard and Wegnez, 1979). The latter proved to consist of one molecule of 5 S rRNA and a protein of 40,000 daltons, and the former contained four subunits, each formed on one molecule of 5 S rRNA, three of tRNA, one of the preceding protein, and two of a protein of 50,000 daltons (Picard *et al.*, 1980). Similar particles were demonstrated to be present in a teleost fish, with comparable compositions, except that the protein of the 7 S particles was lighter in weight (Denis *et al.*, 1980). Apparently, the precise nature of the proteins and sedimentation characteristics of the RNP particles varied with the species to some degree, for the molecular weights were found in *Triturus cristatus* to differ from those of *Xenopus* (Kloetzel and Sommerville, 1981), although the 1 : 3 ratio between 5 S and tRNA remained the same.

The proteins bound to mRNA to form RNP particles have been found to be of at least eight major species in *Xenopus* and to be specific for the oocyte

(Darnbrough and Ford, 1981). Four very abundant ones were of an extremely basic nature and had molecular weights in the range of 50,000 to 59,000; two of this group were confined to immature oocytes, while the others were present throughout oogenesis but absent from adult cells. The remaining four were less fully characterized, but two were larger molecules, with weights of 75,000 and 100,000, while two were smaller, at least one of which appeared to lack a poly(A) segment.

The origins of the mRNAs have been followed during oogenesis in the milkweed bug *Oncopeltus fasciatus,* a species having a meroistic type of ovary. In this type, unlike that of *Drosophila* the trophocytes are confined to the germarium, their nutrient products passing via a nutritive tubule connected to each oocyte (Capco and Jeffery, 1979). As the latter cells underwent maturation, poly(A)-bearing RNA was found to accumulate in the trophocyte cytoplasm and also to pass through the nutritive tubules to the egg cells. Although the numerous follicle cells that surrounded the respective oocytes similarly showed high levels of polyadenylated RNA, no evidence was encountered suggesting its passage into the egg cells. In early oocytes that were transcriptionally inactive, similar nucleic acids accumulated rapidly, obviously from exogenous sources. Then later the level of this substance continued to increase after the formation of the chorion, when the nutritive tubules no longer transported mRNA, strongly intimating an internal origin for the nucleic acid. Uniform distribution of mRNA within the oocyte prevailed except towards the close of vitellogenesis, when the poly(A)-bearing RNA became more abundant at the anterior and posterior polar portions of the cytoplasm than elsewhere.

The poly(A) segments themselves have received attention recently in mature and ovulated oocytes in *X. laevis*. Following exposure of the oocytes to progesterone, the mean poly(A) length was found to increase by 10 to 20 nucleotides, largely as a result of extension of preexisting poly(A); in addition, the number of such sequences increased by around 10% (Darnbrough and Ford, 1979). When germinal vesicle breakdown subsequently occurred, poly(A) was degraded over a 10-hr period, resulting in losses of between 35 and 50% of such segments; however, the segments that remained appeared to be undiminished in length. Since similar changes in poly(A) content occurred also in oocytes that had been denucleated prior to exposure to progesterone, the changes were believed to be programmed by the cytoplasm, with poly(A) polymerase the enzyme active in the processes (Slater and Slater, 1979).

Oocyte-Specific RNA. Few partial, let alone complete, sequences of gametic macromolecules have as yet been established, one of the exceptional examples being the terminal portions of genes for 5 S RNAs from two species of *Xenopus* (Korn and Brown, 1978). As the sequences of somatic counterparts from *X. borealis* and *Drosophila* also have been determined, a comparison of the sections and adjacent 3′ spacers is of interest (Table 1.1). Examination of the two gene sequences from oocytes shows them to be identical; however, the

Table 1.1

Comparisons of Oocyte (o) and Somatic (s) 5 S RNA Gene
Terminal Portions from Diverse Sources[a]

X. laevis$_o$	GGT TAG TAC CTG GAT GGG AG– ACC GCC TGG GAA TAC CAG GT
X. borealis$_o$	GGT TAG TAC CTG GAT GGG AG– ACC GCC TGG GAA TAC CAG GT
X. borealis$_s$	GGT TAG TAC TTG GAT GGG AG– ACC GCC TGG GAA TAC CAG GT
Drosophila$_s$	GAT GGG GGA CCG CTT GGG AAC ACC GCG TGT TGT TGG CCT CG
X. laevis$_o$	GTC GTA GGC TTT TCA AAG TTT TCA ACT TTA TTT TGC CAC AG
X. borealis$_o$	GTC GTA GGC TTT TAG ACT TTT GCC AGG TCA AAG TTT TGC AG
X. borealis$_s$	GTC GTA GGC TTT TGC ACT TTT GCC ATT CTG AGT AAC AGC AG
Drosophila$_s$	TCC ACA ACT TTT TGC TGC CTG CTG CCT GCT GCC TGC TGC C

[a]Based on Korn and Brown (1978).

spacers indicate differences at 16 of the 30 sites, a correspondence of under 50%. The oocyte and somatic genes from *X. borealis* are comparable, a different nucleoside occurring only at the 10th site, yielding a value of 98% homology. Surprisingly the corresponding spacers differ at three fewer points than do those of the two oocyte genes, there being only 13 discrepancies or a 60% homology.

The fruit fly and toad somatic genes are homologous only at 22 of the 52 sites, that is, there is but a 40% agreement between them on a point-to-point basis. The spacers are somewhat more widely divergent, showing different nucleosides at 21 of the 30 sites, for a 30% homology. Perhaps, when the remainder of the genes and adjacent spacers have had their sequences determined, these various distinctions and similarities will become of greater significance, but the data are too sparse now to permit drawing meaningful conclusions. On the basis of the gene sequence, the two oocyte genes appear to be more closely related than are those of the oocyte and somatic cells from a single source. Yet the corresponding spacer differences indicate that the two gametic genes are more remote from one another than are the two from different tissues of *X. borealis*.

Protein Synthesis. Specific details of proteins synthesized during oogenesis are still less thoroughly documented than are those of RNA; consequently, broad quantitative aspects necessarily provide the major portion of the present discussion. But the oocyte contains the enzymatic requirements for complete processing of proteins, for even foreign proteins of unrelated species were completely processed after being injected into *Xenopus* oocytes (Lane, 1981). In *Rana pipiens*, it has been demonstrated that the rate of protein formation in full-grown oocytes was between two and four times as great as in young cells (Ecker, 1972; Shih, 1975), and similar results have been obtained with *Xenopus* female gametes (Woodland, 1974; O'Connor and Smith, 1976). To the contrary, in mouse oocytes, the absolute rate decreased, becoming reduced from 43 pg/hr per oocyte to 33 (Schultz *et al.*, 1978b). The rate of one of the major proteins synthesized in mouse oocyte, tubulin, has been shown on the average to be 1.3% of the total; its absolute rate of synthesis was decreased from 0.61 to 0.36 pg/hr per oocyte during meiotic maturation, the β subunit being formed at twice the rate of the α, despite the two being incorporated into microtubules in a 1 : 1 ratio (Schultz *et al.*, 1979a). However, polymerization of the tubulin into microtubules was inhibited, at least in part through a residue of tyrosine being inserted into the carboxyl terminus of the α subunit (Preston *et al.*, 1981).

It is of interest to note that enucleation of full-grown oocytes of amphibians does not affect the rate of protein synthesis (Ecker, 1972). On the other hand, inhibition of protein synthesis prevents the maturation of oocytes, puromycin being a particularly effective inhibitor (Smith and Ecker, 1969). Since synthesis was resumed when nuclear sap from mature germinal vesicles was injected into the treated oocytes, it was proposed that one protein synthesized by these maturing oocytes was a maturation-promoting factor, without which maturation was not induced (Wasserman and Masui, 1975). Not all laboratories have secured comparable results, however (Drury and Schorderet-Slatkine, 1975). Nevertheless, synthesis of other proteins seems to be essential, too, especially for germinal vesicle breakdown (Wasserman and Smith, 1978).

Another unexpected aspect of protein synthesis during oogenesis that has come to light concerns an increase of phosphorylation of those substances during maturation. When ovulation was induced in *R. pipiens* or *X. laevis*, a marked increase in phosphorylation was exhibited (Morrill and Murphy, 1972; Maller *et al.*, 1977). In the ovulated eggs of the latter species, increased activity of a cAMP-stimulated protein kinase was also described, as well as of a cAMP-independent one (Tenner and Wallace, 1972). Later a second cAMP-dependent type was found, which, although highly specific for histones, seemed to induce maturation (Wiblet *et al.*, 1975). It is pertinent to note in this connection that the cyclic nucleotide level in the frog eggs is now known to become reduced by 60 to 80% during maturation of the oocyte (Kostellow and Morrill, 1977).

Several specific proteins have been found that are particularly favorable for isolation and identification, permitting their synthesis during oogenesis to be traced. In one investigation using high-resolution two-dimensional gel electrophoresis, rates of incorporation of [^{35}S]methionine into each of 12 ribosomal proteins were measured during mouse oogenesis (LaMarca and Wassarman, 1979). These proved to be synthesized at all stages of oogenesis that were examined. Although equimolar amounts of the various types were consistently found in the ribosomes, they were always produced in nonequimolar quantities, the respective rates differing at times by as much as one order of magnitude. During oogenesis the relative rate remained close to 1.5% of the total protein production, as it did also in the mature oocyte; however, following ovulation it dropped to 1.1%. During the transition from the primary oocyte to the secondary, the absolute rate of synthesis of these proteins decreased by 40% from its earlier rate, compared to a 23% drop in total protein production.

　　Histone Synthesis. In somatic cells and unicellular organisms, histone production typically is closely coupled to synthesis of DNA, an observation correlated to the two substances being intimately associated with the formation of chromatin. Thus, histone mRNA is present only during the S phase in somatic cell cultures and is degraded with the onset of G_2 (Perry and Kelley, 1973). Since maturing oocytes do not replicate their DNA, histone synthesis does not appear to be a likely activity, yet it now has been thoroughly documented as occurring in sea urchin and *Xenopus* eggs (Benttinen and Comb, 1971; Cognetti *et al.*, 1974; Woodland, 1979). In oocytes undergoing vitellogenesis, basic proteins, both histonal and nonhistonal, were produced that had a property profile similar to those of early (pregastrula) embryos, particularly the arginine-rich histones (Johnson and Hnilica, 1971). These were produced in quantities sufficient to supply the needs of the early embryo. Some qualitative aspects of histone synthesis in *Xenopus* oocytes have also been presented (Woodland, 1979). Although histone H3 resembled that of somatic cells in exhibiting the same proportions of acetylated- and phosphorylated-forms, H4 existed primarily in a diacetylated condition. Thus, what is a transitory stage in the transport of this histone in somatic cells was in a steady-state phase in the oocytes. However, when the oocyte had matured into the ovulated egg, histone synthesis increased up to 50-fold (Woodland and Wilt, 1980a,b). These two cited articles also reported that histone mRNA was stored primarily in the nonadenylated state in oocytes, although small quantities of adenylated also occurred.

　　If recombinant plasmid DNA is injected into the germinal vesicle of *X. laevis* oocytes, it undergoes seemingly normal transcription and translation (Mertz and Gurdon, 1977; Etkin, 1978; Kressmann *et al.*, 1978). When two plasmid (pSp2 and pSp102) of a sea urchin, each containing the DNA fragment that embraces the histone H1, H2B, and H4 coding regions and adjacent spacers, were injected into the germinal vesicles of *X. laevis* oocytes, transcriptional products proved to comigrate with authentic sea urchin H1 and H2B (Etkin and Maxson, 1980). Because the H4 product was indistinguishable from the *Xenopus* histone of the same type, its synthesis could not be confirmed. The injected genes were transcribed at a rate approximating 0.1 transcript/gene per hr, representing about 0.1% of the total transcriptional activity.

1.2.6 Oogenesis in Metaphytans

　　Among the flowering plants in general, oogenesis displays a number of traits that contrast to those of the metazoans. First, the production of the egg cell takes place in a greatly reduced sexual generation, while an asexual spore-producing generation is predominant. Second, the production of the spore involves meiosis, so that oogenesis is carried out by ordinary mitotic division. Unfortunately, exploration of these processes has been conducted nearly exclusively by the light microscope, so that ultrastructural changes that might accompany them remain to be discovered. Yet the development of the egg into full-fledged plants holds so much invaluable information for the entire topic of embryogenesis that a review of the available facts, familiar though they largely may be, is essential.

Within the ovary of the pistil are contained one or more megasporangia, known as ovules, that are usually covered by two integuments. Each of these encloses a megaspore mother cell, which soon divides twice meiotically to give rise to four megaspores. Three of these products degenerate, leaving the fourth to become the megasporophyte. Much variation exists in the steps beyond this point, depending upon the species, but the essential features include, first, the growth of the megasporophyte to fill much of the megasporangium. Hence, at the end only the single layer of the latter, known as the nucellus, remains. After the growth of the megasporophyte is thus completed, its nucleus undergoes division by mitosis, the two resulting daughter nuclei being moved to opposite ends of the cell. There they divide twice by mitosis, sometimes accompanied by cell wall formation. Of the eight nuclei or cells thus produced, one from each end, referred to as polar nuclei, migrates to the center of the former megasporophyte, now called the embryo sac, thereby leaving a group of three near each pole. That group at the inner end, the antipodals, eventually disintegrates, while the central one of those lying near the micropyle becomes the egg cell or nucleus, the lateral two being synergids.

1.3. SPERMATOGENESIS

For the greater part, the processes of forming male gametes, spermatogenesis, differ little from those of oogenesis, except that in higher vertebrates and in many invertebrates they occur within a tube. However, toward the close of the set of maturation events, the developmental changes are so strikingly distinct that they frequently are given the special term spermiogenesis, or occasionally spermateliosis. Possibly because of the pronounced characteristics gained by the maturing spermatozoon, more attention has been devoted to these gametes than to those of the female.

1.3.1. The Generations of the Cells

Spermatogenesis in Higher Vertebrates. The early history of spermatogenesis in vertebrates parallels that of oogenesis closely (Clermont, 1970),

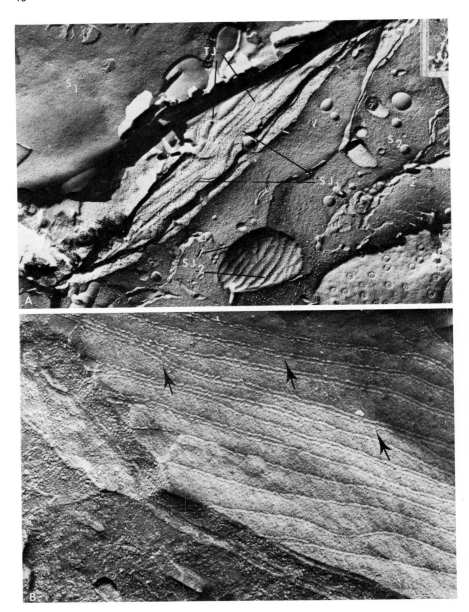

Figure 1.18. Junctions between Sertoli cells. (A) Between these two Sertoli cells (S_1 and S_2), a septate junction (SJ_1) graduating into a tight junction (TJ) is shown in this freeze-fracture replication, and a second septate junction (SJ_2) is close by. 25,000×. (B) At higher magnification a similar preparation reveals the presence of double rows of particles (arrows) located in grooves on the E face of the septate junction. 57,500×. (Both courtesy of Connell, 1978.)

except that the medullary portion of the ovotestis persists, rather than the cortical. During the early stages, this region, enclosed by the tunica albuginea, contains a number of cords of primordial germ cells. Later these solid columns become hollow, as the sex cells, now known as primary spermatogonia, move to the periphery to form a lining. The tubes then are the elementary seminiferous tubules in which the sperm develop; in addition to the sex cells are a number of Sertoli cells, that form irregular-sized pockets in which spermatozoa develop. Since complex septate gap and tight junctions, as well as desmosomes exist between adjacent Sertoli cells (Figure 1.18A,B), they are thought to provide the blood–testis barrier and serve as a seal between the interstitial and seminiferous fluids (Connell, 1978, 1980; Hinrichsen and Blaquier, 1980; Marcaillou and Szöllösi, 1980). Recent investigations have disclosed a number of complex ultrastructural features to develop between the sperm and Sertoli cells, that become altered as the primordial cells undergo maturation (reviewed by Russell, 1980). But as the precise roles are not established as yet, the details cannot be included at this time.

As in oogenesis the stem cells proliferate extensively by means of ordinary mitosis, except that division is always so oriented that one daughter cell in each instance is directed towards the center of the lumen. The peripheral products of these divisions remain as part of the lining and there continue to divide indefinitely in the same fashion (Figure 1.19). Three types of these spermatogonia can be recognized, two of which are known as type A spermatogonia,

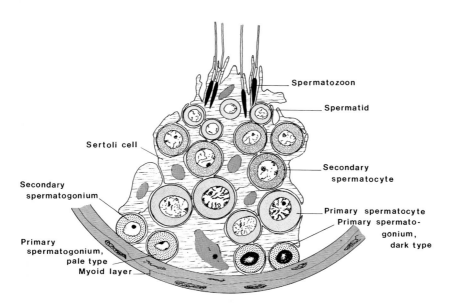

Figure 1.19. Association between Sertoli cells and the various stages of spermatogenic cells.

one the dark (Ad) and the other the pale (Ap). In the first of these, the nucleus is ovate and encloses deeply stained, finely dispersed chromatin, except centrally where lightly stained material predominates. In addition, one or two nucleoli are present, usually closely applied to the nuclear envelope. Contrastingly, type Ap has the nucleus either ovoid or discoid, with the fine-grained chromatin entirely pale-stained; one or two nucleoli similarly can be noted associated with the nuclear envelope. In the third category of these cells, type B, the nucleus is spherical, with distinct particles or clumps of dark-stained chromatin, especially around the periphery. Moreover, the nucleolus appears to be free of the nuclear envelope, often being centrally located. According to some electron microscopic investigations, a fourth class may be present, but its actuality has not been confirmed.

The more proximal product of this mitosis, the primary spermatocyte, now begins to enter into meiosis, usually beginning in these advanced vertebrates with a preleptotene stage. As prophase I progresses, the cell increases in size to some extent, while the nucleus becomes greatly enlarged. However, no meiotic arrest occurs as during oogenesis; instead the cells complete the entire division cycle without interruption to produce two equal-sized secondary spermatocytes. The latter continue the meiotic processes immediately, carrying out the second maturation division in such a relatively short span of time that this stage is not frequently observed in sections of seminiferous tubules. Since this division is likewise equal, each primary spermatocyte ultimately gives rise to four identical products called spermatids. Because of the centripetal orientation of daughters in each generation of cells, the spermatids as well as the spermatozoa into which they mature lie adjacent to the lumen.

Before tracing the metamorphic changes undergone by the spermatid in becoming transformed into a spermatozoon, the several classes of spermatogonia need additional attention. In man and a number of other mammals, it has been established that the dark type A is the primary spermatogonium, which can divide either into two others of the same kind or two of the pale type A, either category of which can undergo mitotic division to form type B, the secondary spermatogonium. The latter then undergoes a similar type of division, resulting in preleptotene primary spermatocytes (Clermont, 1966a,b). In man the entire set of processes through the formation of sperm requires only 16 days (Clermont, 1970), whereas in such cold-blooded vertebrates as the salamanders of the genus *Plethodon*, the two meiotic divisions alone require 26 days (Morgan, 1979).

Spermiogenesis. The gross aspects of spermiogenesis, the processes through which a spermatid is transformed into a spermatozoon, are relatively few in number and superficially of no great complexity (Franzen, 1970; Phillips, 1980). Possibly the first event that can be noted is the formation of a flagellum on one of a pair of flagellar centrioles that appears beneath the spermatid plasmalemma. After this swimming organelle has attained a moderate length, the entire structure with the attached centriole is moved inwards to the nucleus. The nucleus itself then can be observed to become denser as it loses much of its aqueous content along with all its RNA and much protein. While it thus becomes reduced in size and much more compact, it undergoes great changes in shape, first becoming ovate and finally acquiring a nearly rodlike form, the entire cell elongating concurrently. In the meanwhile, the mitochondria, which originally were scattered throughout the spermatid, become congregated at one side of the nucleus close by the centrioles. As the entire spermatid becomes still more elongated, it begins to lose cytoplasm in large droplets called blebs. Bleb formation continues until very little cytoplasm remains around the nucleus and basal portion of the now fully elongated flagellum.

Ultrastructural investigations have added considerable detail to the basic events just enumerated. The flagellum has proven to be quite varied in structure; in urodele amphibians, for instance, it is placed laterad to a central rod (Barker and Baker, 1970). The mitochondria, which are usually ovate throughout spermatogenesis, gradually elongate and align themselves in a number of spiraling rows around the basal region of the flagellum to form the midpiece. In each species of mammal, the number of such rows and spirals in the midpiece is quite specific (Threadgold, 1976; Phillips, 1977; Gould, 1980; Dillon, 1981, pp. 397–399). A complex sheath also develops around much of the remainder of the flagellum, leaving a bare whiplash free at the apex; the dense fibers that are embedded within the sheath have been shown to have a helical conformation (Paddock and Woolley, 1980). The centrioles remain at the very base of this apparatus, pressed against or into the nuclear envelope, one member of the pair bearing the flagellum. The other, proximal member remains inert until fertilization; then in the egg it aids in the formation of the first mitotic spindle. The latter observation adds emphasis to the point established elsewhere (Dillon, 1981, pp. 177–179) that the flagellar organelles frequently referred to as "basal bodies" and the centrioles that engage in mitosis are merely two aspects of one and the same organelle. The endoreticulum also plays an active role in spermiogenesis, becoming very extensive until the final phases, when it regresses (Clermont and Rambourg, 1978).

The Golgi apparatus is especially active during the development of the spermatozoon. Although at first it is located at what eventually becomes the anterior region of the sperm, it moves laterally as it produces a large number of vesicles. The latter structures then migrate to the apex, where they ultimately fuse to form the acrosome (McMaster-Kaye and Kaye, 1980a,b), a type of lysosome belonging to the recently named class pungisome (Dillon, 1981, pp. 177–181). Its function is that of assisting in the penetration of the ovum, as discussed in the section on fertilization (Chapter 2, Section 2.1).

Ultrastructure of Vertebrate Spermatogenesis. Some aspects of spermatogenesis become clear only when the fine structure of all generations of the male sex cells are reviewed, for the discussion of which the South Af-

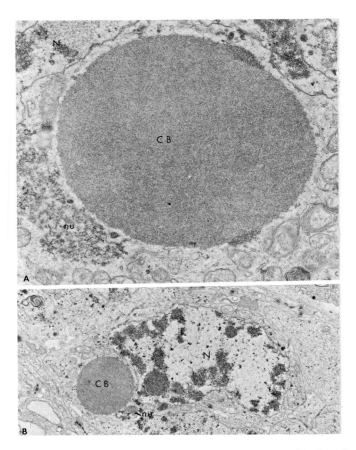

Figure 1.20. The chromatoid body in *Xenopus*. (A) A chromatoid body (CB) lies adjacent to the nucleus (N) and a mass of nuage (nu) in a primary spermatogonium experimentally treated *in vivo* with actinomycin D. 18,000×. (B) In the secondary spermatogonium, the chromatoid body is much reduced in size; a small patch of nuage lies nearby in association with mitochondria. 11,800×. (Both courtesy of Kalt *et al.*, 1975.)

rican clawed toad, *X. laevis*, provides the model (Kalt, 1973, 1976, 1977; Kerr and Dixon, 1974; Kalt *et al.*, 1975). One of the most distinctive features of these cells throughout most of the spermatogenic events is the chromatoid body (Figure 1.20A). In primary spermatogonia, there are one to four rounded masses of coiled fibrillar material that is so fine and uniform as to appear in cross sections as moderately electron-opaque, minute particles. Similar bodies have also been described in mammalian male gametes (Bawa, 1975; Söderström, 1981). At that stage these organelles average about 2.5 μm in diameter, a dimension that decreases to about 1.5–2 μm after division into secondary spermatogonia has taken place (Figure 1.20B). Reduction in size continues throughout spermatogenesis, primary spermatocytes having only one such body, now reduced to about 0.2–0.5 μm in diameter. By pachytene of meiosis I, the chromatoid body becomes somewhat vesicular, which condition continues into the early spermatid. Then further degeneration takes place, the body eventually disappearing in the cytosol or being lost with the cytoplasmic blebs. In these animals the chromosomes at pachytene lack the lampbrush modification found in oocytes, the chromatin being in loose tangles rather than loops (Figure 1.21A, B). Denser clumps of strands are found along the axis that have been thought to correspond to chromomeres (Comings and Okada, 1975).

Another distinctive feature of amphibian and mammalian spermatogonia or earlier cells is the presence of nuage or germinal plasm (Figure 1.22), found also in oogonia of these animals. As in those cells, this is diffuse, strongly electron-opaque material, in anurans but not mammals closely associated with clusters of mitochondria (Kalt *et al.*, 1975). As in female amphibians, nuage decreases in abundance with the onset of prophase I of meiosis (Kalt, 1973). During the closing phases of rat spermatogenesis, the nuage has been noted to move to the chromatoid body (Figure 1.23) and become attached to it (Söderström, 1981). Except for the movement of the various organelles already described, little of note is to be found in these developing cells, perhaps the only additional pertinent feature being the abundance of vesicular endoreticulum of both rough and smooth varieties. While not especially extensive in primary spermatogonia, an increase in these organelles is initiated in spermatocytes that becomes strongly marked in early spermatids (Bawa, 1975). An interesting variant in the structure of completed spermatozoa of vertebrates has been described in detail recently (Folliot, 1979). In toads of the genus *Bufo*, much of the propulsion of sperm was shown to be provided by a broad, undulating membrane that extended throughout the length of the flagellum on one side (Swan *et al.*, 1980). In certain other toads, including members of the genus *Bombina*, the sperm proved to have the flagellum entirely replaced by the undulating membrane, the centrioles being located just posterior to the acrosome (Furieri, 1975).

Spermatogenesis in the Onychophora. Considering that spermatozoa of all species carry out the same basic functions, those of contacting the egg and penetrating it, an amazing amount of variation in morphology exists in the male gamete of metazoans. Although whole books have already been published on the comparative aspects (Franzen, 1956; Afzelius, 1975; Baccetti and Afzelius, 1976; Fawcett and Bedford, 1979), much additional information is coming to light continually. Thus, it is possible here to provide only a few examples, but these have been selected to show both the overall similarities and some of the diversity that exists among invertebrates.

One of the numerous invertebrate taxa whose processes of producing sperm

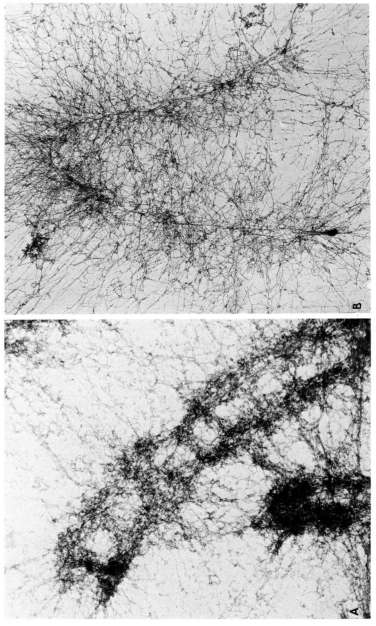

Figure 1.21. The nature of chromosomal pairing and banding. Chromosomes removed from male Chinese hamster V-79 cells *in vitro* after treatment with actinomycin D. (A) Paired sister chromatids from a metaphase cell, stained with uranyl acetate, show strong interdigitation of fibers at banded regions 17,800×. (B) A pachytene chromosome, unstained, has areas of condensation that correspond to chromomerelike regions. 9400×. (Both courtesy of Comings and Okada, 1975.)

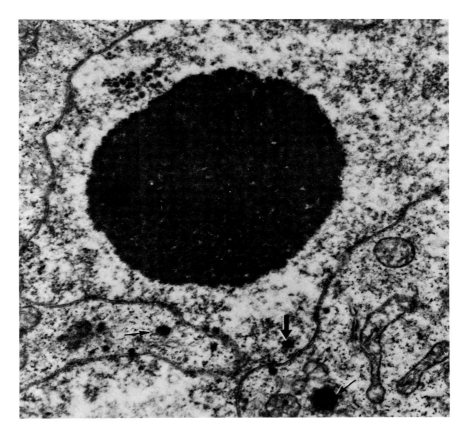

Figure 1.22. The possible source of nuage in *Xenopus*. Because granular material within the nucleus (heavy arrow) has a similar appearance and density as those in the cytoplasm (thin arrows), it was suggested that the material for the latter is formed in the nucleoplasm. 47,000×. (Courtesy of Kerr and Dixon, 1974.)

have received recent attention is the Onychophora, whose affinities seem to be with the Arthropoda, particularly the Diplopoda and Chilopoda (Camatini *et al.*, 1974, 1977, 1979; Baccetti *et al.*, 1976; Lavallard, 1976; Baccetti and Dallai, 1977). In *Peripatopsis capensis* the large, ovate testes enclose an extensive cavity, in which cells at various stages of differentiation are contained. At the earlier stages, little of importance is to be observed, except that cleavage of spermatocytes frequently is incomplete. The resulting intercellular bridges often persist until the close of the second meiotic division with the formation of spermatids. However, the cells do not mature in synchronous fashion, even at the same level in a given testis; consequently, all stages of development including primary spermatogonia may be found in all levels of the testicular

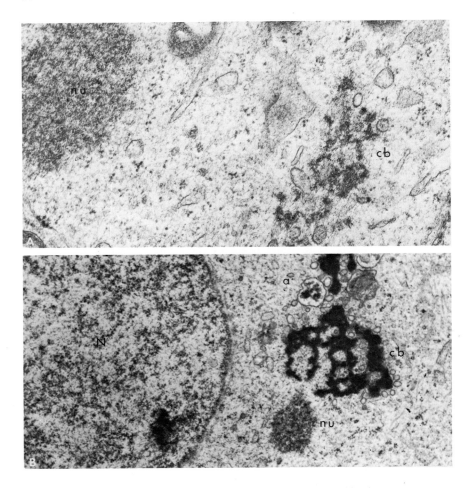

Figure 1.23. Nuage and chromatoid bodies of mammals. (A) In this midpachytene spermatocyte of the rat, a newly formed, small chromatoid body (cb) is located at some distance from nuage (nu). 28,000×. (B) Later as in this spermatid, the chromatoid body is much larger than the nuage and both become located near the nucleus (N). A proacrosomal vesicle (a) also lies adjacent. 9500×. (Both courtesy of Söderström, 1981.)

lumen and even in the vasa efferentia. In the spermatids, a single relatively broad dictyosome is present during much of spermiogenesis, consisting of about 20 cisternae of typical metazoan form, the proximal ones concave, sometimes deeply so. The principal product of this body consists of vesicles that contain spherical masses of an electron-opaque substance; after reaching mature size they migrate to the periphery of the cell where they eventually form a regular series beneath the plasmalemma (Figure 1.24A; Camatini *et al.*, 1979). Later these structures leave the peripheral region to congregate and fuse into a mass many times the size of the nucleus, the contents becoming vesicular and losing much of its opacity as fusion proceeds (Figure 1.24B). Finally, the degenerate mass is sloughed off along with the other cytoplasm, providing material for formation of the spermatophore. Thus, these Golgi vesicles, although developed in typical fashion, do not form the acrosome so characteristic of many other metazoan spermatozoa but enter into the formation of an enveloping body.

Contrastingly, in the sperm of another member of the same genus, *P. moseleyi*, an acrosome has been reported to be present (Ruhberg and Storch, 1976). Perhaps the most characteristic feature of the sperm of the present species is the manchette of microtubules that spirals around the nuclear envelope, even in the early spermatid, a development that parallels an event of oogenesis. A single layer of rather close-set microtubules may be seen at that stage in the perinuclear region, distad to which is a series of inflated endoreticular cisternae. At later stages the latter become fused into a single continuous cisterna which encloses nearly the entire nucleus and to which the microtubules, now even more densely placed, connect by way of bridges. Still later, after the flagellum has developed nearly to completion, the coiled manchette becomes prolonged posteriorly over the midpiece, where it lies just beneath the outer membrane of the sheath.

Spermatogenesis in Coelenterates and Annelids. Several species of the familiar genus *Hydra* have been the subject of spermatogenic investigations. The gametes develop from interstitial cells, not primordial germ cells set aside early in embryogenesis as is typical of most metazoans. In these simple animals, development takes place in testes, or spermaria, produced on the exterior surface of the stalk by outpocketings in the epithelial layer. The wall of these organs is a single-celled layer, which encloses a large cavity, loosely subdivided by extensions of a few epithelial cells. Within these partially separated chambers, the forming male gametes are arranged in five or six layers, each of which represents a different generation of cells, all in a given layer being in a like stage of development. The spermatogonia form the deepest layer and lie at the mesogleal lamella (Brien and Reniers-Decoen, 1951), whereas the late spermatids are located at the distal surface. An individual testis appears capable of releasing spermatozoa in small numbers at intervals of 5 to 60 min over an extended period of time (Zihler, 1972). Apparently in some species, secondary spermatocyte division is incomplete, so that the spermatids remain attached in groups of four until maturation has made considerable progress. In contrast, in *Hydra attenuata* the spermatogonia but not the spermatids are interconnected by cytoplasmic bridges (Stagni and Lucchi, 1970).

In a related colonial hydroid, *Eudendrium racemosum*, an unusual condi-

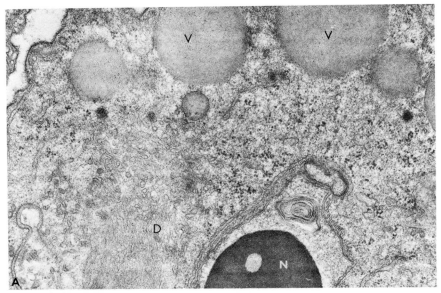

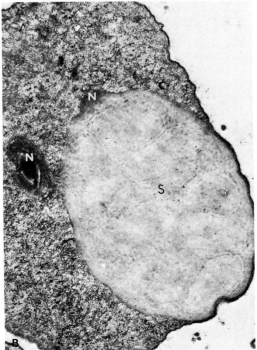

Figure 1.24. Fate of Golgi vesicles in *Peripatopsis*. In the members of this genus of onychophorans, the sperm lack an acrosome; in place of the latter the Golgi vesicles are ejected from the sperm to become part of the spermatophore wall. (A) In this late spermatid the vesicles (V) derived from the dictyosome (D) are arranged at first around the periphery of the cell, at some distance from the nucleus (N). 30,000×. (Courtesy of Marina Camatini, unpublished.) (B) Later the vesicles fuse to produce a sperule (S), which is soon cast out of the cell. 21,000×. (Courtesy of Camatini *et al.*, 1979.)

tion has been reported (Hanisch, 1970). When spermatogonia changed into primary spermatocytes, they became reduced in size, the nucleoli were lost, the chromatin developed a distinctive pattern, and a short flagellum was produced. Then in the secondary spermatocyte, a flagellum grew at both ends of the cell, one going to each spermatid at the close of the second meiotic division. Primary spermatocytes, as well as spermatogonia, were united to others of their respective generations by intercellular bridges.

In most species of earthworms, certain features recall parallel events that were noted during oogenesis. Spermatogenesis in these annelids begins in the testes but is completed either in testis sacs or in seminal vesicles. Generally, all spermatogonia and spermatocytes remain associated with their respective generations as they undergo division synchronously; thus, when division is complete, the resulting 128 (rarely 256) spermatids are grouped together (Jamieson, 1978; Jamieson and Daddow, 1979). Each member of the group is sttached by a bridge to a cytophore, a central cytoplasmic mass devoid of nuclei, the entire combination being known as the sperm morula. Beyond this point, the metamorphic processes of converting the spermatid into the complex spermatozoon offer no remarkable features.

Spermatogenesis among Arthropods. Spermatogenesis in spiders has been shown to involve several unusual characteristics. In the first place, sex determination among the araneans falls into three categories, the largest of which is comprised of X_1X_2O males and $X_1X_1X_2X_2$ females. However, about 10% of spider species have XO males and XX females and 5%, $X_1X_2X_3O$ males and $X_1X_1X_2X_2X_3X_3$ females. During spermatogenesis, leptotene and pachytene stages are rare or absent, and synaptonemal complexes have been found in only a few species, including *Dysdera crocata* (Benavente and Wettstein, 1980). Further, typical early prophase stages have been largely replaced by a long and well-defined diffuse stage, in which only nucleoli and sex chromosomes can be identified. In metaphase the holocentric sex chromosomes rarely can be recognized.

Perhaps the most marked specializations during spermatogenesis are found among such fungus gnats as those of the genus *Sciara*. The early stages of the processes do not need to be detailed here, but the particulars are to be found in Metz *et al.* (1926), Metz (1927, 1938), and Metz and Schmuck (1931). In brief, among the distinctive features is the behavior of the nucleus of the primary spermatocyte; this structure does not divide meiotically, since bivalents are not formed; moreover, nuclear division is unequal and is accompanied by equally asymmetrical cytokinesis. Consequently, only a single (or in some cases two) spermatid is produced per primary spermatocyte. In the related genus *Miastor*, for a concrete example, each testicular cyst of the early larva prior to the last premeiotic division (White, 1946) contained four spermatogonia, each with 48 chromosomes, the octoploid number. By metamorphosis these had undergone division, so that a cyst enclosed eight primary spermatocytes. Each of the latter then divided, producing two secondary spermatocytes, one having 6, the other 42 double chromosomal pairs. The first of these underwent division, producing two spermatids, each with six chromosomes, while the second degenerated. Quite frequently there are unisexual broods, some females having all male progeny, others all female (Roosen-Runge, 1977).

The ultrastructural features of the processes of spermiogenesis in these gnats also display some unique characteristics. As the spermatid matures, the several mitochondria accumulate a great quantity of proteinaceous material and then fuse to form a single, greatly elongated mitochondrion (Doyle, 1933; Phillips, 1966). The latter reference also devotes attention to the unusual centriole. Instead of its wall being composed of a circlet of nine triplet sets of microtubules, as in the somatic tissue of this insect and almost all organisms, in the early spermatid it is oblong-ovate and contains 70 singlet microtubules (Figure 1.25A). From these, 70 doublets then develop, as the entire organelle is moved from its anterior location to the posterior. The doublets elongate, extending down the length of the flagellum in place of the usual 9 + 2 pattern; toward the posterior region, the originally ovate conformation opens and then folds to form one or more loose spirals (Figure 1.25B).

General Patterns of Sperm Specializations. Some generalizations regarding adaptive value of form have been drawn from sperm structure (Afzelius, 1955, 1972; Franzen, 1956, 1970), to which numerous exceptions can obviously be expected. Primitively, spermatozoa, like ova, seem to have been deposited in an external aquatic environment, as so many representatives of invertebrate phyla still do today (Baccetti and Afzelius, 1976; Afzelius, 1977). As a rule, such primitive male gametes have radially symmetrical conical heads, or even rounded ones, with a single, long, active flagellum. Since energenic metabolites are usually absent from the milieu, the sperm derive energy from intracellular deposits. In certain sea urchin sperm, for instance, the chief source of energy is from oxidation of phospholipids deposited in the mitochrondria (Afzelius and Mohri, 1966), whereas those of *Paracentrotus* draw upon stored glycogen (Anderson, 1968; Anderson and Personne, 1976).

In cases in which fertilization is internal, the spermatozoa are often modified for the prefertilization environment, particularly in those instances in which that milieu has a viscosity distinctly greater than that of water. Among the modifications that have been reported are additions of microfilaments to the typical flagellar axoneme; these may be of various sorts, including actin and myosin, and apparently serve to increase the effectiveness of the propelling apparatus (Anderson and Personne, 1976). Moreover, in these advanced types modification of head shape and arrangement of the mitochondria into extensive midpieces also occur, several examples of which have been described in earlier paragraphs. In some cases dimorphism of spermatozoon structure exists, two notable examples of which are provided by internally fertilized prosobranches

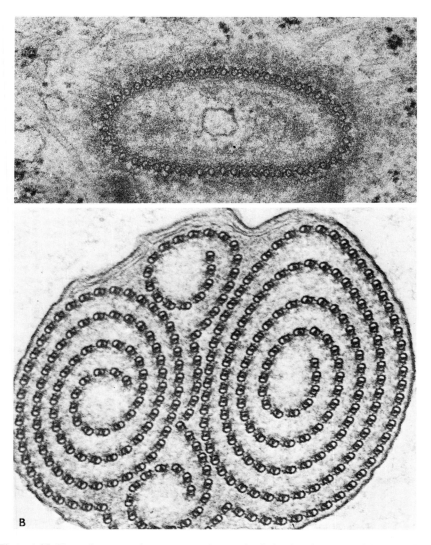

Figure 1.25. Unusual structures in gnat sperm. Among the distinctive ultrastructural features of the sperm of such gnats as *Sciara* is a centriole (A) whose wall consists of about 70 single microtubules instead of nine sets of triplets as elsewhere. 65,000×. (B) In place of the familiar 9 + 2 pattern of most flagella, those organelles in the members of the genus *Rhynchosciara* contain multiple spirals of microtubules. 90,000×. (Both micrographs unpublished, courtesy of David M. Phillips.)

of various genera. In *Pomacea*, long-headed, but otherwise typical, eupyrene*
sperm are produced together with oligopyrenic cells, which are of much greater
length and bear clusters of 8 to 16 flagella (Meves, 1903; Pollister and Pollister, 1943). Although the oligopyrenic types are introduced in large numbers
into female reproduction receptacles along with the others, they do not fertilize
eggs but undergo rapid degeneration. Because of the latter habit, they have
been suspected of serving as nurse cells for the eupyrenic spermatozoa (Hanson
et al., 1952). In representatives of a second genus, *Opalia*, and their relatives,
the multiflagellated sperm attach by hundreds to the surface of the normal sperm
that are produced, and accordingly they have been claimed to serve in place of
a penis in transporting the sperm during breeding, thus eliminating the need for
copulation (Fretter, 1953; Wilson and Wilson, 1956). However, such a role has
not been observed by other investigators (Bulnheim, 1962). Still another example of dimorphism is provided by the pond snails of the genus *Paludina*, in
which two types of sperm have long been known to exist; the normal eupyrene
sperm is multiflagellated in this instance, whereas the apyrene type is simply
uniflagellated.

   Epididymal Maturation. In cyclostomes, teleost fishes, and frogs, the
sperm when released from the testis are immediately capable of actively swimming and fertilizing the ovum, but in mammals of all types, the testicular product is immotile. To gain motility and the capability for fertilization, the spermatozoa in marsupial and placental forms must undergo maturation in the
epididymus (Bedford, 1979). The course followed by these cells then is from
their point of origin in the seminiferous tubules first to the rete testis to which
the latter connect; thence they travel through the vasa efferentia to the caput
epididymis, the first of three divisions of this organ (Figure 1.26). The other
two divisions, the corpus and cauda, are passed through before the sperm reach
the vas deferens ready for ejaculation. All epididymal regions consist of a highly
convoluted tubule, estimated to be about 25 m long in men and up to 70 m in
stallions (Bishop, 1961).

   During their passage through that organ, the sperm mature at various rates,
some completing the process in the caput, others in the corpus, and the remainder in the cauda. In the boar, for a case in point, 25% of the sperm taken from
the first region were motile, whereas 75% of those removed from the corpus
and 92% of those of the final region were active. One change that could be
observed to occur early is the posterior migration of a cytoplasmic droplet from
the sperm head towards the tail, where it was finally lost (Jones, 1975). Another involved the condensation of the acrosome, a third, similar changes in

---

*Meves (1903) proposed the term eupyrene for sperm containing the full complement of chroma-
tin, oligopyrene for those with subnormal amounts, and apyrene for gametes that lacked it completely.

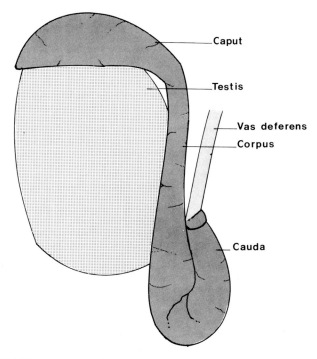

Figure 1.26. Epididymis of a rat. This characteristic organ of male mammals consists of a very long, tortuous tubule in which the sperm undergo maturation as they pass from the testes to the vas deferens.

the perforatorium, and fourth, alterations in the properties of the plasma membrane, in addition to the acquisition of motility already mentioned. About 7% of the boar sperm were observed to undergo degeneration in the epididymis (Jones, 1971). After becoming mature, mammalian spermatozoa may retain their capacity for fertilization for various periods, ranging from about 20 days in rats and guinea pigs, around 35 days in rabbits, and up to 7 months in certain bats (Racey, 1972, 1975; Jones and Glover, 1975).

In opossums, as the acrosome became modified in the corpus and cauda regions of the epididymis, the membranes of adjacent sperm heads interacted in such a manner that the sperm were united into pairs by their anterior ends (Figure 1.27B; Krause and Cutts, 1979). All were thus combined by the time they were ready to leave the epididymis. Among monotremes like the echidna (*Tachyglossus aculeatus*), the epididymis is poorly differentiated (Figure 1.27A); although five regions of the excurrent duct can be recognized histologically, the distinctions from one region to another often are not pronounced (Bedford and Rifkin, 1979). The sperm are quite simple, being threadlike as in the birds and reptiles; in ultrastructure they are even simpler than the male gametes of the turtle. A rostral cleft is lacking and little of the subacrosomal material characteristic of most mammals and reptiles is present. In keeping with its general simplicity, the spermatozoon undergoes very little maturation in the epididymis (Bedford and Rifkin, 1979), the only changes that have been detected being the acquisition of motility and loss of the cytoplasmic droplet.

In the placental mammals one function of the epididymis is that of absorbing the fluid produced by the testis; about 90% of that substance is absorbed, cells bearing microvilli along the entire length of the tubules being involved in the process (Levine and Marsh, 1971; Wong et al., 1978, 1979). During absorption, the ionic and hormonal contents of the fluid undergo changes, as does the pH also, the latter decreasing from 7.3 in the seminiferous tubules to about 6.5 in the caput (Howards et al., 1979). The hormonal changes involve, first, the replacement of the principal hormone in the testes, testosterone, by dihydrotestosterone in the epididymis, and second, the concentration of both of these androgens then decreasing still more in the distal region. Of metabolites present for possible maintenance of the sperm, lactic acid, perhaps produced by the glycolytic activities of the lining cells, seems to be the most important (Brooks, 1979).

One investigation into the nature of the events that led to motility of the spermatozoon examined the phosphorylation of the axoneme microtules in rat sperm (Tongkao and Chulavatnatol, 1979). Despite the gametes from both caput and cauda regions possessing protein kinases (Hoskins et al., 1974) and forming phosphoproteins, the tubulin of the cells from the former region was not phosphorylated while that from the latter was. Thus, the tubulin undergoes some sort of modification en route through the epididymis, permitting its accessibility to the enzyme action, or the specific requisite kinase is confined to the cauda.

A number of alterations in properties of the surface and plasmalemma of the head also have been described. For example, ferritin–wheat germ agglutinin was found to bind strongly to the acrosomal and postacrosomal regions of the spermatozoa taken from the caput epididymis, while it did so only sparingly to those of the cauda, except at the extreme apex of the head, and scarcely at all to the ejaculated cells (Nicolson et al., 1977; Nicolson and Yanagimachi, 1979).

Various techniques employing ^{125}I- or ^{3}H-labeling revealed the presence of several proteins on the heads of sperm cells from the cauda that were absent on those from the caput, most of which, including a sialoglycoprotein, had molecular weights in the neighborhood of 35,000 to 39,000, but one was close to 59,000. In contrast, a galactoprotein of the smaller size was shown to occur on caput sperm but was absent in those of cauda origin (Nicolson and Yanagimachi, 1979). Such differences are reflected in part also in the results of anti-

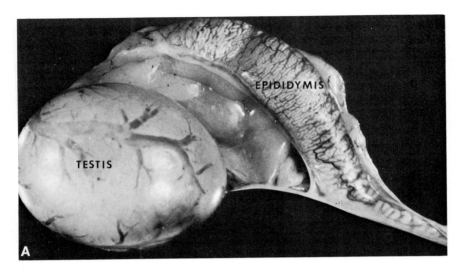

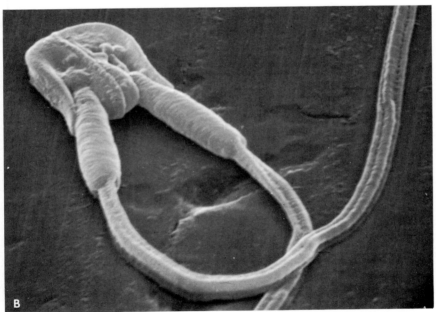

Figure 1.27. Reproductive features among monotremes and marsupials. (A) In the echidna, the epididymis is far simpler than that of eutherians (Figure 1.26) and lacks external division into regions. Five histologically distinct regions, however, are discernible in the interior, four near the upper portion, the last one close to the vas deferens. (Courtesy of Bedford and Rifkin, 1979.) (B) In the American opossum, the sperm when mature fuse by their heads to form pairs. 5000×. (Courtesy of Krause and Cutts, 1979.)

genic investigations. When antibodies were prepared against mature pachytene spermatocytes or later stages, virtually no reaction was obtain with leptotene or zygotene spermatocytes and earlier stages, whereas all later cells reacted strongly (O'Rand and Romrell, 1980). When antibodies against secondary spermatogonia were prepared, about 2,000,000 sites per cell were quantified for all early spermatogenic stages through mature pachytene spermatocytes; this figure decreased to about half that level in early spermatids and to 3000 in spermatozoa from the vas deferens (Millette, 1979). Other studies have yielded comparable effective demonstrations of the changes in protein composition experienced by the sperm as it undergoes differentiation and then maturation (Romrell and O'Rand, 1978; O'Rand, 1979).

cAMP has been strongly implicated in the processes whereby sperm become motile, but the exact site of its occurrence is not firmly established. Apparently, from foregoing reports, movement of the flagelium commences in the cauda epididymis, and then is furthered during ejaculation by exposure to male accessory gland secretions (Harrison, 1975). While a role for cAMP appears secure, the mechanism for its action has not been determined. Further changes in spermatozoa take place after deposition in the female genital tract, where capacitation occurs. In part this involves a secretion of the sperm acrosome called acrosin, which aids in penetration of the zona pellucida of the ovum as described under fertilization. The presence of this important biochemical is complicated by the existence of protein trypsin-inhibitors in the seminal fluid which bind with the acrosin on a one-to-one irreversible basis (Laskowski and Sealock, 1971). Hence, it has been speculated that this inhibitor may play a role in eliminating faulty or damaged acrosomes, thus permitting only intact spermatozoa to reach the ovum surface (Suominen and Setchell, 1972).

1.3.2. Macromolecular Aspects of Metazoan Spermatogenesis

Quite in contrast to the ultrastructural and cytological aspects of spermatogenesis, the macromolecular facets have not received as much attention as they have in oogenesis, yet a fair quantity of data on the subject has accumulated. As in oogenesis, the synthesis of RNAs has been particularly well explored.

rRNA during Spermatogenesis. Early studies using autoradiographic techniques concluded that rRNA synthesis was either absent or virtually so in mammalian spermatogenesis (Utakoji, 1966; Muramatsu *et al.*, 1968), but more recent investigations have proven this conclusion to be erroneous (Stefanini *et al.*, 1974; Tres, 1975; Söderström and Parvinen, 1976; Monesi *et al.*, 1978). Through use of semithin sections and electron microscopic autoradiography, it was demonstrated that the nucleoli incorporated labeled precursors of RNA during meiosis in men, male rats, and mice (Kierszenbaum and Tres, 1974; Stefanini *et al.*, 1974; Tres, 1975). The pattern of labeling suggested that a stepwise increase in rRNA transcription occurred until midpachytene, after which there was a gradual decline, leading to a complete halt during the most advanced stages of meiosis (Stefanini *et al.*, 1974). After transcription, however, maturation of the products appeared to be slower than typical in somatic cells of metaphytans and metazoans (Parchman and Lin, 1972; Sconzo *et al.*, 1972).

Other RNA Synthesis. The transcription of other genes follows a well-marked path during spermatogenesis in mammals. During the leptotene to early pachytene stages of meiosis, the rate of incorporation of [^{3}H]uridine was found to be quite low (Monesi, 1964, 1965; Monesi *et al.*, 1978), but beginning toward the middle of the latter period it rose rapidly to reach a strong peak just before the termination. Then in diplotene, it began a decline again, a gradual process that attained its original low level only by mid-diakinesis; it then ceased entirely during the remainder of meiosis. In early spermatids it was briefly resumed, only to cease once more in elongated spermatids and spermatozoa. Similar patterns of RNA synthesis have also been reported in orthopterans (Muckenthaler, 1964).

In the spermatocyte of vertebrates, the irregular, laterally projecting loops and tangles of chromatin, rather than the axis, have been found to be the sites of RNA transcription during meiosis. Most of the transcripts have proven to be DNA-like hnRNAs of unusual stability (Monesi, 1964, 1965); the majority of these products remained associated with the chromosomes for a long period, except for a small fraction that broke down with the nucleus or was slowly released into the cytoplasm. The largest portion remained intact within the nucleus until late diakinesis or prometaphase, when it was rapidly moved into the cytosol. Thus, most of the RNA present in spermatids represents molecules synthesized during diplotene or diakinesis. A sizable fraction of the RNAs were polyadenylated and consequently may be considered to represent mRNAs (Geremia *et al.*, 1977).

Changes in Chromatin Structure. That the ultrastructural aspects of chromatin changes might be extremely profitable to investigate is made clear by two similar studies, whose results are in direct conflict. In the house cricket during early and much of middle spermiogenesis, the chromatin fibers were shown to bear closely paced nucleosomes, quite like those of somatic cells (McMaster-Kaye and Kaye, 1980a). Before the thick fibers of late spermatids began to form, however, the nucleosomes were lost, one at a time and seemingly in random fashion (Figure 1.28A, B). Since the histones had earlier been shown to remain throughout these stages, they were thought to become incorporated into other types of nucleoprotein complexes. Quite to the opposite in the dogfish, the beaded appearance of chromatin usually attributed to the presence of nucleosomes was reported to persist through the spermatid stage into the sperm (Gusse and Chevaillier, 1980). However, the proteins associated with the DNA underwent alteration, in that three different fractions became complexed with the nucleic acid in the nuclei of sperm; these proteins appeared at

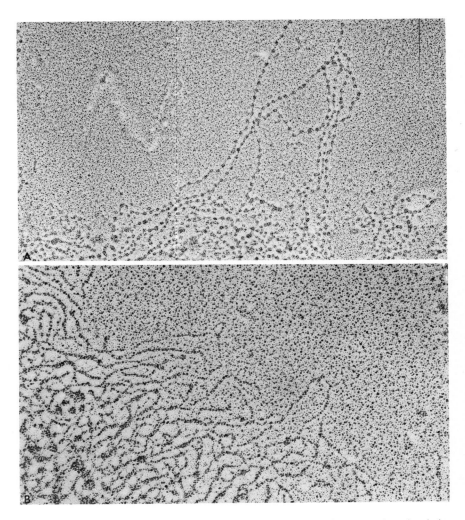

Figure 1.28. Chromatin changes during condensation. As chromatin undergoes condensation during spermiogenesis in the cricket, it loses its earlier characteristics. (A) Up to the midpoint in sperm formation, the chromatin of the spermatid nucleus retains its typical beaded appearance. 66,000×. (B) By the time the nucleus has elongated, the fibers have lost most of the nucleosomes, yet the chromatin retains the usual quantities of histones. 105,000×. (Both courtesy of McMaster-Kaye and Kaye, 1980a.)

Table 1.2
Primary Structure of Three Species of
Protamines from Rainbow Trout[a]

Protamine 1a	PRRRR--SSRPVRRRRRRPRRVSRRRRRRGGRRRR
Protamine 1b	PRRRRRRSSSSRPIRRRR-PRRVSRRRRR-GGRRRR
Protamine 2	PRRRR--SSSRPVRRRR-ARRVSRRRRRRGGRRRR

[a] Based on Ando and Watanabe (1969).

the termination of differentiation, when the gametes had become fully elongated. Subsequently, two of the fractions underwent modification, for only one remained acid soluble. If the latter were extracted, no change in nucleosomal structure was observed.

Doubtlessly some of the protein changes just noted might be correlated to the substitution of protamines for histones, a phenomenon known to occur during spermatogenesis among higher vertebrates in general, including mammals (Avramova *et al.*, 1980). Several aspects of the processes that are involved have been thoroughly explored in the fishes, particularly rainbow trout, which are especially favorable for such studies because of the seasonality of spermatogenesis (Iatrou and Dixon, 1978). Hence, needed cell populations can be obtained by treatment with pituitary extracts that stimulate the testicular cells to undergo maturation. The protamines in this species are a group of three or four polypeptides with chains of only 32 or 33 amino acid residues (Ando and Watanabe, 1969; Davies *et al.*, 1976). As may be observed in Table 1.2, about two-thirds (21 or 22) of the sites are occupied by arginine residues, four by serine, and two or three each by proline and glycine, the remainder being filled by valine or isoleucine. The structural likeness of the three components listed in the table is also an obvious feature, all of which are synthesized only in the spermatid on characteristic pairs of ribosomes (Ling *et al.*, 1969; Ling and Dixon, 1970). The brevity of the polysome chain may perhaps result from the messenger's being too short to bear more than that number at any given time. After synthesis, the polypeptides move into the nucleus and there, as they are combined into complexes with DNA, undergo phosphorylations and dephosphorylations of the four serine residues. The resulting chromatin, called nucleoprotamine, is in a highly condensed state that proved inactive as a template for RNA polymerase from *E. coli* (Marushige and Dixon, 1969). Experimental evidence suggested that the nucleoprotamine must have lacked the typical nucleosome particles (Honda *et al.*, 1975), but this deduction is in conflict with the observations made on dogfish chromatin discussed in the preceding paragraph, if it too contained protamines. Both poly(A)-bearing and -deficient mRNAs for protamine occur (Iatrou and Dixon, 1977); more recently, four size

classes of these mRNAs were described, which persisted even after removal of
the poly(A) tracts (Iatrou *et al.*, 1979). Although translation of these mRNAs
was confined entirely to the spermatid, transcription was found to occur in
primary spermatocytes (Iatrou *et al.*, 1978), an especially pertinent sequence
of events. Mammalian protamines are much longer, in bull sperm containing
45 amino acid residues, and although similarly arginine rich, include a wider
range of other amino acids, including six cysteines (Dixon *et al.*, 1977).

More critical examination of nucleosome structure during spermatogenesis
is imperative; simple determination of the presence or absence of these particles
fails to reveal much pertinent data. This statement is supported by a recent
reinvestigation into the structure of chromatin in sperm and in embryo and adult
somatic cells in a sea urchin (Keichline and Wassarman, 1977, 1979). While
the size of the repeat length was uniformly 222 base pairs in embryos and in
adult intestine, compared to 199 in mouse liver, they were much longer in
sperm chromatin, containing 250 base pairs. The sperm chromatin also contained a unique species of histone H1 (Ozaki, 1971), and H2A and H2B were
demonstrated similarly to differ from those of adult tissues (Simpson and Bergman, 1980). Changes in structure of insect sperm chromatin have likewise not
escaped observation. In the house cricket (*Acheta domesticus*) the chromatin of
those early spermatids that are just beginning to elongate was in the form of
thicker and straighter fibers than those of somatic cells (Kaye and McMaster-
Kaye, 1975). These threads were oriented nearly perpendicularly to the inner
wall of the nuclear envelope, but finer, more irregular ones filled much of the
nuclear interior (Figure 1.29A). As additional nuclear elongation occurred, the
bases of the fibers became thickened still further, leading to fusion of adjacent
components and a resulting decrease in numbers. These processes of thickening
and fusion continued until the peripheral chromatin was in the form of a continuous, broad, electron-opaque band from which a few, folded thick fibers
extended proximally. The interior portion then similarly underwent condensation so that in the mature sperm the entire nucleus was an opaque mass (Figure
1.29C, D). During these processes, in addition to the five of somatic tissues,
two new histones developed that were absent in somatic cells and also the testes
of young nymphs. Moreover, they were present in adult testes only after the
initial stages of spermiogenesis and appeared to replace the somatic histones

Figure 1.29. Changes in chromatin organization in the house cricket. The appearance of chromatin
in these insects undergoes remarkable changes as the sperm is formed. (A) After the nucleus has
elongated to a degree, the chromatin fibers are thick and nearly straight, projecting at right angles
from the nuclear envelope. 35,000×. (B) Later the bases of the fibrous masses thickened, reducing
the number of individual components through fusion. 14,500×. (C, D) As the sperm develops
during the successive later stages shown by these cross sections, the chromatin continues to condense.
These structural changes are accompanied by the appearance of new types of histones, as discussed
in the text. C, 49,000×; D, 51,000×. (All courtesy of Kaye and McMaster-Kaye, 1975.)

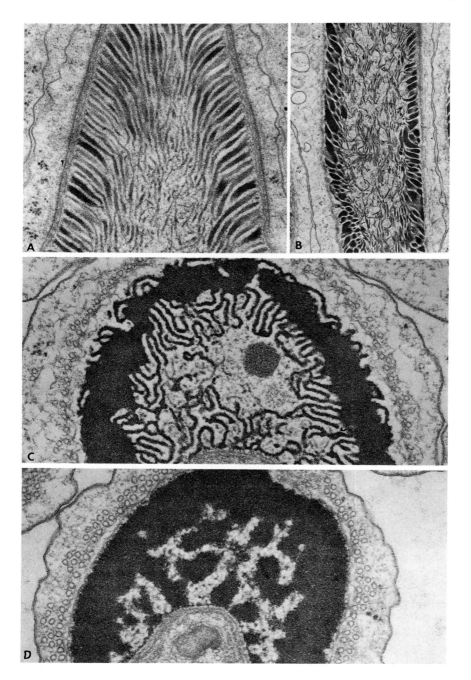

during the late stages of nuclear elongation in the spermatid—80% of the histones present in the latter were ascertained to be of the new types.

Protein Changes during Vertebrate Spermatogenesis. In view of the changes in structure during spermatogenesis that have just been described, it is to be expected that correlated alterations in protein constituents should also be equally marked. However, only a bare beginning has been made towards following the time sequence of the appearance and regression of any one particular species, most investigations having dealt with classes of these substances. Tritium-labeled leucine was injected intratesticularly into mice, and epididymal sperm were extracted on alternate days over a 32-day period; the latter were digested and fractionated into SDS-soluble and -insoluble proteins (O'Brien and Bellvé, 1980a,b). The soluble fraction was found to be translated chiefly during meiosis and early spermiogenesis, but the distribution of radioactivity on SDS-polyacrylamide gels showed both quantitative and qualitative changes in the several generations of cell types. The SDS-insoluble proteins from the head of the sperm fell into four categories: acidic, moderately basic, protamine, and residual, each of which was synthesized at specific time periods during the spermiogenic processes. Protamines were most actively synthesized during middle and late spermiogenesis, whereas the acidic and moderately basic classes were produced near the termination of spermiogenesis after transcription no longer was detectable.

As indicated in connection with chromatin structural changes, the synthesis of histones during spermatogenesis in the rat has recently received attention. In mammals two species of histones are present in testicular cells that are absent in somatic ones; these testis-specific ones, designated as TH1 and TH2B, are closely related in molecular weight and amino acid content to the somatic counterparts, H1 and H2B. Both of these, as well as the full somatic complement, were present in all stages through the early spermatid but were absent from the fully elongated sperm (Brock *et al.*, 1980). Synthesis of TH1 and TH2B continued through pachytene of the primary spermatocyte but had ceased in early spermatids. Moreover, synthesis of H2B did not occur in pachytene or subsequent stages. Since injection of hydroxyurea *in vivo* reduced DNA synthesis in the testis to 1% of control values but did not affect the production of TH1, H1, or TH2B, it was demonstrated that the synthesis of these proteins was not dependent on DNA production.

In actuality, the sperm of mammals contains a large number of proteins not found in other cell types (Goldberg, 1977), among which are unique isozymal variants of phosphoglycerate kinase, diaphorase, hyaluronidase, and lactate dehydrogenase. The last is probably the best characterized of these enzymes and has been the subject of a number of thorough investigations. In mice, the isozyme is referred to as LDH-X and is a tetramer comprised of four identical C subunits encoded by a gene that is active only in the testes; in all other tissues the enzyme consists of A and B subunits. The earliest activity of LDH-X was detected 14 days postpartum and was most abundant in late pach-

ytene spermatocytes and round spermatids (Wieben, 1981); with further maturation the isozyme decreased to about half its earlier activity. Actin is another
protein whose synthesis has been followed during the course of spermatogenesis but in this case largely in invertebrates. In a cranefly, actin was abundant
in the spermatocyte and spermatid but was undetectable in mature sperm (Strauch
et al., 1980). Moreover, its characteristics underwent changes correlated to
development, being 80% sedimentable in the earlier cell generation but only
20% in the spermatid. Quite in contrast, actin was found in mature spermatozoa
of the colonial hydroid, *Hydractinia*, closely associated with the flagellar centriole (Kleve and Clark, 1980).

Thus far, few investigations have focused on the changes that occur during
spermatogenesis in the total profile of protein synthesis, one current exception
being devoted to such processes in the mouse (Boitani et al., 1980). Three
stages were analyzed by isoelectric focusing and autoradiography in middle to
late pachytene spermatocytes, round spermatids, and transitional spermatids.
As might be expected, the greatest diversity in polypeptide species was in the
earliest of these stages, in which at least 250 different fingerprints were detected (Figure 1.30). In contrast, while but a slight diminution was to be noted
in the rounded spermatids, the transitional ones showed only about 100 species
being synthesized (Figure 1.31A, B). However, the changes in synthesis were
varied in expression. Protein D, for example, was confined strictly to the sper-

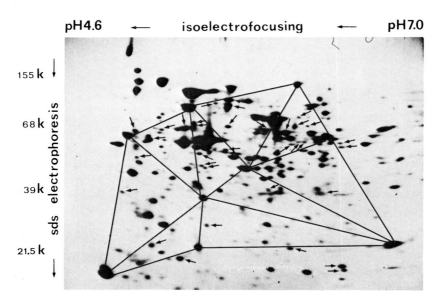

Figure 1.30. The polypeptides of middle to late pachytene spermatocytes of the mouse. Fingerprints
of about 250 species are present. (Courtesy of Boitani et al., 1980.)

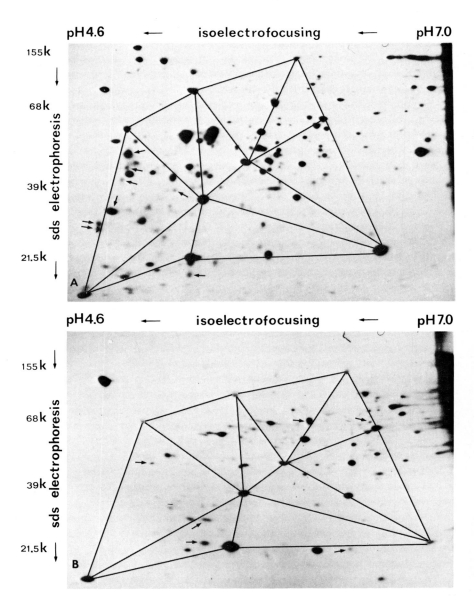

Figure 1.31. Changes in protein profile during spermatogenesis. (A) Even in this round spermatid the number of polypeptide species present is greatly reduced relative to that of the spermatocyte (Figure 1.30), and still greater reduction is obvious in the protein profile of transitional spermatids (B). (Both courtesy of Boitani *et al.*, 1980.)

matocyte, and B was formed most abundantly in that stage, but it continued into the early spermatid in decreased abundance and was absent from the transitional spermatid. In contrast, protein C was absent from the spermatocyte but became increasingly synthesized with advancing development, while F was far more marked in the round spermatid than in either of the other stages.

1.3.3. Male Gametogenesis in Metaphytan Taxa

In taxa outside the Metazoa the male gamete probably has been a much greater favorite with investigators than the relatively poorly-differentiated ovum, for it has often proven to be quite as complex structurally as that of the animals, especially in many higher plants. Because of this complexity, more attention similarly has been paid to the finished product or its immediate predecessors than to the early stages, so ultrastructural features and biochemical properties of developmental phases as a whole remain for the future to disclose. Undoubtedly the most thoroughly explored areas of this field are represented by the mosses and ferns, but a sufficiency of other types has been examined to provide an aspect missing among the metazoan sperm, that is, a firm basis for an insight into the phylogenetic history of this gamete. To avoid intimating functional or behavioral differences where none exist, the zoological term spermatozoon is here employed as in the foregoing section, rather than the botanical name spermatozoid, and for the same reasons metazoan terminology is applied to developmental stages insofar as is warranted.*

Spermatogenesis in Bryophytes. Except for the absence of meiosis, which processes had occurred earlier during the formation of the microspore that gave rise to the gametophyte, a surprising number of correspondences are to be noted between the plant cell generations of spermatogenesis and their animal counterparts. The developmental stages in mosses are selected as the first model, because they have been treated in a particularly thoroughgoing account of spermatogenesis in those plants (Lal and Bell, 1975). As the young antheridium develops, the cells of its wall, which stain strongly with oxmium, give rise to an internal layer of spermatogonia (spermatogenous cells of botanists), which remain unstained. Moreover, while the chloroplasts of the antheridial cells are well developed and functional, those of the spermatogonia remain as proplastids; ribosomes are plentiful, although only occasional polysomes can be found. These cells undergo a period of proliferation by mitotic division, one result of which is the formation of several blocks per antheridium, division being synchronous within but not between blocks. Moreover, favorable sections often show intercellular bridges connecting the spermatogonia by way of perforations in the cell wall.

---

*Unfortunately, too few molecular and ultrastructural details have become available of algal sperm development to permit a meaningful discussion (Moestrup, 1975).

The later stages of spermatogenesis have not been reported in mosses, but possibly are similar to those of liverworts (Carothers, 1975). In the latter plants the penultimate division of the spermatogonia results in a pair of spermatocytes, the most distinctive features of which are: the presence of two pairs of centrioles near the plastids and simple mitochondria virtually devoid of cristae. Following a series of structural changes, the spermatocyte undergoes a final mitotic division to form spermatids, after which differentiation begins. The earliest change then noted is the retraction of the protoplast from the cell wall, a process that becomes increasingly marked as differentiation proceeds. Concurrently the nucleus is moved to one side, while most of the remaining organelles become concentrated at the opposite. However, one chloroplast and usually a single mitochondrion, which like the others has developed swollen cristae, becomes closely applied to the nucleus laterally where the two bodies remain even in the mature spermatozoon. This nucleus-associated chloroplast undergoes marked alteration, developing a few thylakoids and crystalloid deposits of lipoproteins, so that it eventually resembles the prolamellar body of higher plants. This lateral arrangement of cell parts appears to be more frequent among diverse species of bryophytes (Bonnot, 1967; Genevès, 1968), than does the polar arrangement described by Paolillo et al. (1968a,b).

After these maturational changes have been completed, metamorphosis of the spermatid begins, processes that consist of a series of remarkable alterations in structure of several organelles. Among those showing modification are the Golgi bodies, which become more abundant and display a high level of activity that persists until late in the metamorphic processes. No acrosome develops from the resulting vesicles, however; instead, the latter seem to contribute to the thick layer of mucilage that covers the completed spermatozoon (Lal and Bell, 1975). Within the nucleus, several changes also are noted, even early in the transformation of the cell. First the nucleolus disperses, while the chromatin gradually condenses, in the initial stages forming scattered patches of electron-opaque material and later numerous opaque rods distributed throughout the nucleoplasm. After considerable condensation has occurred, the nucleus begins to elongate, eventually becoming quite long and slender; then near the close of the processes, it curves to assume a sickle shape, while the chromatin becomes completely condensed. Externally, in the meanwhile, a manchette of microtubules that has formed in the cytoplasm moves into contact with the nucleus; this flat band has been thought to be implicated in the changes in nuclear shape. Since in the ferns of the genus *Pteridium*, this structure has been shown to be a complex with the envelope that eliminates the perinuclear space (Bell, 1978), it may prove to be similarly constructed in these mosses. Whether the nuclear envelope remains intact throughout metamorphosis or becomes fragmented has not been determined.

Undoubtedly the most marked metamorphic changes involve the development of the flagellar apparatus. Except perhaps in liverworts, centrioles usually have been absent throughout the spermatogonial and spermatocytic periods to this point, but now a pteridoplast (often called a blepharoplast; Dillon, 1981, pp. 191, 192) develops *de novo*, and differentiates into the precursor of the tetriole (multilayered body) and two centrioles.

The tetriole, described in detail previously (Dillon, 1981, pp. 189–191), in mosses consists of only three layers as in ferns, not four as in liverworts (Carothers and Kreitner, 1967). This body then becomes associated with a single specialized mitochondrion and migrates with it to the anterior end of the nucleus. Here the mitochondrial part embeds in a pit in the nucleus while the tetriole completes differentiation. After the basic structure has been finished, the microtubules that form the distal layer increase in length, extending beyond the underlying plates until they reach about two-thirds around the nucleus. At the same time a pair of flagella, produced on the centrioles, grow posteriorly nearly paralleling the microtubular ribbon just described. After the flagella have elongated until they extend well beyond the body of the cell, the cytoplasm becomes reduced in quantity, perhaps by bleb formation as in metazoans, until the spermatozoon is completed, ready for release.

Spermatogenesis in Other Lower Embryophytes. The foregoing discussion has already brought out the chief distinctions of the liverwort spermatogenic processes, including the earlier appearance of centrioles and the presence of four layers in the tetriole, rather than three. However, in the pteriodophytes and relatives a number of novel features are to be noted.

In such fern allies as the horsetail rushes (Duckett and Bell, 1977) and club mosses, as well as in the ferns themselves, the pteridoplast first appears in the spermatocytes; it then divides into two before these cells cleave into two spermatids, rather than in the spermatid stage as in the mosses (Duckett, 1975; Vaudois and Tourte, 1979). Also as in that taxon, the individual subunits of the pteridoplast break apart to form numerous procentrioles as the rudiments of the tetriole become visible in contact with the granular remnants (Robbins and Carothers, 1978). At this time, only the outer microtubular band and the inner lamella are discernible, but the specialized mitochondrion lies against the latter, continuing around one end to reach the microtubular region. However, this continuation is absent in horsetail rushes (Duckett, 1973). The microtubules overlie the lamellar plates at an angle between 35 and 45°, a point that has much bearing on the future shape of the gamete.

Beyond this initial stage, the tetriole increases rapidly in size, growth of the lamellar strip being coordinated with increase in the number of microtubules, so that lamellar profiles lacking tubules are never encountered. The lamellar plate soon attains its ultimate length of 5–10 μm in ferns and 15–20 μm in *Equisetum*, as the microtubules gain their final number (around 150 in the ferns and 300 plus in the horsetail rushes). As the microtubules now undergo elongation until they extend far beyond the plate, the shape of the spermatid nucleus changes from its original spherical to an arcuate droplet form, becoming increasingly elongate, slender, and spiral as metamorphosis proceeds. In the end it forms about four complete gyres in *Pteridium* spermatozoa, but the structure is so arranged within the cytoplasm that the overall form of the gamete is spherical. As development progresses, the former procentrioles, now fully mature centrioles, become situated along the external surface of the tetriole, where they give rise to flagella. With these developments the lamellar strip separates from the nucleus and moves anteriorly, remaining attached to the nuclear surface by only the microtubular band. Thus in the ferns the tetriole is at the anterior end of the spermatozoon, while the nucleus occupies the posterior nine-tenths. The latter is associated with microtubules, while the anterior half in addition is accompanied by one or more elongate mitochondria.

A similar coil, comprised of the tetriole, mitochondria, nucleus, and microtubules, develops during spermiogenesis in such specialized ferns as *Marselia*, but the spiral is deeper, involving around 10 gyres. Of these only four or five are actually occupied by the nucleus, whereas the mitochondrion is found in nine (Myles and Bell, 1975; Myles and Hepler, 1977). Moreover, the flagella are much more abundant, about 100 to 120 being present, attached to a like number of centrioles; the motile organelles are distributed over the entire length of the coil, not just over the lamellar plate. At first, the flagella are enveloped by cytoplasm, but as the gamete approaches maturity, they become exposed through the shedding of cytoplasm to gain the pear shape characteristic of the spermatozoon. Chloroplasts are to be found in the posterior part of the cytoplasmic mass, but this entire portion, along with part of the nuclear membrane, is shed after the sperm has been released but prior to its reaching the egg.

Because it has not been widely realized by plant cytologists concerned with lower embryophytes that the processes of gametogenesis really encompass three distinctive cell types, the two early stages are usually grouped together under the term spermatogenous tissue in the stoneworts as in the mosses and others. Consequently, it is not known whether in the stoneworts the centrioles first appear in the spermatogonial, spermatocytic, or spermatid generations. In members of the genera *Chara* and *Nitella*, it is clear, however, that they are absent from somatic tissues and that they appear either in the early spermatid or possibly the spermatocyte (Figure 1.32A; Pickett-Heaps, 1968; Turner, 1968). Within the antheridium, the spermatogonia undergo multiple mitotic divisions to form long threads which fill the lumen of the chamber as a tangled mass, divisions within a given thread being synchronous. These male gametic cells are interconnected by intercellular bridges through pores in the walls. Since procentrioles are observed when the threads are quite short, those organelles obviously are formed *de novo* in early spermatogonia; however, they do not attain their mature structure until the cessation of mitosis, that is, in the early spermatid (Figure 1.32B; Pickett-Heaps, 1968). When differentiation of the latter into the spermatozoon commences, the nucleus moves to one end of the

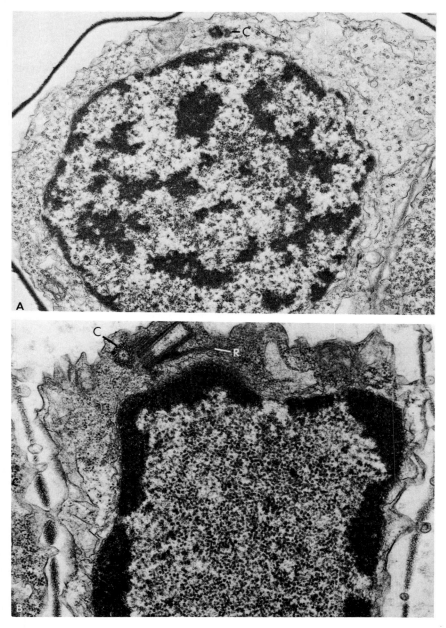

Figure 1.32. Changes in chromatin structure in a stonewort. In *Nitella*, the organization of the chromatin becomes strongly condensed around the periphery by the time the early spermatid stage has been attained. (B) The centrioles, which appeared *de novo* in prophase in the mitotic form (A), have now acquired their flagellar configuration, along with a rhizoplast. A, 16,000×; B, 30,000×. (Both courtesy of Turner, 1968.)

cell, and the chromatin starts to condense beneath the nuclear envelope. Concurrently the cytoplasm becomes more dispersed as it begins to retract from the cell walls (Figure 1.32B). Chloroplasts lack complete thylakoids and resemble prolamellar bodies, and the rare mitochondria tend to show a degree of vesicularization such as that which marks those of higher green plants. The Golgi bodies are quite active and display the intercisternal elements likewise so characteristic of higher plants (Dillon, 1981, pp. 239–242). Later as these trends continue and the cytoplasm becomes still more widely removed from the walls, a flagellum is formed on the larger of the two centrioles. The latter in the meanwhile has become associated with a mitochondrion and together the pair are moved to one end of the nucleus, with which the mitochondrion provides the actual contact. Soon afterwards a manchette of eight microtubules can be noted, while the nucleus becomes more elongate. To this band an increasing number of microtubules is added until a total of about 27 is attained. At the same time a layer of dense amorphous material accumulates proximal to the manchette, underlain by a less opaque lamella; undoubtedly these layers represent precursors of the tetriole of higher forms, but in the stonewort they have not yet gained their highly structured form. The nucleus elongates and coils somewhat, perhaps aided by the manchette of microtubules that covers one side, as in the mosses. As it coils it becomes arranged behind this protetriole, followed by a cytoplasmic sac containing the plastids and other remaining organelles, to form an elongate, very slender, slightly spiraled, biflagellated spermatozoon.

   Spermatogenesis in Cycads and Ginkgoes. In cycads, the microspores, which are produced meiotically within a microsporangium, are not shed when mature but are retained to begin development into the male gametophyte. Enclosed within the spore coat, the microspore divides by mitosis to form a one-celled prothallus and an antheridial initial cell. After the latter has undergone a second mitotic division to produce a generative cell and a tube cell, the resulting three-celled gametophyte, or pollen grain, is ready for release. Probably by wind action, pollen may be deposited onto a drop of mucilagelike material (the pollination droplet) at the entrance of the micropyle of the megastrobilus and is drawn into the pollen chamber of the microsporangium, or nucellus, when the droplet is retracted. After several months, the male gametophyte develops a pollen tube, within which the generative cell divides mitotically to produce two spermatozoa. These sperm develop in a back-to-back orientation and, when mature, rank as the largest among the metaphytans, ranging up to 0.5 mm in diameter (Norstog, 1975). As in ferns, a pteridoplast gives rise to numerous procentrioles, that in turn develop into centrioles on which 10,000 to 12,000 flagella are produced (Mizukami and Gall, 1966). The centriole–flagellum combinations are arranged along a tetriole coupled to the nucleus as in ferns, but in this case the entire structure is confined to the anterior half of the sperm. Aside from the formation of the tetriole, few ultrastructural features of spermatogenesis have received attention in these organisms.

The processes in *Ginkgo*, including the *de novo* formation of a pterido-plast, are quite similar to those of cycads, except for minor details. When mature, for example, the pollen grain contains two prothallial cells, one of which has degenerated (Gifford and Larson, 1980). Then after pollination has been achieved, the generative cell divides mitotically to produce a sterile cell and a spermatogenous cell. The latter then undergoes division to produce two spermatozoa oriented back-to-back.

Spermatogenesis in Flowering Plants. The reduction of the male ga-metophyte to a pollen grain in the cycads and the intracellular production of sperm introduces some of the features of spermatogenesis in their more ad-vanced relatives, the flowering plants. In these organisms the microsporangia are the pollen sacs enclosed within the anther. The sacs, lined with a tropho-cytic layer called the tapetum, are filled with pollen mother cells, each of which undergoes meiotic division twice to produce a cluster of four microspores. After a wall consisting of two layers (the exine and intine) has developed around the spore, the enclosed cell germinates, dividing mitotically, typically without cy-tokinesis, to form a syncytium containing two nuclei. One of these is the tube nucleus, representing the remnants of the ancestral prothallus and the other is the generative nucleus. Thus mature, the microgametophyte, or pollen grain, is ready for release. Following pollination, the pollen grain produces a pollen tube that grows down the pistil to reach the embryo sac, the tube nucleus remaining near its growing tip. The generative nucleus descends the tube's length behind the tube nucleus, and eventually undergoes division into two sperm nuclei en route. Thus, there are neither spermatozoa nor spermatids.

Possibly because of the absence of marked differences between cell gen-erations, changes in ultrastructure that might accompany the development of the sperm nuclei do not appear to have attracted much attention. However, some progress has been made regarding the proteins involved in the formation of the microsporocyte wall. During their early proliferation stages, the pollen mother cells are interconnected by cytoplasmic bridges, so that division is syn-chronous, recalling a characteristic of spermatogonia. When ready to undergo meiosis, each of these meiocytes (mature pollen mother cells) deposits a wall of callose (β-1,3-linked glucan) about itself, sealing off the cytoplasmic bridges in the processes. Within this wall, the equivalent of a primary spermatocyte commences meiotic division, during prophase I of which the ribosomes are lost along with other organelles. Then in the secondary spermatocyte, the ribosome complement is restored and the other organelles replaced (Dickinson and Hes-lop-Harrison, 1970)—one would suspect interesting differences to exist be-tween the lost set and their replacements. The endoreticulum develops in as-sociation with the future germinal-aperture sites within each component of the resulting tetrad enclosed by the callose wall (Heslop-Harrison, 1968; Knox, 1976). Then a layer, which serves as a precursor to the exine proper (the pri-mexine), and consists largely of cellulose, is laid down beneath the callose; on the exterior of this layer are arranged the first elements of the pattern that will characterize the pollen grain. When that precursorial structure has been completed, it becomes coated with sporopollenin, most of which is secreted by the tapetum; as the exine is thus brought into existence, all its knobs and other distinctive traits ultimately become completed with this deposit.

During wall formation, part, but not all, of the pattern is dependent upon the presence of microtubules, for such inhibitors of microtubule formation as colchicine have been shown to interfere with the full development of the design. Once this coat is complete the trophocytes of the tapetum break down (Santos *et al.*, 1979), and the callose coat over the tetrad is degraded, freeing the microspores into the pollen sac. Following their release, the exine is completed, beneath which the microspores commence secreting the intine; during these secretory processes, the cytoplasm of most microspores concurrently becomes filled with vacuoles. Only after vacuolization is finished do the microspores undergo a mitotic division to form the ripened pollen (Raghavan, 1976, 1978, 1979). When cultured, such vacuolized grains cannot develop embryoids; only those that do not contain vacuoles can undergo transcription of their DNA and eventually produce such bodies.

The formation of the spore coat has been elaborated here for only one reason—extremely important proteins are embedded within it that play a role in pollination. Although the normal function of the various enzymes is that of providing intraspecific-recognition mechanisms, they are also the agents that induce hayfever and similar allergies in vertebrates of many types. Among the proteins that are known to be confined to the intine are a ribonuclease and acid phosphatase, while succinic acid and NADH dehydrogenases, cytochrome oxidase, and a protease are found only in the exine (Knox, 1976). In addition, the two layers share a number of proteins, including allergens, phosphorylase, amylase, esterase, and polygalacturonase and other hydrases of carbohydrates. As a result of the presence of certain species-specific substances, foreign pollen can be rejected from the stigma or, later, in the style by inhibition of the growth of the pollen tube. Moreover, in some species, similar processes provide for self-incompatibility, pollen from a given individual plant being prevented from fertilizing its own ovules but remaining capable of doing so with other members of the same species. The genetics of these properties have been shown to involve multiple alleles at two or more loci in rye, tobacco, cherry, and a number of other species (Linskens and Kroh, 1967).

1.4. GAMETOGENESIS IN VARIOUS EUKARYOTES

A number of eukaryotes have complex life cycles, often involving asexual alternating with sexual generations, especially among fungi and red and brown algae. Since it is generally recognized that differentiated gametes probably were derived evolutionarily from undifferentiated swimming spores (zoospores), it is essential, too, to view one or more instances of the latter's formation. Because the gametes, whether male or female, are typically provided with flagella, this discussion is associated with spermatogenesis rather than oogenesis.

In advanced organisms like fish and even seed plants, ultrastructural and macromolecular aspects of meiosis and maturation have been incompletely explored; accordingly, it is to be expected that descriptive accounts of the events in lower organisms would be even more sketchy. Here as in the discussion pertaining to the metaphytans, an attempt is made to apply metazoan terms for cell types and the like wherever possible, in order to make similarities and differences more apparent and meaningful.

1.4.1. Gametogenesis in Fungi

In general, gametogenesis in the various types of fungi does not lend itself to comparisons with metazoan and metaphytan processes, for the structure of the organisms differs so radically as to preclude the existence of true tissues, let alone well-developed organs. Consequently the larger part of ultrastructural studies have concentrated on the zoospore or gamete itself, rather than on the precursorial stages. Thus, few analyses of the biochemical changes that must occur in the cells as they mature and associated macromolecular events during gamete production have been documented.

Gametogenesis in the Phycomycetes. One of the simpler groups of fungi is the class Phycomycetes, whose members are constructed of tubular cells arranged into long hyphae and rhizoids. A number of studies on zoospore morphology of these molds have been made during the past decade, so that the fine structure of the cell from a diversity of representatives is known. In one of the simpler types, *Synchytrium endobioticum* (Lange and Olson, 1978), some of the more characteristic features of advanced forms are lacking. The flagellar centriole is situated at the base of the flagellum just beneath the plasmalemma rather remote from the nuclear envelope; no mitochondrion is directly associated with this organelle, but one or two lie at some distance. To one side of the nucleus is a substantial so-called side-body complex, consisting of a large mitochondrion lying close to the nucleus and a short series of cisternae of rough endoreticulum. As in the majority of organisms, the ribosomes are distributed fairly uniformly throughout the cytoplasm.

However, in most members of the taxon, these minute bodies become concentrated into an electron-opaque nuclear cap, a body larger than the nucleus (Figure 1.33A), that is enclosed in membranes derived from the nuclear envelope, as in *Catenaria* (Olson *et al.*, 1978). In the members of this genus, the flagellar centriole is in contact with a flattened region of the nucleus as among metazoans and is closely associated with several mitochondria. This association includes the extremely long mitochondrion of the side-body complex, which extends thence anteriorly to reach over much of one side of the

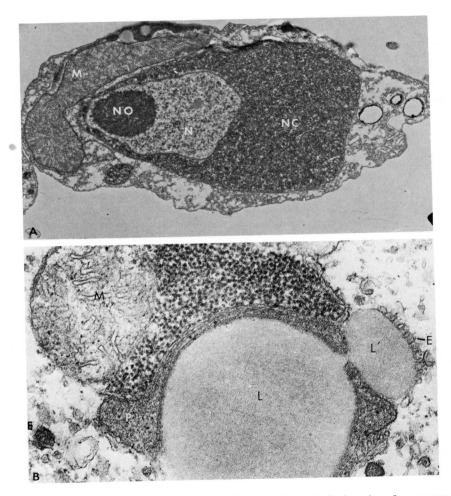

Figure 1.33. Characteristics of fungal zoospores. (A) In this longitudinal section of a zoospore head of *Blastocladiella*, a nuclear cap (NC) is present, that has an appearance not unlike the acrosome of metazoan sperm; here it nearly encloses the slightly elongate nucleus (N), in which a nucleolus (NO) remains intact. A portion of the mitochondrion (M) that is associated with the side body also is shown. 10,944×. (Courtesy of J. S. Lovett, 1975.) (B) The ribosomal nature of the nuclear cap is evident in this section of a *Phlyctochytrium* zoospore; the association between the cap and the side body complex is apparent. The latter structure consists of a large lipid body (L), here connected to a small continuation (L′) that forms part of the eyespot (E) and to a mitochondrion (M) and peroxisome (P). 60,000×. (Courtesy of Lange and Olson, 1977.)

nuclear cap. In this genus the complex is more advanced than in *Synchytrium*, as it includes several liposomes and a peroxisome lying beneath cisternal endoreticulum of the smooth type. In *Phlyctochytrium* the liposome forms by far the greater part of the side body (Figure 1.33B), for it even exceeds the nucleus in size (Lange and Olson, 1977). The meiospore (zoospore produced meiotically) has the same structure as that resulting from mitosis.

Knowledge of the details of sporangium development and zoospore and gamete formation at best is of a preliminary nature. Typically the hyphae were found to consist of cylindrical or spherical cells that contained several nuclei; thus, they were syncytia, while the rhizoids were anucleate (Lessie and Lovett, 1968). In *Blastocladiella*, the spherical body became separated from the rhizoidal portion by formation of a septum, while its several nuclei underwent mitotic division. How often division took place was not specified in that article, nor were cellular changes reported until the onset of the differentiation processes that correspond to spermiogenesis in other taxa. During mitotic proliferation, each nucleus had been provided with paired centrioles at both spindle poles, the second, smaller (daughter) organelle being uniformly oriented at right angles to the mature one (Dillon, 1981, pp. 397–399). The latter had been situated in a depression in the nucleus throughout the proliferation stage but as metamorphosis began, a flagellum developed upon it. As this process proceeded, a distinctive type of vesicle appeared in the cytoplasm, which fused with another to create an ever-increasing vesicle surrounding the flagellar core. The inner membrane of this cylindrical vesicle became the flagellar sheath, while the outer soon was continuous with the plasmalemma; thus, the vesicle represented a sort of cleft in which the flagellum elongated. In the meanwhile, one group of mitochondria became associated broadly with one side of the nuclear envelope as the first step in forming the side body; concurrently, ribosomes were moved to an anterior position, where they ultimately became concentrated into the nuclear cap. Changes in nuclear structure likewise accompanied these developments, its original spherical configuration becoming modified into a conical form as an electron-dense body gradually appeared within it. This opaque structure was identified as the nucleolus, but more probably it represented condensed chromatin as in other advanced eukaryotes.

Gametogenesis in Other Fungi. No satisfactory ultrastructural or macromolecular accounts of gametogenesis seem to be available for members of the Ascomycetes and Basidiomycetes. In the former taxon, the male gamete often is merely a branch of a hypha, which upon contact with a female branch of a neighboring hypha of the same species donates one or more nuclei to the latter, but in some cases, flagellated sperm (called spermatia) are produced which reach the female gamete by various means to effect fertilization (Dring, 1975). Basidiomycetous fungi have similar hyphal gametes, with many variations and specialized structures (Kemp, 1975), but here, too, while the meiotic processes are well known (Huffman, 1968; Lu and Raju, 1970), molecular biological information is sparse.

1.4.2. Gametogenesis among Algae

Gametogenesis among Brown Algae. Fortunately, the processes of gamete formation have been followed more adequately at the ultrastructural level in the brown algae, even though macromolecular information is virtually absent. In advanced members of the taxon, there is an alternation of asexual and sexual generations, and, as in the metaphytans, the sporophyte is the principal generation, the gametophyte typically being a small, flat thallus or perhaps only a few hyphal cells (Fritsch, 1952). In *Cutleria*, the fan-shaped thallus bears arcuate rows of sori on its surface, in which the female gametangia (really ovaries) are produced (LaClaire and West, 1978). The first step in producing these structures was reported to be the appearance of a knob laterally on a filament cell, which had developed from an epidermal cell; this single-celled protuberance increased in size and then became separated from the parent cell by means of a septum. During growth, the cell underwent two transverse divisions mitotically to become a four-celled series; later each of these products divided vertically twice, so that in the end each ovary contained four tiers of four cells each. The protoplasmic mass of the cells then withdrew from the walls, as a flagellum developed. The spermatogenic processes in the same species were found to differ little from those of oogenesis, except that more cytoplasm was shed and the flagellar apparatus was better developed (LaClaire and West, 1979). Unfortunately, the changes in cell structure that probably occurred during gametogenesis were not followed in either case.

A more complete account has been provided by an investigation into zoo-sporogenesis in another member of the group. *Chorda tomentosa* (Toth, 1974). Unlike the gametogenic processes just described, the formation of the asexual zoospores involved meiosis, so that its several cell generations might be thought to correspond more closely to those of metazoans. According to this report cited, the cells of the external layer of the elongate tubular body, the meristoderm, ceased dividing vertical to the surface to enlarge the plant body diameter, but underwent division parallel to the exterior so as to produce two new cell types on the external surface. One of the pair grew into a sterile hair called a paraphysis, while the other served as the mother cell of the future sporangium. The latter first increased in size before entering into meiotic division, during which processes the nucleolus persisted until late prophase, well-developed synaptonemal complexes being present (Toth and Markey, 1973). Other characteristics included the presence of typical mitotic centrioles at each pole, the breakdown of the nuclear envelope at metaphase I, and the absence of cytokinesis, so that the end result was a four-celled syncytium. As further growth occurred, numerous synchronous mitotic divisions took place, similarly not accompanied by cleavage; however, the chloroplasts divided in concert with the nuclei, and as growth continued, assumed positions adjacent to the sporangial wall (Figure 1.34A). A nucleus later was moved into position to the proximal side of each plastid, at first at random points, but with further development a

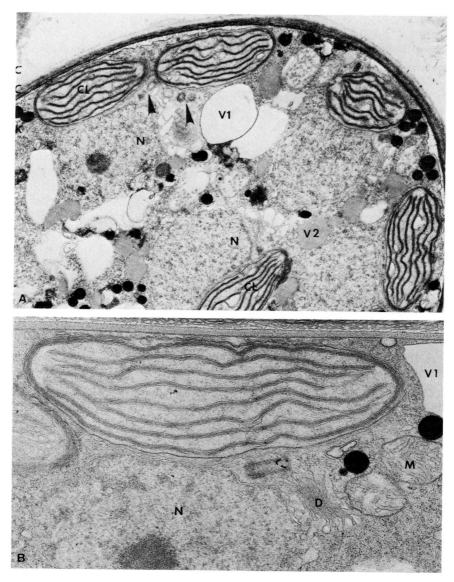

Figure 1.34. Zoospore formation in a brown alga. After meiotic division of the spore mother cell
into four nuclei, subsequent mitotic divisions lead to the formation of a multinucleated syncytium
in a thick-walled sporangium, as shown in (A). The association of each nucleus (N) with a chloroplast
(CL) and a pair of centrioles (arrowheads) is an especially striking feature. In addition, two types
of vesicles may be noted, V1 and V2. 10,000×. (B) In this enlarged view, the nucleus–chloroplast–
centriole association may be perceived also to include mitochondria (M) and a dictyosome (D).
The centriole (C) may be observed to be of the flagellar type. 26,300×. (Both courtesy of Toth,
1974.)

side-by-side orientation was acquired. Between these two organelles, paired centrioles subsequently appeared, one of each pair then elongating into the typical flagellar type, while a dictyosome, several mitochondria, and diverse vesicles gathered into the vicinity (Figure 1.34B). Mitosis ceased when 128 nuclei had been produced, followed by retraction of the protoplast from the sporangial wall; cleavage then occurred, resulting in that same number of individual spores. During the later stages, the nucleus became somewhat more electron-opaque and, towards the termination, dark deposits of condensed chromatin could be noted as flagella developed.

Gametogenesis among Red Algae. In the red algae, spermatogenesis has been somewhat more thoroughly studied than oogenesis, but knowledge of the subject is still at an elementary level. The processes take place within a bulbous axial organ of the sporophyte, known as a conceptacle, the same term being applied to the female organ. Within the lower half of this chamber is a fertile layer, composed of basal calls (Figure 1.35A), which apparently are modified vegetative cells (Peel and Duckett, 1975; Cole and Sheath, 1980; Kugrens, 1980); however, their actual origins do not seem to have been followed as yet. Since the same type of cell lines the interior of the female conceptacles, they may be viewed as primary germ cells until they develop sexual orientation; after that event they may be considered here in the male conceptacle to correspond to spermatogonia, but whether more than one type of those cells exists as in the metazoans is unknown. These cells divide mitotically to produce "spermatial mother cells"—really spermatocytes (Figure 1.35B) whose meiotic processes had already taken place in production of the sporophyte. These spermatocytes then divide mitotically to give rise to two spermatids (referred to as spermatia), which then undergo metamorphosis into spermatozoa.

Under the electron microscope, the spermatogonium showed a moderate-sized nucleus, throughout which were a number of small electron-opaque aggregates, and a cytoplasm that was somewhat vesicular and fairly electron-transparent. While mitochondria were not abundant, chloroplasts in the proplastid condition were well represented. The latter organelles persisted throughout the entire processes but degenerated at the end, so that the completed spermatozoon was colorless, a striking characteristic among chlorophyll-bearing organisms. Perhaps the most outstanding trait of the spermatogonium was the thick microtubular bundle that lay along one side of the nucleus. In the sper-

---

Figure 1.35. Spermatogenesis in red algae. In *Corallina officinalis*, development of the gametes occurs in special organs called conceptacles, the lumen of which is lined with fertile so-called basal cells. (A) The basal cell, really a spermatogonium, has the chromatin dispersed in the nucleus (N), a marked nucleolus (No), and a few chloroplasts in a proplastid (P) state. 29,000×. (B) In the spermatocyte (spermatial mother cell), the chromatin has commenced to condense, the proplastids (P) have lost some of the thylakoids, and a few mitochondria (M) are present. 29,300×. (Both courtesy of Peel and Duckett, 1975.)

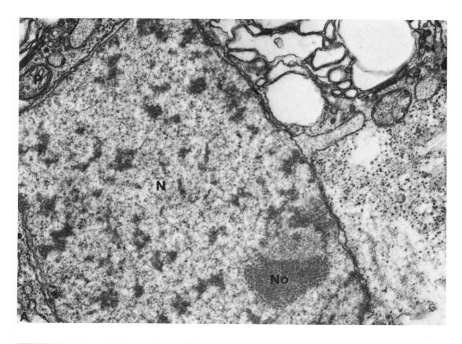

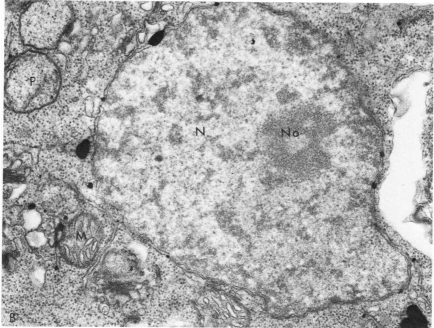

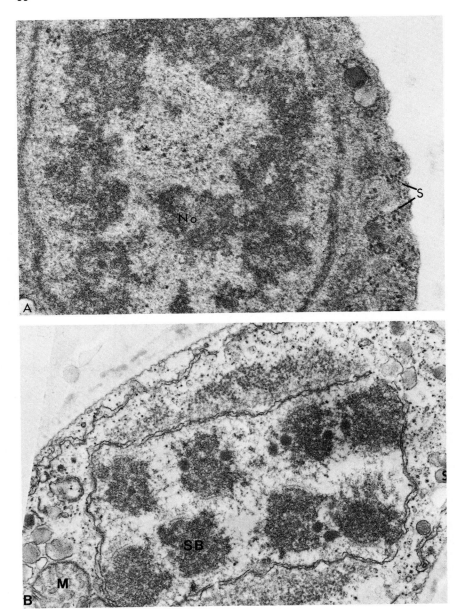

Figure 1.36. Late stages in sperm development in *Corallina*. (A) A spermatid still attached to the lining of the conceptacle, in which the chromatin has condensed to form an oblong mass enclosing the nucleolus. A few starch grains (S) are visible in the cytoplasm. 52,000×. (B) After their release into the lumen, the chromatin of mature spermatids condenses to form "spheroidal bodies" (SB). Mitochondria (M) have now acquired a more typical structure, and starch grains (S) are also visible in the cytoplasm. 26,000×. (Both courtesy of Peel and Duckett, 1975.)

matocyte, which was smaller than the foregoing type, the cytoplasm lost much of its former vesicular nature and showed an increase in electron-opacity, contrasting to the more transparent nucleus. Within the latter, the chromatin had condensed to a slightly greater extent than earlier, while the mitochondria remained ovate as previously and contained somewhat swollen tubular cristae. Spermatids (Figure 1.36A) were characterized by the heavy particles of condensed chromatin within the nucleus, which became increasingly elongate as the cell underwent metamorphosis; these particles eventually congregated into a small number of oblong areas in which were rounded opaque structures (Figure 1.36B). While elongation of the cell and nucleus proceeded, the mitochondria increased in size as they were moved to one end. Just before the completion of metamorphosis, the chloroplasts disintegrated, as floridean starch granules developed to become quite abundant in the completed spermatozoon. The finished gamete never acquired a flagellum but had an elongate posterior appendage, exhibiting limited powers of undulation. The real nature of this distinctive apparatus still remains to be elucidated.

2

Gene Action Changes during Fertilization

Once the two types of gametes have completed the necessary maturation steps, they are capable of uniting to form a zygote and initiating embryogenesis. As may be suspected from the complexity just observed in the steps of generating the eggs and sperm, neither the union of those gametes nor the formation of the embryo is a simple event, with little variation from taxon to taxon; rather, both are as complex and varied as the major groups of organisms themselves. Yet a number of features common to all are found to pervade most of the sexually reproducing biotic world. Because of their abundance, size, ease of culture, synchronous division, and other favorable attributes, echinoderm eggs have provided the basis for the great bulk of the investigations into these phases of development, but studies on vertebrates and metaphytans have served to enrich the literature to a considerable extent. In the present chapter, the penetration of the sperm into the ovum and related events are followed, while the development of the early embryonic stages and then their subsequent differentiation are the respective provinces of the following two chapters.

Fertilization involves three separate and distinct steps: first, insemination, the attachment of the sperm to the ovum; second, the physical penetration of the egg plasmalemma and other membranes by the male gamete; and third, the fusion of the two contrasting nuclei to form the primary nucleus of the zygote (Wilson, 1925). While from a functional viewpoint, only the last of these events should be considered to be fertilization, to which the other two are preliminary steps, the literature in this field has not generally recognized the triple nature of gametic union, especially in investigations at the molecular level. As in gametogenesis, numerous changes in gene expression are evidenced as the sperm enters the egg and combines with the nucleus, but the reader must deduce for himself that new proteins underlie the altered behavior or structure, for their actual existence has as yet been finally demonstrated biochemically in relatively few instances. However, what has been actually ascertained at the molecular level is presented in a separate section.

2.1. ATTACHMENT AND PENETRATION

After insemination, obviously the actual steps in penetration of the ovum depend in each instance on the nature of the covering protecting it and accordingly are subject to extensive variation. In many cases, the female gamete is naked, being protected solely by the plasmalemma or having only a single additional membrane known as the vitelline membrane or chorion. In other organisms, it may be provided further with one or more thick or resistant coats, as in many mammals, amphibians, and various invertebrates.

2.1.1 Attachment of the Sperm

Under the category of attachment of the sperm to the egg can also be included those preliminary events that lead to the actual attachment per se. Among those activities are agglutination, the acrosome reaction (Figure 2.1) described elsewhere (Dillon, 1981, pp. 291–293), and cell recognition, as well as any chemotactic influences that guide the sperm to the egg and even the activation of the male gamete discussed in Chapter 1, Section 1.3.1. Some, such as cell recognition and attachment, are general phenomena and receive attention again in later chapters, but for the greater part, each is unique or else is largely confined to egg and sperm interaction.

Chemotactic Influences. Chemotaxis, the movement of cells either towards or away from a greater concentration of a given chemical in a gradient, has rarely been successfully demonstrated among metazoans as an active influence in orienting the sperm towards the egg. Reported exceptions are confined to two remotely related taxa, the Cnidaria and Tunicata, the former containing the more thoroughly documented cases. In the colonial hydroid *Campanularia*, cinephotomicrography was employed to demonstrate conclusively that the sperm swam toward female gonangia or gradients of extract from such organs (Miller and Nelson, 1962). Later, the same phenomenon was shown to exist in five hydroid genera in which fertilization was internal (Miller, 1966) and, more recently, in a species of *Hydractinia* in which the eggs are spawned and bear only a gelatinous coat (Miller, 1974; Metz, 1978). The effects, which proved to be incompletely species specific, appeared to result from the presence of perhaps five active agents in the eight species that were tested. One of the reactants was shown to be a small basic peptide with a molecular weight of around 1000 (Miller and Tseng, 1974). Current investigations indicate that in

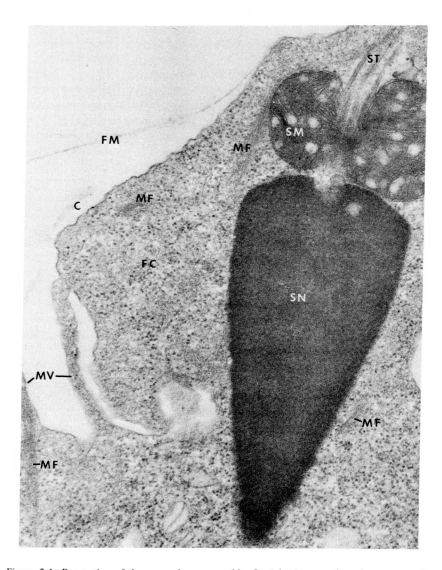

Figure 2.1. Penetration of the sperm in a sea urchin. In *Arbacia punctulata* the sperm nucleus (SN), midbody mitochondria (SM), and base of tail (ST) are completely enclosed by the fertilization cone (FC) within 1 min after insemination. Parts of the fertilization membrane (FM), and three microvilli (MV) are also shown; the presence of several bundles of microfilaments (MF) is of importance to a later discussion (Section 2.4.2). 68,000×. (Courtesy of Longo, 1980.)

the Leptomedusae, the chemotactic factors have a molecular weight of 5000 or less, whereas in the higher groups, Anthomedusae, Limnomedusae, and Trachymedusae, they have weights between 10,000 and 15,000 (Metz, 1978).

Among the tunicates, chemotaxis is not mediated by polypeptides but by lowered pH. For example, in *Ciona intestinalis* and several species of *Styela*, the sperm respond to the pH gradients by swimming in the direction of greater acidity (Miller, 1977), and therefore, the response is not species specific to any degree.

Chemical Attractants among Various Eukaryotes. Chemotactic responses have been known in the spermatozoa of certain types of plants for many years (Pfeffer, 1884; Machlis and Rawitscher-Kunkel, 1967) and have received attention in a broad spectrum of types ranging from unicellular algae to seed plants and fungi (Paolillo, 1981). Among isogametous algae, plus and minus strains of various species of *Chlamydomonas* have been the center of focus, with varying results. When capillary tubes, which contained cell-free filtrate from *C. moewusii* var. *rotunda* minus-strain cell cultures, were placed in a suspension of plus cells, the latter aggregated about the open tip and inside the tube, but no similar reactions were obtained with other combinations of types (Lewin, 1950; Hutner and Provasoli, 1951). When a suspension of minus cells was placed in the capillary, they did not leave the tube when it was immersed in a plus culture; on the other hand, when a plus culture-containing capillary was dipped into a minus culture, the plus cells swam out of the tubule and formed clumps with minus cells in the open suspension. Four other species of the genus displayed comparable chemotactic responses (Tsubo, 1961); however, the supernatant of *rotunda* minus strain was found to attract plus cells of *C. moewusii* s. str. and *C. eugametos*, but not those of *C. reinhardi*. The chemotactic agent was shown to be heat stable to 130°C and highly volatile but was not further identified.

Somewhat more striking results have been obtained in cases in which the gametes are isogametous in being of equal size and bearing like flagella but are anisogametous in behavior, a condition referred to as physiological anisogamy (Hartmann, 1934). In *Ectocarpus silviculosis*, for instance, some members of a suspension of the isogametes become nonmotile and attract considerable numbers of those that are still actively swimming. Although similar behavior has been reported for the green algae *Hydrodictyon reticulatum* (Mainx, 1931) and *Chlamydomonas paupera* (Pascher, 1931), the brown algae *Cladostephus* and *Cutleria* (Schreiber, 1931), and two species of the fungal genus *Synchytrium* (Köhler, 1930; Kusano, 1931), only in water mold of the genus *Allomyces* has substantial experimental evidence been provided that suggests the existence of a chemotactic agent (Machlis, 1958a,b). The latter, however, is not completely isogametous, for the male gametes are orange and highly active, whereas the females are colorless and sluggish. Subsequently a hormone named sirenin has been isolated and partially characterized (Machlis, 1963; Machlis *et al.*, 1966);

it was described as an oxygenated sequiterpene, with a molecular weight of 236.

Among more advanced types of protistans in which male and female gametes are clearly differentiated into sperm and eggs, a large number of chemotactic responses and agents have been demonstrated, for summaries of which reference should be made to Machlis and Rawitscher-Kunkel (1967). Among the mosses, ferns, and liverworts, no apparent instances of hormones or species-specific substances have been reported, but only such general reagents as malic and maleic acids, rubidium salts, and sucrose. Even crushed cells from a variety of sources, including such animal parts as fly legs, sometimes served as attractants for the sperm.

Chemical substances, distinguished as chemotropic agents, may also induce directional growth in hyphae, pollen tubes, or other plant parts lacking flagella and thereby facilitate fertilization. When hyphae of such molds as *Rhizopus nigricans* and *Mucor mucela* of contrasting plus and minus strains approach one another on a culture, protuberances called zygophores develop on each, commencing before actual contact is made (Blakeslee, 1904). As these then grow toward one another, the tip of each becomes removed, permitting fusion and eventual fertilization to occur. These two processes much later were found to be controlled by separate hormones (Plempel, 1960). In the first place, each strain produces a hormone called a gamone; that from the plus strain induces zygophore formation in minus mycelia and vice versa. Secondly, as the protuberances develop, they produce zygotropic hormones, each of which is active on the growth of zygophores on mycelia of the opposite side from the hormonal source. Extensive tests showed that the hormones are gaseous, unstable substances that are readily oxidized in air.

Chemotropic responses were first demonstrated for pollen tubes in the late 19th century; now it appears that at least two separate systems are present (Linskens, 1969). One water-soluble and heat-sensitive factor has been isolated from the ovules, placentae, and inner ovary epidermis of the lily pistil (Noack, 1960), and was shown to have a molecular weight of 600. The present concept is that it acts largely by maintaining wall growth of the pollen tube tip (Rosen, 1961, 1964). In contrast, the second chemotropic agent is heat stable and probably is calcium (Mascarenhas and Machlis, 1962). In addition to these isolatable substances, a gradient in pH has been demonstrated to exist in the style, the stigma having pH 5.5, while the tissue below it increases gradually to 7.0 (Britikov, 1952). More importantly to present concerns, the pH of the cytoplasmic contents of the pollen tube itself changes as it passes through this region, becoming strongly acid after it has penetrated the stylar tip.

Attachment in Mammals. Through the *in vitro* use of rodent eggs denuded of the cumulus oophorus and zona pellucida, a clear picture of the events of sperm attachment in mammals has emerged. For about 5 sec after contact has been made with the egg, the flagella of free-swimming sperm beat vigorously, after which they beat more slowly, completely ceasing within 15 to 25 sec (Yanagimachi, 1979). The binding of the sperm head is in part facilitated by the numerous microvilli that coat the entire egg surface, except the area where the second polar body will be extruded later. In the hamster, this region is relatively small, whereas in the mouse egg, it covers about 20% of the total surface (Yanagimachi and Noda, 1970a). *In vivo*, by the time the sperm has become bound to the egg it has already undergone the acrosome reaction (Bedford, 1968, 1972; Yanagimachi and Noda, 1970b; Zamboni, 1971). Three glycoproteins have been identified in the zona pellucida, that known as ZP3 being involved in binding of the sperm (Bleil and Wassarman, 1981). Unreacted ones can also adhere to the ovum in the same fashion but can carry the processes of fertilization no further (Noda and Yanagimachi, 1976). The events in sperm and egg interaction that follow attachment, being more appropriate to the discussion of penetration, are related in the following section.

2.1.2. Penetration among Echinoderms

In certain pioneering studies on fertilization of echinoderm eggs (Lillie, 1913, 1914), it was observed that the seawater in which sea urchin eggs had been standing induced agglutination of sperm introduced into it and also increased their motility. As a result, it was postulated that the unfertilized ova secreted a substance, which was called fertilizin, that entered the gelatinous coats covering the eggs, secretion of which ceased at the moment of fertilization. More recent exploration, however, has demonstrated that while it is the egg coat which possesses these properties, the secretions are not produced by the ovum but probably by the ovary during oogenesis (Tyler, 1948, 1960).

Agglutination and the Gelatinous Coat. The gelatinous coat of echinoderm eggs consists of one or more glycoproteins, the major one of which in *Arbacia* has a molecular weight of around 300,000 and contains about 20% amino acids on a dry weight basis (Vasseur, 1949; Tyler, 1956). In the same genus, the carbohydrate portion consists of glucose, galactose, mannose, and fucose, but in other genera xylose and fructose may also be present. Because each type of sugar in the glycoprotein becomes esterified with sulfuric acid, up to 25% of the dry weight may stem from the sulfate radicals that are present (Vasseur, 1947). Moreover, several small polypeptides, consisting of 9 or 10 amino acid residues, aid in activating the penetrating sperm (Suzuki *et al.*, 1981).

When spermatozoa contact ova of their own species, they become agglutinated in clusters by means of a reaction that occurs between their heads and the coat. In the case of members of the genus *Arbacia*, this reaction is induced mainly by interactions between the principal carbohydrate constituent, fucose, and binding sites present on the sperm head (Hathaway, 1959; Hathaway and Metz, 1961). After a short period, the agglutinated clumps break up, releasing individual sperm whose ability of fertilization has been strongly reduced. Experiments with eggs matured in the presence of $^{35}SO_4^{2-}$ ions have shown that the dissociation of the sperm clumps, mediated by a sulfatase, results in the release of about half the radioactivity (Tyler and Hathaway, 1958). Hence, the loss of ability to fertilize eggs is thought to result from the retention on the sperm head of only half of each original molecule with which it had interacted in the egg coat, the other half being released into the environment.

The activating effects of the gelatinous coat have been most strikingly demonstrated through employment of aged sperm. Aging of male gametes leads to their gradual loss of motility, but contact with a solution of the egg coat results in greatly enhanced rate of beating on the part of the flagellum, which movement continues for a protracted period. In old sperm this response has been shown to be accompanied by an increased respiratory rate mediated by an egg-secreted substance whose other properties remain unknown (Hathaway, 1963). A third response of the sperm upon contact with the egg coat is centered in the acrosome (Figure 2.1), as mentioned in Chapter 1 and described more fully elsewhere (Colwin and Colwin, 1964; Dillon, 1981). In the present organisms and in many other invertebrates, the reaction results in the production of a short, rather thick, anteriorly directed filament or rod (Dan *et al.*, 1964).

Penetration of the Egg Coat. Even the earliest thorough studies reported the interconnection of the sperm and egg by way of the filament just mentioned (Fol, 1879). These also observed the formation of a broad hyaline protrusion from the egg that appeared to meet the spermatozoon and then engulf and transport it into the interior of the ovum (Figure 2.1). However, later investigations demonstrated that this ''fertilization cone'' actually formed after, not before, the male gamete had penetrated the membrane (Chambers, 1933) and that it then crept up the filament and over the sperm head (Colwin and Colwin, 1955, 1956). Since these and the remaining processes of sperm penetration appear to be identical in most of the higher metazoans, a more lucid account can be provided by abandoning the comparative approach temporarily and combining the results of many researches on a diversity of animals.

In metazoans in general, the acrosomal vesicle and granule break down upon contact of the head with the fertilization cone, releasing one or more enzymes that digest a short path partly through the vitelline membrane (A. L. Colwin and Colwin, 1961; L. H. Colwin and Colwin, 1961). The action of these enzymes, along with other unknown factors, actually creates a tubule through that covering (A. L. Colwin and Colwin, 1963; L. H. Colwin and Colwin, 1963), while the plasmalemma covering the sperm head undergoes degeneration, usually after it has fused with that of the egg (Tyler, 1964). Often the compact sperm nucleus then becomes greatly elongated and narrow as it is moved through the tubule into the egg cytoplasm and is followed by the basal mitochondria and part of the flagellar apparatus. However, in the annelid *Hydroides hexagonus*, no change in nuclear shape occurs as the sperm traverses the vitelline membrane (A. L. Colwin and Colwin, 1961; L. H. Colwin, and Colwin, 1961). Nevertheless, the most outstanding feature, the entry of the nucleus only after it has become denuded of cytoplasm, does appear to be a consistent feature of the metazoan processes, for it has been described also from mollusks, rats, and rabbits (Szöllösi and Ris, 1961; Pasteels and de Harven, 1962; Hadék, 1963). This seems to be an essential feature of the normal processes of fertilization, because live spermatozoa introduced by a micropipet into unfertilized eggs not only failed to undergo the usual changes shown by normal sperm but also did not activate the ovum (Hiromoto, 1962). After penetration is completed, the plasmalemma of the egg undergoes many changes in organization (Wolf *et al.*, 1981).

  Cross-Fertilization Experiments. Experiments involving the insemination of sea urchin eggs with sperm from members of other classes or phyla were quite popular in the early portion of the present century (e.g., Giard, 1900; Boveri, 1903), the results of which have been summarized by Hertwig (1936). As the latter reference points out, the first stages of fertilization exhibit little species specificity even to the point of nuclear fusion. In a more recent investigation along these lines, sea urchin oocytes were inseminated with either mussel or nemertine spermatozoa, the results of which are especially pertinent to the present account (Afzelius, 1972a). Sperm from either source were able to reach the surface of the oocyte and attach but could not do so with mature eggs. Penetration in each case was abnormal, in that the nemertine (*Malacobdella grossa*) gametes were taken in by processes resembling phagocytosis, whereas the sperm of the mussel (*Cyprina islandica*) entered by the more standard procedures of contact by microvilli and fertilization cones. Later electron microscopic studies (Afzelius, 1972b) showed tht the sperm had experienced the acrosomal reaction and that, following penetration, the sperm centrioles developed asters after the nucleus had rotated in normal fashion. However, the sperm nucleus in each case lacked the usual appearance of a penetrated sperm and was visible only as a fibrous mass. In earlier experiments when the pronuclei came into mutual contact, fusion frequently did not occur; in those instances where fusion was achieved, all the paternal chromosomes or a large portion of them were later ejected (Hertwig, 1936).

2.1.3 Penetration in Other Organisms

  Few detailed accounts of egg penetration are available for other metazoans, one of the exceptions being provided by studies on mammalian processes. Two especially fine series of researches have been conducted, one of which treats the denuded rodent egg and the other intact ones. In addition, Zamboni (1971) and his co-workers (1970) have presented the ultrastructural events in the mouse, and Bedford (1972), in the rabbit. Although electron microscopic studies of penetration in plants have been conducted, the results are

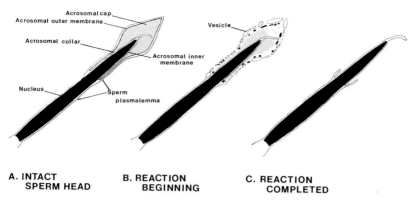

A. INTACT   B. REACTION   C. REACTION
   SPERM HEAD   BEGINNING   COMPLETED

Figure 2.2. The acrosome reaction in mammaliam sperm. In this sperm of the rabbit as in those of many metazoans, activation involves the breakdown of the anterior plasmalemma and outer acrosomal membrane, thereby releasing the enzymatic contents of the acrosomal cap (A, B) that aid in penetration of the egg coat. Subsequently these membranes are completely destroyed, leaving only the inner acrosomal membrane, which then becomes continuous with the posterior plasmalemma (C), with several characteristic appendages. (Based on the electron micrographs of Bedford, 1968.)

still incomplete relative to those of metazoans, but what has been ascertained is of great interest.

Penetration in Mammals. Since the investigations using rodent eggs denuded of their investing coverings continue a discussion begun under the topic of attachment, presenting their results first offers considerable advantage (Section 2.1.1). Although, as shown there, the acrosomal reaction (Figure 2.2) is an absolute requirement of sperm penetration, the processes of invasion differ sharply from those of echinoderms (Kopečný and Fléchon, 1981). Here no acrosomal filament develops, as in those of many other animals, nor does the acrosomal inner membrane undergo changes of any detectable type (Colwin and Colwin, 1967; Bedford, 1972). Use of colloidal iron hydroxide particles, which bound to the plasmalemma of the egg but not to that of the sperm head, made it possible to follow some of the steps involved in penetration (Yanagimachi *et al.*, 1973; Yanagimachi, 1979). A low sort of fertilization cone extended outwards to the sperm head, which paralleled the egg's surface; it then spread over it, beginning near the middle and progressing toward each end until it was completely engulfed (Figure 2.3 I–K). During these steps, the membrane of the sperm was gradually replaced by that of the egg, to judge from its increased ability to absorb iron hydroxide particles. As a general rule among mammals, the entire flagellum is taken into the egg in similar fashion, but in the Chinese hamster and voles (*Microtus*), the tails detach from the heads and consequently do not become incorporated into the ovum (Austin, 1961). In those forms in which it does enter, the entire flagellum, including the mito-

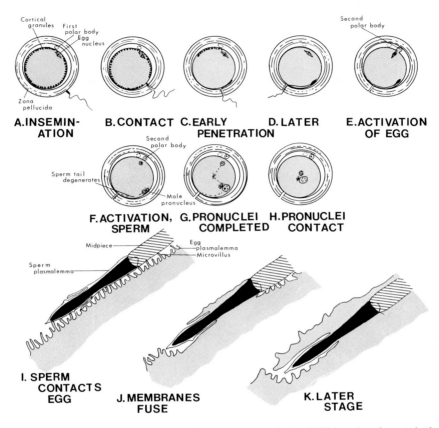

Figure 2.3. Penetration and fertilization of the egg in mammals. (A–H) This series of events in the rat processes begins (A) after the sperm has penetrated the cumulus oophorus and reached the zona pellucida; the egg nucleus is in metaphase at this time. It is not until the sperm has entered the egg completely that meiosis of the ovum nucleus resumes (E). (Based on Austin, 1965.) (I–K) Steps in the penetration of the sperm into the egg in the hamster. (Based on Yanagimachi, 1979.)

chondria of the midpiece, later gradually disintegrates, as do the organelles of the head, except the nucleus and centrioles. Thus, the mitochondria of the resulting individual eventually show the traits characteristic of the mother alone.

Because of the technical difficulties involved, similar complete ultrastructural studies on intact mammalian eggs have not been made, so for the present an account of penetration through the several protective coverings observed under the light microscope must suffice (Austin, 1965; Pikó, 1969). First, the sperm must penetrate through the cumulus oophorus (Figure 2.3), but this appears to be readily accomplished by the proteolytic enzyme hyaluronidase that is carried by the sperm (Austin and Walton, 1960). Upon reaching the zona, the head attaches vertically, in which orientation penetration takes place by processes generally believed to involve a lysin called acrosin, supplied by the acrosome (Stambaugh *et al.*, 1969; Zaneveld *et al.*, 1971). However, recently evidence has been advanced which suggests that penetration results from a drilling action (Bedford and Cross, 1978), with the aid of peptides released at this time (Hartmann and Hutchison, 1981). After passing through this covering, the sperm arrives at the plasma membrane, initiating a stimulus that signals the activation of the cortical granules. These are discharged in succession, beginning at the point of the sperm's contact and proceeding about the surface in all directions to the opposite pole to complete the formation of the fertilization membrane. Before this reaction is quite finished, the sperm head has become arranged parallel to the plasmalemma of the egg, penetration then continuing as just described.

Penetration in Other Chordates. Although the processes followed during sperm penetration into the mammalian egg are largely typical of the vertebrates as a whole, a number of distinctions are to be noted from one class to another. Among avians, including the domestic fowl, the sperm experiences the acrosomal reaction as it passes through the outer layer of the vitelline membrane, which is still undergoing development in the most anterior portion of the oviduct (Okamura and Nishiyama, 1978a). It then dissolves a passageway through the inner layer, possibly by acrosomal enzymes, thus reaching the perivitelline space and the plasmalemma of the egg. Contact, made at about a 45° angle, leads to the formation of a pitlike impression in the egg surface and results in rupture of both the plasmalemma and the inner acrosomal membranes, which then fuse. The pit possibly is an invagination of the egg cortex, as reported below in fish eggs (Figure 2.4). No microvilli or fertilization cones

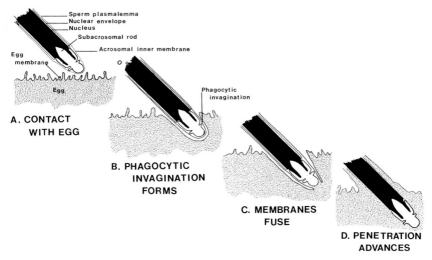

Figure 2.4. Penetration in the chicken ovum. In some accounts the phagocytotic invagination is referred to as a pit. (Based on Okamura and Nishiyama, 1978b.)

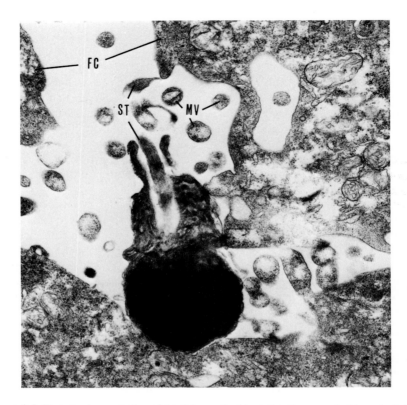

Figure 2.5. First step in penetration of the fish egg. In this section the sperm had inseminated the egg just 10 sec prior to fixation. The sperm head, midbody, and portions of the tail (ST) are seen to be in close proximity to a fertilization cone (FC) and a number of microvilli (MV). 16,800×. (Courtesy of Iwamatsu and Ohta, 1978.)

appear to be involved in sperm penetration, but a narrow zone of ovum cytoplasm does come to extend along the penetrating male gamete as far as the midpiece of the tail (Okamura and Nishiyama, 1978b). In some instances the sperm may be brought in by phagocytotic activities on the part of the egg (Koyanagi and Nishiyama, 1980).

Penetration into the fish ovum has also been followed recently in an ultrastructural investigation (Iwamatsu and Ohta, 1978). Using polyspermic medaka eggs denuded of their chorions, the researchers found that the sperm were secured by numerous microvilli of the egg surface or by fertilization cones, as in mammals (Figure 2.5). Since these sperm lack an acrosome, the plasmalemmae of the two gametes lie in direct contact but do not fuse immediately. Within a minute after insemination, the egg has formed a narrow deep invagination in which the sperm becomes engulfed (Figure 2.6), after which the plasmalemmae

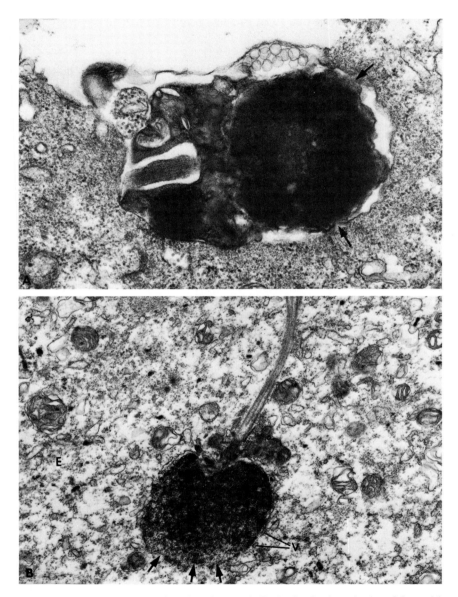

Figure 2.6. Later steps in penetration of a fish egg. (A) By 1 min after insemination of the medaka egg, the spermatozoon has become enclosed by cytoplasmic protrusions from the ovum and lies within a shallow invagination. Arrows indicate regions where fusion of the plasmalemmae has commenced. 28,000×. (B) Two minutes later the sperm has completely penetrated the egg and its nuclear envelope has begun to undergo vesicularization (V) and the chromatin to disperse (arrows). 14,000×. (Both courtesy of Iwamatsu and Ohta, 1978.)

fuse in such a fashion that the male gametes become denuded. The entire spermatozoon is thus brought into the egg, including the midpiece and tail.

Penetration in the Acanthocephala. So many features of penetration
among the invertebrate phyla are similar to those of either the chordates or the
echinoderms that little is gained by elaborating the details. The Acanthocephala, however, are exceptional in a number of ways, both in the structure
of the gametes and in the processes resulting in their union. The eggs of the
animals are in the form of syncytia referred to as ovarian balls, the gametic
constituents of which remain as primary oocytes until fertilization (Marchand
and Mattei, 1980). These balls are located within the body cavity, where fertilization occurs. Upon insemination, the spermatozoa, which have the flagellum directed forward, move through the various egg coats and attach to the
oocytes by means of that organelle and then penetrate the female gamete quite
deeply within a narrow but rapidly deepening invagination (Figure 2.7; Marchand and Mattei, 1976). Before penetration occurs in *Neoechinorhynchus*, the
flagellar apex becomes swollen at the point of contact and the ovarian ball
undergoes a cortical reaction (Marchand and Mattei, 1979). In all genera studied, since the sperm has a mean length of 60 nm and the oocyte a diameter of
only 10 nm, the former gamete becomes greatly folded as it enters the latter
still enclosed within the elongate phagocytotic vesicle (Figure 2.7A). After the
sperm has been completely phagocytosed in this fashion, the phagocytotic pocket
breaks down and the sperm tail becomes detached.

Penetration in Seed Plants. In seed plants the processes of fertilization
are exceptionally complex and still remain incompletely described. Entry may
be made through the chalaza or even through the lateral walls (Linskens, 1969),
but by far the more frequent path to the embryo sac is by way of the micropyle.
The pollen tube carrying the sperm nuclei is conducted into this opening, guided
by special temporary structures called obturators, which are derived from the
placenta or inner integument (Maheshwari, 1950; Kapil and Vasil, 1963). Once
through the micropyle, the pollen tube grows between the two synergids and
egg cell, which are arranged as a three-parted cylinder. This growth continues
through a filiform apparatus to about the center of the cluster of cells, where
the tip of the pollen tube ruptures, releasing its contents into one of the synergids. The filiform apparatus is derived from the thickened outer walls of the
synergids, as a result of their having degenerated by this time into a slimy
mass. After being thus penetrated, the invaded synergid bursts, but whether
following or preceding the rupture of the pollen tube has not been determined.
Nevertheless, it rapidly degenerates, with large vacuoles developing in the cytoplasm and the nucleus becoming shriveled (van Went and Linskens, 1967),
while the second synergid usually remains intact for about 1 week (Jensen,
1965).

Accounts of penetration of the sperm nucleus are not entirely clear, but
one sperm nucleus enters the egg cell from the synergid, evidently along with

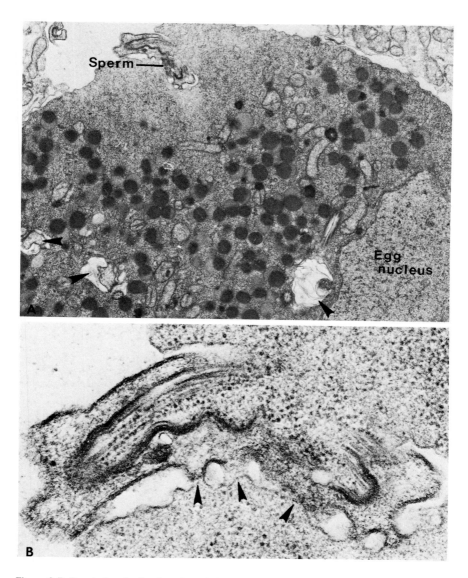

Figure 2.7. Penetration in the Acanthocephala. (A) The sperm of *Breizacanthus* has entered by way of a deep phagocytotic invagination, sections of which may be seen around the sperm head and fragments of tail indicated by arrowheads. 16,000×. (B) Enlargement of part of (A). Fusion of the plasmalemmae has begun to take place as indicated at the arrowheads. 55,000×. (Both courtesy of Marchand and Mattei, 1980.)

a relatively small quantity of cytoplasm from the pollen tube (Richter-Land-mann, 1959). The precise fate of the cytoplasm also is obscure, but it has been established that it does not become intermixed thoroughly with that of the egg until the first cleavage (Linskens, 1969). The sperm nucleus then moves toward the egg nucleus, by processes that at one time were claimed to be amoeboid (Steffen, 1953), but more recently it has been proposed to drift to the point where the egg nucleus had been located (Gerassimova-Navashina, 1960, 1961). More than likely, movement is provided by the same means as in the metazoan cells, by the egg cytoplasmic constituents under the guidance of the cytosolic genetic mechanism. In the meanwhile, the second sperm nucleus has left the synergid near its proximal end and has gained the polar nuclei, unaccompanied by pollen tube cytoplasm. Whether either male nucleus undergoes any changes in structure during migration does not seem to have been noted.

 Fertilization in Plants. In seed plants three types of nuclear fusion have been described (Gerassimova-Navashina, 1960). The first, called the premi-totic, resembles the processes in the sea urchin in that the two pronuclei unite through fusion of the nuclear envelopes, followed later by mitotic division. It is found in the brown seaweeds like *Fucus* and in grasses and composites. However, it is not completely identical to that of metazoans, because the plant sperm pronucleus develops a nucleolus, a structure never lost by the egg counterpart. After combining with the egg pronucleus, the male no longer reacts to the Feulgen reagents, although its parts remain visible and readily recognizable (Steffen, 1951; Vazart, 1958).

 The second, or postmitotic, type is similar to the mammalian to the extent that the two pronuclei do not fuse but remain separate entities until metaphase of the first cleavage divisions (Figure 2.8). There the resemblances cease, however. In the first place, both nuclei either retain or develop nucleoli, as in the foregoing. Secondly, the sperm nucleus does not seem to undergo alteration until after it has contacted that of the egg; then it acquires a nuclear envelope and increases in size until it is of the same dimensions as that of the female. After both nuclear envelopes then disintegrate, the chromosomes of each become aligned on the metaphase plate. The preceding type is characteristic of the pines and of a number of genera in the lily family, while the third, or intermediate, is known from the genus *Impatiens*. As in the first variety, the sperm nucleus enters that of the egg without seeming to undergo prior modification, except in entering prophase. There it remains distinct for some time, depending on the species, until the female structure finally also enters prophase. Even after both organelles have thus embarked on mitotic division, the chromosomes may not completely merge. Indeed, if a common spindle does form, the chromosomes may remain in separate groups, but quite frequently two spindles are present (Cooper, 1940).

 The union of the second sperm nucleus with the polar nuclei apparently proceeds more rapidly than any of the foregoing types. The typical procedure

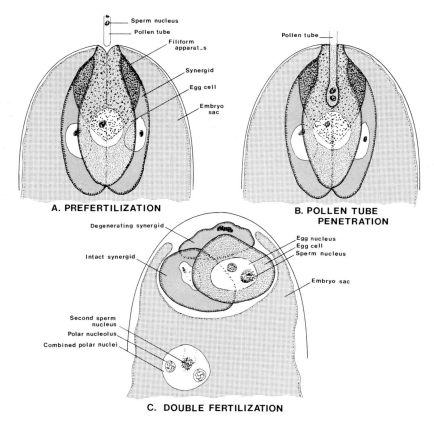

Figure 2.8. Fertilization in seed plants. The major steps alone are indicated; three variations have been described, based on the time of occurrence of the mitotic events. (Based in part on Linskens, 1969.)

after contact has been made is for the three nuclear bodies to lie in mutual contact, with the sperm partially between the other two. Then the former penetrates one of the polar nuclei, possibly by union of the nuclear membranes, the second polar nucleus soon following suit. This triplex nucleus then enters prophase of the first endospermal division.

2.2. POSTPENETRATION EVENTS

Immediately after the spermatozoon has penetrated the egg coat, or sometimes upon contact of the sperm with the egg, a number of structural or other changes can be noted. Among metazoans where they have been most thoroughly documented, the reported modifications are predominantly surface phenomena, most of which result in the formation of the so-called fertilization membrane or are at least associated with that event.

Formation of the Fertilization Membrane in Echinoderms. The formation of the fertilization membrane in echinoderms involves the vitelline membrane and those cortical granules described in the preceding chapter as lying just beneath the plasmalemma of the egg. Although in starfish the vitelline membrane is a thick structure, as implied in the discussion of sperm penetration, in sea urchins it is quite thin and closely applied to the egg plasmalemma, a structural difference that is reflected strongly in fertilization-membrane formation. Originally this process was most thoroughly investigated in sea urchins. In these latter animals, upon entry of the sperm nucleus, the cortical granules are moved to the surface of the ovum in contact with the plasmalemma, which then fuses with that enclosing each of its granules to form a mosaic membrane, while the granules themselves become greatly distended. This distention terminates with their rupture, expelling a major constituent, the "dark bodies," outward against the vitelline membrane, which in the meanwhile has moved away from its former close proximity to the plasmalemma (Afzelius, 1956; Endo, 1961). The ejected dark bodies then become spread out over the inner surface of the vitelline membrane and eventually are modified into a continuous layer. This new structure, together with the vitelline membrane, forms the fertilization membrane.

Concurrently, the remaining content of the cortical granules, termed the hemispherical globules, form a coat over the vesicular remnants, together with which they become modified into the hyaline layer around the periphery of the ovum, an observation that is shown in a later paragraph to be subject to some doubt. Between this new layer and the fertilization membrane is the perivitelline space which contains a sulfated mucopolysaccharide (Immers, 1961).

In starfish the thick vitelline membrane that covers the ovum is penetrated by numerous broad microvilli that project outward for about 0.2 nm from the cytoplasmic surface. Within a few minutes after penetration, the microvilli become still longer, reaching lengths of 0.5 to 1.0 nm (Mazia *et al.*, 1975; Eddy and Shapiro, 1976). This increase in length has been referred to as the first burst of elongation (Schroeder, 1978, 1979). As in sea urchin eggs, the dark bodies then erupt from the cortical granules, followed by a corresponding sequence of events (Monroy, 1965). All of these activities have been shown to be energy dependent, for they are inhibited by reagents that uncouple oxidative phosphorylation (Okazaki, 1956a,b; Dillon, 1981, pp. 324–328). Late in fertilization, in sea urchins as well as starfish, just prior to the first division the microvilli undergo a second burst of elongation, during which they attain lengths up to 10 nm (Figure 2.9; Burgess and Schroeder, 1977; Schroeder, 1978).

Another surface event that follows quickly after insemination is the development of a hyaline layer which persists in intimate contact with the early

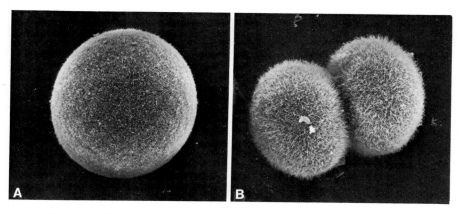

Figure 2.9. Surface changes of ova following fertilization. (A) Denuded sea urchin egg after first burst of microvillar elongation. At this time (12 min postinsemination) the microvilli have grown from the 0.2 μm length of the unfertilized egg to 0.5 μm. (B) A similar egg 180 min after fertilization; following the second burst of elongation, the microvilli now average 1.8 μm in length. Both 540×. (Courtesy of Schroeder, 1978.)

embryo through the gastrula. It contains a single major proteinaceous constituent, called hyalin, that is precipitated by calcium (McBlaine and Carroll, 1980). This forms within 20 min after insemination and on the basis of ultrastructural and biochemical evidence has been assumed to be a product of the cortical granules (Kane and Hersh, 1959; Anderson, 1968; Yazaki, 1968; Kane, 1970). Recent data from a study on unfertilized eggs of *Strongylocentrotus* using lactoperoxidase-catalyzed radioiodination have demonstrated clearly that either a precursor or the protein itself is present prior to fertilization (McBlaine and Carroll, 1980). But whether the substance was then localized in the cortical granules or elsewhere was not explored.

Postpenetration Events in Mammals. Because an extensive review of mammalian cortical granule structure, formation, and function has recently appeared (Gulyas, 1980), it is possible to confine attention here to the more immediately pertinent aspects of the subject. As in the sea urchin egg, these are membrane-enclosed rounded, bodies largely lying just beneath the plasmalemma and filled completely with an electron-opaque substance; however, the electron density of the particulate matter varies from species to species and often within the same ovum in some mammals (Austin, 1961; Zamboni and Mastroianni, 1966; Baca and Zamboni, 1967; Gulyas, 1974, 1976). In most mammalian eggs, the granules are not distributed entirely over the egg but tend to be absent in the region overlying the meiotic apparatus. Moreover, the egg surface is covered with short microvilli, except over the cortical granule-free areas (Gulyas, 1976; Nicosia *et al.*, 1977); occasional association between a granule and a microvillus has been reported (Szöllösi, 1967; Zamboni, 1974).

Basically the cortical reaction that occurs at attachment of the sperm differs little from that just presented in the preceding section. As there, the plasmalemma fuses with the membrane of each cortical granule in turn, releasing their contents into the perivitelline space (Bedford and Cooper, 1978). However, the expelled substance does not rise and form a layer beneath the vitelline membrane, but spreads over the surface of the plasmalemma (Gulyas, 1980). Moreover, the zona pellucida, perhaps as a consequence of that distinctive action, does not become the fertilization membrane; rather the plasmalemma itself does, at least in the rabbit (Szöllösi, 1962, 1967). The membrane is not the only protective device against supernumerary sperm, however, for excess ones that succeed in penetretion are resorbed by the cytoplasm of the zygote (Yu and Wolf, 1981).

Postpenetration in Other Metazoans. In the anuran amphibians the eggs are protected by two coverings, the vitelline membrane in contact with the plasmalemma, acquired before leaving the ovary, and the jelly coat, deposited in several layers over the vitelline membrane during passage through the oviduct (Miceli *et al.*, 1977). During penetration of *X. laevis* eggs, the cortical granules do not release their contents into the perivitelline space as in mammals but through the vitelline membrane beneath the jelly coat (Grey *et al.*, 1974; Wolf, 1974a,b). However, in such fish as *Fundulus heteroclitus*, the action resembles that of mammals (Brummett and Dumont, 1981).

In the case of the amphibians, the deposited substance interacts with materials released from the inner layer of the jelly coat (Wolf *et al.*, 1976) to form an electron-dense layer, thereby transforming the vitelline membrane into the fertilization membrane in both *Xenopus* and *Bufo* (Miceli *et al.*, 1977).

Except in the echinoderms already discussed, the cortical reaction in invertebrates has received relatively little attention from biologists, having been described only from cnidarians, annelids, and a few arthropods (Hudinaga, 1942; Pasteels, 1965; Dewel and Clark, 1974). What has been noted in shrimp of the genus *Penaeus* is particularly striking (Hudinaga, 1942; Clark *et al.*, 1980). In these animals the cortical granules are in the form of stout rods densely placed throughout the entire cortex beneath the plasmalemma, the latter being invested by a vitelline membrane. At spawning as the sperm penetrate the ova, the rods are strongly ejected from the egg, carrying the vitelline membrane outwards from the surface for some distance. Here the granular contents become converted into the gelatinous mass that ultimately attains a total diameter about three times that of the egg proper. This coat persists intact until the formation of the second polar body, after which it gradually disintegrates. After its disappearance at about the second cleavage, a hatching membrane is formed in its stead (Clark *et al.*, 1980).

2.3. PRONUCLEAR INTERACTION

Strange as it may appear, the most important step in the formation of the zygote, the fusion of the male and female nuclei (pronuclei), has received almost no attention at the molecular and ultrastructural levels, and exceedingly little even from light microscopic studies. Two principal types of immediate response following penetration are recognizable, depending on the organism: (1) the two nuclei approach one another immediately and fuse, or (2) the male nucleus remains relatively inert, while that of the female gamete completes meiotic division, usually accompanied by polar body formation. Only then do the nuclei approach one another and fuse.

Early Nuclear Events in Echinoderms. In sea urchin eggs, which are of type 1 behavior, the sperm nucleus enlarges as its chromatin decondenses; then as a nuclear membrane forms, it moves toward the interior of the cell, followed soon afterward by similar movement on the part of the egg nucleus (Mar, 1980). During its migration, the male pronucleus, as it now is called, undergoes a rotation of approximately 180°, so that the paired centrioles leave their former posterior location to assume an anterior one (Flemming, 1881). Since the centriole possesses neither flagella nor pseudopods and accordingly is incapable of autonomous movement, it certainly cannot "lead the way" for the nucleus as formerly claimed (Boveri, 1888). Furthermore, as shown elsewhere (Dillon, 1981, p 526), microtubules of spindles and asters exhibit no stress of any sort during elongation or shortening, and therefore are not involved in the movement as once proposed (Chambers, 1939), despite the aster's being formed during nuclear migration. This absence of involvement is further indicated by the migration of the egg nucleus toward that of the sperm, even though it lacks asters as well as centrioles.

The first sign of activation on the part of the egg pronucleus is its becoming enlarged or swollen, even though it may be surrounded by a broad region of nonactivated cytoplasm or experimentally drawn into a capillary tube (Allen, 1954). However, its migration does not begin until the surrounding cytoplasm has become activated; therefore, it is obvious that the two activities, swelling and movement, are the consequences of at least a pair of different factors. Or if viewed more closely, swelling is a response on the part of the egg nucleus, whereas its movement is strictly a cytoplasmic activity under the control of the supramolecular genetic mechanism. Movement of the egg pronucleus is the most rapid of all these activities (Schatten, 1981).

Nuclear Events in Mammals. In intact rat eggs, which are of type 2, light microscopic investigations have provided a clear view of the major events that follow the penetration of the egg by the sperm (Austin, 1965). Shortly after the completion of the fertilization membrane, the egg nucleus finishes the second meiotic division, breaking the second meiotic arrest (Chapter 1, Section 1.2.1), while the sperm nucleus remains inactive for about 15 min (Colwin and

Colwin, 1967). After that lapse of time, the latter begins to undergo decondensation, a process that requires somewhat under an hour to complete. In the meanwhile, the second polar body has been formed, and the egg nucleus has swollen to assume its status as a pronucleus. At this time, the sperm nucleus has similarly developed a nuclear envelope, enlarged into the male pronucleus, and rotated 180° to bring the centriole into a proximal location. Both pronuclei then are moved from their peripheral sites toward the center, the sperm derivative developing an aster as it does so. When the pair comes into contact, the chromosomes become aligned on a megaphase plate, and, the process of fertilization now being complete, the resulting zygote is ready for the first cleavage. The time of occurrence of the several events has now been followed in naturally ovulated mouse eggs (Krishna and Generoso, 1977). The first evidence of penetration was observed 1¾ hr after coitus and pronuclei developed about 1 hr later. However, DNA synthesis did not commence for another 3 to 4 hr, and the first cleavage followed in approximately 2 hr.

Molecular Events in Sperm Nucleus Transformation. Further details of the transformation of the sperm nucleus into the male pronucleus have been provided by a number of ultrastructural and molecular studies on the fertilization of lower vertebrate and invertebrate eggs (Figure 2.10). Although many differences, largely temporal and developmental, but some structural, exist from taxon to taxon, the sea urchins of the genus *Arbacia* may well serve as the basic model (Longo, 1973a,b; Longo and Kunkle, 1978). In the first place, it should be recalled that during spermatogenesis when the chromatin of the spermatid underwent condensation, most of the RNA and much of the protein content had been lost (Chapter 1, Section 1.3.1). Thus, to regain its former relaxed state, at least the proteins must be reacquired (Gurdon, 1974, 1975; Harris, 1974). Part of the increase in size may therefore be assumed to be derived from the acquisition of such substances (Gurdon, 1975), water and solutes from the cytoplasm probably accounting for much of the remainder.

In *Arbacia punctulata,* the nuclear envelope of the sperm breaks down rather rapidly after entry into the egg. The specific fate of the resulting vesicular remnants is unknown, but it is not likely that they merely become lost among the other membranous structures of the zygote, as has been proposed (Longo and Kunkle, 1978). More probably they undergo complete degeneration (Figure 2.11), the resulting molecules being recycled in common with those of most other components of the cell (Dillon, 1981, pp. 65–67). As the envelope disintegrates, the condensed chromatin of the nucleus commences to relax, the compact electron-opaque material gradually dispersing into numerous fine threads as the entire body increases in volume. After the chromatin has become fully relaxed, a new nuclear envelope is formed by steps corresponding to those described in detail elsewhere (Dillon, 1981); only about 15% of the new envelope consists of components from the sperm nuclear covering (Longo, 1976a,b). With its development thus completed, the male pronucleus is moved toward the center of the zygote where it encounters its female counterpart (Fig-

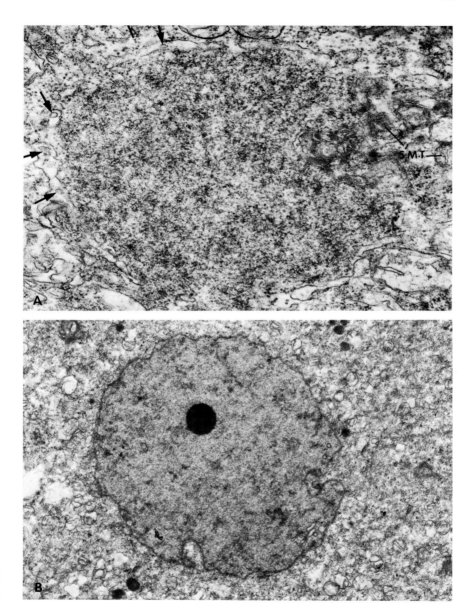

Figure 2.10. Development of the male pronucleus. (A) Male pronucleus of medaka 5 min postinsemination. Vesicles, some including secondary bodies (arrows), have developed along the dispersed chromatin. A centriole (C) and sperm mitochondria (SMT) also are evident. 28,000×. (B) By 25 min postinsemination, the male pronucleus has become greatly enlarged, the magnification being only one-fifth that of (A). It has also acquired a nuclear envelope and a distinct nucleolus. 5600×. (Both courtesy of Iwamatsu and Ohta, 1978.)

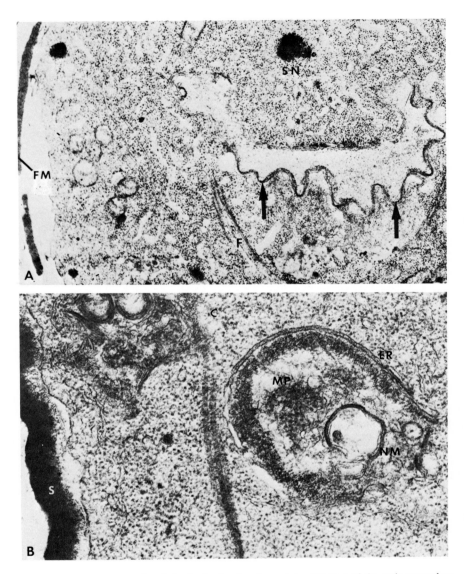

Figure 2.11. Sperm pronuclear behavior in the Acanthocephala. (A) Part of the male pronucleus after completion of penetration into the ova of *Breizacanthus*. A remnant of the nuclear envelope has become undulant (arrows) as it leaves the remnants of the sperm nucleus (SN). Parts of the sperm flagellum (F) and fertilization membrane (FM) also are shown; the latter represents the first element in the formation of the acanthor shell. 19,000×. (B) In a later stage after the acanthor shell (S) has thickened, the male pronucleus (MP) shows a more electron-opaque chromatin, in which bits of the nuclear membrane (NM) still persist. The smooth endoreticulum vesicle (ER) that partly encloses the male pronucleus is reminiscent of that which surrounds organelles of other cells. 35,000×. (Both courtesy of Marchand and Mattei, 1980.)

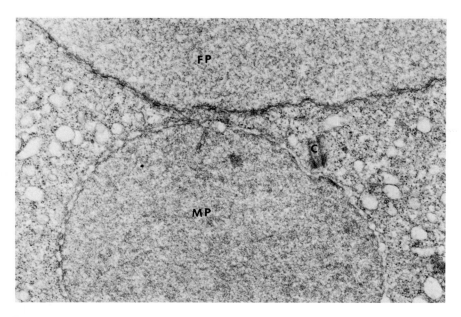

Figure 2.12. Pronuclei of a sea urchin zygote. The mature male pronucleus (MP) has just arrived at that of the egg (FP), just prior to nuclear envelope fusion. It is obvious that the former is somewhat more electron-dense than the latter. Slightly to the right is one of the centrioles (C) of the sperm that preceded the male pronucleus during its migration. 22,000×. (Courtesy of Longo, 1980.)

ure 2.12). Unlike the mammalian processes in which the envelopes of both pronuclei break down, in these organisms they fuse, thus forming a continuous covering over a single zygote nucleus. This remains intact then until the first mitosis of cleavage.

Control of Nuclear Behavior. Although it is now thoroughly established that cytoplasmic factors are active in the control of the conversion of sperm nuclei after they have penetrated the egg membranes, the nature of the substances and the precise extent of their influences are still in a state of confusion. The condition of the cytosol of the egg has long been known to influence the behavior of the sperm nucleus (Wilson, 1925; Longo, 1973a, 1976a), and, more recently, the latter's transformation into a pronucleus has been demonstrated to occur in eggs deprived of maternally derived chromatin (Skoblina, 1974; Longo, 1976b). One or more factors in hamster and rabbit eggs have been clearly demonstrated to be responsible for the decondensation of the sperm nuclear chromatin (Thibault and Gerard, 1970; Yanagimachi and Usui, 1972). Furthermore, much evidence points to the presence of a substance or substances in the egg that are active in the development of the male pronucleus. It is believed to be an egg component that appears when the germinal vesicle breaks down, for male pronucleus formation failed to occur in enucleate toad oocytes (Katagiri, 1974; Skoblina, 1974; Katagiri and Moriya, 1976). According to the results of investigations that reinseminated either zygotes or two-cell embryos, the mature egg components active toward this end disappear or are inactivated shortly after fertilization has occurred (Yanagimachi and Usui, 1972; Usui and Yanagimachi, 1976), because no male pronuclei developed. However, contrary results have been obtained with sea urchin embryos and *Xenopus* eggs (Sugiyama, 1951; Graham, 1966), as well as from experiments attempting insemination of cultured somatic cells. In some cases the sperm nuclei failed both to form pronuclei and to synthesize DNA (Sawicki and Koprowski, 1971; Bendich *et al.*, 1974; Phillips *et al.*, 1976), whereas in others chromatin decondensation occurred or DNA was synthesized (Gledhill *et al.*, 1972; Gabara *et al.*, 1973).

Incorporation of supernumerary sperm has also led to the conclusion that an egg factor was necessary for male pronucleus formation in pig and surf clam (*Spisula*) eggs. Moreover, multiple sperm incorporation has indicated that the factor may be present in limited supply, for only the earlier spermatozoa showed signs of maturation (Hunter, 1967; Longo, 1973b). Similar polyspermy experiments with *Arbacia* eggs at various stages of development demonstrated that only those that had completed meiosis could induce sperm nuclei to transform (Longo and Kunkle, 1977; Longo, 1978).

Cross-fertilization experiments, although limited in number, have produced some particularly pertinent results. In brief, the researches, based on insemination of *Arbacia* eggs with mussel (*Mytilus*) sperm, have led to the conclusions that the sperm nuclei are capable both of forming pronuclei and of combining with the female pronucleus (Giudice, 1973) Longo, 1976b). However, the foreign *Mytilus* pronucleus resembled that of the normal male pronucleus in being smaller than that of the female, not larger as when it had penetrated into a mussel egg. Moreover, although the pronuclei met centrally and united, the union did not involve the fusion of nuclear envelopes as is usual in sea urchins; instead the male and female pronuclei aligned ready for the first cleavage mitosis (Longo and Kunkle, 1978).

2.4. MACROMOLECULAR EVENTS ACCOMPANYING FERTILIZATION

Generally speaking, mature unfertilized eggs are metabolically repressed, but penetration of the sperm and postpenetration events are typically accompanied by a pronounced series of ionic and metabolic changes. Early attention was devoted largely to differences in rates of oxygen consumption or protein synthesis, but lately more specific contrasts in activities have been brought to light. As has already been shown, the factors involved in stimulating cellular activity are largely of maternal origin, since the sperm contributions to the zygote are limited almost entirely to the nucleus and centriole.

2.4.1. Changes in Metabolic Rates

Cell Respiration. The metabolic change first reported to take place at fertilization was in cellular respiration, when Warburg (1910, 1911) described the severalfold increase in oxygen consumption that occurred in newly inseminated sea urchin eggs. For example, with *Hemicentrotus pulcherrimus* ova, measurements of O_2 consumption showed that the rate remained relatively constant at about 1.1–1.2 μl O_2/hr per mg of unfertilized eggs (Ohnishi and Sugiyama, 1963; Yasumasu and Nakano, 1963), but within a few minutes after insemination (corresponding approximately to completion of penetration), the rate jumped to about 3.8 μl and increased exponentially thereafter. Actually previously, with *Psammechinus miliaris* eggs, the respiratory jump had been demonstrated to be even more dramatic (Laser and Rothschild, 1939). In this case, O_2 consumption nearly doubled within 5 min after sperm penetration, whereas CO_2 evolution more than tripled; during the ensuing like period of time, both activities returned to nearly the prefertilization rates and then began the exponential increases reported above. The basis for these respiratory phenomena has been attributed in part to the low levels of all glycolytic intermediates and hexose phosphates that have been found to exist in the unfertilized ovum (Aketa *et al.*, 1964), despite the presence of large quantities of glycogenlike substances. Thus, it was suggested that the metabolic pathway leading from glycogen to glucose-6-phosphate was blocked before fertilization and that sperm penetration released the block. These researchers were then able to demonstrate that the hexose-monophosphate shunt became activated at fertilization and resulted in a large increase in the level of NADPH* in the developing zygote (Krane and Crane, 1960). Additionally, an inhibitor of cytochrome oxidase activity in unfertilized ova has been reported, which is lost in the new zygote (Maggio and Monroy, 1959). Although the inhibitor is known to act on sulfhydryl groups and to be located in the cytoplasm rather than in mitochondria (Cooperstein, 1963), it has not been determined as to how it is released or becomes inactivated by penetration of the sperm.

Protein Synthesis. Despite the large quantities of mRNA present in the unfertilized egg (Chapter 1, Section 1.2.2), protein synthesis proceeds very slowly. Moreover, the movement into the cell of labeled amino acids is at a low rate (Hultin, 1953a,b; Giudice *et al.*, 1962). However, within 5 to 10 min after insemination, protein synthesis increases 5- to 30-fold, and amino acid

---

*Reduced nicotinamide adenine dinucleotide phosphate, an important energy-transferal substance.

transmembrane transport is greatly enhanced (Hultin, 1952; Epel, 1967; Humphreys, 1971; Reiger and Kafatos, 1977). Permeability to amino acids was found not to be a limiting factor, for although [^{14}C]glucose was metabolized into various amino acids by the ovum, the products were not incorporated into proteins until fertilization had occurred (Monroy and Vittorelli, 1962).

Later it was shown that the ribosomes of the egg were free in the cytoplasm, rather than in the form of polysomes (Monroy and Tyler, 1963), so it seemed that the mRNA was somehow unavailable to the ribosomes until after fertilization, when polysome formation proceeded rapidly. More recently, it has been found that the increase in protein synthesis (translation of the mRNA) could be elicited by weak bases applied to unfertilized eggs, leading to the hypothesis that increase in intracellular pH led to the rapid production of proteins. Moreover, it was also clear that fertilization led to an elevation of the zygote pH (Steinhardt and Mazia, 1973; Epel *et al.*, 1974; Johnson *et al.*, 1976; Winkler and Grainger, 1978). Still more recently, a series of experiments revealed that intracellular pH did indeed control translation rate in the sea urchin egg and early embryo (Grainger *et al.*, 1979). However, artificial raising of the intracellular pH in unfertilized eggs required at least 30 min longer than fertilization to achieve the same level of protein synthesis. Since translation of mRNA did not continue at the same rate during early cleavage but decreased in spite of the elevated pH, it was concluded that other unknown factors also are involved in control. While the mechanism has not been revealed that induces the elevation of the pH, a discussion in a following paragraph suggests one possibility.

Ion Distribution. The metabolism of various ions also undergoes marked changes at fertilization, some of which might be related to the elevation of pH just described. The rate of ^{32}P utilization is almost zero in unfertilized sea urchin eggs, at which level it remains for about a 15-min lag period following sperm penetration; it then increases rapidly for 30 to 60 min at which time it reaches a maximum (Litchfield and Whiteley, 1959). If anaerobic conditions or dinitrophenol are added during the lag period, the phosphate rate of increase is retarded, but these agents are ineffective after the lag period has been passed.

Membrane potential changes also have been recorded that vary with the species. In starfish eggs, potentials ranging from -5.2 to -40 mV (inside negative) have also been found, which dropped about 5 mV with the completion of penetration, only to rise about 10 mV within a few minutes (Tyler *et al.*, 1956). Similar changes have also been demonstrated in the egg of the cyprinid fish, *Oryzias latipes* (Maeno *et al.*, 1956; Ito, 1962); however, in *Fundulus* no potential was detected either before or after fertilization (Kao, 1955). The potentials were shown not to be essential in the medaka egg for either the blocking of polyspermy or activating the egg (Nuccitelli, 1980a,b). Accompanying these changes in membrane potential are similar alterations in conductance properties, potassium transport being especially facilitated (Steinhardt *et al.*, 1972; Jaffe and Robinson, 1978). This increase in K^+ conductance, which involves a requirement for ATP and the formation of new channels, was shown to be independent of calcium release but was dependent on the rise in pH (Shen and Steinhardt, 1980). Further, this study indicated that the pH increase was induced through membrane ATPase activity.

Extensive changes in the cellular distribution and total content of Ca^{2+} and Mg^{2+} ions have also been described, one of the earlier reports (Mazia, 1937) indicating a release of the former substance from a bound to an ionic condition 10 min after fertilization. Later studies showed that an actual loss of Ca^{2+} into the environment also followed penetration by the sperm (Örström and Örström, 1942; Monroy Oddo, 1946), and the later of these articles also revealed a similar loss of Mg^{2+}. In *Lytechinus pictus*, between 2.5 and 4.5 μM free calcium was released within 45 to 60 sec after fertilization, while cortical granules *in vitro* required 9 to 18 μM Ca^{2+} for discharge (Steinhardt *et al.*, 1977). Furthermore, fertilization of mouse eggs has been demonstrated to be highly dependent on the presence of Ca^{2+} ions (Shellenbarger and Shapiro, 1980).

2.4.2. Changes at the Macromolecular Level

While the dramatic change in protein synthesis just described has attracted the majority of investigations at the molecular level of fertilization events, the number of reports devoted to other aspects is slowly increasing. Nevertheless, beginning the discussion with those related to protein generation offers a number of advantages. Obviously each change in a protein or RNA represents a specific instance in gene expression and is a part, therefore, of the problems to be explained before this book is completed.

mRNA in Protein Synthesis Changes. To explore the question of whether the nature of the mRNA was responsible for the blockage of translation in the unfertilized egg, a study was made of the requirement for a certain modified guanosine residue at the 5' terminal (Hickey *et al.*, 1976). Many viral and cellular mRNAs bear a 7-methylguanosine at that location, linked by way of a nucleoside triphosphate, without which ''caps'' globin mRNA cannot be translated (Griffin, 1975; Muthukrishnan *et al.*, 1975). However, mRNA from eggs of *L. pictus* denuded of cap structures proved to be freely translatable, indicating that this facet of the messenger molecule was not involved in protein synthesis suppression. Quite to the contrary, mRNA from mouse eggs could not be translated when denuded of their caps, but no difference in degree of capping was found between mRNA from unfertilized versus fertilized ova (Schultz *et al.*, 1980).

The attachment of poly(A) sequences to RNA takes place within the nucleus of cells as a whole, because both hnRNA and its cytoplasmic derivative, mRNA, exhibit this trait (Adesnik *et al.*, 1972; Darnell *et al.*, 1973; Weinberg, 1973). However, a large increase in poly(A) synthesis has been noted both in fertilized eggs and in parthenogenetically activated enucleated egg fragments (Slater *et al.*, 1973; Wilt, 1973). Hence, the postfertilization increase in this activity appears to take place in the cytoplasm, using mRNA of oogenic origin. This supposition has now been confirmed through use of [^{3}H]adenosine and [^{14}C]uridine on fertilized ova and early embryos of *L. pictus* (Slater and Slater, 1974). Moreover, a poly(A) polymerase has been found in the cytoplasm, suggesting that polyadenylation might also take place outside the nucleus (Slater *et al.*, 1978). In fact, later studies have shown that until the late blastula stage, the largest portion of poly(A) polymerase activity is cytoplasmic but becomes nuclear in later stages (Egrie and Wilt, 1979).

These poly(A) tracts have been employed as a marker of mRNA in determining the distribution of the messages between polysomes and free RNP particles (Lovett and Goldstein, 1977). In unfertilized eggs, 58% of the poly(A)$^+$ RNA and 72% of the ribosomes were found not to be in polysomes, which figures were altered within 1 hr after insemination to 51% of the poly(A)$^+$ RNA and 48% of the ribosomes. By 7 hr postinsemination, the quantities reached plateaus at 30% of each not being in polysomes. The poly(A)-bearing RNAs did not change size during postfertilization events but remained the same as in the unfertilized egg, ranging from 30 S to 70 S, with a mean of 50 S (but compare Kaumeyer *et al.*, 1978). The poly(A) segment itself ranged from 50 to 200 nucleotides in length, with a mean of 115; only 1 to 2% of the total RNA present bore poly(A) segments.

In a recent investigation into the rate of synthesis of RNA in the sea urchin egg (Dworkin and Infante, 1978), most of this nucleic acid was reported to be synthesized in the nucleus and to have sedimentation coefficients between 16 S and 30 S. As just discussed, most of the material was present as RNP but was unstable, reaching a steady state with a half-time of about 30 min. The rate of accumulation did not change with fertilization but remained at the level of the unfertilized egg, 1.4×10^{-14} of RNA/min per egg. Although this represents 10-fold greater rate than that found later in the blastula, it was shown to equal 3×10^{-13} of potential mRNA at fertilization or only about 10 to 15% of its requirements at that time. Thus, synthesis of RNA was demonstrated not to be a factor in the increase of protein production.

DNA Synthesis. Several laboratories have investigated the possible role of DNA synthesis and its relations to pronuclear events following insemination. In studying the chemical changes in *Arbacia punctulata,* one team of researchers found that production of one of the ingredients of DNA, thymidine triphosphate, was initiated about the time penetration was completed (Longo and Plunkett, 1973). Synthesis of this TTP continued at an increasing rate thence through pronuclear migration until prophase, about 40 min later. Production of DNA itself commenced prior to pronuclear fusion, 10 or 15 min after penetration (Anderson, 1969); even the pronuclei of supernumerary sperm began synthesis of this substance, substantiating the claim that fusion of the pronuclei is not a prerequisite for its onset. Through use of puromycin to inhibit protein synthesis, it was found that the first period of DNA formation was unaffected but was inhibited following the first cleavage (Black *et al.*, 1967; Young *et al.*, 1969). However, in *Urechis*, inhibition of protein formation within 55 min of fertilization prevented the first DNA production and first cleavage (Blankstein and Kiefer, 1977). After that it only affected the second cleavage.

Using pronase-treated frog sperm injected into toad oocytes matured with and without germinal vesicles, Skoblina (1976) was able to demonstrate that the nucleoplasm was involved in initiating DNA synthesis. Sperm nuclei behaved normally in nucleated eggs, swelling, synthesizing DNA, and dividing. Production of the nucleic acid was detected first at the metaphase II stage. To the contrary, sperm introduced into eggs that had been matured in the absence of a germinal vesicle failed both to enlarge and to produce DNA. Once suspected of involvement with activation of replication, DNA polymerase activity has been shown to be insufficient for it to play such a role (Ford and Woodland, 1975). Whatever the factor may ultimately prove to be, it is effective on sperm nuclei from many sources—even nuclei from embryos of the fruit fly *D. melanogaster* synthesized DNA when injected into *Xenopus* eggs (Smith *et al.*, 1980).

Chromosome Condensation. A topic indirectly related to the synthesis of DNA, the condensation of chromosomes, has been explored by several laboratories recently. When sperm nuclei were permitted to fertilize immature sea urchin eggs that had been artificially activated by ammonia, premature chromosome condensation in the male nucleus was induced. In other words, the male chromosomes became condensed in company with those of the female as the egg nucleus matured through meiotic division. Since even enucleated egg halves (merogons) as well as nucleated ones had the same capacity (Krystal and Poccia, 1979), a cytoplasmic factor appeared to be involved; however, in enucleated merogons, the life of that activity was only 5 to 10% of that of nucleated ones. Transcription was found not to be essential, but translation of stored maternal mRNA was needed prior to the G2 stage of the activated egg. Similar results have also been obtained with echiuroid and frog eggs (Bataillon and Su, 1930; Das and Barker, 1976).

A second factor has also been uncovered that had a related but different function (Meyerhof and Masui, 1979). This substance, known as cytostatic factor, was first discovered when brain nuclei from adult *Xenopus* were injected into mature oocytes. These nuclei were observed both to undergo chromosome condensation and to be associated with spindles and asters (Gurdon, 1968). Subsequent investigations have made it clear that this factor does not actually induce chromosome condensation by itself, but arrests the cell cycle at metaphase and maintains the conditions of that phase in the cytoplasm, which in turn induce the actual chromosome condensation. Two components with cyto-static activity were detected, one of which was Ca^{2+} sensitive, the other insensitive to that cation (Meyerhof and Masui, 1979).

Protein Synthesis. The proteins which become associated with the sperm chromatin after penetration have also been suspected of playing a part in the dramatic changes undergone by the male nucleus in form and organization. To investigate this possibility, polyacrylamide gel electrophoretic analyses were made of the proteins from zygote and sperm nuclei and from pronuclei of both sexes (Kunkle *et al.*, 1978a). The results demonstrated marked changes both in solubility traits and peptide profiles in the sperm nuclei after penetration. Among the proteins acquired was one of a molecular weight in excess of 80,000 and, as a whole, a protein composition similar to that of the female pronucleus. However, there are sperm-specific variants of histone H1, that gradually give way to those of the early cleaving embryo (Poccia *et al.*, 1981). The zygote nucleus, in contrast, showed greater similarity to the combined pronuclei, but differences could be noted, including the presence of several polypeptides absent from pronuclear extracts. Moreover, a recent investigation has revealed that histone repeat transcripts accumulate in this central body of the female gamete (Venezky *et al.*, 1981).

Experiments involving incubation of isolated sperm nuclei in the cytosol extracted from the eggs showed that the nuclei underwent enlargement and became spherical as during fertilization (Kunkle *et al.*, 1978b). During this incubation about 30% of the acid-soluble fraction of the nuclear proteins was removed, whereas the other fractions displayed great increases in polypeptides, a large percentage of which had molecular weights exceeding 60,000. Some unknown component of the egg cytosol appeared necessary for the enlargement of the sperm nuclei. Perhaps the extensive phosphorylation of proteins and the 40 S ribosomal subunit that have been demonstrated also are important to these processes (Ballinger and Hunt, 1981).

Tubulin and Microfilaments. A current investigation, concerned with the microtubules and microfilaments, combined treatment with cytochalasin B (which interferes with actin) with transmission electron microscopy (Longo, 1980). The results showed that the chemical inhibited the formation of microfilaments, in the absence of which the microvilli of the surface did not elongate nor did a fertilization cone form (Figure 2.13). Furthermore, the reagent prevented the penetrated sperm nucleus from rotating as it migrated, but did not interfere with its migration or its fusion with the female pronucleus. In untreated fertilized eggs, the microvilli were noted to undergo reorganization when the sperm had attached; further, their movement as well as the development of the fertilization cone were demonstrated to be dependent upon the presence of bundles of microfilaments.

In a second series, use of cleared material, stained with a methylene blue–azure II combination, permitted the observation of the development of a spiral

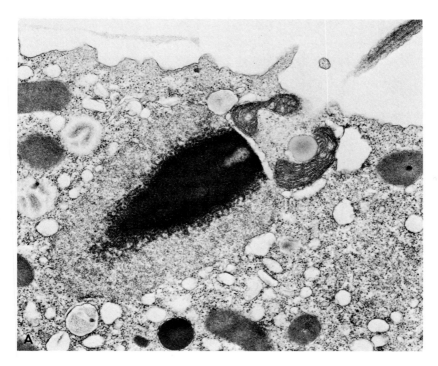

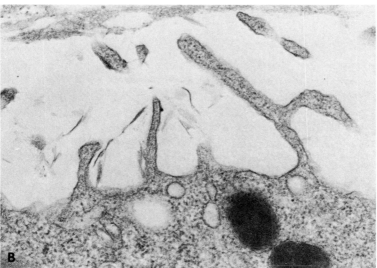

Figure 2.13. Results of actin inhibition. Treatment of *Arbacia punctulata* eggs with cytochalasin B 1 min after insemination inhibited the production of actin and thus of many microfilaments. (A) As a result the fertilization cone so evident in Figure 2.1 failed to form. 22,000×. (B) Although microvilli formed, they are seen to be devoid of microfilaments. 65,000×. (Both courtesy of Longo, 1980.)

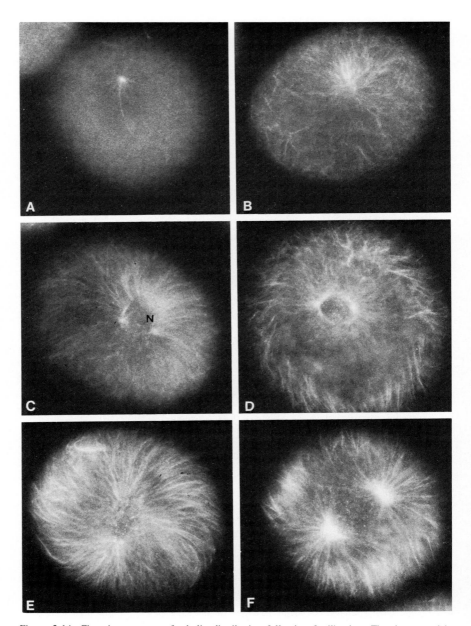

Figure 2.14. Changing patterns of tubulin distribution following fertilization. The time stated in the following sequence of *Strongylocentrotus purpuratus* zygotes is the period elapsed since insemination. (A) At 9 min a starlike point of tubulin deposits marks the site of sperm entry. (B) Four minutes later tubulin-staining fibers have extended through much of the subsurface cytoplasm.

system of microfilaments in *Strongylocentrotus purpuratus* zygotes (Harris, 1979). Within 10 min after insemination, the eggs showed the presence of the sperm aster in association with a pronucleus that had already undergone considerable migration. At the same time, pigment granules that had been distributed throughout the cytoplasm prior to fertilization began to be moved to the surface, whereas the interior of the cell was permeated by a meshwork of fine fibers. After the passage of a second 10-min period, the male pronucleus and its monaster had nearly reached the female pronucleus at the center of the cell, from which point a great number of fibers radiated to the egg surface. Within a third like period, the cortical fibers, assumably consisting of actin, had acquired a spiral arrangement, which remained intact for approximately 30 min while the pronuclei were fusing. Then as the amphiasters formed and enlarged, the cortical fibrils broke down and disappeared. The cortical fiber system appears to correspond to that observed in fertilized and butyric acid-activated eggs of *Lytechinus* (Mar, 1980).

In a further set of investigations from the same laboratory (Harris *et al.*, 1980a,b) immunofluorescence microscopy was employed, largely with tubulin antibodies (Figure 2.14). These studies demonstrated that the spiral cortical fibrils actually were microtubules, rather than actin microfilaments as originally suspected, for antibodies to this protein gave no reaction as long as the spiral system persisted. Moreover, the timetable of major events was refined to some extent. Pronuclear fusion was found to occur at 30 min postinsemination, and interphase asters at 50 min, while the streak stage lasted until 75 min (Figure 2.14E). The cortical microtubule system appeared at about 12 min and endured to the streak stage. After 90 min the extremely large asters that had formed earlier became greatly reduced during early prophase of the first cleavage mitosis (Figure 2.14F), but reexpanded widely in the metaphase that ensued.

Postfertilization Waves. Waves of contractions resulting in dark–light–dark zones have been observed in salamander zygotes, more recently in those of *Xenopus* (Hara, 1971; Hara *et al.*, 1977), and even in anucleate fragments of *Tubifex* zygotes (Shimizu, 1981). In all cases, the exact time of their appearance was dependent upon the temperature. Two sets, each dual in nature, were described originally. At 24°C, the first wave of the "postfertilization" set occurred about 15 min after insemination, followed within 10–15 min by the second, both of which originated at the point of sperm entry. As a rule, the latter was less pronounced than the first, sometimes to the extent that it could not be observed at all. The second set, the "surface contraction waves," began

---

(C) At 25 min tubulin fibers of the monaster extend from two organizing centers on opposite sides of the nucleus (N). (D) After an additional 5 min, the monaster microtubules have disappeared from the central part of the cell, but remnants persist near the cell periphery. (E) This micrograph taken at 76 min represents the streak stage. (F) Largely, microtubule loss progresses outward, except for some that remain associated with the aster centers. All 575×. (Courtesy of Harris *et al.*, 1980a.)

just 15 min before the first cleavage furrow appeared, each being initiated at the point where that cleft would first form. In this series, too, the second wave was much less conspicuous than the first, which it followed by about 7 min. Later the discovery was made of an additional wave; this appeared at the time of penetration, beginning almost immediately at the point of sperm entry (Hara and Tydeman, 1979) and was like the others in consisting of dark–light–dark zones. Thus, three sets of waves, two dual and one single, are known to be propagated over the surface of the egg after it has been fertilized. Even when mitosis is prevented chemically, these waves are developed in synchrony with cleavage in untreated eggs (Hara *et al.*, 1980), demonstrating the presence of a clock mechanism even in these lower levels of organization.

Nuclear Transplantation. No discussion of fertilization would be truly representative that failed to include the results of nuclear transplantation experiments (e.g., Gurdon, 1976; Ellinger and Carlson, 1978). In pertinent experiments of this type, unfertilized eggs are employed after removal of the nucleus; then a nucleus from a specialized cell, either somatic or embryonic, is introduced into the enucleated one. If successful, this combination develops into a normal individual, whose traits are always those of the nuclear, not the cytoplasmic, strain or subspecies (Gurdon, 1961). In recent years the procedures have been improved somewhat by use of serial transplants, in which a young embryo, that is itself the result of a nuclear transplant, is broken into its cellular parts to serve as a source of nuclei for further experiments. The advantage obviously is that thus a large number of genetically identical nuclei becomes available (Gurdon, 1976). To date, success has been obtained only with various amphibians, insofar as use of nuclei from differentiated cells is concerned. However, the unspecialized cells of blastoderm have been employed as a source of nuclei with *Drosophila* eggs (Illmensee, 1972). From each such experiment only a few normal individuals can usually be obtained, the majority developing inviable abnormalities. The failure to undergo normal development has been claimed to ensue from chromosomal damage that results from the differences in division rates that exist between the nucleus and recipient cell (Gurdon, 1976), but the phase of the cell cycle at time of removal of the donated nuclei also plays a role (von Beroldingen, 1981). Thus, the conclusion was reached that all animal somatic cells possess pluripotent nuclei, that is, are capable of leading to the normal differentiation of tissues. Pluripotentiality of nuclei should not be identified with pluripotentiality of cells, which topic receives attention again in the subdivision that follows.

Rather than the division rate differences between nucleus and cytoplasm just offered in explanation of the small percentage of successful transplants, some more fundamental process might more probably be the underlying factor. In all cells the nucleus and cytoplasm necessarily differentiate together, as shown by this type of experiment as well as those using cell fusion (Harris, 1974), perhaps through mutual feedback mechanisms. Thus, the egg cytoplasm of an

though in synchrony with them and at a corresponding level. At the fourth cleavage, the upper tier containing the four animal blastomeres divides latitudinally to produce a double layer containing eight moderate-sized products called mesomeres (Figure 3.1E), while concurrently the lower tier divides extremely unequally, pinching off four minute cells near the vegetal pole. These micromeres eventually give rise to the primary mesenchyme, while their large sister macromeres become the gut and part of the larval epidermis. The complete cleavages, representing the holoblastic type, are indicative of the presence of a yolk content too low to interfere with cell division. Cleavages also should be noted to be radial, their planes being either meridional or parallel to the original equator (Stearns, 1974).

The mechanics of producing the unequal divisions that result variously in macro- and micromeres or the ovum and polar body have received some attention in the literature. In sea urchins, the few investigations have been especially concerned with the asters of the dividing blastomeres. In those that divide equally, such as the animal mesomeres, the asters at each end of the spindle are of similar size and shape, both being of the radiate type, with rays projecting in three dimensions. At the fourth cleavage involving the vegetal blastomeres of the sea urchin, the spindle forms just beneath the cell surface. Whereas the aster at the proximal end of the spindle is radial and of normal size, the distal one is daisylike in form, all the rays lying on a single plane across the axis of the spindle (Dan and Nakajima, 1956; Dan, 1978). Similar asters occur in *Spisula solidissima* when the first cleavage gives rise to small animal cells and large vegetal ones (Dan *et al.*, 1952). When these unequal cleavages are observed by phase microscopy, the nuclei of the eight cells formed by the third cleavage of sea urchin zygotes may be noted to be located centrally, but before the fourth division, the nuclei of the vegetal cells rotate, each bringing one centrosome toward the vegetal pole. Headed by those centrosomes, the nuclei are then moved to the plasmalemma close to that pole; hence, when the asters form, the distal ones are unable to send out other than laterally directed rays because of their proximity to the external membrane (Dan, 1978). If sodium lauryl sulfate is added to the medium at the four-cell stage, nuclear migration does not occur, resulting in equal cleavage and the production only of normal three-dimensional astral rays.

As a result of these observations, it has been proposed that the cause of unequal division is the migration of the nucleus to a distal location when undergoing mitosis (Dan, 1978). This conclusion, however, mistakes an effect for cause. As pointed out in relation to the movement of pronuclei prior to fusion (Chapter 2, Section 2.3), nuclei have no means of locomotion. Hence, the positioning of the nuclei of the vegetal blastomeres is dependent upon the supramolecular genetic mechanism, which also is responsible for establishing the site of cytokinesis (Dillon, 1981, pp. 556–558). In the treated eggs, the sodium lauryl sulfate inhibits this genetic mechanism from moving the nucleus to a peripheral location and also from localizing the microfilaments beneath the plasmalemma in the subpolar position. Thus, mitosis occurs centrally in each cell and cytokinesis is equatorial.

Cleavage in Lancelets. In the fertilized egg of such lancelets as *Branchiostoma*, the vitelline membrane persists during much of early cleavage (Conklin, 1932), the animal pole being marked by the second polar body, which remains within the perivitelline space. After a sperm has penetrated the egg, usually toward the vegetal pole, and has become converted into a pronucleus, it is moved toward the center to meet the female pronucleus as usual. But as it is moved, much of the cytoplasm also is rearranged by the supramolecular genetic mechanism, the end result being the formation of a crescent of cortical material adjacent to the point of the sperm's entry (Manner, 1964). Because this crescent marks the location of the future mesoderm, it is possible to draw a fate map of the cellular parts even at this early zygote stage (Figure 3.2).

The first cleavage, which occurs within 1½ hr after fertilization, is meridional and passes through the animal and vegetal poles as well as the midpoint of the mesodermal crescent (Figure 3.3). The second is not fully meridional but is displaced slightly posterior to the central axis, thereby producing two

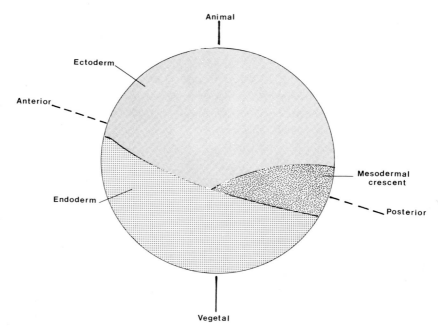

Figure 3.2. Zygote and fate map in lancelets. The mesodermal crescent is a marked feature of the fertilized zygote in *Branchiostoma* and other lancelets. At this time the animal–vegetal pole actually exists, whereas the anterior–posterior axis corresponds only to that of the later embryo.

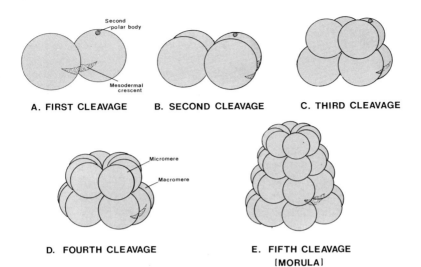

A. FIRST CLEAVAGE   B. SECOND CLEAVAGE   C. THIRD CLEAVAGE

D. FOURTH CLEAVAGE   E. FIFTH CLEAVAGE
[MORULA]

Figure 3.3. Cleavage in lancelets. Cleavage in lancelets like *Branchiostoma* is complete (holoblastic) but somewhat unequal, so that two size classes of micromeres, which correspond to the mesomeres of the sea urchin, and two of macromeres are the result.

slightly larger anterior and two smaller posterior blastomeres, on the latter of which the crescent is located. Similarly the third cleavage is subequatorial and is unequal, the resulting vegetal blastomeres being somewhat larger than the animal. Thus, this 8-cell stage consists of 4 vegetal macromeres and 4 animal micromeres, the anterior members of each set being larger than the posterior. The fourth division is meridional, double, and also not quite equal; this is followed by a double horizontal fifth cleavage, resulting in a 32-cell morula stage, beyond which synchrony of division is lost.

Early Stages of Amphibian Embryogenesis. Not infrequently in frog eggs the animal hemisphere is darkly pigmented, while the vegetal hemisphere, in which the rather abundant yolk is concentrated, is pale. These polar distinctions are accompanied by clinal contrasting distributional relations at the ultrastructural level; ribosomes, mitochondria, and fat bodies gradually increase in abundance toward the animal pole, while yolk platelets show an increasing gradient toward the vegetal (Brachet, 1977). Moreover, the egg nucleus is located beneath the former. The sperm enters on the animal hemisphere usually within 60° of the pole, thereby activating the egg to complete meiosis, terminating the second meiotic arrest established at oviposition. After penetration has been completed and the male pronucleus has developed, the latter is moved toward the female pronucleus, along with some of the pigmented cortical cytoplasm. In concert with this migration, a gray crescent often becomes visible

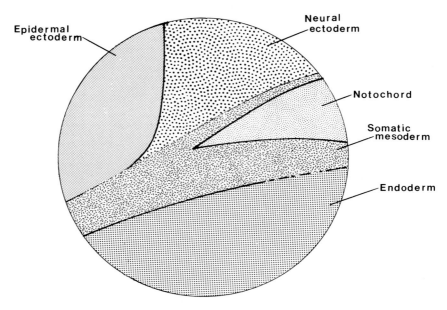

Figure 3.4. Fate map of the urodele amphibian egg. (Based in part on Vogt, 1929, and Landström and Løvtrup, 1979.)

that marks the future site of the blastopore and half of the future dorsal region of the adult (Figure 3.4).

The gray crescent also is an important indicator of the plane of embryonic and adult bilateral symmetry, for the plane of the first cleavage passes through it and the animal and vegetal poles (Brachet, 1977; Sussman and Betz, 1978; Kirschner and Gerhart, 1981). After a second equal meridional cleavage has occurred at right angles to the first, division becomes unequal, being strongly influenced by the abundant yolk. Hence, the third cleavage takes place horizontally, well above the equator of the zygote, dividing it into four animal micromeres and four much larger vegetal macromeres. The fourth is double and meridional, and the fifth, also double, is quite unequal, resulting in 16 each of micromeres and macromeres, beyond which point cleavage no longer is regular. It should be pointed out that cleavage through the yolk-bearing macromeres is much slower than in the micromeres, so that the former may be only partly subdivided long after the latter have completed cytokinesis.

Early Cleavage in Turtles and Birds. Cleavage patterns in reptilians and avians are sufficiently similar to permit their discussion as a single unit. Both types of organisms have eggs of a heavily telolecithal variety, so that cleavage, of the meroblastic type, is confined to a small area called the germinal disk. The first two cleavage planes pass through the animal pole, but it has not been determined whether the orientation of the first of these is corre-lated to the point of sperm entry (Eyal-Giladi and Kochav, 1976). These in-complete cleavages are then followed by two double ones, the third one parallel to the first, the fourth parallel to the second. Thus, only the central cells are completely delimited from the yolk. In birds, the cleavages are less uniform than in turtles, the furrows often being irregular; in both types of organisms continued cleavages result in a mound of cells referred to as the blastoderm. The characteristics of the various stages in cleavage may be found in more detail in Table 3.1.

Cleavage in Mammals. In mammals, the early stages of embryonic de-velopment take place within the zona pellucida and are extremely simple, being of the holoblastic equal type. The first two cleavages are meridional, passing through both poles but whether or not in relation to sperm entry does not appear to have been established. As usual, the third is horizontal and, in this case, is equatorial. The fourth is double and meridional, whereas the fifth is horizontal and likewise double, continued divisions ultimately resulting in a solid ball of cells called the morula.

A Spiral Type of Cleavage. Not all metazoans undergo the regular ra-dial type of cleavage that has thus far characterized the discussions; quite a few invertebrates undergo a spiral variety, in which the rows of cells of the third and following cleavages are off center from one another (Costello and Henley, 1976). Included among the taxa that exhibit this type are the polyclad Turbel-laria, Annelida, Rhynchocoelia, Mollusca (except the Cephalopoda), Echiuro-idea, and Sipunculoidea. Acoel Turbellaria likewise have a modifed form of this pattern, as do also the Cirripedia (Crustacea) and Rotifera.

Although, not unexpectedly, details vary with taxon, the processes in the Mollusca as represented by *Crepidula* (Conklin, 1897) provide a reasonable model that has been especially thoroughly explored (Figure 3.5). In these ani-mals the first two cleavages are equal and meridional, producing four equal blastomeres referred to as A, B, C, and D that characterize the four-quadrant type of spiral cleavage. However, before each division, including the initial one, the cells rotate around the egg axis slightly, first to the left and then to the right, alternating in this fashion throughout the cleavage stages. Thus, the odd-numbered divisions have a right-handed (dexiotropic) inclination, the even-numbered a left-handed (laeotropic or laevotropic). One net result of these ro-tatory movements is that the opposite cells contact one another at only one pole. While the spindles are arranged diagonally in the first two cell divisions, only with the third cleavage does it become clear that the division pattern is actually spiral. At this time cytokinesis occurs oblique to the equator and is greatly unequal, resulting in four micromeres (1a–1d) at the animal pole (Fig-ure 3.5C) and four first-generation, yolk-laden macromeres (1A–1D) at the vegetal pole. Successive similarly unequal cleavages of the macromeres pro-duce two additional quartets of micromeres, leaving four macromeres in the

Table 3.1

Stages of Development in the Chick Embryo[a]

Stage	Uterine Age (hr)	General stage	Characteristics
I	0-1	Cleavage	All or most cells open externally; cytoplasm with large vacuoles.
II	2	Cleavage	14-16 cells closed laterally, encircled by open ones. Blastomeres elevated above germ; vacuoles smaller.
III	3-4	Cleavage	Blastoderm reduced in breadth but thickened; 80-90 closed blastomeres. Lower surface with 10-16 cells.
IV	5	Cleavage	250-300 blastomeres above and 80-90 ventrally; blastoderm as in stage III; subblastodermal cavity forms.
V	8-9	Cleavage	Blastomeres equally developed on dorsal and ventral surfaces; subblastodermal cavity enlarged, reaching nearly to periphery.
VI	10-11	Cleavage	Cleavage stage completed; blastomeres small, forming an epithelial sheet of uniform thickness.
VII	12-14	Area pellucida	Some cells shed from lower surface at posterior half of the germ plasm; these rest on the yolk in the subgerminal cavity; area pellucida begun posteriorly.
VIII	15-17	Area pellucida	Area pellucida has spread toward both sides, forming a sickle-shaped area.
IX	17-19	Area pellucida	Area pellucida spreads forward; area opaca not sharply delimited.
X	20; oviposited	Area pellucida	Area pellucida completed; the area opaca sharply marked off.
XI	---	Hypoblast	A horseshoelike concentration on blastoderm posteriorly marks the beginning of the hypoblast.
XII	---	Hypoblast	Hypoblast lines half of the lower surface of the area pellucida, but is not continuous.
XIII	---	Hypoblast	Hypoblast completed.
XIV	---	Hypoblast	Hypoblast has well-defined borders; a cellular bridge is begun between hypoblast and area opaca.
2[b]	---	Primitive streak	Primitive streak begins to form anterior to the bridge of stage XIV.

[a] Based on Eyal-Giladi and Kochav (1976).
[b] Stage 2 of Hamburger and Hamilton (1951).

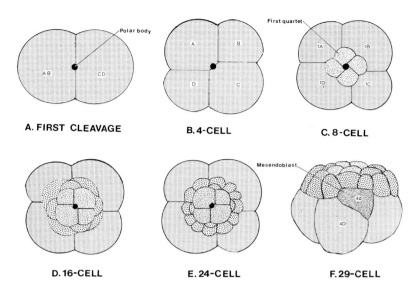

A. FIRST CLEAVAGE   **B. 4-CELL**   **C. 8-CELL**

D. 16-CELL   **E. 24-CELL**   **F. 29-CELL**

Figure 3.5. A spiral type of cleavage in a mollusk (*Crepidula*). All are dorsal views of the dividing zygote, except (F) which is a lateral view. At the four-cell stage (B), on the ventral surface metameres B and D contact one another as A and C do in the present aspect. (Based on Conklin, 1897.)

16-cell stage. These unequal divisions continue through a 28-cell stage; then one of the posterior macromeres (4D) alone divides, producing the mesendoblast and thereby creating a 29-cell embryo (Figure 3.5F). These cells then divide again, in company with others, so that at the 68-cell stage, the mesendoblast has given rise to the mesoblast completely separate from the endoblast (Clement, 1976; Costello and Henley, 1976). Among variations of the spiral type of cleavage is the occurrence of decidedly unequal divisions beginning with the very first one, as in *Nereis* (Wilson, 1892), or with the second, as in *Polychoerus* (Costello, 1961).

Development in a number of mollusks and annelids is characterized by an additional peculiarity, the formation of a polar lobe. This broad knoblike part actually appears and disappears on four occasions, initially at the time of formation of the first polar body, when it is in the form of a low, broad protrusion at the vegetal pole. Following retraction shortly thereafter, it reappears when the second polar body is produced as a larger but irregular knob but located as before. After being resorbed once more, it develops again just prior to the first cleavage, eventually becoming nearly as completely separated from the embryo proper as the two blastomeres that are then formed; it may be seen to be attached to the CD blastomere, to which it is subequal in size. The third resorption then occurs to make its final appearance in company with the second cleavage as a broad but low protrusion; it then becomes incorporated into the D blastomere to serve as the major organizing region of the developing embryo.

The slight interconnection that exists between the polar lobe and the embryo proper invited its removal by early investigators (Crampton, 1896; Wilson, 1904a,b), as well as recent ones (Clement, 1952, 1971; Verdonk, 1968; Morrill *et al.*, 1973; Cather and Verdonk, 1974; Newrock and Raff, 1975; Cather *et al.*, 1976; Guerrier *et al.*, 1978). Early experiments with similarly spirally cleaving embryos had indicated the existence of extensive powers of self-differentiation on the part of individual micromeres and macromeres (Wilson, 1904b), so that this type of development was often considered to represent a mosaic of independently differentiating cells. Eventually, however, the polar lobe was found to be a determining as well as an organizing center (Wilson, 1929), resulting in a modification of previous concepts to the new view that mosaicism was merely a variant of induced development.

When the third polar lobe is removed, neither mesendoblast nor mesoderm bands are formed, and bilateral symmetry never develops, nor are the foot, operculum, shell, and eyes produced. Embryos halved at first cleavage develop differently, according to whether the polar lobe is attached to the given part or not. That half consisting of the future A and B quadrants that lack the lobe develop into incomplete embryos, all the parts being absent that are wanting in lobeless whole embryos, whereas those that consist of the future C and D quadrants on which the lobe is left intact produce embryos with eyes, shell, and the foot (Cather *et al.*, 1976). In *Dentalium* the dorsoventral polarity of the embryo has also been shown to be dependent on the presence of the polar lobe (Guerrier *et al.*, 1978). Experimental studies on other mollusks, especially on those that lack a polar lobe, have confirmed the observation noted above, that so-called mosaic development is not really distinct from the inductive type except in degree. All types of embryogenesis appear to involve interactions between and within cells, never sharply defined, predetermined destinies (Guerrier and van den Biggelaar, 1979; van den Biggelaar and Guerrier, 1979).

3.1.2. Molecular Events during Cleavage

Investigations into the molecular events that take place during the cleavage stages tend to be unevenly distributed as to subject matter. For a rather protracted period, the RNAs, particularly the messenger variety, held the center of attention, but more recently the histones have attracted the efforts of an increasing number of investigators.

Histone Synthesis. Because of the rapid rate of cell division that occurs during embryogenesis, histone synthesis is an especially significant aspect of embryonic development. The production of these proteins must keep pace with that of DNA, as the two are partners in the formation of the great quantity of chromatin needed. During the 40 hr required to produce the gastrula from the fertilized egg, no fewer than 800 new nuclei must be developed. Shih *et al*. (1980) imply that certain proteins reported to be present in the nuclei of oocytes and synthesized in the cytoplasm (Smith and Ecker, 1970; Ecker and Smith, 1971) had been identified as histones only through the researches of Adamson and Woodland (1974, 1977), but there had been earlier reports. For example, histones and histone mRNAs had been described previously in sea urchin embryos [Cognetti, Spinelli, and Vivoli, 1969, unpublished results (see Cognetti *et al*., 1974); Johnson and Hnilica, 1971; Kedes and Birnstiel, 1971] and their synthesis during oogenesis and early embryogenesis demonstrated (Cognetti *et al*., 1974).

By extracting newly synthesized histones from *R. pipiens* oocytes or cleavage-stage embryos that had been injected with tritium-labeled lysine or arginine, it has been possible to calculate the rates of their synthesis (Shih *et al*., 1980). Rates in two-cell embryos were found to be at least 10-fold higher than in maturing oocytes, a trend that continued throughout cleavage; thus, at the blastula stage an additional 3-fold gain had been attained in the form of a rise from 1200 to 4500 pg/hr per embryo. The production of the various types was not uniform, synthesis of H4 being barely detectable; however, a pool of that type equal to about 74 ng was found in the oocytes, an amount stated to be sufficient to permit development to the blastula stage (Cognetti *et al*., 1974). The disproportion in H4 synthesis just mentioned is difficult to comprehend in light of the nature of histone gene organization in sea urchins (Kedes *et al*., 1975; Weinberg *et al*., 1975; Cohn *et al*., 1976; Wu *et al*., 1976; Holmes *et al*., 1977). In adults the genes for all five histones are located in a repeating structue, with a modal length of 6000–7000 bases and several hundred copies (Kedes and Birnstiel, 1971; Skoultchi and Gross, 1973; Arceci *et al*., 1976); consequently it is likely that the entire set of genes is transcribed as a unit, producing large precursors which are then processed into definitive mRNAs (Kunkel *et al*., 1978). However, in late-cleavage-stage embryos (128-cell), no high-molecular-weight histone transcripts were found, all falling in the range of 7 S–12 S. Contrastingly, in the late (mesenchyme) blastula transcripts were in the range of 18 S.

Although earlier studies had indicated that the histones produced during early embryogenesis were qualitatively identical to those of the adult (Byrd and Kasinsky, 1973, 1974), it was soon discovered that this was not the case. One of the first instances described more accurately involved sea urchin embryos in which a distinctive form of histone H1 of the morula gave way to another that proved to be entirely characteristic of the gastrula (Johnson and Hnilica, 1971; Easton and Chalkley, 1972; Seale and Aronson, 1973; Ruderman and Gross, 1974; Ruderman *et al*., 1974). However, these reports are in conflict with other studies which showed that histones from oocytes and cleavage-stage embryos were indistinguishable in electrophoretic motility (Lifton and Kedes, 1976) and in cell-free protein synthesis systems (Gross *et al*., 1973; Arceci *et al*., 1976);

the former do agree with later studies which demonstrated that several shifts in histone phenotypes occurred during cleavage. Although histones H3 and H4 appeared to be homogeneous classes and remained unchanged in these early periods of embryogenesis, histones H1, H2A, and H2B were found to be represented by at least nine types, all of which were identified species (Childs *et al.*, 1979). Some of the early cleavage types continued to be synthesized into gastrulation, but certain new ones appeared in the blastula and gastrula, as pointed out later. However, the mRNAs for these might have been formed many hours before the proteins themselves could be detected. The cleavage-stage histones were shown to be transcribed from different sets of genes than those of the later embryos.

But even the conservative histones, H3 and H4, have proven to be modified in early development. In mature chromatin, H4 contains only a single acetylated amino acid residue, an α-N-acetylserine located at the N terminus. Since H1 and H3 also bear similar α-N-acetyl groups, it is conventional to overlook this type of modification and to consider them "nonacetylated" forms nevertheless (Woodland, 1979). Mature chromatin contains non-, mono-, di-, and more highly-acetylated forms of H4, but the newly synthesized histone of early embryogeny is still more abundantly acetylated when first incorporated into chromatin (Louie and Dixon, 1972; Jackson *et al.*, 1976). Contrastingly, H3 is mainly in an unsubstituted condition when freshly synthesized, gaining modifications with the passage of time (Jackson *et al.*, 1975). Since the histones H3 from the cytoplasm and nucleus of oocytes are similar in their modifications, attachment to DNA is thereby shown not to be requisite for such substitutions to occur.

Tubulin and Microfilaments. As pointed out previously (Chapter 1, Section 1.2.2), tubulin is one of the proteins made most abundantly by the oocyte and early embryo, accounting for 1.3% of total translation. After a decrease in amount during meiotic maturation in the mouse oocyte, it has been found to increase to some extent in the zygote and still further in the eight-cell embryo (Schultz *et al.*, 1979). In the axolotl, changes in chemical properties of the tubulin have been noted during embryogenesis (Raff and Raff, 1978). Electrophoretic analyses showed that the protein from oocytes, eggs, and embryos of that salamander differed from the same substance of adult brains and testes, the patterns of proteolytically derived peptides being especially distinctive between oocytes and testes, in which the α subunit was even more diversified than the β.

mRNA during Cleavage. The dramatic increase in protein synthesis that follows fertilization has stimulated only a small amount of interest in the molecular aspects during the early cleavage stages. Most investigations have recorded the more contrasting conditions found in the gastrula and later embryos, while the relatively few devoted to the present stages have been confined to qualitative and quantitative changes in mRNA levels. During sea urchin cleavage, early researches based upon enucleated eggs or radiation- or actinomycin-treated embryos demonstrated clearly that transcription was not essential, the maternal mRNA present being sufficient for the needs through cleavage (Gross and Cousineau, 1963; Denny and Tyler, 1964; Gross et al., 1964). However, it was then reported that, while maternal mRNA made up the great bulk of these nucleic acids as "heavy" polysomes, newly synthesized mRNA was also present in the form of "light" polysomes and RNP particles (Spirin and Nemer, 1965; Dworkin et al., 1977). These distinctions appeared to arise from differences in protein content, the oogenetic mRNPs bearing a greater proportion of polypeptides than the newly formed (Young and Raff, 1979). Among the poly(A)$^+$ mRNAs in sea urchin, as well as other animal cells, is one type referred to as the complex or rare mRNA class (Lewin, 1975a,b; Davidson and Britten, 1979). These terms refer to the group consisting of a large number of diverse sequences, approximating 10,000 per cell, each of which is represented by only a few copies (Galau et al., 1974; Lev et al., 1980). Transcripts prepared that were complementary to two cloned genomic single-copy sequences of maternal mRNAs in the egg were found virtually to disappear by the end of the cleavage stage. One of the two was detected in cytoplasmic RNA from the intestinal cells of adult sea urchins but in low levels (Lev et al., 1980).

Synthesis of mRNA has also been reported to occur in early mouse embryos according to evidence from several lines of investigation. Use of radiolabeled precursors of RNA resulted in the detection of newly transcribed mRNA at the 4- and 8-cell stages of cleavage (Ellem and Gwatkin, 1968; Church and Brown, 1972) and even in the 2-cell (Church, 1970). Moreover, blockage of such synthesis by means of α-amanitin inhibited further development of cultured preimplantation embryos (Golbus et al., 1973; Levey et al., 1977). However, the most compelling evidence has come from studies involving paternal genetic characteristics. For example, the paternal isozyme for glucose phosphate isomerase was detected in the 8-cell embryo (Chapman et al., 1971; Brinster, 1973) and that for β-glucuronidase was found in the 4-cell stage (Wudl and Chapman, 1976). Still more recently the proportions of newly transcribed mRNA were determined and reported in the 2-cell, 8- to 16-cell, and blastocyst stages as 6.7, 3.5, and 3.3% of the whole, respectively (Levey et al., 1978). Furthermore, the decline in amount of maternal poly(A)$^+$ mRNA present has been followed through the entire cleavage period in these mammals (Bachvarova and DeLeon, 1980).

Ribosome-Related Activities. Also indirectly implicated in protein synthesis, production of ribosomal proteins and RNA has received occasional attention along several avenues of investigation. One line has devoted efforts to studies of the development of the nucleolus, in which the rRNA precursors are produced. Apparently throughout the Metazoa as a whole, the nucleolus is absent from ovulated eggs and from the male and female pronuclei after fertilization, a condition that persists in most species which have been studied until the gastrula stage or even later. However, some exceptions have been known for some time, most notable among which are the mammals, in whose embryos it reappears at the four-cell stage (Mintz, 1964; Ellem and Gwatkin, 1968; Woodland and Graham, 1969; Pikó, 1970). More recently, a selective silver-staining technique has been developed that stains only those regions of chromosomes that serve as nucleolus organizers and are active in the synthesis of at least 28 S rRNA (D. A. Miller *et al.*, 1976; O. J. Miller *et al.*, 1976; Croce *et al.*, 1977). Through its use, nucleolar-organizer centers have been shown to be active in two-cell and older embryos of mice, but not in earlier stages (Hansmann *et al.*, 1978). Chick embryos, too, have been found to have nucleoli develop at a fairly early stage, although not so early as in mammals, for several laboratories were able to detect nucleoli in uterine eggs developed to stage VII (Eyal-Giladi and Kochav, 1976; Raveli *et al.*, 1976).

Measurements of absolute rates of synthesis of ribosomal proteins likewise indicate the early formation of new ribosomes in mammalian embryos. By the eight-cell stage in mice, this class of substances accounted for 8.1% of total protein synthesis in the growing organism, representing an 11-fold increase from fertilization (LaMarca and Wassarman, 1979).

DNA Synthesis during Cleavage. Varied aspects of the replication of DNA during the cleavage stages of development have been explored, albeit not abundantly, for DNA synthesis is, of course, a prime requirement for the rapidly repeated mitoses of the early embryo. In investigating the source of the nucleosides for DNA replication in sea urchin embryos, it was disclosed that exogeneous as well as endogenous deoxyribonucleosides were employed (Villee *et al.*, 1949; Abrams, 1951; Nemer, 1962). Although at one time it had been suggested that one of the main regulatory steps in DNA synthesis was the rate of production of thymidine triphosphate (Roth, 1964), such has been demonstrated not to be the case, because this triphosphorylated nucleoside in cleavage stages of two sea urchins was found to be produced in quantities 10 times greater than actually incorporated into DNA (Suzuki and Mano, 1974). Phosphorylation of the other three common deoxyribonucleosides, while different from that of thymidine, also occurred in much greater quantities than needed for DNA replication.

The DNA polymerases of eukaryotic cells have not been explored as thoroughly as have those of such prokaryotes as *Escherichia coli*, in which the most abundant of these enzymes, DNA polymerase I, has proven not to be the primary replicative enzyme (Dillon, 1978, p. 85–90). In eukaryotes, polymerase-α is frequently considered to be chiefly responsible for this function, for in rapidly growing protistans only an enzyme similar to the vertebrate DNA polymerase-α is present (Wintersberger, 1974; Crerar and Pearlman, 1976; Loomis *et al.*, 1976). Since *D. melanogaster* embryos contain large quantities of DNA polymerase (Margulies and Chargaff, 1973; Loeb, 1974), this material has now been employed to provide more direct evidence as to the nature of the replicative DNA polymerase (Brakel and Blumenthal, 1977). It was found to be more heterogeneous than previously reported (Karkas *et al.*, 1975) but in the main to resemble DNA polymerase-α of vertebrates. One fraction was described as sedimenting at 7.3 S and another at 9.0 S.

Energy-Related Compounds. Despite glycogen's being the primary source of energy during early embryogeny (Gussek and Hedrick, 1972), relatively few explorations have been made into its metabolism (Gipson, 1974; Eyal-Giladi *et al.*, 1979). In general, production of the carbohydrate appeared to be carried out largely during the later stages of oogenesis, ceasing with maturation of the egg (Bergami *et al.*, 1968; Brachet *et al.*, 1970; Huebner *et al.*, 1975). Then at ovulation or fertilization intensive catabolism of the substance began (Yurowitzky and Milman, 1972). In eggs removed prematurely from the chicken, two waves of glycogen synthesis and breakdown have been described (Eyal-Giladi *et al.*, 1979). The products of the first wave, which occurred during late oogenesis, were degraded within vesicles during the first hours in the oviduct. Then just prior to the onset of cleavage, a second wave of production began within other vesicles and continued to the miduterine period; this cycle of glycogen was catabolized rapidly in still another type of vesicle, consumption terminating just prior to area pellucida formation.

3.2. THE BLASTULA AND SUBSEQUENT EMBRYONIC STAGES

Although some specializations of blastomeres became evident during the cleavage stages just described, these are largely expressed fully only in the later stages that follow. Hence, in sea urchins, the macromeres may be considered differentiated from the mesomeres and micromeres to a degree. However, if a vegetal half of an eight-cell embryo is separated from its animal counterpart as well as from the micromeres, it develops into a normal larva. If the micromeres are left on such a half, only an incomplete larva results, lacking a stomodaeum and ciliary tufts. By itself, the animal half develops only to a blastula, but if micromeres are grafted onto these mesomeres, a nearly normal larva is produced (Stearns, 1974). These patterns of changes are explained as the result of induction, the evoking of specific activities in one tissue by a second, a characteristic of most metazoan development. However, much more marked specializations of cell type are found in later stages of the embryo described in the present section and even more in the chapter on differentiation that follows. Each such specialization or modification, whether in size, shape, or molecular activity, reflects a change in the expression of one or more genes and provides the type of data especially sought in the present undertaking.

3.2.1. Postcleavage Stages in Echinoderms

Blastula Formation. In sea urchins, the embryo begins to assume a spherical form perhaps with the 128-cell stage, but it does not attain the full status of blastula until the 10th cleavage when it consists of better than 1000 cells. At this time it is spherical, with a large blastocoel surrounded by a single layer of cells (Figure 3.6A, B). The cavity is filled with a gel, containing fibrous material and a colloidal substance, possibly a mucopolysaccharide (Monné and Hårde, 1951; Wolpert and Mercer, 1963). As the spherical form is acquired, cilia develop on the surface of the embryo that rotate the embryo within the fertilization membrane that encloses it (Figure 3.6C). By this time the sphere has been polarized with respect to future morphogenesis and for immediate developments, the animal pole being marked by the thicker and longer cilia located there in the form of a tuft. Generally two axes are present, the animal–vegetal axis thus indicated and a dorsoventral one, located at an angle of about 45° from the other. The ventral side is the surface on which the

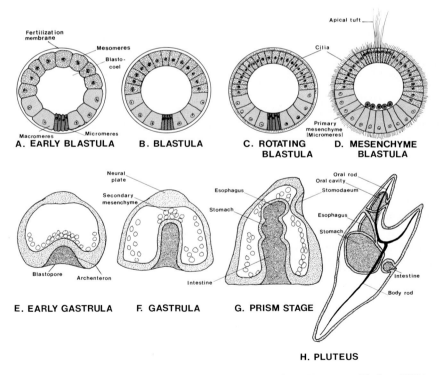

Figure 3.6. Postcleavage stages in sea urchin development. (Based in part on Giudice, 1973.)

blastopore opens (Hörstadius, 1939). A plane passing through both axes divides the embryo symmetrically into right and left halves.

About 3 hr after the ciliary pattern has been completely developed, that is, around 10 hr postinsemination, the fertilization membrane is broken down by enzymatic action, and the embryo becomes a free-living larva (Giudice, 1973). Some evidence has been presented which indicates that the hatching enzyme is contained in a system of membrane-bound vesicles (Yasumasu, 1960, 1963), that possibly represent the type of lysosome recently named the exophagosome (Dillon, 1981, p. 273). Following a period of around 6 hr the blastula becomes flattened at the vegetal pole, the cells thereby acquiring a more strongly columnar shape, and that tissue becoming thicker than the animal. At the same time, the micromeres, which previously had formed part of the vegetal cell layer, move into the blastocoel (Figure 3.6D), where at first they accumulate as unattached individual cells. These are then considered to be primary mesenchyme cells and for a time remain in the vicinity of the vegetal pole, but they later migrate around the sides of the cavity by means of pseudopods, which are often of the filopodial type. This unusual stage between the typical blastula and gastrula is referred to as the "mesenchyme blastula"; it is especially striking in that active tissue differentiation is thus initiated, rather than in the gastrula as in most animals.

The mechanism of forming the blastula in echinoderms has attracted considerable discussion. Originally the hyaline membrane was assigned an important role in the developmental processes of both this and the stage that follows (Dan, 1960). Purely mechanical activities were envisioned to suffice, which ensued from the elastic properties of the membrane and the changes in the manner by which the blastomeres were attached to it. Later the concept was amended by addition of a supposed increase in adherence between the cells as a significant factor (Wolpert and Gustafson, 1961), postulated in part to result from the septate desmosomes that the electron microscope had revealed (Wolpert and Mercer, 1963). However, experiments using fertilized eggs of the starfish (*Asterina pectinifera*) that were denuded of the fertilization membrane have produced somewhat contrasting results (Dan-Sohkawa and Fujisawa, 1980). The first few cleavages produced blastomeres that were virtually unconnected to one another, but after the 8th division, the cells began to become tightly appressed and arranged in a compact sheet. Then after the 9th or 10th cleavage, the free edges of the sheet turned upwards, so that by the time another division occurred, it had become folded into a hollow but irregular blastula. Septate desmosomes first appeared concurrently with the formation of the compact sheet, but the basement membrane was laid down only after completion of the blastula.

Formation of the Gastrula. Although begun to a slight extent in the mesenchyme blastula, differentiation becomes a pronounced feature of the embryo only with the advent of the gastrula. According to Gustafson and his co-workers (Gustafson and Kinnander, 1956a,b; Gustafson and Wolpert, 1961a, 1962, 1963, 1967), who employed cinephotomicrography, the archenteron begins to invaginate shortly after the primary mesenchyme has completed migration (Figure 3.6E, F). The early processes, which appear to be autonomous, result in infolding of the ventral region to about one-third of the ultimate length of the primitive gut. Among the major activities that produce this structure are continuous pulsations on the part of the cells, accompanied by changes in shape at critical points. After this early phase has been completed, small cells, the secondary mesenchyme, are budded off the tip of the invaginated structure; these attach by filopodia both to the roof of the latter and to the inner surface of the animal pole cells (ectoderm) that lies dorsally. It is claimed that subsequent invagination of the primitive gut is accomplished by contractions of the pseudopodia (Dan and Okazaki, 1956; Dan, 1960), but undoubtedly further cell divisions are likewise involved that result in its growth, for isolated vegetal plates continue to invaginate (Moore and Burt, 1939). Furthermore, no comparable pseudopodial activity has been observed in early gastrulae of *Lytechinus* (Trinkhaus, 1965).

    The Prism and Pleuteal Stages. When the archenteron has become fully invaginated, the larva undergoes a radical change in shape, while internally the skeletal parts begin to develop. As the cells around the animal pole become more columnar to form a so-called animal plate, a flattening occurs along the dorsoventral axis, so that in longitudinal section, the larva appears triangular, ushering in the prism stage. The thickening continues for a time, resulting in a caplike conformation of the animal pole, while just ventrad to this cap an invagination appears that marks the location of the future mouth, or stomodaeum. The upper edge of this infolding together with the apical tuft forms the ciliary band. The archenteron in the meanwhile has commenced a series of developments, the earliest of which is the constriction of the animal portion into a vesicle, which is the first rudiment of the coelom (Figure 3.6G). Then, apparently through the action of the pseudopodia of the secondary mesenchyme and coelomic cells, the primitive gut bends toward the forming stomodaeum, assuming an inverted J shape as a consequence. While the growing coelom produces a sac on each side that makes direct contact with the ectodermal wall, two constrictions form on the archenteron, dividing it into three parts, the esophagus, stomach, and intestine (Hörstadius, 1939), and the blastopore undergoes modification into the anus.

    Concurrently with the above changes, the first skeletal elements begin to be produced in the form of triradiate spicules secreted by primary mesenchyme cells. Series of such spicules are synthesized and consolidated into skeletal bars. In greater detail, skeletal bar formation commences when several rows of cells within the blastocoel attach by their filopodia, which fuse into syncytial cables. Then calcite is precipitated within the cables and conducted to an intersection involving three cables, at which point the triradiate spicule just mentioned is then formed. Further deposition of calcite leads to growth of the spicules to result in the long rods (Okazaki, 1956, 1962, 1965; Bevelander and Nakahara, 1960; Karp and Solursh, 1974). The completed skeleton consists of a pair of such structures, each of which has three main branches, called the body, oral, and anal rods.

Although the next larva, the pluteus (Figure 3.6H), is strikingly distinct from the prism stage in external morphology, very simple processes are involved in its production. The first appearance of the ensuing changes is the formation of four buds located in the ciliary band at the perimeter of the oral region. It has been claimed that these buds have little capacity by themselves for further growth, that they increase in length only when pushed outward by the growing skeletal rods (Gustafson and Wolpert, 1961b; Stearns, 1974). However, this is ascribing the biological function of growth to a mineral substance, calcite, rather than to an active living cellular part of an organism. Moreover, low doses of actinomycin, which inhibit skeletal growth completely, do not hinder the elongation of the arm buds and body apex (Peltz and Giudice, 1967). More likely the processes resemble those of cytokinesis by septum formation described recently (Dillon, 1981, pp. 511–518). That is to say, the buds elongate by cell division, while the skeletal rods are increased in length through further deposits of calcite being made on their tips by the cells of the coelom or mesenchyme. Growth is coordinated in such a fashion that the tip of a rod remains an approximately constant distance from the apex of the arm or other body part through which it extends. This proposed cellular control of skeletal growth is further corroborated by the species-specific nature of the skeletal parts, for the morphology of the various rods and branches provides the chief taxonomic characters for recognizing larvae of different sea urchins. While the skeletal parts are acquiring their full length, the left coelomic sac attaches to the dorsal ectoderm, the point of attachment later becoming the hydropore.

3.2.2. Later Embryological Stages of Chordates

Postcleavage Stages in Cephalochordates. In the lancelets, cleavage results in a cylinder of cells through the central axis of which is a cavity open at both poles, usually considered the blastocoel. As further cleavages reach approximately the 128-cell stage, both openings become closed, and the cells realign to form a hollow blastula, the mesodermal crescent still being evident on the surface. Quite as in the echinoderm blastula, this area marks the location of the posterior pole of the embryo, while the anterior–posterior axis projects from that point at an angle of about 60° to the animal–vegetal axis, which in turn is marked at the animal pole by the polar body. In sections, the three presumptive germ layers may be seen to have already become partly differentiated at this time, the endoderm being represented by the large cells of the anterior and ventral regions, the ectoderm by the smaller cells of the anterior and dorsal sides, and the mesoderm by the crescent.

The first indication of gastrula formation is the flattening of the vegetal surface (Conklin, 1932). At first the flattened area lies parallel to the anterior–posterior axis, but later the posterior region becomes more strongly depressed than the anterior as the entire embryo elongates and becomes subdepressed. Invagination then begins close to the posterior end of the ventral flat section, but soon involves the entire ventral surface as the archenteron deepens. As the latter structure becomes more strongly invaginated, its dorsal wall soon reaches the ventral surface of the ectodermal cells, against which it becomes firmly appressed. The embryo as a unit becomes more strongly arched until ultimately it has nearly reacquired its earlier spherical form, while concurrently the blastopore is constricted somewhat as it assumes a triangular form. Externally, this opening is abutted against almost exclusively by ectodermal cells.

The embryo now elongates along its anterior–posterior axis, the blastopore having attained as much a posterior as a ventral position; later its location becomes dorsoposterior as the dorsal surface first becomes flattened and then depressed over a broad area called the neural plate. Still later an elongate triangular slot, the neural groove, forms centrally in that plate, accompanied by an ingrowth of the ectodermal edges of the plate. Concurrently the corresponding cells of the ventral lip of the blastopore grow dorsad, closing off the pore. Slowly the cells from the sides and rear completely close over the neural plate and groove, both of which in the meanwhile have been undergoing a folding movement. Together these activities result in the formation of the neural tube that characterizes the neurula stage of all chordates.

Postcleavage Embryonic Stages in Amphibians. Among amphibians, the blastula is formed almost entirely by the very rapid mitotic divisions of the animal cells, in contrast to the much slower ones of the vegetal macromeres. By continuations of these processes, perhaps accompanied by some rearrangement on the part of the blastomeres, the blastocoel is developed. In section this is seen to lie beneath the animal pole and to be entirely in the animal hemisphere, the vegetal half of the embryo being completely filled by large yolk-bearing cells (Figure 3.7A). Each part of this blastula now has a prospective fate (Figure 3.4), but the regions can be mapped more clearly after the blastopore has been formed in the very early gastrula (Landström and Løvtrup, 1979).

The blastopore that marks the onset of gastrulation at about the 15th cleavage appears just below the gray crescent (Hara, 1977; Hara and Boterenbrood, 1977). As may be seen in longitudinal sections, were invagination to occur in this original orientation, the primitive gut would pass ventrad to the blastocoel (Figure 3.7B). However, two opposing sets of movements, neither of which involves invagination, are active in gastrulation. One set, referred to as epi-

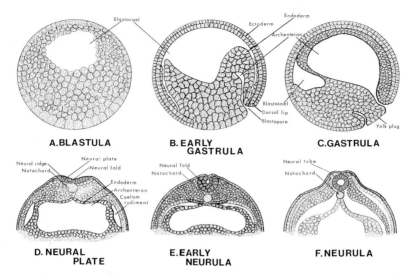

Figure 3.7. Further development in the frog.

boly, centers around the rapid growth of the animal cells, so that those of the surface flow down and around the remainder of the embryo, the processes of which have recently received attention with the scanning electron microscope (Keller, 1980; LeBlanc and Brick, 1981). This superficial movement ceases as it reaches the dorsal lip of the blastopore, an area once occupied by the gray crescent, where it becomes transformed into migratory movements into the interior. Eventually this inward-directed flow, or involution, results in the production of the archenteron (Figure 3.7C). As in the lancelets, the blastopore is at first large, but not nearly so voluminous as in those cephalochordates, and later becomes constricted and largely blocked by vegetal cells in the form of a yolk plug. While these surface migrations are proceeding, the second set of internal movements results in an anteriorly directed relocating of the blastocoel, so that by the time the archenteron has developed fully, it has acquired a position directly opposite the blastopore. However, by now the cavity has become greatly reduced in size and, not much later, disappears entirely, just as in the lancelets.

On the surface of the gastrula there appears an elongate, flattened area, the neural plate, which is soon set off by low continuous elevations, the neural ridges (Figure 3.7D). These increase in height and, as they do so, they move mesad toward one another; accompanying this development is the formation of a narrow neural groove along the midline of the neural plate. The groove deepens, while the sides of the neural plate curve over top of it, bringing the ridges closer toward one another, movements that continue until a neural tube covered by ectoderm has been brought into existence (Figure 3.7E, F). Concurrently, beginning in the early neurula on the anterior surface or below the neural plate, a sense plate had developed; by the time the late neurula has been completed, this structure gives rise to optic vesicles, below which is a rudimentary stomodaeum, bordered by mucous glands and gill plates.

Before continuing into postcleavage events in the chick and mammal, it is well to examine the epibolic and involutive movements of the cells more closely. In the first place, the cells cannot move merely by flowing movements induced by pressures resulting from cycles of cell division and growth, as Berrill and Karp (1976) point out. The movement of cells over the surface is not to be questioned, for the pigmented area of the animal hemisphere can be observed to spread over the surface to an increasing extent. Consequently epiboly is an actual event, but the mechanism that produces it needs to be examined critically. In the first place, increasing the number of cells would tend only to enlarge the diameter of the embryo, for the lateral pressure ensuing from cell multiplication can in no way be transformed into involutive ones. The forces generated by growth could much more simply be alleviated by the formation of a bulge over the rather extensive blastocoel. Secondly, the vegetal cells, now referred to as endoderm, do not remain passive, but stream upward into the interior of the embryo, assisting in the reduction of the blastocoel. Third, there is the problem of the reduction in surface area as movement takes place from the greatest circumference, at the equator of the embryonic sphere, toward the smallest circumference at the pole where the blastopore is located.

Reexamination of the fate map of the early gastrula makes the problem clear, for it is self-evident that the width of the blastopore can in a mechanical fashion accommodate the ingress of only a single row of cells of its own breadth at any given moment. But since the circumference of the embryo far exceeds that of this opening, many times this amount of cells needs to penetrate it from all directions. Yet, since the fates of the several surface areas can be marked off on the blastula, it follows that entrance into the blastopore must be a very orderly process, not in a random and inconstant fashion as would occur if numerous rows of cells were by mere chance to converge and enter through this small passageway into the interior. Undoubtedly the motive forces are of a simple enough nature, but they will never be disclosed and understood unless they are sought. And as long as this seemingly satisfactory, but impossible, concept is accepted, the necessary researchers will not be conducted.

Later Embryonic Stages in the Chick. By the time the cleavage period of the chick embryo has terminated, the germinal disk (blastodisk) is an arched plate of very fine cells extending to the edge of the yolk (Hamburger and Hamilton, 1951). As further cleavages continue, the blastodisk becomes free of contact with the underlying yolk, forming the blastocoel as a result. From above, the blastodisk that forms the roof of that cavity appears paler than that part which remains in contact with the yolk; accordingly the former region has become known as the area pellucida and the latter, the area opaca (Rosenquist, 1966). Actually, the area pellucida originally becomes free of the yolk surface toward the posterior region of the blastodisk, the blastocoel enlarging in a forward direction with the passage of time (Eyal-Giladi and Kochav, 1976).

When the area pellucida has nearly attained its full dimensions, cells leave the blastodisk, either by infiltration or delamination, and spread over the surface of the yolk to form the basement of the blastocoel. At first these multiply in irregular patches, but later congregate in the posterior part of the blastocoel to produce a sheet of cells overlying the yolk. This sheet then spreads by multiple cell divisions over the entire basement of the cavity; this layer is distinguished by the term hypoblast, whereas its older counterpart overlying the blastocoel is now called the epiblast. Once these layers have been completed, an elongate groove bordered by a ridge on each side develops on the posterior half of the area pellucida. This primitive streak and its bordering primitive folds widen slightly at their anterior ends to form the primitive pit. Anterior to this is a short, arcuate raised area called Hensen's node, which corresponds to the dorsal lip of the blastopore in amphibians. The primitive streak appears to result from inductive activities of the hypoblast, which layer in turn is influenced by the marginal zone of the epiblast (Azar and Eyal-Giladi, 1979, 1981).

There is some controversy as to the exact nature of developments beyond this point. One view is that involution of the epiblast occurs along the primitive streak by cells produced in a proliferation center located around Hensen's node (Derrick, 1937; Manner, 1964; Rosenquist, 1966), but the actual mechanism is in doubt (Spratt and Haas, 1962). At any rate, whether from the epiblast, hypoblast, or primitive streak, a sheet of cells, the mesoblast, grows outward from the latter between the epiblast and hypoblast to form the mesoderm, while an extension of this layer grows forward centrally beneath Hensen's node, eventually to become the notochord (Meier, 1979, 1981). In the meanwhile, the mesodermal sheet splits on each side longitudinally to form the coelomic sacs, during which processes the primitive streak regresses rapidly in a posterior direction. After the gastrula has thus been brought into existence, the hypoblast is recognized as endoderm, and epiblast as ectoderm. No archenteron exists at this time.

The first step toward development into the neurula stage is the thickening of the ectoderm over the forming notochord to produce the neural plate. The edges of this plate then round up and thicken into neural folds, which elevate and grow toward one another as in other vertebrate embryos. Growth mesially is more rapid at some distance anterior to Hensen's node, so the middle portions of the neural folds meet and fuse first, from which point completion of the neural tube proceeds both cephalad and caudad. Anteriorly the last region of the tube to close is known as the neuropore, while posteriorly at the primitive streak is the sinus rhomboidalis, where involution still continues to occur for a time. Almost as soon as an area of the neural tube becomes completely

closed, somites appear along it, the entire stage reaching completion in somewhat under 24 hr.

In following the development of the mesoblast with the scanning electron
microscope, it was found to be patterned from the time of its inception at the
primitive streak (Meier, 1979). Metameres appeared to develop as they tra-
versed Hensen's node, each of which consisted of two paraxial regions (the
somitomeres) and an enclosed axial region. In the endoblast lying beneath the
two rows of these tripartite structures was a series of similarly sized and arranged circular patches. At first each somitomere was a squat cylinder containing a slight cavity, but at neurulation all were first converted to triangular wedges
before they finally became condensed into cubes, as they began to form the
metameric somites. The formation of collagen fibers has proven to be vital to
somite formation, possibly by anchoring the cells and thereby providing tension

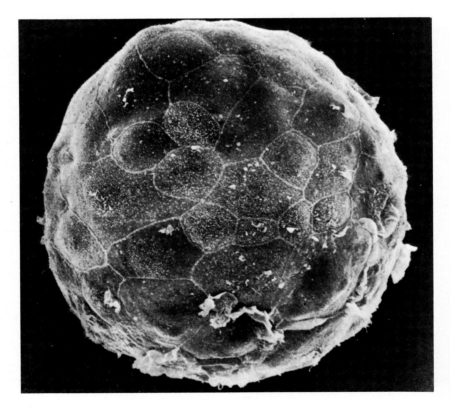

Figure 3.8. A mouse blastocyst in the preimplantation stage. This scanning electron micrograph is
of a specimen flushed from the uterus on the fourth day of pregnancy. The surface of the cells is
not bulged and microvilli are nearly absent. 1000×. (Courtesy of Sherman *et al.*, 1979.)

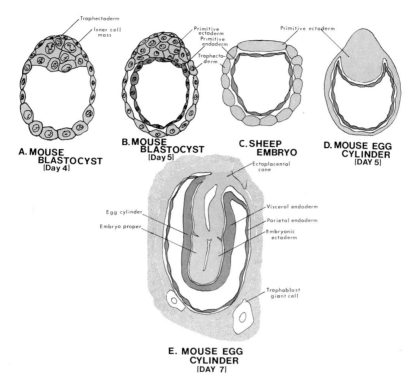

Figure 3.9. Postcleavage events in mammalian development. Implantation usually occurs at either of the stages represented by (C) and (D). (Based in part on Rossant and Papaioannou, 1977.)

(Bellairs, 1979; Bellairs and Veini, 1980), but fibronectin also plays an active role (Ehrismann *et al.*, 1981).

Further Embryonic Stages of Mammals. A number of traits unique to mammalian embryogenesis appear during the development of the morula into the next more advanced stage (Figure 3.9). First the blastomeres of the morula secrete a fluid that collects in the blastocoel. As this liquid accumulates, the cells are forced outward to the zona pellucida, where they form a single cell layer, the trophectoderm (formerly trophoblast) enclosing the blastocoel (Figure 3.9A). However, an undispersed mass of cells remains at the animal pole, known as the inner cell mass (earlier called the embryonic disk or epiblast) which is the main body of the embryo. The resulting hollow structure is referred to as the blastocyst (Figure 3.8) until after implantation, that is, through the gastrula. Beyond this blastula stage, development parallels that of the chick and reptiles in many of its features, despite the absence of yolk in most modern types (Rossant and Papaioannou, 1977). Usually the zona pellucida breaks down while a monolayered sheet of cells develops in all directions from either the center of the inner cell mass or the trophectoderm (Dalcq and Jones-Seaton, 1949; Mulnard, 1955). Growth of this hypoblast, or endoderm, continues until the cells form a sac, the archenteron or endocoel, reducing the blastocoel to a narrow cavity just under the trophectoderm (Figure 3.9B).

The end of the blastocyst stage is usually accompanied by implantation, after which either of two different courses of procedures may be followed, depending on the taxon. In the first of these, characteristic of most mammals, the inner cell mass does not undergo invagination, so that further development is as described in the following paragraph (Figure 3.9C). In the second alternative, found in a number of such advanced rodents as the mouse, rat, and guinea pig, the inner cell mass grows down into the embryo, compressing the archenteron and becoming covered over by the formation of a thick layer of extraembryonic ectoderm (Figure 3.9D; Selenka, 1884; Huber, 1915; Jolly and Férester-Tadié, 1936). This results in the so-called egg cylinder, at the very apex of which is the ectoplacental cone. Around the opposite end, the trophectoderm differentiates into trophoblast giant cells by endoreduplication of the DNA without cell division, as discussed later (Zybina, 1961, 1970; Hunt and Avery, 1971; Barlow and Sherman, 1972; Nagl, 1972). In addition, the primitive endoderm of the blastocyst increases in extent over the inner surface, while a layer of parietal, as well as one of visceral, endoderm eventually covers the entire egg cylinder.

In the majority of mammals, once the early gastrula has been completed as described in the preceding paragraph, its further development commences with the thickening of the inner cell mass into a "concrescence" or primitive streak (Daniel and Olson, 1966). Then as in the chick, involution of the embryonic disk (epiblast) possibly occurs along this line, resulting in the production of a flat sheet of cells toward each side and an anterior projection that develops into the notochord (Snow, 1977). A proliferation center around Hensen's node has been postulated to exist at this time, quite as in avian development (Daniel and Olson, 1966; Snow, 1977, 1978); further resemblance to the chick can be noted in the mesoderm layers forming double sheets except centrally to provide the forerunners of the coelomic cavity. Although earlier studies had indicated that the epiblast consisted of a homogeneous population of undifferentiated cells, all of which are pluripotential (Gardner and Papaioannou, 1975; Skreb et al., 1976), precise cell counts of division rates suggest that regionalization to some extent does exist (Snow, 1977).

Formation of the neurula also recalls that of the chick in most of its particulars. The portion of the embryonic disk overlying the notochord is modified into the neural plate, whose edges thicken, roll up, and grow toward the mid-dorsal line in typical fashion. Here, too, the neural tube is first closed near its center, further closure continuing thence in both directions, producing a neural pore anteriorly and a sinus rhomboidalis posteriorly, while somites appear as each given sector of tube is completed.

That more extensive ultrastructural investigations of developmental stages could be profitable is indicated by studies that have been conducted on a variety of mammalian embryonic sources, including blastocysts of rabbit, preimplantation embryos of the house mouse, and trophoblast of sheep (Davies and Wimsatt, 1966; Calarco and Brown, 1969; Hoffman and Olson, 1980). Light microscopic researches earlier had indicated crystalline inclusions to be present in the cells of these and others of a similar nature in various reproductive and glandular tissues (Figure 3.10). The bodies have now been shown to be bundles of microtubules, which conclusion reached by electron microscopic procedures was confirmed by electrophoretic analysis.

Another of the fine structural studies focused mainly on implanted egg cylinders of mice (Batten and Haar, 1979). In the pre- and definitive primitive-streak stages, the ectoderm surrounding the proamniotic cavity consisted of tall, pseudostratified columnar cells having large nuclei and prominent nucleoli, whereas the embryonic portion of the endoderm that surrounded it was squamous and more strongly basophilic, and the extraembryonic part highly columnar. In addition, the cells of the latter tissue had a prominent border of microvilli, between the bases of which were numerous micropinocytotic vesicles and vacuoles. Their nuclei were often deeply lobed and occasionally contained what appeared to be lipid droplets. Among the other ultrastructural features which could be noted were abundant rough endoreticulum and some swollen cristae in the mitochondria. In contrast, the ectoderm cells were largely free of cytoplasmic organelles but showed a few profiles of rough endoreticulum; the occasional mitochondria had mostly tubular cristae; and numerous free ribosomes were present. However, gap junctions appeared between cells as the primitive streak stage was entered. Following the advent of that stage, after the mesoderm first formed, its cells proved to be stellate and loosely connected to one another by means of filopodia. Although mitochondria were sparse, rough endoreticulum was not uncommon, and occasional dictyosomes were noted.

Implantation Events. Largely through use of tissue culture techniques, some of the changes in and requirements of the growing blastocyst are beginning to emerge. Up to the time of blastocyst formation (approximately the 64-cell stage), mouse embryos can be grown in any one of several simple media (Biggers *et al.*, 1971), but after emergence from the zona pellucida that encapsulates the early stages, a richer medium containing amino acids and serum is essential (Gwatkin, 1966; Hsu, 1973, 1980; Sherman, 1975). Further development to the trophoblast or egg cylinder stage then can proceed to the equivalent of the 7th, or even 8th day of pregnancy. Such cultured embryos have been shown to gain giant nuclei as already described for normally grown ones and to produce Δ-5,3-β-hydroxysteroid dehydrogenase and thus convert pregneno-

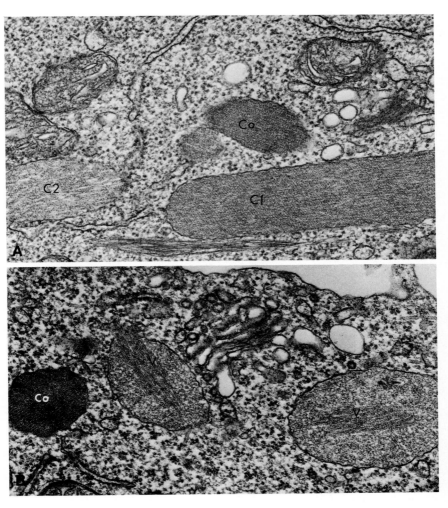

Figure 3.10. Trophoblast cells of the rabbit embryo. (A) In the cells of the blastocysts of many mammals, crystalline inclusions are present, consisting of arrays of microtubules as may be seen in the longitudinal section of a bundle (C1). A second bundle in oblique section (Co) and a loosely arranged one (C2) may also be noted. 42,000×. (B) Two vacuoles (V) containing tubular elements are present, in addition to the crystalline deposit (Co). 40,000×. (Both courtesy of Hoffman and Olson, 1980.)

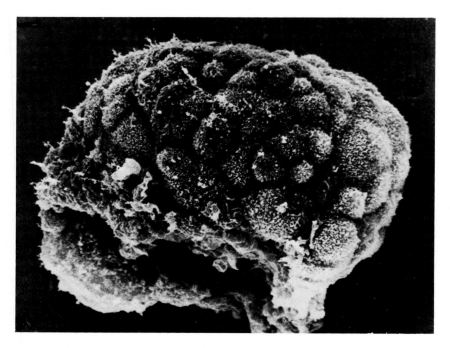

Figure 3.11. A mouse blastocyst at implantation. As the embryo approaches the implantation stage, the cell surfaces bulge outward and develop long microvilli. Compare with Figure 3.8. 1000×. (Courtesy of Sherman *et al.*, 1979.)

lone to progesterone (Rizzino and Sherman, 1979; Sellens and Sherman, 1980). In several studies on either cultured blastocysts or on those removed from uteri, transmission and scanning electron microscopy have made clear that the embryo undergoes a series of expansions and contractions at this time (Sherman and Wudl, 1976; Shalgi and Sherman, 1979; Sherman *et al.*, 1979). Before the embryo breaks out of the zona pellucida, the individual blastomeres bulge outwards on the surface and are densely covered with microvilli (Figure 3.11). Then, after liberation of the embryo from that membrane ready for adhesion to the uterine lining, the cells are flattened and separated from one another by low ridges, while only minute microvilli sparsely populate the surface. Still later, at the time of trophoblast outgrowth, the blastomeres bulge above the surface once more and become densely coated with microvilli that are longer than at the earlier stage.

Formerly a popular area of research (reviewed by De Feo, 1967, and Nalbandov, 1971), the possible involvement of histamines in implantation subsequently fell into disuse until the discovery that two kinds of receptors for those chemicals exist both in blastocysts and endometrial cells (Black *et al.*, 1972;

Dey *et al.*, 1979a). Accordingly a recent investigation explored their possible involvement by examining the histamine-synthesis capacities of rabbit blastocysts and endometrium (Dey *et al.*, 1979b). This was approached by means of measuring one of the enzymes involved in its synthesis, histidine decarboxylase. None of this enzyme was detected in endometrial extracts, whereas significant amounts occurred in 5- to 7-day blastocysts, especially in 6-day embryos. Furthermore, inhibitors of this enzyme interrupted implantation when injected intraluminally into the uterus on day 5.

3.2.3. Early Development in Other Organisms

It is beyond the purposes of the present work to review every type of early development that has been described. However, several organisms whose developing embryos diverge in habit from all the preceding are necessary, either because they have been subjected to much pertinent experimentation or because they contribute in other ways to the total picture of gene changes during embryogenesis.

Development of the Fruit Fly. In the majority of insects, including the fruit flies of the genus *Drosophila*, the developmental processes appear to resemble those of no other metazoan, but actually are a highly modified variety of the spiral type—a relationship particularly lucidly shown by the intermediate variations found in such crustaceans as *Lepas*. After fertilization has been fully consummated, the nucleus of the fly zygote undergoes division but during the early period is not accompanied by cytokinesis (Figure 3.12); hence, there are no cleavage stages (Sonnenblick, 1950; Bownes, 1975; Turner and Mahowald, 1976; Zalokar and Erk, 1976). During the first several nuclear divisions, the nuclei are confined to the anterior half of the zygote, the posterior portion remaining devoid of those bodies until the 4th division (Figure 3.12A, B; Parks, 1936). Furthermore, the products of nuclear divisions, which occur synchronously at mean intervals of 9 min at 25°C, remain central until after the 8th division (Figure 3.12C, D). At that time the majority move into the cortical cytoplasm, forming the "syncytial blastoderm," those that remain centrally being referred to as vitellophages. However, all have assumed a peripheral location by the 10th division cycle. With the 9th division, polar cells are developed posteriorly exposed on the surface. Later these are invaginated into the embryo, where about half of them become the primordial germ cells; the remainder have no other major fate as sometimes proposed but merely degenerate or are excreted (Mahowald *et al.*, 1979; Underwood *et al.*, 1980).

Approximately 6000 nuclei develop within 2½ hr after fertilization (Figure 3.12F); then during the following hour, a plasmalemma is formed around each nucleus, bringing the "cellular blastoderm" stage into existence (Figure 3.12G; Schubiger and Wood, 1977). This is soon followed by gastrulation and germband formation (Rickoll, 1976), during which cytoplasmic continuations be-

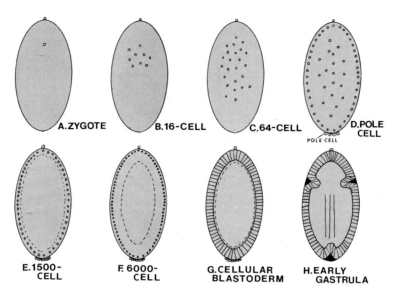

Figure 3.12. Major stages in the development of a fruit fly. (Based in part on Schubiger and Wood, 1977.)

tween the blastoderm and yolk sac persist. One of the peculiarities of higher insect embryogenesis is the formation during larval development of folded single-layered epithelial tissues, known as imaginal disks, which are precursors of various cuticular adult body parts (Bryant, 1979).

While the development of insects is generally considered to be deterministic and even mosaic as in other spiral-cleaving types, the degree of these qualities has not been fully established (Lawrence and Morata, 1979; Nüsslein-Volhard, 1979).

Evidence has been presented that cells of the imaginal regions in the cellular blastoderm are restricted in their potentialities, at least to broad anterior or posterior regions (Chan and Gehring, 1971). Furthermore, experimental injuries to the egg gave rise to larval or adult abnormalities that correlated with the induced defects (e.g., Bownes and Kalthoff, 1974); however, the extent, specificity, and mechanism of the determination are not understood. Nonetheless it is becoming clear that mosaic behavior becomes manifest only at the blastoderm stage (Kauffman, 1977; Schubiger and Wood, 1977).

Early Development in the Angiosperms. Development in angiosperms is represented by a diversity of types, only two of which merit close attention here (Jensen, 1963). The first variant is represented by the common carrot (*Daucus carota*), a species which has served as the subject for much experimental embryogenic research. Although the triploid nucleus resulting from

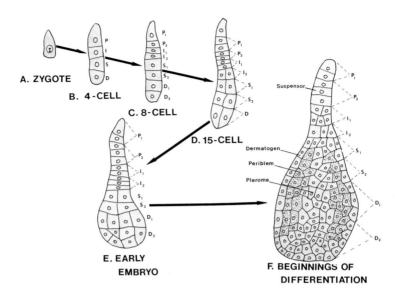

Figure 3.13. Early embryogeny of the carrot. (After Borthwick, 1931.)

the union of the two polar cells and one sperm nucleus undergoes concurrent development to form the endosperm (McClintock, 1978), only the events in the zygote proper are focused upon in the following discussion (Figure 3.13). In the carrot the first two cleavages are transverse, resulting in a linearly arranged series of four cells designated D, S, I, and P from distal to proximal end (Figure 3.13A, B; Borthwick, 1931). The next set of cleavages, too, is transverse, so that the embryo at this time consists of a regular row of eight cells, which are denoted as D_1 and D_2, S_1 and S_2, I_1 and I_2, P_1 and P_2. While the latter four cells then each undergo an additional transverse division, the first four divide vertically (Figure 3.13C, D). Further cleavages are irregular, but the embryo proper is produced entirely from the products of D and S, whereas the suspensor results from the cell progeny of I and P. The cells of the embryo in the strict sense continue to replicate, first forming the "globular embryo," the outer layer of which becomes the epidermis (Figure 3.13E, F).

After the globular embryo has developed to a point where it contains perhaps 1000 cells, it elongates by continuing divisions into the early "heart-shaped" stage and the suspensor is lost. Within the later heart-shaped embryo, lobes are produced laterally on the distal end, accentuating the cordiform configuration; these two lobes are precursors of the cotyledons that characterize this group of plants. At the same time the cells of the interior are undergoing differentiation into a procambial cylinder. Later the body of the embryo elongates still more strongly, acquiring a torpedo shape, while the cells of the procambial cylinder become differentiated to a greater degree, further steps in which processes are examined in a later chapter.

In embryoids derived from cultured tissues of the carrot, only two of the four early types of cells are considered to develop from the somatic parent, namely D and P (Street, 1976). Even as early as the second cleavage, D may undergo vertical division and P often does so with the third one. A globular mass therefore soon is produced, but the products of the latter typically result only in a short suspensor, leaving D as the progenitor of the embryo proper. This and similar experiments on cultured cells have demonstrated that many cells of mature plants are totipotent and can therefore give rise to normal embryoid offspring under the conditions of cell culture.

Early Embryogeny of Maize. A number of correspondences can be noted in the development of the maize zygote (Figure 3.14) and that of the cultured somatic embryoid of the carrot just described. However, the first division is highly unequal, the distal cell (D) being only a fourth or less the dimensions of the proximal (P). Typically P undergoes a second transverse division, followed by a few vertical ones, ultimately forming a short suspensor that is lost late in embryogeny (Randolph, 1936). In the second cleavage of D, however, division is usually vertical; the two products of this cell have been shown by radiation-induced genetic markers to indicate the left and right halves of the resulting plant, dividing each leaf along the middle of the midrib and continuing up through the midline of the tassel (Steffenson, 1968). Since these are the first two cells of the embryo proper, what these experiments clearly demonstrate is that there is no regional movement of cells such as characterizes animal embryogenesis, the only migrations being those produced obliquely, vertically, or horizontally by the regularity of the cleavages. No globular or heart-shaped stages are attained during the development of this monocotyledon-

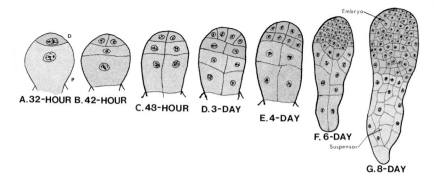

Figure 3.14. Early embryogeny in maize. Note that the figures are inverted relative to those of Figure 3.13. (Based in part on Randolph, 1936.)

ous species such as mark the dicotyledonous ones. As shown in a discussion on differentiation (Chapter 5, Section 5.3), the anlage for the plumule is laid down much later in embryogenesis, when the other embryonic parts become distinguishable.

3.3. MOLECULAR ASPECTS OF LATER DEVELOPMENT

In older stages of embryogenesis, which are larger or more readily collected in sufficient quantities or grown under controlled conditions, the molecular aspects have received more detailed attention than in earlier, less accessible stages. Ultrastructural studies along comparative lines seem to be in less than desired numbers, whereas molecular ones are somewhat more abundant but never providing a plethora of material for synthetic studies. Here the molecules, rather than the type of organism, provide the organization centers for discussion.

3.3.1. Changes in the Nucleic Acids

DNA and Chromatin Changes. Although a relatively small number of observations of changes in DNA and chromatin during the later embryonic periods have been reported, several are of special note. Among those that investigate plant materials is a group concerned with suspensor cells, the brief life history of which includes three stages: (1) A proliferation stage, in which these cells multiply by ordinary diploid mitosis in company with the rest of the proembryo; (2) a differential stage, during which the number of cells in the suspensor remains constant while the genomes undergo endoreduplication, accompanied by mitotic cell division in the embryo proper; and (3) a functional stage, during which the suspensor tissue carries out its several roles (Nagl, 1970). In *Phaseolus coccineus* this structure has attained its definitive cell number and size by the globular stage of the embryo, after which it undergoes differentiation into two regions. Of these are knoblike micropylar portion contains about 20 giant cells, whose chromosomes have undergone nine endoreduplications; thus, the DNA of each consists of nearly 8200 chromosome equivalents (Brady, 1973). Replication, however, is not uniform in each of the polytene chromosomes, for many segments have been described as experiencing disproportional DNA synthesis, or DNA amplification (Cremonini and Cionini, 1977). Moreover, in other plants, including members of the genus *Tropaeolum*, certain heterochromatin regions have been found to be underreplicated (Nagl *et al.*, 1976). More recently in a study of two nucleolar organizer chromosomes (S_1 and S_2) in the red bean, no correlation in extent of either amplification or underreplication of even adjacent bands could be detected (Forino *et al.*, 1979). In other words, each region is replicated independently of the others.

The genomes of the giant trophoblast cells of certain rodent embryos undergo similar endoreplication, one of the few instances in mammalian cells in which this phenomenon is known to occur (Kalf *et al.*, 1980). Consequently, each nucleus contains many times the haploid amount of DNA (Zybina, 1961, 1963; Barlow and Sherman, 1972). These giant cells may be considered to be in permanent interphase, with one S phase following another, thus leading to polyploidy and greatly enlarged nuclei (Pearson, 1974). In a recent investigation of the problem, giant nuclei of rat trophoblast cells were isolated and cultured for periods of 2 hr or more while the processes of incorporating tritiated dTTP into the DNA were observed. The system proved to be highly dependent on the presence of ATP, Mg^{2+}, and the four deoxyribonucleoside triphosphates and was stimulated by addition of monovalent cations, such as K^+ (Kalf *et al.*, 1980). Although DNA polymerases α, β, and γ were present, use of selective inhibitors demonstrated that the replication of the genome was carried out largely, if not exclusively, by the last of these types.

X-Chromosome Expression Changes. It is well known that only a single X chromosome is functional in the somatic cells of man and other mammals (see Lyon, 1972, for a review). This inactivation of one such sex chromosome in females takes place during embryogenesis, but its precise point of occurrence is still controversial. However, since some cells of heterozygotes express the maternal allele, while others the paternal one, the resulting mosaicism has provided a means for analyzing certain of the events during development (Migeon, 1978). One set of alleles that has proven especially valuable is that which specifies two known varieties of glucose-6-phosphate dehydrogenase, A and B, which differ in electrophoretic mobility and therefore are readily identified. Through their use it has been established that each clonal population derived from skin cells of heterozygous individuals express only a single variety of the enzyme, indicating not only that one X chromosome alone was active, but also that all the descendants of the single original cell had the corresponding one functional (Davidson *et al.*, 1963). In hybrid fused cells, such as mouse + human, it has been revealed that two X chromosomes could function in the same cell and that the presence of one such chromosome neither inactivates an active mate nor activates an inactive one (Migeon, 1972; Migeon *et al.*, 1974). Moreover, the functional state of either one remains unaltered by use of such chemicals as various hormones, polyanions, dimethylsulfoxide, and bromodeoxyuridine, and even simian virus 40 (Romeo and Migeon, 1975).

The mouse embryo has been a favored subject for investigations into developmental aspects. Employment of X/X and X/O mouse embryos permitted the observation of evidence for dosage compensation in the X-linked gene for phosphoglyceric acid kinase (Kozak and Quinn, 1975). During the preimplantation stages of development X/X individuals exhibited a much higher level of synthesis of the enzyme than did the X/O counterparts, producing it at a rate of 2.55–2.71 nM/hr per embryo during the first 48 hr compared to 1.4 nM/hr per embryo in X/O specimens. Then by 72 hr the rate in the first type dropped to 1.44 nM/hr per embryo, while that of the latter decreased to 0.9 nM. However, the differences between the two disappeared by the egg cylinder stage (150 hr), increasing to 193 nM for X/X and 183 nM for X/O embryos. Although the latter results were interpreted in terms of gene compensation, they could equally signify the inactivation of the second X chromosome in X/X examples, thereby eliminating the dosage differences that existed in earlier stages.

Changes in staining properties of one X chromosome have been followed during development, using quinacrine mustard fluorescence and acetic saline Giemsa techniques (Takagi, 1974). Whereas during early cleavage both X chromosomes showed the same banding pattern as that from adult male fibroblasts, around the 50-cell stage, one began to stain uniformly throughout its entire length. At the same time a gradual change in replicatory behavior became manifest, the uniform-staining one finishing replication after the other; this slow change was only completed by the ninth day of gestation, when the adult condition was totally acquired. Of even greater interest is the discovery that it is the maternal X chromosome that remains active in a number of instances. Such nonrandom expression of the maternal sex chromosome has been described in yolk sac and chorion of the mouse and yolk sac of the rat (Takagi and Sasaki, 1975; Wake et al., 1976; Takagi et al., 1978). More recently, studies employing the phosphoglyceric acid kinase variants discussed earlier have shown that this nonrandom suppression of the paternal chromosome can be noted as early as in the trophoblast stage of heterozygous female embryos (Frels and Chapman, 1980).

tRNA and rRNA Changes in Later Embryos. In addition to those already detailed as occurring in cleavage stages, changes in tRNAs have also been recorded in the mesenchyme blastula of *S. purpuratus* (Zeikus et al., 1969). The differences that were found were largely of a quantitative nature; for example, the embryonic leucine $tRNA_1$ was about equal in relative quantities to that of the egg, whereas leucine $tRNA_2$ was almost absent in the former and nearly as abundant as the first type in the latter. More striking results were obtained with lysine $tRNA_1$, the egg showing only types I and III and the blastula having a large proportion of type II in addition to the other two. Although in earlier reports it had been believed that tRNAs were not synthesized by sea urchin embryos until this stage of development (Glišin and Glišin, 1964; Gross et al., 1965; O'Melia, 1979a), more sensitive fractionation procedures permitted the demonstration of newly produced tRNA and 5 S RNA during cleavage (O'Melia and Villee, 1972; O'Melia, 1979b). Synthesis of tRNAs also has been shown to occur in early cleavage in the rabbit (Manes, 1971; Schultz et al., 1973), but qualitative changes have so far been found only in blastocyst and later stages (Clandinin and Schultz, 1975). The only major distinction detected, however, was that the tRNAs from preimplantation embryos were distinctly deficient in methylated nucleoside residues relative to those of later stages.

An associated activity is also of interest at this point. An enzyme known as tRNA nucleotidyltransferase catalyzes the incorporation of AMP and CMP from the corresponding triphosphates into the 3′ termini of tRNAs, but the precise function of this activity *in vivo* remains obscure. Nevertheless, activity of this enzyme was demonstrated to increase markedly following fertilization in *X. laevis* to reach a maximum level at gastrulation, after which it underwent a dramatic decrease (Paradiso and Schofield, 1976). No stage-specific inhibitors of this enzyme could be detected. Since the enzyme therefore seemed to be of special importance during early development, it was suggested that it may play other roles than maturation of precursor tRNA.

A group of three enzymes important in the synthesis of RNA in general also have been investigated in the same organism. This triplet of RNA polymerases, designated by Roman numerals, is engaged in the transcription of the several classes of RNA, polymerase I being active in the production of rRNA, II in hnRNA, and III in 4 S and 5 S RNA. Each species is maternally produced during oogenesis, the levels remaining constant after fertilization through the blastula stage but increasing gradually thereafter (Roeder, 1974). However, total synthesis declined during embryogeny, and extents of activities during the various stages underwent marked changes (Thomas *et al.*, 1980). Although it constituted the major portion of free RNA polymerase present in the blastula, virtually no polymerase I was found to be bound to the DNA, but with further development it slowly gained the leading role in transcription until it represented 90% of the transcriptive-active protein in young tadpoles. Both free and bound molecules of species I were shown to be localized in the nucleoli, as expected if it synthesizes rRNAs. Much of the decline in RNA synthesis resulted from changes in the activity of the other two polymerases. For example, polymerase II represented 75% of the total transcription in the blastula but decreased greatly thereafter.

Because the rate of production of rRNA is so slight compared to the synthesis of other types, it has become possible only recently to establish firmly that this class of nucleic acid was produced to some extent (Surrey *et al.*, 1979). Results varied with the species of sea urchin tested. In *S. purpuatus* the rate was identical in blastula and late gastrulae, at 40 copies of nuclear precursorial rRNA molecules/min per cell, whereas in *L. pictus* blastulae 16 copies and in gastrulae 23 copies of the transcript were made per minute per cell. Hence, contrary to a belief that prevailed in some quarters, ribosomal genes are not quiescent prior to gastrulation, nor is their activation a necessary concomitance to the formation of the gastrula. However, at that time there may be an enhancement of the rate of processing the transcripts to produce the definitive rRNAs.

The precursors to various types of RNAs being thus known to be synthesized and processed in the nucleus (Darnell, 1968), it has been thought that perhaps protein synthesis might be regulated by way of transport of the various transcripts through the nuclear envelope into the cytoplasm (Singh, 1968; Ho-

gan and Gross, 1971; Shiokawa and Pogo, 1974; Duncan *et al.*, 1975; Shiokawa *et al.*, 1977). In the last report cited, it was made clear that tRNA,
mRNA, and 18 S rRNA were transported to the cytoplasm in *Xenopus* neurulae
prior to 28 S rRNA. The tRNA fraction followed a complex curve of abundance, suggesting that it was turned over rapidly after leaving the nucleus
(Abelson *et al.*, 1974). More recently, it has been ascertained in the clawed
toad that 5 S rRNA had a history similar to that of the 28 S variety, being
delayed for transport to the cytoplasm concomitantly with the latter (Shiokawa
et al., 1979). A reason for the transport of 18 S rRNA preceding the large
variety could not be ascertained, but similar results had been reported earlier
for mouse and chick fibroblasts (Horiuchi *et al.*, 1972; Johnson *et al.*, 1976).
One explanation that has been offered is that the processing time is more prolonged for 28 S rRNA (Darnell, 1968; Edström and Lönn, 1976), but this
would certainly not apply to the 5 S species.

Under unfavorable environmental conditions, *Artemia* (brine shrimp) embryos develop into gastrulae and then encyst and remain dormant until favorable conditions are restored. Upon the resumption of development, RNA synthesis increased rapidly at first but declined to 80 or 90% of the early levels during
the nauplius stage (Bagshaw *et al.*, 1980). Concurrently with those changes,
comparable increases and decreases were observed also in the nuclear RNA
polymerases. Although RNA polymerase II was synthesized during all stages,
it declined strongly in the nauplius to resume again before metamorphosis.

Some years ago treatment of 16-cell-stage sea urchin embryos by the
Giemsa technique had shown that the staining abilities of the micromeres fluctuated during the cell cycle (Agrell, 1958), while those of the meso- and
macromeres remained constant. These results, interpreted as reflecting changes
in RNA content, were later confirmed through use of azure B (Cowden and
Lehman, 1963). More recently microphotemetric measurements of the specific
staining properties have been made, which also largely confirmed the earlier
results (Dan *et al.*, 1979). It was shown that the micromeres stained more
deeply than the others, not only during interphase, but throughout the cycle,
albeit to a lesser degree during mitosis. Further, it was demonstrated that the
micromeres contained the same density of ribosomes as the yolk-free areas of
the other types of blastomeres but differed in lacking the yolk-rich cytoplasmic
areas. Hence, there was greater apparent dilution of the staining in large than
in small cells. The ultrastructural aspects of this later study also revealed that
the ribosome-rich area surrounded the nucleus in all cells; these perinuclear
cores were also the location of the bulk of the endorecticulum and mitochondria
but were free of yolk granules.

mRNA Changes following Cleavage. As in earlier stages, the dramatic increase in protein synthesis that follows fertilization has attracted the
lion's share of investigations in the postcleavage embryo at the molecular level.
It is of interest to note that the encysted gastrulae of *Artemia* resemble the early

stages of embryos and unfertilized eggs in containing a large store of poly(A)$^+$ mRNA, mostly present in the form of RNP particles (Felicetti *et al.*, 1975). These ranged in size from 4 S to 80 S and were efficiently translated in a wheat germ system into proteins having molecular weights from 8000 to 40,000. However, in the encysted embryos polysomes were nearly absent but increased in number greatly within 1 to 4 hr after development had been resumed (Amaldi *et al.*, 1977).

The diversity of the mRNA in oocytes of *Drosophila* (Goldstein and Arthur, 1979), previously reported to be in the range of 15,000 different sequences (Chapter 1, Section 1.2.2), has been followed into the gastrula (3½ hr) and late embryo (17½ hr) stages (Arthur *et al.*, 1979). In the gastrula 2.5%, and in the late embryo 5.3%, of these had disappeared, and 7.7% of the sequences found in the gastrula and an additional 4% present in the late stages were not detected in the oocyte sequences. However, the rate of poly(A)$^+$ RNA production was very high, accounting for 14% of the total present at the end of the blastoderm stage (Anderson and Lengyel, 1981). Thus, while new mRNAs are produced during the gastrula and later, the majority that occur in the oocyte are retained throughout embryogenesis. Contrasting results have been obtained with the oocyte mRNA of midges of the genus *Smittia* (Jäckle, 1979), in which insects the maternal poly(A)$^+$ mRNA was rapidly degraded after formation of the blastoderm.

In sea urchins, it has been found that the amount of poly(A) attached to mRNA doubles after fertilization and, more importantly, that this increase results predominantly from polyadenylation occurring in the cytoplasm (Slater *et al.*, 1972, 1973; Wilt, 1973; Dolecki *et al.*, 1977); in adult mammalian cells this activity, it will be recalled, is largely a nuclear function (Jelinek *et al.*, 1973; Lewin, 1975a,b; Brandhorst, 1976). Unlike the condition first reported for dipterans, the mRNAs of mesenchyme blastulae and gastrulae in these echinoderms are newly synthesized, not maternally derived (Galau *et al.*, 1977); nevertheless, the poly(A) segments were demonstrated to have been added within the nucleus, with little further elongation occurring later in the cytoplasm (Brandhorst and Bannet, 1978). These observations are correlated to those made earlier, that, while the total synthesis of hnRNA plus mRNA increases 2-fold between cleavage and the pluteal stages, the rate per nucleus actually decreases severely (Kojima and Wilt, 1969; Emerson and Humphreys, 1970). In addition, it has been shown that the amount of hnRNA decreases to one-half or one-third from cleavage to the gastrula and that a further reduction occurs at the pluteus stage; concurrently, persistent mRNAs decrease 20-fold at the gastrula stage, but no additional reduction occurs later (McColl and Aronson, 1978). A contrasting condition appears to prevail in mammalian embryos, however, for in the mouse the amount of poly(A) in the egg (1.9 pg) decreased to 1.0 pg in the fertilized egg and to 0.68 pg in the two-cell embryo before increasing to 3.8 pg in the blastocyst (Levey *et al.*, 1978).

Two classes of mRNAs have been recognized in pregastrula embryos, which were similar in all properties except in the presence or absence of the poly(A) segment, 90% falling into the poly (A)$^-$ category (Nemer et al., 1974; Dworkin and Infante, 1976). The presence or absence of the poly(A) appeared to have no relation to the type of proteins that were encoded, for both poly(A)$^+$ and poly(A)$^-$ mRNAs coded for the same abundant proteins in blastulae (Brandhorst et al., 1979). However, this is in conflict with other reports that show a lack of sequence homology and translational properties between the two types in vivo (Milcarek et al., 1974; Nemer et al., 1974; Fromson and Verma, 1976; Surrey and Nemer, 1976). Use of anucleolar mutants of X. laevis, which do not produce 18 S and 28 S rRNAs, facilitated the study of poly (A)$^\pm$ mRNA in this amphibian (Miller, 1978), the maternal supply of ribosomes sufficing to the swimming tadpole stage (Wallace, 1960). It was thus found that about 80% of the mRNA either lacked poly(A) segments entirely or had segments too short to bind to oligo(dT).

A small number of investigations have been concerned with aspects of the mRNA other than the extent of polyadenylation and have examined the heterogeneous nuclear population as well as the cytoplasmic. In the neurula and subsequent larval stages, the nuclear RNA hybridized to extents of 11.3 and 12.1%, respectively, to single-copy DNA, and mixtures of the nuclear and cytoplasmic fractions hybridized to a nearly equal extent, indicating a large amount of sequence homology (Shepherd and Flickinger, 1979). The results also intimated that some mRNA sequences which occurred on polysomes of neurulae were not found there in larvae but were present in the nuclei. The converse of this was also true, for mRNAs found on larval polysomes occurred in the nuclei of neurulae, even though they were absent from the polysomes of that stage. With normal blastulae of this clawed toad, poly(A)$^+$ mRNA was found to be synthesized at a higher rate on a per cell basis than in later stages, one-third of the amount produced being transported rapidly into the cytoplasm (Shiokawa et al., 1979). Synthesis of small nuclear RNAs was initiated also at the blastula stage.

In a current report, the changes in steady-state populations of poly(A)$^+$ mRNAs were followed from oogenesis to organogenesis in developing Xenopus embryos (Sagata et al., 1980). The total poly(A) content was described as decreasing from 1.8 ng/oocyte to 1.0 ng/matured egg; following fertilization, it then increased to 1.7 ng/embryo at the blastula stage. This was followed by a further steady increment, so that by the heartbeat stage a level of 6 ng/embryo was attained. The size classes of poly(A) present were also determined. Only two types were detected in oocytes, having mean lengths of 60 and 20 nucleotides, respectively, whereas eggs and all embryonic stages contained three, with mean lengths of 100, 80, and 20 nucleotides. While the largest class occurred equally in the nucleus and cytoplasm, poly(A)$_{80}$ was found mainly in the nucleus, and poly(A)$_{20}$ exclusively in the cytosol. Much of the postgastrula increase resulted from the poly$(A)_{100}$, the proportional quantity of which became much greater after that stage. It was concluded that these results indicated: (a) a possible deadenylation of a population of maternal poly$(A)^+$ mRNA during maturation of the oocyte; (b) followed after fertilization by polyadenylation of an mRNA population, perhaps that previously deadenylated; (c) possible destruction of maternal mRNA during gastrulation; and (d) the existence of predominantly newly synthesized mRNA after the neurula stage.

Certain recent discoveries of RNA structure do not seem to have attracted the attention they deserve. At first it appeared that oligomeric segments of adenylic and uridylic acids were properties confined to hnRNAs, especially those of embryos (Molloy et al., 1972; Nakazato et al., 1973; Dubroff and Nemer, 1975; Dubroff, 1977). On the basis of various combinations of these segments, three different categories containing five species were described (Dubroff and Nemer, 1976). In the α class, segments of 25 nucleotides and others of 12 nucleotides of adenylic acid [oligo$(A)_{25}$ and oligo$(A)_{12}$] were present but no poly(A); it included two species, $\alpha_U$hnRNA which also contained oligo(U)-enriched regions and $\alpha_N$hnRNA which did not. The β class had no oligo$(A)_{25}$ but contained a poly$(A)_{175}$ segment and a region of oligo$(A)_{12}$; β_U also included oligo(U)-enriched stretches, whereas β_N did not. The γ class lacked the poly$(A)_{175}$, oligo(U), and oligo$(A)_{25}$ segments but had the oligo$(A)_{12}$ sections in common with the others. During development of the sea urchin early blastula to the mesenchyme blastula, the proportion of the β class of hnRNA, as well as of poly$(A)^+$ mRNA increased greatly. In contrast, the proportion of the persistently most abundant γ class reached a peak at the early blastula, when DNA and histone syntheses also were at a maximum, while the α class reached its peak at midblastula. More recently, however, the oligo(U) sequences have been found to be conserved to some extent in cytoplasmic mRNAs, whereas few, if any, oligo(A) segments are (Dubroff, 1980). In a subsequent discussion, it is brought out that some of the oligo(U)-bearing types are considered to be "transcriptional control RNAs," that function in selective protein synthesis.

By use of the electron microscope to observe the stage-specific patterns of transcription in sea urchin embryos (Busby and Bakken, 1979), several new features of nuclear RNA production have been revealed. Of the active regions of chromatin visualized in Strongylocentrotus gastrulae, the great majority (82%) was represented by only a single fibril, whereas 18% contained multiple fibril arrays of these transcriptional units, the highest number noted being 14 in one instance. Nucleosomes were detected on actively transcribed regions as well as on inactive, a density between 24 and 27 per nanometer of chromatin being found in both types of fibers (Figure 3.15). All the ribonucleoprotein being synthesized was considered to be nonribosomal in nature, ribosomal genes being rarely active in these gastrulae. A subsequent study revealed that transcript lengths were similar in gastrula- and prism-stage embryos but were distinctly

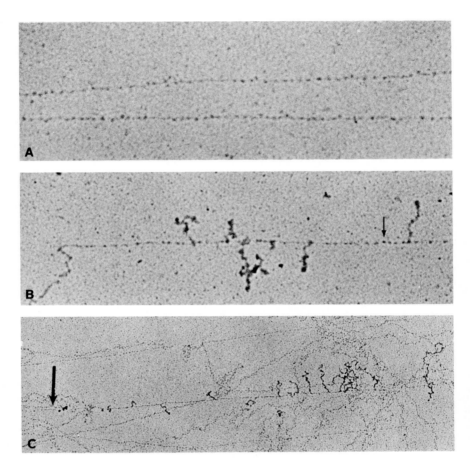

Figure 3.15. Sea urchin chromatin strands. Nucleosomes (arrow) may be noted both on the nontranscribed (A) and on the transcribed strand (B), the latter bearing a number of fibrils of ribonucleoproteins. Thus, transcription does not involve removal of the nucleosomes. Both 66,000×. (C) That transcription of a chromatin strand was initiated near the point indicated (arrow) is suggested by the increasing lengths of the transcripts with distance from it. 22,000×. (All courtesy of Busby and Bakken, 1979.)

shorter during cleavage (Busby and Bakken, 1980). In addition, the cleavage-stage chromatin contained a class of short, repeated RNP fibrils not found elsewhere.

3.3.2. Changing Patterns of Protein Production

Protein Synthesis and Related Changes. Rates of protein synthesis relative to those of unfertilized eggs and possible controls have been popular subjects for researches on older embryos, too. In one study with sea urchins in which labeled leucyl-tRNA was employed, the rate of incorporation in gastrulae was observed to be more than 100 times as high as in unfertilized eggs (Regier and Kafatos, 1977), with very little difference between the early cleavage, blastula, and gastrula stages. As far as control of synthesis is concerned, neither the methylation of tRNAs in rabbits (Clandinin and Schultz, 1975) nor the protein content of ribosomes in *Bufo* (Senatori *et al.*, 1979) appeared to be significant. However, in cell-free systems, ribosomes from eggs were always less active than those from blastulae (Danilchik and Hille, 1981).

It should be noted, however, that only quantitative aspects of the ribosomal proteins were considered in the Senatori report, for some, although unknown, ribosomal factor appears to be involved, according to researches on *Artemia* embryos. One investigation employed high-salt-washed ribosomes from both encysted and advanced embryos in various combinations with cytosol from the same two contrasting sources (Sierra *et al.*, 1974). Endogenous protein synthesis was observed only with ribosomes from the advanced embryos, regardless of the nature of the cytosol, but since the activity was suppressed with the elongation inhibitor, edeine, the translation of mRNAs in this system was deduced to involve only elongation of previously initiated chains. In addition, cytosol from developed eggs was found to be essential in translating mRNA from brome mosaic virus or rabbit globin mRNA, whereas the source of the ribosome exercised no influence. Hence, the cytosol appeared to contain an essential initiation factor, and the cysts seemed to lack mRNA. Similar rate-limiting influence by initiation factors has been demonstrated also in echinoderms (Hille *et al.*, 1981).

Qualitative changes in protein synthesis have attracted several investigations, autoradiographs of polyacrylamide slab gels showing large differences between cleavage and blastocyst rabbit embryos (Van Blerkom and Manes, 1977). In midges of the genus *Smittia*, for instance, mRNAs of the embryo were found to replace those from internal sources during the blastoderm stages, and several new proteins appeared that were not detected prior to blastoderm formation (Jäckle, 1979; Jäckle and Kalthoff, 1979). In addition, patterns of protein synthesis during the early developmental stages of *Xenopus* were analyzed by two-dimensional gel electrophoresis (Figure 3.16; Ballantine *et al.*, 1979). Through the termination of the blastula stage, no newly synthesized protein was revealed that had not been present also in the oocyte, but during gastrulation several new species appeared, and even more were added during neurulation (Figure 3.17). Similar results have also been obtained by other techniques (Bravo and Knowland, 1979; Woodland and Ballantine, 1981).

In greater detail, early oocytes were reported to produce a larger number of proteins than those that had been induced to mature by progesterone, and unfertilized ova made fewer than the latter. However, some were present before fertilization that were also in the unmatured oocyte but not in the matured. Two of the identifiable ones that were entirely or virtually missing from the

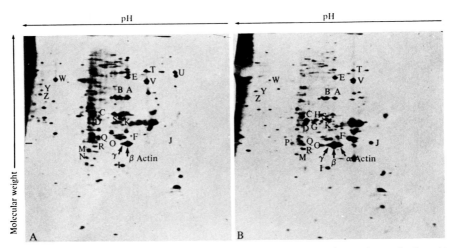

Figure 3.16. Protein profile changes during development. The numerous changes in proteins brought about during development of *Xenopus* are made clear by these autofluorographs of two-dimensional gel separations from oocytes before maturation (A) and tail-bud tadpoles (B). The absence of α-actin in the former and its appearance in the latter are especially noteworthy events. (Courtesy of Ballantine *et al.*, 1979.)

egg but occurred in both types of oocytes were γ- and β-actin; similarly α-actin did not appear in oocytes or embryos until the gastrula stage was attained (Sturgess *et al.*, 1980). Several experiments were also run in which each embryo was sectioned into two or more parts before isotopic labeling and analysis. In this way the proteinogenic processes of the ectodermal–somitic mesodermal portion were compared to the endodermal splanchnopleural. Although the contrasting parts largely synthesized identical proteins, α-actin was found only in the ectodermal portion, along with such others as that denoted as protein D. When neurulae were treated in like fashion, the ectodermal section produced a number of proteins that were absent from the endodermal, the converse being equally true. However, α-actin was present only in small quantities in the endodermal sections.

The changes that occur in the synthesis of the protein known as acid phosphatase-1 have been followed during embryogeny in *D. melanogaster* (Yasbin *et al.*, 1978). In the first place it was demonstrated by use of mutant forms that the enzyme during the embryonic stages was strictly of maternal origin, having been synthesized during oogenesis. Moreover, the maternal enzyme persisted until the third larval instar. At fertilization several isozymes were detected, but all except one of these disappeared during the early stages of development. Secondly, through employment of ultrastructural histochemistry, a related investigation disclosed a much earlier time for expression of paternal genes than had previously been proposed (Sawicki and MacIntyre, 1978). Eggs from females that lacked the gene for acid phosphatase-1 were crossed with males

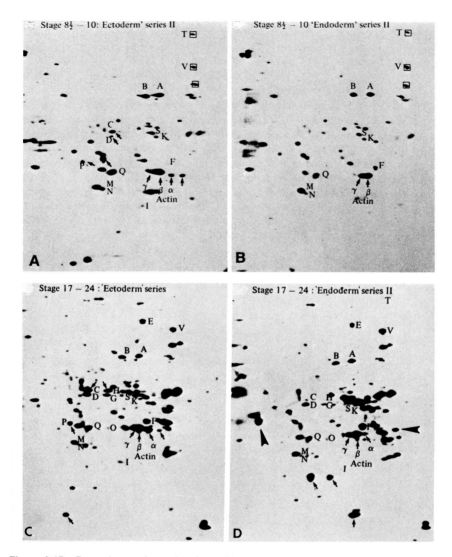

Figure 3.17. Comparisons of proteins from different regions of *Xenopus* embryos. (A, B) Autofluorographs of two-dimensional gel separations of the ectodermal (A) and endodermal (B) portions of the same late blastulae. The absence of α-actinin in the latter portion is especially noteworthy, but many other differences may be observed. (C, D) Corresponding portions from later stages, on which arrowheads and small arrows indicate particularly prominent differences. (Courtesy of Ballantine *et al.*, 1979.)

possessing genomes heterozygous for various isozymes of the enzyme. No lead phosphate deposits were found in thin sections until the fifth hour postfertilization, that is, about the time of cellular blastoderm formation. Both in these embryos and in earlier ones from wild-type females, the enzymatic activity appeared to be associated with lysosomes, often in contact with the membranes enclosing α-yolk granules. Among mollusks, multiple species of acid phosphatases appear and disappear during development but are not sufficiently characterized to discuss in detail (Moon and Morrill, 1979).

A study of sea urchin development has been made to determine whether the synthesis of proteoglycan was implicated in the changeover from maternal mRNA usage in blastulae to embryonic mRNA in gastrulae. Inhibition of proteoglycan was accomplished with three different reagents used separately; one prevented coupling between the protein and polysaccharide moieties, another interferred with sulfation of the polysaccharide, and the third inhibited elongation of the polysaccharide chain (Kinoshita and Saiga, 1979). Regardless of the inhibitor or its time of application to cleavage embryos, development ceased at the blastula stage. Hence, this substance appears to be essential for development to the gastrula and more advanced stages, a conclusion that coincides thoroughly with observations made during late embryonic periods discussed in the next chapter.

Since microtubules and microfilaments are so abundant in cells of many types, including eggs and early embryos as already described, it is inevitable that these structures should play important roles in later development. Through use of colcemid, which inhibits microtubule formation, it was revealed that the presence of these structures is requisite for blastocoel formation in the mouse (Wiley and Eglitis, 1980). In untreated late morulae, the blastomeres contained numerous vesicles, at first scattered through the cytoplasm, which then became aligned beneath the surface on the sides in contact with other cells. These vesicles gradually diminished in number, apparently emptying their contents as they disappeared just before blastocoel formation (cavitation). In treated morulae, however, the vesicles neither aligned normally nor emptied their contents, cavitation failing to take place as a consequence. Since in theory, the antimicrotubule chemical should also have interferred with mitotic division, the cell number of treated blastocysts was compared to untreated, but the results surprisingly showed no difference. Hence, it was concluded that the microtubules participating in cavitation differed from those involved in mitosis or cytokinesis.

Histone Synthesis. As described earlier (Sections 3.1.2), the transcripts of histone genes from cleavage stages were in the range of 7 S to 12 S in size, but beginning with the mesenchyme blastula, high-molecular-weight transcripts were found (Kunkel *et al.*, 1978). Moreover, new H2A, H2B, and H1 subtypes appeared at this stage (Cohen *et al.*, 1975), encoded by different genes (Kunkel and Weinberg, 1978; Newrock *et al.*, 1978). As the histone 2A family has recently been reported to include at least eight different species, even greater heterogeneity may later prove to be present (West and Bonner, 1980).

Studies of histone changes in postcleavage embryos of sea urchins from two independent laboratories appeared in print nearly concurrently, each of which provided details of the patterns from differing standpoints but with sufficient overlap to add mutual corroboration (Brandt *et al.*, 1979; Childs *et al.*, 1979). In addition, those reports were in harmony with portions of earlier studies (Cohen *et al.*, 1975; Sures *et al.*, 1976, 1978; Grunstein and Grunstein, 1977; Newrock *et al.*, 1977; Grunstein, 1978). At least three species of sea urchins, representing the same number of genera, were employed in these investigations, *Parachinus angulosis*, *S. purpuratus*, and *L. pictus*, suggesting that the results are characteristic of sea urchins as a whole, and perhaps of other echinoderms and even chordates.

The study by Childs and his co-workers (1979) focused on the histone mRNAs by way of two approaches. By means of one of these the number of nucleoside residues contained in the various messengers was determined in "early" (blastulae, 8 hr) and "late" embryos (gastrulae, 42 to 48 hr), each of which proved to be at least 100 sites longer than actually needed to code for the protein. Moreover, the nucleic acid and all five classes of histones underwent a decided change from the early to late embryos. In both *S. purpuratus* and *L. pictus* the mRNA for H1 was of only one species in the early extracts, but two were present in the late, each about 35 nucleoside residues longer than before. This species of histone has been demonstrated clearly to stabilize the structure of nucleosomes, which are absent when it is extracted (Thoma *et al.*, 1979). Similarly, only one species was found in early embryos for each of the other classes of histones, except H4 (Figure 3.18); that was represented by two species, as was all of the gastrular material, with one exception—three types of H3 were determined to be present. The messengers for H1 were the only ones that were longer in the gastrula than in the blastula, all others being 30 to 60 nucleoside residues shorter.

In the second approach that was employed, autofluorograms or gel electrophoretic analyses were made of the histone mRNAs at the two stages. Autofluorograms of each of the five categories of histone mRNAs from the two contrasting age-classes of embryos arranged side-by-side showed marked mobility differences in all cases and in H2B and H3 also in numbers of bands present (Figure 3.19). Greater accuracy was obtained by first preparing labeled translation products of the blastula histone mRNAs in a wheat-germ cell-free system and then making comparisons with histones of late embryos. By these means four species of H2A and three of H2B were determined as being present in the blastula, and an additional species of the first type in the gastrula.

The investigation by Brandt and colleagues (1979) determined partial amino acid sequences of histone H2B from sea urchin sperm and two age groups of embryos and compared them to somatic histones from the adult and other sources

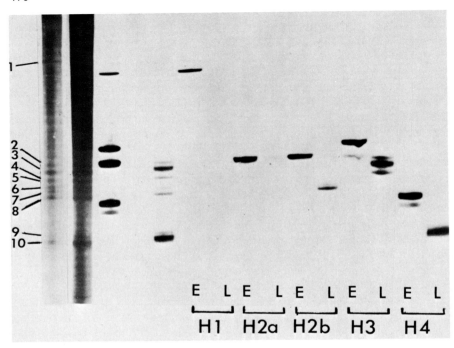

Figure 3.18. Changes in histone mRNAs during development of a sea urchin (*Strongylocentrotus purpuratus*). Autofluorograms of the various species of histone mRNAs of early (E) and late (L) embryos. The early stage is from 8-hr blastulae and the late from 42- to 48-hr gastrulae. (Courtesy of Childs *et al.*, 1979.)

(Table 3.2). Two of the three histone H2B species from the sperm agreed at most points but differed markedly from species 1, especially in the N-terminal segment; in that sector less than 50% homology was found to exist between species 1 and 2, whereas 2 and 3 showed 100% homology there (Figure 3.20). As indicated by the table, even more pronounced differences in this N terminus exist between sperm H2B and early blastula histones of the same type. Only 25% of the 15 sites that are shown correspond to one another; in addition, it is obvious that a 4-site segment of the sperm has been deleted from the embryonic protein. Too little has been determined in the terminal sequences to permit meaningful comparisons, but only 33% of the sites can be noted to be homologous between these early and late blastula histones. The sequences from adult somatic tissues of the mollusk and calf differ both from one another (about 25% homology) and from the embryonic types (33% homology), but each histone from adult sources resembles the embryonic species more closely than it does those from the sperm. Sperm species 1, being by far the most divergent in primary structure, probably represents the ancestral form of the protein.

Table 3.2
Partial Sequences of Histone H2B from Sea Urchin Developmental Stages

	N-Terminal region	Central region
Sperm[1]	PSQKSPTKRSPTKRS	MSVMNSFVNDVFERIAAEAGRLT
Sperm[2]	--PRSPAKTSPRKGSPR	MSVMNSFVNDVFERIAGEASRLT
Sperm[3]	--PRSPAKTSPRKGSPR	MSVMNSFVNDVFERIASEASRLT
Early blastula[1]	----APTGQVAKKGSKKAV	MSIMNSFVNDIFERIAGEASRLT
Early blastula[2]	----APTGQVAKKGSKKAV	MSIMNSFVNDVFERIAGEASRLT
Late blastula[1]	----APTGQVA	MSIMNSFVNDIF
Late blastula[2]	----PAKAQVAGA	MSVMNSFVNDVFE
Late blastula[3]	----AAKAQGAGA	MSIMNSFVNDVFE
Adult gut	a	MSLMNSFVNDVFERIAAEASRLT
Mollusk adult[b]	----PPKVSSKGA--KKAGKA	MSIMNSFVNDIFERIAAEASRLA
Calf thymus[c]	---PEPAKSAPAP--KKGSP	MBVMNSFVNDIFERIAGEASRLA

[a] N terminus is blocked.
[b] *Patella*: van Helden *et al*. (1979), on which sequence the numbering of the central sites is based.
[c] Iwai *et al*. (1972). All others from Brandt *et al*. (1979).

The histones of the unfertilized egg and zygote unfortunately were not examined in the foregoing study. However, results of electrophoretic analyses have indicated that the histones of the fertilized egg are identical to those before fertilization and that those of the sperm are never present in the embryo pattern (Carroll and Ozaki, 1979). Moreover, none of the embryonic types occur in the fertilized egg. In addition, it has been shown that in blastomeres which were isolated from early blastulae, changes from early to late histones were made at appropriate times, thus demonstrating that the changing expression of genes is strictly an intracellular function (Arceci and Gross, 1980). In *Strongylocentrotus*, the maternal and blastula histone H4 were identical or nearly so, but were replaced in later stages by a highly divergent form (Grunstein *et al.*, 1981).

Microtubules and Microfilaments. Because of their possible involvement in the shapes of individual cells, microtubules and microfilaments, including those of actin, have received attention in the postcleavage stages of embryogenesis as well as in the earlier ones (Merlino *et al.*, 1981). In the micromeres of the early blastula, the microtubules appear to diverge from points, called satellites, closely associated with the flagellar centriole, and then descend along

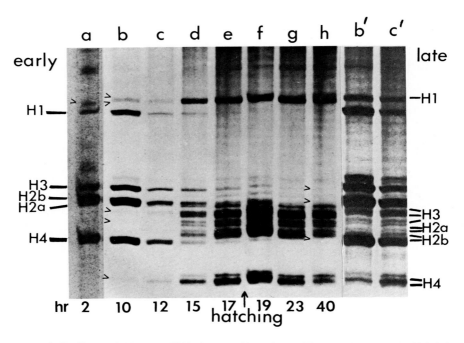

Figure 3.19. Changes in histone mRNAs in sea urchin embryos. These autofluorograms of labeled histone mRNAs in embryos of various ages have the species of early stages indicated on the left, those of late stages on the right. Lanes b' and c' are longer exposures of b and c, respectively. (Courtesy of Childs *et al.*, 1979.)

the sides. Later as these cells commence to migrate into the blastocoel to become the primary mesenchyme, they lose the cilia and become spherical (Gibbins *et al.*, 1969). However, the microtubules remain associated with a centriole, but whether that organelle was of the mitotic or flagellar type was not clear. After entering the blastocoel, the cells change shape once more, becoming amoeboid and bearing slender pseudopodia containing large numbers of microtubules. When these cells join their pseudopodia to fuse into those "cables" believed to be involved in archenteron extension, the microtubules become arranged parallel to the long axis of the cable, and no longer are associated with centrioles.

Although the present consensus holds that a preformed pool of tubulin prevails at a constant level from oogenesis through development in vertebrates and invertebrates alike (Burnside *et al.*, 1973; Raff and Kaumeyer, 1973; Green *et al.*, 1975; Raff, 1975, 1977), recent evidence from embryos of *Ascaris suum* seems to militate against the universality of that condition (Friedman *et al.*, 1980). Use of specific binding properties of the protein to colchicine and prop-

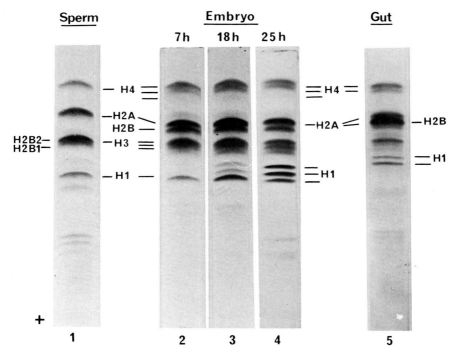

Figure 3.20. Comparisons of histones from the sperm, various stages of the embryo, and gut of the adult of the sea urchin. Both qualitative and quantitative distinctions are shown by the electrophoretograms of sea urchin histones during development. (Courtesy of Brandt *et al.*, 1979.)

erties of the resulting tubulin–colchicine complexes revealed a number of differences between the tubulins of eight-cell embryos and gastrulae. Thus, the members of this protein class present in embryos may be as heterogeneous as those of adult metazoans (Dillon, 1981) and may undergo changes from one age group of embryos to another.

3.4. INDUCTANCE AND OTHER DEVELOPMENTAL FACTORS

3.4.1. Inductance and Competence

Inductance. One of the earlier deductions that has provided some basis for an understanding of the mechanisms of embryogeny was that the presence of one tissue may induce a second one to undergo differentiation. For example, Spemann and Mangold (1924) discovered that when the dorsal lip of the blastopore from the gastrula of a salamander egg was transplanted into another gastrula in either a ventral or lateral location, a second embryo was induced to develop. In this case, more than induction was actually involved, for the transplanted region (graft) supplied much of the notochordal mesoderm (chordamesoderm) while the recipient (host) supplied the nervous system. But the principle of one tissue influencing another was clear. However, the role that determination plays simultaneously should not be overlooked. In a recent set of experiments, somitic mesoderm from *Xenopus* neurulae was treated and transplanted into several contrasting locations, but all grafts developed normally regardless of location and whether they had been placed on ectoderm or endoderm (Forman and Slack, 1980). Other studies, including UV-irradiated embryos, have cast further doubts as to the complete validity of inductance (Youn and Malacinski, 1981).

The Chemical Nature of Induction. With the discovery of inductors or ''organizers,'' a search was soon begun for the specific chemicals that might be involved. At first, various proteins, including nucleoproteins, were implicated, followed shortly by sterols. But these efforts were soon lessened when the discovery was made that while dorsal-lip transplants were the only living tissue that could induce primary embryonic events, almost any tissue from an animal of any type could do so, providing it was denatured by heat or alcohol. Even organic compounds like sucrose, inorganic substances as iodine and kaolin, and local mechanical injury were found to be effective inductors. In short, it became evident that organizers do not actually induce another tissue to differentiate in a certain way, but merely serve as triggers that initiate or release a built-in response (Løvtrup *et al.*, 1978). However, the role that determination plays simultaneously should not be overlooked. This observation received recent support from the results of a study that used heparin solutions on the ventral halves of developing frog gastrulae (Flickinger, 1980). The treated partial embryos were found to produce a number of characteristic dorsal tissues and organs, including brain, skeletal muscle, and nephric tubules. Moreover, the chemical was noted to stimulate the accumulation of labeled DNA and RNA within the embryos.

Yet most embryonic tissues that are active inductors can be chemically separated into fractions that induce different specific reactions (Saxén and Toivonen, 1962). Further chemical analyses have shown that fractions which organize the archencephalon (the forebrain, eyes, and nose) differ in composition and chemical properties from those that induce such mesodermal structures as muscle or kidney, as well as from others which lead to the origin of the spinal cord. Perhaps the more sophisticated electrophoretic and chromatographic procedures available today would permit the isolation of inductive substances that escaped detection in the earlier investigations with less precise and sensitive techniques. Beginnings toward this end have been made in the chick embryo; for example, use of tritiated phenylalanine permitted it to be found that two proteins that appeared in the hypoblast at the time of primitive streak initiation occurred in the epiblast at later stages (Eyal-Giladi et al., 1975).

Ions as Inductors. One of the working hypotheses that emerged from the search for specific factors is that regional changes in ion concentration or pH might alter gene action or energy-yielding systems in such a manner that cell differentiation was thereby induced (Barth and Barth, 1968; McMahon, 1974). Experiments with presumptive epidermis of frog gastrula have shown in the absence of other tissue that the development of nerve and pigment cells was dependent on the concentration of free Na^+ cations. Moreover, the normal induction of these cells in this tissue by mesoderm from dorsal-lip explants was likewise demonstrated to be dependent on the external concentration of sodium, the effect occurring at a concentration of 0.088 M NaCl in the culture medium. If reduced to 0.044 M NaCl, the mesoderm differentiated into muscle and mesenchyme, but neural and pigment cells were not formed. Similar production of neurons from presumptive epidermis was induced also by such cations as Li^+ and Ca^{2+}, and later treatment with any of the three ions triggered the neurons to differentiate into pigment cells, but the cells first had to become neurons before they were competent to become pigment cells.

Competence. The ability of a tissue to react in a specific morphogenetic manner to an inductive influence has been given the term competence, two varieties of which are recognized, the first of which is referred to as primary. For a case in point, if the ectoderm from various developmental stages of amphibian embryos ranging from blastula to early neurula are transplanted, a gradual loss of ability to respond in the normal fashion of forming a neural tube is revealed. Ectodermal transplants from late gastrulae, by way of illustration, no longer are able to form brain structures, and those of the late neurula stage cannot form any part of the nervous system. Still older ectoderm that has begun differentiating into epidermis cannot be induced to alter that course of action.

However, the epidermis from late neurulae is able to respond to other inductors. For instance, if placed under the influence of an eye vesicle, it can differentiate into the lens, or if associated with hindbrain, it can develop into an ear vesicle, or even into nasal pits if forebrain inductive influences can be brought to bear upon it. This new responsiveness, absent at earlier stages and acquired with increasing age, is referred to as secondary competence. Such changes in response to influences appear to be part of the normal processes of differentiation, at these early as well as later stages. The region of the amphibian embryo just discussed, that which gives rise to the nervous system, has been shown to undergo a whole succession of competence phases. As the blastula develops, the most intense capacity is that for forming mesoderm; however, with the late blastula, this ability falls off rapidly, whereas neural competence quickly increases for a time (Gebhardt and Nieuwkoop, 1964). The mesodermal derivatives continue their mesodermal and endodermal direction of differentiation, but neural competence is lost with the early gastrula being replaced by one for transformation into the various parts of the brain and spinal cord.

3.4.2. Positional Effects and Ovostatification

Positional Effects. Inductance and competence, as important and exciting as they are as factors in embryogenic events, are only two facets of the whole problem of development of the zygote into the adult. Among those that have long been recognized is the location in the embryo of a specific blastomere or tissue. Such positional effects imply local specific circumstances, currently poorly understood. They often do not carry precise instructions for the formation of any particular structure, but rather they appear to influence groups of cells, which are still uncommitted to any particular destination, to organize into one of the numerous patterns permitted by their genomes. This property has been renamed positional information or signaling (Wolpert, 1969) and receives attention in more than one ensuing discussion.

One of the more striking examples of positional effects or information is provided by cross-transplants between frog and salamander embryos. The former type has a pair of adhesive suckers below the mouth that consists entirely of epidermis, while the latter possesses a pair of rodlike, so-called balancers, which epidermal structures contain a core of cartilage (Berrill and Karp, 1976). When competent ectoderm from a site on a salamander embryo remote from the balancers is transplanted on a site on a frog embryo where suckers otherwise would develop, the salamander type of organ develops instead. To the contrary, when similar competent epidermis from a frog embryo is grafted onto an embryonic salamander in the corresponding position, adhesive suckers are formed. Thus, while each tissue responds to the position into which it has been transplanted, its response is that of its species, that is, of its own specific genomic constitution. However, rather than merely responding to the position, there remains a possibility that the ectodermal explants might actually be interacting with an underlying inductor which triggers the formation of an organ in each case, modified by the specific genetic information carried.

More clear-cut examples of positional effects are generally overlooked in the literature, possibly because of the obviousness. In developing amphibians, the ectodermal cells of the early blastula migrate by epiboly into the interior of the embryo and there form a different fundamental cell layer, the primary distinction of which being one of location. Similarly the cells of the epiblast of avian and mammalian embryos involute along the primitive streak to become mesoderm and notochord in their new situation. Even these two derivatives of the same involuted epiblast cells differentiate in diverse ways according to their particular site, those centrally located becoming notochord, the laterally situated ones, general mesoderm. In addition there may be other factors, including inductors, that influence the directions of specialization followed by the external and internal or central and lateral cell layers, but if they exist, they have not been demonstrated as yet.

This concept receives support from experiments on developing eggs of the free-living soil nematode *Caenorhabditis elegans*. The results indicated that the differentiation of blastomeres is determined to some degree by internal factors that become differentially distributed during early cleavages, whereas the patterns of cleavage are guided by internal cues (positional effects) as well as by internal determinants (Laufer *et al.*, 1980). Through investigations on nemertine embryogeny, Freeman (1979) has drawn similar conclusions, for his results indicated that during the cleavage stages, determinants may become localized at specific sites in the several blastomeres under the regulation of the cell cycle. The point of view is that with each cell division, a certain amount of progress is made toward localizing a given determinant within each specific blastomere until eventually it becomes confined to its definitive site. To make the concept of more general application, extension is necessary to allow for gradients of determinants, such as those in certain insect embryos (Kalthoff, 1979). Thus, it might be viewed as including the clinal distribution of a specific determinant, greater amounts becoming concentrated in a given region than in adjacent ones and still less in each successively more distant sector.

Ovostratification. In many eggs, especially the telolecithal variety like those of amphibians, a yolk-containing vegetal pole is readily distinguished from the yolkless animal pole. Moreover, the latter is characterized by the presence of the polar body of meiosis and by a heavy pigment layer. Although these traits thus obviously mark the polarity of the amphibian eggs, they appear to be indicators that are secondary to a more basic, less visible organization of the protoplasm. It will be recalled, for instance, that the animal pole of mammalian eggs is established early in oogenesis by their being attached to the ovarian cortex. Another illustration is provided by eggs of the brown seaweeds of the genus *Fucus*, in which no signs of polarity are evident at and following fertilization. Then beginning about 10 hr later, RNA becomes concentrated at one side of the nucleus, along with cytoplasmic organelles, marking polarity of an internal nature. Within 2 hr beneath this point externally, the egg bulges and becomes pear-shaped, the protrusion indicating the beginnings of a rhizoid. About 6 hr later, a cleavage plate develops, dividing the egg into two unequal parts, the smaller one being the rhizoid cell and the larger, the prothallus. While the *Fucus* egg itself is devoid of inherent polar properties, a number of factors can induce their formation. If a beam of light strikes the fertilized egg, the rhizoid and RNA concentration form on the opposite side from the source, and if an electric current is applied, the rhizoid appears toward the anode (Jaffe, 1966, 1968). A similar situation exists in certain mollusks and annelids which develop a polar lobe, as described earlier. This always appears on the vegetal pole and seems to contain highly specific cytoplasm (Clement, 1976; Dohmen and Verdonk, 1979).

The clear-cut polarity of the amphibian egg that has been mentioned in several earlier discussions has long attracted the attention of embryologists (Løvtrup *et al.*, 1978). Distinctions have been made between primary polarities of the unicellular egg, such as the animal–vegetal and dorsoventral polar axes, and the definitive polarities of the embryo that appear during development, including the craniocaudal, definitive dorsoventral, and mediolateral polar axes (Nieuwkoop, 1977). In the egg, the animal–vegetal polarity is made obvious by the distribution of pigment, yolk, and cell organelles, while the dorsoventral-polarity axis is established by the formation of the gray crescent. Correctly the latter should not be thought of as establishing this axis, but as an external manifestation of fundamental internal changes. For example, in both *Discoglossus pictus* and *X. laevis* eggs, gray-crescent formation follows the appearance in the center of the zygote of an area of clear, nearly yolk-free cytoplasm that soon becomes transferred toward the future dorsal side (Klag and Ubbels, 1975; Ubbels and Hengst, 1978).

This zygotic dorsoventral polarization is then followed by a secondary one. Rotational experiments revealed that in the blastula, the original dorsoventral polarity no longer resides in the animal portion of the embryo, because no influence of the gray crescent could then be demonstrated (Nieuwkoop, 1969). This polarization is not represented by a distributional gradient but rather by a center of dominance, the entire mass having already been established as endoderm. Somewhat later the inductive influences lead to the formation of mesoderm at the periphery of the animal portion, where the latter contacts the vegetal part, particularly at the dorsal lip of the blastopore. This germ layer thereby acquires what may be referred to as the tertiary dorsoventral-polarity axis, which ultimately leads to the definitive one (Nieuwkoop, 1977). More recently, however, parts of the preceding concept have proven to be invalid, for dorsal cells transplanted from blastulae or gastrulae into the blastocoels of intact embryos induced secondary axes of dorsoventral polarity in the recipients (Malacinski *et al.*, 1980).

Polarity in fertilized ova is just one aspect of a broader feature of organization, that often is referred to as stratification. Since this term has other uses in biology, it is proposed here that the name ovostratification be employed to designate the phenomenon. One especially clear example has already been described in the discussion of the early divisions of sea urchin embryogenesis. Here the eggs are organized into five strata, subdividing the animal–vegetal axis (p. 130; Figure 3.1). During cleavage, then, each stratum becomes a definite type of cell, the lowermost the micromeres, followed by two sets of vegetal macromeres, and at the upper pole, two sets of animal mesomeres. In turn each set has different presumptive destinations, the micromeres becoming the primary mesenchyme, the macromeres the endoderm, and the mesomeres the ectoderm. Even though yolk is moderately sparse in those organisms, the animal pole had been marked by the polar body and a distinct impression in the jelly coat, and the yolk concentrated at the opposite side.

However, centrifugation experiments have shed further light on the fundamental nature of ovostratification. If sea urchin eggs are centrifuged in random orientation with respect to the centrifugal field, the component organelles become stratified at various angles relative to the original animal–vegetal axis. First cleavage is frequently meridional to the new axis of stratification, as is the second also. Further, the third is horizontal, as in untreated zygotes, but the fourth, which produces the micromeres, always occurs at the original vegetal pole (Morgan, 1927). Later, gastrulation takes place at the same point, quite as in normal eggs. Thus, although the visible components can be restratified physically and the accompanying modified orientation of the nucleus may realign the first several mitotic divisions, the fundamental axis of stratification resists such alteration. In fact, in many metazoans, even the original orientations of the early cleavages remain unaltered after centrifugation.

Cleavage orientation leads into an aspect of cytokinesis that was not presented in an earlier discussion (Dillon, 1981, pp. 511–525), as it is more appropriate here. When hydrostatic pressure was applied to cleaving sea urchin eggs, the progress of the furrow was halted and even reversed in direction (Marsland and Landau, 1954; Marsland, 1956). If the pressure was released, cleavage resumed, unless the pressure was maintained for periods in excess of 15 min. In the latter case cytokinesis was omitted, even though the nuclei had divided normally, but what is especially remarkable is that double cleavage occurred at the next division, so that the normal four cells resulted. Since these experiments were performed before the widespread activities of actin in the cell had come to light, various interpretations of the observations were offered. Now that actin fibers are known to be deeply involved in cleavage-furrow formation and to be moved from site to site within the cell during a normal cell cycle, as well as in polar lobe formation and cleavage in the mollusks of the genus *Ilyanassa* (Schmidt *et al.*, 1980), some of the mystery surrounding the missed furrow and the ensuing double cytokinesis has been removed.

What the overtaking of cleavages does clearly demonstrate is that what was then called the cellular genetic mechanism (Dillon, 1981, pp. 313–316, 556–558) is indeed a genetic apparatus, bearing the responsibility for completing normal embryological development when conditions permit (Nüsslein-Volhard, 1979). Thus, the cytokinetic event was missed under prolonged pressure, because the constantly changing demands of a cell during a normal cycle necessitated the removal of the actin fibers from adjacent to the furrow to another site. Then when a new cycle of division rolled around again, the actin fibers could be placed in accordance with both the needs of the normal division due at that time and the one that was omitted previously, the genetic instructions still having remained intact.

If one then reexamines ovostratification events in this light, it likewise becomes evident that the animal–vegetal-pole-centered organization of the animal ovum, too, is a responsibility of the cellular mechanism. Inheritable information is built into this apparatus which upon a cue from the environment, such as a point of attachment to another tissue, orients the protoplasmic contents of the egg (aside from the organelles) into fundamental relations that cannot be disturbed by artificially induced movements of the yolk or membranous compartments (Hirsh, 1979). In short, unknown components of the cytosol and nucleoplasm, together and separately, carry hereditary information through means of which the embryo begins the complex processes of development.

4

Gene Action Changes during Vertebrate Differentiation

After the stages in embryogenesis beyond those described in the preceding pages have been attained, the embryos undergo development in such complex manners that delineation of their further progress in complete detail becomes undesirable. Instead of descriptions of the elaborating of all the organs in a restricted number of embryonic types, present needs are better served by selecting representative structures that have been more thoroughly explored at the molecular as well as embryonic levels. In some cases, information from sources other than embryology is employed, too, to make as clear as possible the gene action changes involved. Data from various vertebrates, particularly amphibian, mammalian, and avian representatives, provide the basis for discussion in the present chapter, both because invertebrates have received less attention experimentally and because the details of their morphology are less familiar to the majority of biologists. Then in the following chapter a few aspects of differentiation in selected protistan and invertebrate types are provided, along with a few facets of developmental changes among the green plants.

4.1. MUSCLE DIFFERENTIATION

Among the more extensively investigated tissues of vertebrates are the various muscle types of the heart and skeletal parts of the body, the visceral type being omitted because it is too poorly characterized to contribute significantly to the discussion (Burnstock, 1970; Gabbiani *et al.*, 1981). Although cardiac muscle thus often interweaves with skeletal in the following section, many valuable aspects of the former tissue are gained later when the differentiation of the entire heart is examined in a separate discussion.

4.1.1. Myogenesis

The development of muscle tissue, or myogenesis, has been a popular subject for investigation by biologists from a variety of disciplines, currently in particular at the molecular and ultrastructural levels. As one consequence, its chief biochemicals, myosin, actin, and their associated proteins, are very well known and have been described in detail elsewhere (Dillon, 1981, pp. 90–113). But differentiation of this tissue also has been abundantly explored, the greater portion of researches having centered on the more abundant and most readily available striated type from the skeleton, particularly of vertebrate sources.

The Major Aspects of Striate Myogenesis. In general among vertebrates, the earliest forerunners of striated muscle tissue, the presumptive myogens,* are derived from the mesoderm of the lateral plate and myotome region of the individual somites. In the neck and head, however, it has its origins in mesenchyme cells that are unrelated to somites. Although these cells, of whatever background, have already been determined to form muscle, they give no ultrastructural indications of their fate at this time, but appear as ordinary mesodermal cells. However, they tend to be round, with an ovate nucleus (Allen, 1978). As differentiation commences, they become elongated and bipolar myogens while they undergo a period of proliferation. The final division of the myogenic lineage is symmetrical, so that no stem cells are produced by asymmetrical cytokinesis (Klingman and Nameroff, 1980a). However, it has been discovered that the myogens are not a homogeneous population but appear to contain a stem-cell fraction which continues to proliferate. Determination toward the nondividing condition does not take place before the last four or five divisions (Klingman and Nameroff, 1980b), but eventually mitosis and cytokinesis cease, when the cells become known as myoblasts. The earliest evidence of further differentiation is manifested by these postmitotic cells fusing to one another in numbers to form the elongate filaments called myotubes, which are syncytia containing numerous nuclei. Once fusion has begun, or even previously when the period of proliferation ends, the nuclei never again undergo division, the cells being fixed in the G_1 stage of the cell cycle.

Formerly it was considered that further differentiation did not commence until fusion had been initiated (Konigsberg, 1971; O'Neill and Stockdale, 1972; Slater, 1976), but it has now been established that such myotube formation is

---

*In the present account, the practice parallels that of gametogenesis, in that the proliferating stages are differentiated by the term myogen from the terminal nondividing, single cellular stage, which is called the myoblast. In the literature the latter term is often applied indiscriminately to all the unicellular progenitors of muscles.

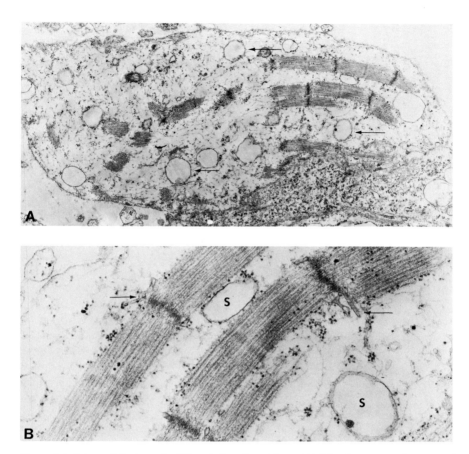

Figure 4.1. Intermediate stages in differentiation of myoblasts. (A) After the myogens have ceased dividing and thereby indicated their having been converted into myoblasts, as in the 14-day chick embryo cells, the contractile fibers become evident, here seen as irregular bundles of fibers replete with Z-disks and A-lines. Sarcoplasmic reticular vesicles (arrows) bearing ribosomes are scattered through the cytoplasm. 11,000×. (B) Later these vesicles become extended into a few tubules located between the myofibrils but still bearing ribosomes. 35,000×. (Both courtesy of Tillack *et al.*, 1974.) See Figure 4.5 for earlier stages.

not a prerequisite (Chi *et al.*, 1975; Holtzer *et al.*, 1975; Moss and Strohman, 1976; Trotter and Nameroff, 1976; Vertel and Fischman, 1976). Since later specialization of structure is totally dependent on the formation of a complex contractile fibrillar system, synthesis of a number of enzymes and structural proteins obviously must commence with the cessation of mitosis, that is, myoblast formation. The thick and thin microfilaments, the myofibrils, replete with Z-disks and A-lines, have appeared by that time, often in irregular fashion and loosely arranged (Figure 4.1A; Tillack *et al.*, 1974). Along with these contrac-

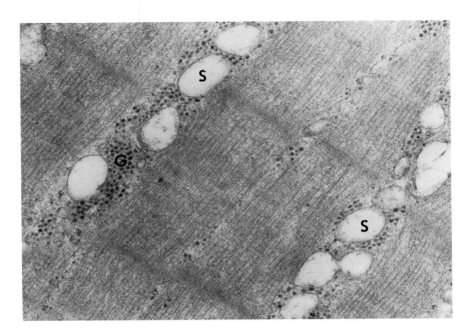

Figure 4.2. Late stage in myoblast differentiation. The myofibrils have now become rearranged, with Z-disks nearly aligned; the sarcoplasmic reticulum is greatly increased in abundance and has lost the ribosomes. 37,000×. (Courtesy of Tillack *et al.*, 1974.)

tile fibers, other characteristic structures of muscular tissue also gradually become evident, including sarcoplasmic reticular vesicles covered with ribosomes externally, and transverse (T-) tubules, associated with the Z-disks (Figure 4.1B). As the myofibrils increase in abundance, the sarcoplasmic reticular vesicles assume their definitive location between them (Figure 4.2), usually in association with glycogen granules, especially late in development (Sommer *et al.*, 1980). It may be noted here that the structure and development of visceral muscle differ from those processes in the skeletal type more in degree than in kind, for the myofibrils are comparably arranged and Z-disks and sarcoplasmic reticulum are similarly present (Amsellem and Nicaise, 1980).

Skeletal Muscle Types. Vertebrate skeletal muscle fibers may be classified in two different fashions, first physiologically, as fast or slow, on the basis of the speed and quality of their reactions, and second morphologically as red or white, depending on the amount of myoglobin present. There is some correlation between the two sets of categories, but it is not always clear-cut. Fast muscle fibers, typically white but occasionally red, have a propagated action potential and a rapid twitch contraction of an all-or-none character, and M-lines described later are present. Usually each is innervated by an axon 12 to 20 μm in diameter, bearing a plate on its single terminus. Slow fibers, always red, have only a junctional potential and react slowly, without an all-or-none trait, and lack M-lines; as a rule innervation is by separate axons 5 to 8 μm in diameter, with multiple branches each ending in a grape terminus. A few muscles, for example the sartorius, consist entirely of fast fibers, whereas the rectus abdominus is comprised solely of the slow variety. As shown in a subsequent discussion, several isozymic differences in certain contractile proteins provide further distinctions between fast and slow fibers (Sarkar *et al.*, 1971; Hoh *et al.*, 1976; Hayashi *et al.*, 1977; Wilkinson, 1978).

Fine Structural Properties. Among vertebrates, the morphological differences between white and red muscle fibers have been especially clearly brought out by ultrastructural investigations on fish and anuran tadpole tails, which are similar both in arrangement and in structure. In each case, the white fibers make up the greatest fraction of the musculature, whereas the red ones occur just below the pigment cells of the skin, largely as a thin superficial layer covering the others (Watanabe *et al.*, 1980). However, in fish as well as the tadpoles, some red fibers are also scattered through the white (Johnston *et al.*, 1975). Both types show the same basic pattern of striation (Figure 4.3), having broad, more electron-opaque regions (A-bands) alternating with much narrower, transparent stripes (I-bands). Each of these contrasting areas is interrupted, the I-band by an extremely opaque Z-disk, the A-band by a narrow pale region (H-band) which is divided into two by a moderately dark M-line. Comparisons of these striations reveal the Z-disks to be broader, more opaque, and irregular in red fibers, whereas those of the white type are quite narrow, less opaque, and generally straight or feebly undulant (Boström and Johansson, 1972; Nag, 1972; Watanabe *et al.*, 1980). In red fibers, the A-bands also are more opaque than in white ones, possibly due to the greater amount of myoglobin present.

A number of other distinctions between the two may be perceived in electron micrographs. The myofibrils of red muscles are much narrower than those of the other type and are also less regularly arranged and more loosely spaced. Moreover, the several regions are not aligned uniformly throughout a red fiber as they tend to be in white, and mitochondria are more numerous in the more abundant cytoplasm (sarcoplasm) of red fibers. Perhaps the presence of a large supply of these organelles accounts in part for the stronger reactivity of red fibers for succinic dehydrogenase and ATPase (Figure 4.4; Korneliussen *et al.*, 1978; Watanabe *et al.*, 1980).

The basis for the striated pattern of vertebrate skeletal muscle is generally taken to stem from the arrangement of thick and thin filaments within the myofibrils. The thin filaments (usually considered to be predominantly actin) are attached individually at one end to a complex of interwoven fibrils, which together comprise the Z-disks, while the free region extends between parallelly arranged thick filaments. The latter are chiefly myosin and provide much of the

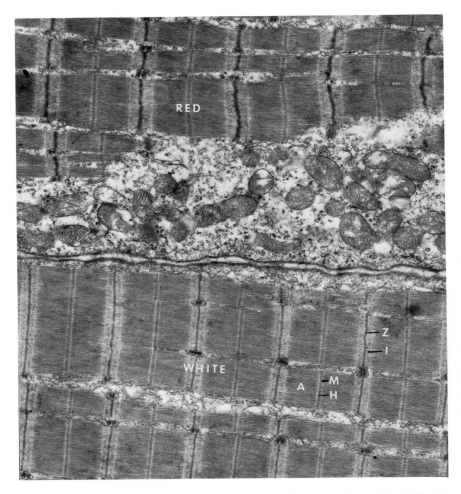

Figure 4.3. Fine structural features of white and red fibers. In the tail of a urodele tadpole, the differences between the white and red muscle fibers are particularly clear. The abbreviations A, H, and I refer to A-, H-, and I-bands, respectively, M to M-line, and Z to the Z-disk, often misleadingly called the Z-line. 20,000×. (Courtesy of Watanabe *et al.*, 1980.)

opacity of the A-band, the more transparent H-band resulting from the failure of opposing thin filaments to meet centrally and the I-bands, from the corresponding absence of thick filaments there. The nature of the M-line remains unelucidated.

Differentiation during Early Myogenesis. Since in a superficial view myogens seem only to undergo multiple cell divisions, little attention has been

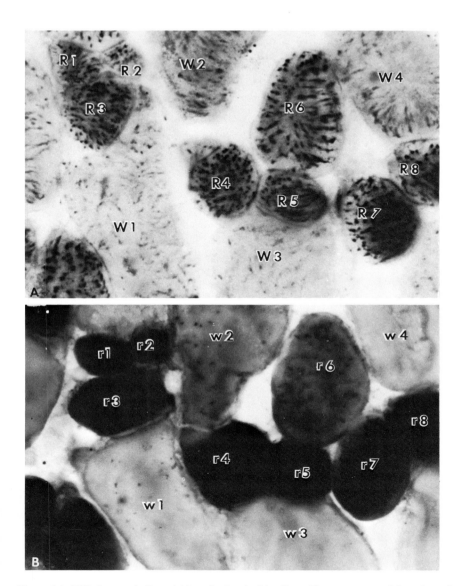

Figure 4.4. Differing metabolic activities of red and white fibers. The transverse serial sections of larval urodele trunk muscle have been treated to show succinic dehydrogenase activity (A) and ATPase activity (B). In both cases, the red fibers (R1–8; r1–8) are far more reactive than the white (W1–4; w1–4). 1600×. (Courtesy of Watanabe *et al.*, 1980.)

paid to the processes of and possible changes during differentiation of muscle tissue until the definitive myoblast stage. As pointed out earlier, fusion into myotubes does not need to occur before some of the distinctive features of muscle fibers are acquired by myoblasts, so that process does not serve as a triggering mechanism as once supposed (Shainberg *et al.*, 1971; Paterson and Strohman, 1972; Loomis *et al.*, 1973). When mononucleated definitive (post-mitotic) myoblasts of the chick were cultured in the presence of phospholipase C to inhibit fusion without affecting recognition or cell cycle parameters, they underwent internal differentiation in the same fashion as fused cells (Trotter and Nameroff, 1976). According to electron micrographs, thick filaments were the first elements of the myofibrils to appear, originating as slightly undulant filaments of varying lengths, placed loosely end to end and with some degree of parallelism (Figure 4.5A). Tubular rough endoreticulum was fairly abundant at this time, as it was later also, but mitochondria were relatively scarce. As more of the contractile proteins were synthesized, the thick filaments increased in abundance and became arranged in loose bundles held together in part by occasional aggregates of an electron-opaque substance that may be assumed to represent precursorial Z-disks. Thin filaments seemed also to be present but were too poorly developed to permit description, except that they were associated with the forming Z-disks. Only a few vesicles were to be noted, aside from the widespread tubular endoreticulum. Later the thick filaments acquired a more compact, regular arrangement to form interrupted series of structural units (sarcomeres), on which precursorial M-lines and H-bands could then be noted. The Z-disk material became more in evidence but had not become condensed into linear arrays, mitochondria were abundant and seemed to be undergoing rapid growth and division, and the vesicles of rough endoreticulum were more numerous. These various developments continued, so that the A-bands became more sharply delineated as the Z-disks condensed into more orderly structures (Figure 4.5B). However, the I-bands remained disorganized for some time (Tillack *et al.*, 1974), while the sarcoplasmic reticular vesicles enlarged and assumed their definitive location between myofibrils.

The formation into myotubes which typically accompanies the foregoing processes has been found to be under the control of several factors. In one study, myogens mostly underwent two cell divisions after being transferred to a plate; the resulting myoblasts then began to fuse about 11 hr after the final DNA synthesis (Slater, 1976). If given fresh medium before the second division, additional divisions occurred, thus delaying myoblast and myotubule formation. On the other hand, if fresh myogenic cells were introduced into medium in which myoblasts had previously undergone fusion, division was inhibited and myotubule formation accelerated, thereby suggesting the presence of a factor that induced tubule formation in definitive myoblasts (Konigsberg, 1971).

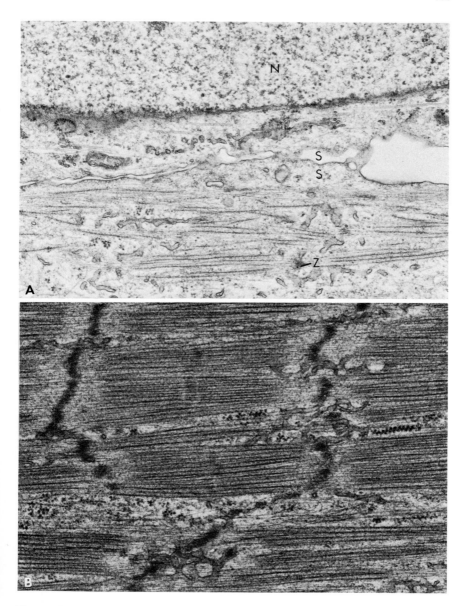

Figure 4.5. Experimentally induced differentiation in embryonic chick myoblasts. When myoblasts are treated with phospholipase C, they fail to fuse but otherwise differentiate normally, as in the stages shown. (A) Myoblast in early stage of forming myofibrils (N, nucleus; S, sarcoplasmic reticular vesicle; Z, forerunner of Z-disk). 19,000×. (B) After removal of the enzyme, the resulting myotubules have developed nearly mature myofibrils, but the Z-disks are incompletely formed. 30,000×. (Courtesy of Trotter and Nameroff, 1976.) Compare Figure 4.1.

4.1.2. Molecular Aspects of Myogenesis

Myosin during Myofibril Formation. At the time myoblasts were shown to be able to undergo differentiation without becoming fused, it was also being demonstrated that synthesis and accumulation of myosin could proceed in the mononucleated myoblasts (Moss and Strohman, 1976; Vertel and Fischman, 1976). Because muscle cells abundantly synthesize numerous contractile proteins in addition to the present one, they are an ideal type for examining the possible presence of coordinate regulation of gene expression during cellular differentiation. Thus, many aspects of the events of producing the very important contractile protein, myosin, have been thoroughly investigated.

At first the major portion of attention was devoted to the heavy chain of this complex substance. This subunit is not synthesized by myogens but is produced in great abundance by late myoblasts, especially at the time of fusion (Emerson and Beckner, 1975; Emerson, 1977). Comparisons have been made of this chain from adult chicken fast white and slow red fibers with adult dystrophic white and embryonic presumptive white fibers, with pertinent results (Figure 4.6; Rushbrook and Stracher, 1979). The peptide maps revealed the greatest differences to exist between the white and red fibers, regardless of the source of the protease, while the dystrophic material differed only slightly from normal adult white fibers. The embryonic peptide pattern, however, although generally similar to that of the other fibers of corresponding types, was quite distinctive, especially in the near absence of bands 2 and 4. A thoroughgoing study of nonmyogenic cells, myogens, and myoblasts cultured to the equivalent of 10-day chick embryos has provided a fuller picture, in revealing that nonmyogenic cells and replicating myogens synthesized similar myogen heavy and light chains that were different from those produced by myoblasts (Chi *et al.*, 1975). Moreover, the products from the two contrasting sources were found to be encoded by different genes. A later investigation then provided additional details in showing that the myotube myosin heavy chain differed from that of the myoblast but was translated from mRNAs that had been transcribed during the myoblast stage (Doetschman *et al.*, 1980).

The light chains of myosin are made more complex than the heavy ones by the existence of isozymes, three of which occur in adult chicken white fibers and two in the slow red (Lowey and Risby, 1971; Frank and Weeds, 1974; Obinata *et al.*, 1976; Matsuda *et al.*, 1977). In embryonic chick white muscle, all five of those isozymes were reported to be produced, whereas none were in dividing myogens (Keller and Emerson, 1980). Only in late myoblasts did the light chains occur, all five types then being represented; however, the smallest of the light chains has been demonstrated actually to be absent in the embryonic chick white fibers (Hoh, 1979) or else rare (Roy *et al.*, 1979a), a condition that prevails also in embryonic red fibers (Rubenstein *et al.*, 1977). Thus, it would appear that red and white fibers do not differ genetically insofar as this

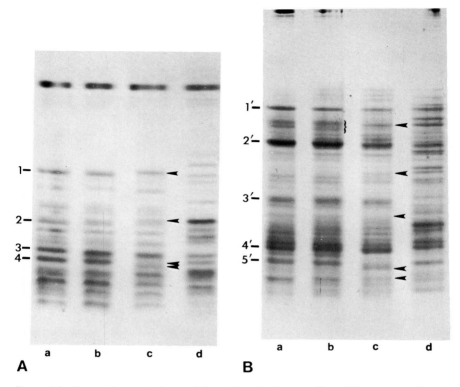

Figure 4.6. Changes in myosin heavy chains during development. Two different preparations of myosin heavy chains from white (a) and red (d) muscle of adult normal chickens, white muscle of dystrophic chickens (b), and presumptive white muscle of 16-day embryonic chicks (c). (A) Digestion of the heavy chains with *S. aureus* V8 protease, whose band is marked with an asterisk. Numerals indicate important peptides for comparison with (B), and arrowheads indicate peptides that differ between normal adult (a) and chick (c) white muscle material. (B) Digestion with papain. (Both courtesy of Rushbrook and Stracher, 1979.)

class of macromolecule is concerned but only in the relative expression of the genes for the various isozymes; in tissue cultures, moreover, both fast and slow muscles synthesized only fast myosin (Rubenstein and Holtzer, 1979). These observations are in accord with the known effects of changes in innervation, which can transform red fibers into white or vice versa (Vbrová, 1963; Pelloni-Muller *et al.*, 1976; Rubenstein *et al.*, 1977; Edgerton, 1978). Thyroidectomy has been shown to have a similar effect, in that white myosin light chains became replaced by those characteristic of red (Johnson *et al.*, 1980). In direct contrast, however, are the results of a study on developing and adult rabbit muscle, which demonstrated that in the fetal mammal there is a distinct class of myosin isozymes, different from those of both types of adult striped muscle (Hoh and Yeoh, 1979).

mRNAs variously specific for the several components of myosin have also served as probes for investigation of the synthesis and nature of this protein in the embryo (Ordahl *et al.*, 1980). Through their use, it has been confirmed that myosin formation in rat muscle paralleled that of the chick in being initiated only in the late myoblast (Benoff and Nadal-Ginard, 1980). The heavy chain component increased from less than 1% of the total proteins to 25% at the time of myotube formation and decreased rapidly after the myotubes had been fully differentiated. These changes were paralleled by similar alterations in the cytoplasmic content of heavy-chain mRNA, except that synthesis of the latter was initiated at least 36 hr prior to myoblast fusion, at a time when all cells in an *in vitro* population were still not committed as to their final fate (Doetschman *et al.*, 1980). One striking feature of this type of mRNA that was produced during differentiation was the abbreviated nature of the poly(A) segment, which had a mean length of under 20 nucleotides, whereas between 100 and 200 is normal.

Other Contractile Proteins during Myogenesis. Not only the myosin constituents vary from one muscle type to another; the proteins that are often considered to be regulators of myosin and actin activities are likewise quite diversified (Dhoot and Perry, 1979). For instance, α- and β-tropomyosin occur in a ratio of 55 : 45 in that order in slow adult skeletal muscle, while they exist in proportions of 80 : 20 in fast (Roy *et al.*, 1979a). Furthermore, each of these fiber types has its own characteristic isozymes of the troponin complex. During embryonic development of both rabbit and chicken, β-tropomyosin has been determined as being the major species in all skeletal muscles examined (Roy *et al.*, 1979a), amounting to 70% of the total in 20-day rabbit embryo tissue. This proportion, however, became reduced to 50% in 26-day specimens and to 45% 1 day after birth (Amphlett *et al.*, 1976). As indicated in an earlier discussion, the physiological and anatomical states also influence the ratios present; continuous stimulation of fast muscle for 3 weeks, by way of illustration, changes the ratio of tropomyosin subunits from the $80\alpha : 20\beta$ of fast fibers to the 55 : 45 of slow (Roy *et al.*, 1979b). Moreover, the thin filaments thmselves have proven to be more complex than commonly believed. Such filaments have been collected in quantities after removal of the myosin from skeletal muscles, the resulting partial myofibrils being referred to as I-Z-I segments (Kuroda and Masaki, 1980). Extraction of protein from such segments yielded 42,000-dalton components, which were found to be of a dual nature when analyzed by isoelectric focusing. The minor band was virtually identical to actin in properties, whereas the major constituent was not identified.

The macromolecular constituents of Z-disks were revealed to be quite complex when they similarly received more thorough investigation. After the components of these lines in chicken myofibrils were extracted by means of rabbit calcium-activated factor, a 95,000-dalton protein corresponding to α-actinin was found to predominate, while a 220,000-dalton component was next in frequency. The heavy constituent was not identified nor were the several other proteins that occurred in lesser quantities (Muguruma et al., 1980), all of which, including the α-actinin, entered into contraction-band formation upon addition of Mg^{2+}-ATP. The Z-disk has an extremely intricate structure in full-face views under the electron microscope (Ullrick et al., 1977a,b). While sensitive to the fixative, the most common pattern is a basket-weave design, possibly induced by the connections of Z- and I-filaments (Figure 4.7A). In cardiac muscle, the pattern is similar, except that it is more open (Figure 4.7B–D; Goldstein et al., 1979, 1980), with somewhat thinner filaments.

Comparisons of the primary structures of actins from a variety of sources proved them to be remarkably uniform. Two from contrasting visceral muscles (bovine aorta and chicken gizzard) were found to differ solely at three sites out of a total of 374, and both were distinguished from skeletal muscle actin at only four sites (Vanderkerckhove and Weber, 1979). Moreover, the protein from cardiac muscle contained only four distinctive points when compared to skeletal muscle, which in turn exhibited the greatest number of differences with actins from nonmuscle sources.

Recently the problems of assembly of the thick and thin filaments during myogenesis have been subject to a number of investigations. In one study of thin filament formation, in which meromyosin-decoration techniques were used, it was revealed that the constituents exhibited the correct polarities and spatial organization relative to thick filaments from the very beginning of myofibril assembly (Shimada and Obinata, 1977). In a later related study, cultured embryonic skeletal muscle cells of the chicken were treated with antibodies to adult troponin and examined by immunoelectron microscopy (Obinata et al., 1979). Since with each type (troponin T, I, and C) the reaction products were distributed along the actin filaments in normal fashion, it was concluded that they, too, are assembled at their definitive sites from the very onset of the processes. This approach, however, leaves unsolved the nature of the several troponins, for troponins T and I have been shown to exist in three isozymic forms, one each for fast, slow, and cardiac muscles (Wilkinson and Grand, 1978; Dhoot and Perry, 1979), while troponin C has two, one in fast muscle and another shared by cardiac and slow (Wilkinson, 1980).

Although the various contractile and associated proteins are products of separate genes, they are synthesized in a highly coordinated fashion. Myosin heavy chains and its two light chains and two subunits of each troponin and tropomyosin were all first detected at the time of fusion and then increased at least 500-fold at nearly identical rates in myotubes and myofibrils (Devlin and Emerson, 1978). α-Actinin also increased but it was produced about three times as rapidly as the remaining contractile proteins, whereas 30 other proteins of a noncontractile nature exhibited different patterns of regulation.

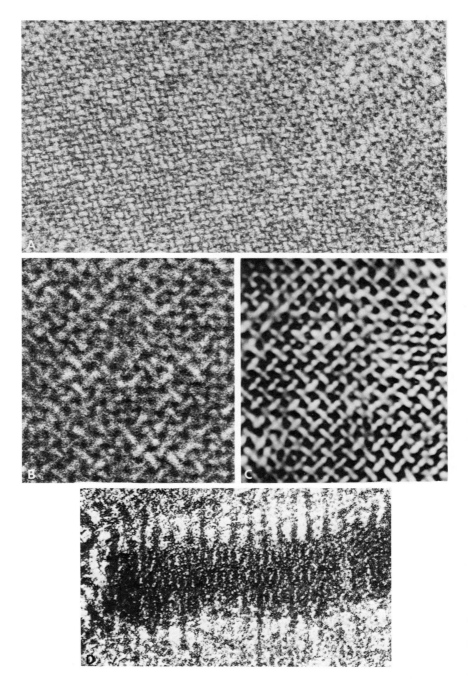

mRNAs of Contractile Proteins. In common with investigations at the early embryogenic levels of development, the important classes of mRNAs have been probed to ascertain indirectly various aspects of muscle protein synthesis during differentiation. Among the earlier studies of this nature was an examination of the relative stabilities of the mRNAs preceding and following myoblast fusion (Buckingham *et al.*, 1974). Whereas in the myogenic cells the half-life of the putative 26 S poly(A)$^+$ mRNA for myosin was 10 hr, it increased to better than 50 hr following fusion, but no other difference between the two could be detected (Bragg *et al.*, 1980). Examination of the total population of mRNAs in the myoblast demonstrated a remarkable diversity of species to exist that underwent a marked reduction in extent following myotube formation. About 60% were messengers for the chief proteins, particularly those of contractile fibers, but the remaining 40% included over 120,000 different species, that were present at a mean rate of one-half copy per cell (Ordahl and Caplan, 1978). However, after the cells had fused to form the multinucleated myotube, the amount of unique-sequence DNA that was transcribed was described as being reduced to 50%. That the mRNAs underwent a successive series of qualitative changes was ascertained through use of hybridization with cDNA from chick embryo myotubes and poly(A)$^+$ mRNAs from myogens and myoblasts (Leibovitch *et al.*, 1979). Hybridization at a 43% level was obtained with the nucleic acids from myogens, 46% from myoblasts, 54% from early myotubes, and nearly 70% with multinuclear syncytial myotubes. Very little, if any, translatable mRNA for contractile proteins was detected in dividing myogens but appeared in the same proportions as detailed earlier under the contractile proteins (Devlin and Emerson, 1979). Other researches similarly employing cDNA–RNA hybridization have shown that mRNA sequences specific for proteins of secondary differentiation accumulated just a few hours before cell fusion (Zevin-Sonkin and Yaffe, 1980).

Somewhat comparable results were obtained in a study involving the use of mRNA and hnRNA from mouse embryonal carcinoma, teratocarcinoma-derived myoblasts, and differentiated myotubes (Affara *et al.*, 1980a). A 30% increase in nuclear RNA complexity was observed in passing from the pluripotential carcinoma cells to the later stages, but these hnRNA sequences were still represented in the corresponding nucleic acids of subsequent embryos. With each successive stage of development, a new group of mRNAs also was found to appear on the polysomes, apparently controlled at the transcriptional level. Among the novel mRNAs in the myotubes were a number of types that encoded

---

Figure 4.7. Fine structure of Z-disks. (A) Z-Disk of frog skeletal (gastrocnemius) muscle, fixed with glutaraldehyde, showing a basket-weave pattern of broad filaments. 105,300×. (Courtesy of Ullrick *et al.*, 1977a.) (B) Z-Disk of canine cardiac muscle revealing a similar pattern but with finer filaments. (C) Same as (B) but printed with masked optics. B, C, 240,000×. (D) This longitudinal section shows the embedment of I-filaments into the lattice of Z-filaments. 182,000×. (B–D, courtesy of Goldstein *et al.*, 1979.)

contractile polypeptides, as might be expected (Affara *et al.*, 1980b). Comparable observations were made on the mRNAs for the light chains of embryonic chick heart myosin, which were represented by chains of 1090 and 980 nucleotide residues in length (Arnold and Siddiqui, 1979). The two chains were shown to comprise 2.0% of the poly (A)$^+$ mRNA and 0.02% of the mRNA of polysomes.

In the preceding chapter (Section 3.3.1) the presence of oligo(U) segments on certain RNAs was reported. Recently it has been demonstrated that at least in some instances these nucleic acids serve as translational control mechanisms and have accordingly been designated as tcRNAs (Bester *et al.*, 1975; Lee-Huang *et al.*, 1977; Zeichner and Breitkreutz, 1978). Purified tcRNA from developing muscle cells has been noted to interact in stoichiometrical proportions specifically with myosin mRNA and inhibit it from being translated, while having little effect on the translation of other species (Heywood and Kennedy, 1976; Kennedy *et al.*, 1978). According to the latter report, association is between the tcRNA and myosin RNPs and not with ribosomes. In addition, it was found that stoichiometric amounts of messenger and control nucleic acids were essential, as well as mixture in the proper sequence.

Other Proteins of Developing Muscle Tissue. One of the first noncontractile proteins detected histochemically in developing muscle has also been the subject of control mechanism investigations. This substance, acetylcholinesterase, has been considered a tissue-specific enzyme of contractile tissues, since it occurs only in the myogenic cells, including those of developing ascidian larvae (Durante, 1956; Whittaker *et al.*, 1977). If embryos of *Ciona* or *Halocynthia* were permanently arrested with cytochalasin B during cleavage up to the 64-cell stage, they were still able to synthesize this histospecific protein at the same time as untreated controls, that is, commencing about 8 hr postinsemination but not at 7 hr (Whittaker, 1973; Satoh, 1979). Even mitotic inhibitors like colchicine and colcemid had the same effect, thus intimating that neither cytokinesis nor nuclear division played roles in the clock mechanism that controlled the appearance of this enzyme and that only activation of appropriate genes did so.

Because fusion of myoblasts into myotubes involves recognition, surface proteins of these cells play an important function in development. Two that have been identified, electrolectin and myonectin, appear to be involved in such activities (Teichberg *et al.*, 1975; Gartner and Podleski, 1975, 1976; Podleski *et al.*, 1979a), while a third, fibronectin, may be involved in attachment of the cells to the substrate (Hynes, 1976; Yamada and Olden, 1978). The latter substance also has been established as promoting cell division and reducing fusion between myoblasts (Podleski *et al.*, 1979b). Electrolectin has been found to occur in two forms, one soluble (s-electrolectin), the other not (p-electrolectin), whereas myonectin is only soluble. In addition the insoluble fraction of the lectin contained another protein that blocked the activity of s-electrolectin (Podleski *et al.*, 1979a). Apparently various other species of the class of surface proteins called lectins play important roles throughout development, to judge from the changes in their binding sites that were observed during ascidian embryogeny (Kawai *et al.*, 1979). In the four-cell stage, the label (ferritin particles) indicated lectin-binding sites to be scattered sparsely and singly over the entire surface, but with the gastrula they had become much more abundant and arranged in clusters. During subsequent stages they unexpectedly became scarcer and were concentrated in greater numbers on the notochord and epithelium than on the muscle cells.

Changes in Nuclear and Organelle Proteins. Several studies have reported on changes that occur in the proteins of the nuclei of chick embryo myoblasts (24 hr), fusing myoblasts (40 hr), and myotubes (66 hr) (Lough and Ingram, 1978; Man *et al.*, 1980a). In the latter article it was shown that most nonhistone nuclear proteins increased appreciably during differentiation in concentration relative to the DNA that was present, one exception being the nuclear actin. Comparisons of these nuclear with cytoplasmic proteins indicated very few correspondences between the two source-classes. A companion paper (Man *et al.*, 1980b) demonstrated that nuclear proteins from developing muscle cells were not phosphorylated to any extent. Radioisotopic phosphorus was incorporated at a greater rate between 24 and 40 hr, but decreased thence to 66 hr, but much variation was exhibited from one protein species to another.

Few investigations seem to have addressed the problem of changes in organelle proteins during development. One of the exceptions has examined hybrid mice embryos that were heterozygous for the multiple subunits of mitochondrial malic enzyme to determine whether mitochondria of multicellular myotubes derive their proteins from one or several nuclei (Friar *et al.*, 1979). Since the results indicated that individual mitochondria can contain the products encoded by several nuclei, the syncytia obviously were not compartmentalized functionally into nuclear domains, the products of all being contributed to the total cytoplasm.

4.1.3. Changes in Mature Muscle

Much of the knowledge concerning gene expression changes in mature muscle has been derived from investigations into regenerating tissue and metamorphosing organisms. At first glance the processes of undergoing differentiation from a larva into the adult form would seem to share little common ground with regenerating damaged or lost tissue, but further thought discloses many overlaps and identity of detail. Both these aspects of differentiation include development of new specialized parts from unspecialized cells, as well as regression of old organs or tissues. In the following account neither of these fields should be expected to be covered in full detail, for space considerations compel restriction to scattered examples that indicate the nature of the alterations which occur and thereby contribute to a fuller picture of gene expression changes during differentiation. Unfortunately, studies on muscle regeneration have been relatively few in number, but the more adequate picture provided later in the discussion of limb regeneration should compensate for this deficiency.

Steps in Muscle Regeneration. Regeneration of a skeletal muscle (the gastrocnemius) in the frog has been particularly clearly detailed by Trupin (1979) and co-workers (Hsu *et al.*, 1979; Trupin *et al.*, 1979). In their investigations the muscle was completely excised and minced by standard procedures (Studitsky, 1963; Carlson, 1968), thereby killing all the muscle fibers but leaving the basal laminae to maintain much of their continuity. The minced tissue was then replaced into the original muscle bed, where at first it induced a light, transient infiltration of neutrophils. Within 3 or 4 days after implantation, three other types of cells had largely replaced those leukocytes, namely typical macrophages, fusiform sublaminar cells, and intermediates that displayed characteristics of both the preceding, all of whose origins become clearer in the discussion of limb regeneration. The fusiform population included at least two classes, presumptive myoblasts and modified macrophages, which could be distinguished by electron microscopy only in that the latter phagocytosed carbon-particle labels and sent out psuedopodia, whereas the former lacked both these properties. All the fibers and plasmalemmae were eventually taken into the macrophages by phagocytosis, but the basal laminae persisted and served in defining the original cell boundaries (Figure 4.8). As the fusiform cells increased in number, largely through local proliferation as suggested by the numerous mitotic figures, they became arranged end to end, forming continuous cuffs around the dead muscle fibers. After about 10 days had elapsed, myogens within the cuffs increased in size and developed into myoblasts having typical euchromatic nuclei containing large nucleoli. These cells soon fused into myotubes and proceeded along the ordinary processes of myogenesis already detailed. Similar steps in muscle regeneration have also been reported in rats (Trupin and Hsu, 1979).

Muscle Tissue Changes during Metamorphosis. Although obviously the topic of muscle regeneration has been covered extremely superficially in the foregoing paragraphs, the essential features shall be found to have been adequately presented. Insofar as the tissue itself is concerned, basically only two sets of activities are involved, destruction of the dead tissue largely by phagocytosis, and production of new muscles by processes quite like those of embryogeny. Nor do these fundamental steps differ during metamorphosis; the old muscular parts must be dismantled in whole or in part and new ones produced by stages resembling those of embryogeny. The regression of the tail in anuran tadpoles is an event too familiar to need description; however, few of the macromolecular changes involved in those processes have been described. Among the exceptions is a series of studies on the acid phosphatase

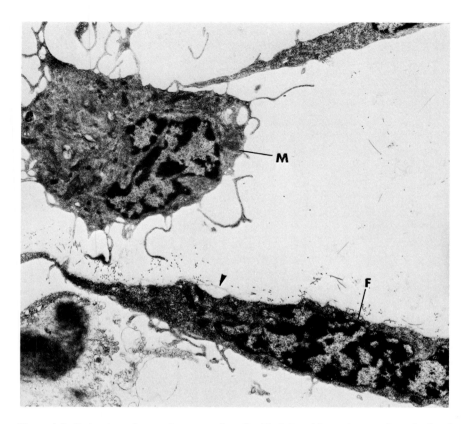

Figure 4.8. Early stages in muscle regeneration. In this 9-day-old muscle transplant, the basal lamina (arrowhead) represents the remnants of the original minced muscle fiber. Beneath it is a fusiform cell (F), some representatives of which type are presumptive myoblasts; above it is one of the macrophages (M), with numerous fine pseudopodia, which consumed the original muscle fibers after their death. 8200×. (Courtesy of Trupin, 1979.)

isozymes of *X. laevis* tadpole tails (Filburn, 1973; Filburn and Vanable, 1973). Regression of the tail, typically induced by thyroxin (Gudernatsch, 1912; Weber, 1962), involved a gradual increase in acid phosphatase activity. During tail resorption, four isozymes (referred to as AP-1 to AP-4) were present, three of which exhibited differential changes in activity as shortening proceeded (Filburn, 1969, 1973). The activity of AP-1, which had a molecular weight of 200,000, changed very little with time, whereas that of AP-4, with a molecular weight of 18,700, decreased. On the other hand, AP-2 (109,000) and AP-3 (40,900) increased substantially in activity during metamorphosis.

Postnatal Changes in Skeletal Muscle. In mammals, the muscles of the newborn young undergo extensive changes in size and in molecular composition. The postnatal growth typically is of a postitive nature but in some instances may be negative; for instance, in the mouse, several muscles are present before or even shortly after birth which later regress and disappear entirely (Jones, 1979). Although the precise pattern of development of the enzyme inventory varied with the taxon, in rodents the fetal isozyme patterns for creatine kinase and lactic acid dehydrogenase underwent transition into that of the adult during the postnatal period (Markert and Urspring, 1962; Eppenberger et al., 1964; Fritz et al., 1975). In other cases, only quantitative changes in enzyme activity have been noted, as in several of the glycolytic series including phosphorylase and phosphorylase kinase (Lyon, 1970; Novák et al., 1972). The activity of the latter protein in mice was demonstrated to increase more than 12-fold during the postnatal period, 80% of which increment occurred during the second week of life (Gross and Bromwell, 1977). Moreover, 6- to 10-day mice had only α', β, and γ subunits, whereas adult skeletal muscles contained the α subunit in addition.

4.1.4. Differentiation in the Heart

Since this is an account of differentiation of the heart, not its embryogenesis, the details of the complex structural changes that occur during development should not be expected in the ensuing discussion. Focus here is on the cellular aspects, where alterations in gene expression may best be perceived. It is sufficient to point out that in the cartilaginous fishes, cyclostomes, and amphibians the organ arises as a tubular cavity in the ventral mesentery of the foregut, about which the cells differentiate directly into the endo- and epicardial coverings and the muscular organ proper, the myocardium. Among the remainder of the Vertebrata, the heart forms from two folds in the splanchnic mesoderm, which are moved mesad and fuse into a tube; in human beings, this early organ is established in the 2-mm embryo having five or six somites. Looping, fusion, outpocketing, and regression of certain parts combine to shape this elementary tube into the definitive complex structure.

Cellular Activities. Despite the many similarities that exist in appearance, the origins of the cardiac muscle tissue that forms the myocardium are quite different from those of the skeletal type. Among the first steps is the fusing of splanchnic mesodermal cells end to end to form irregular branching chains. Because the plasmalemma between cells in such chains is extremely thin, it was originally believed that the latter comprised a continuous syncytium, but the electron microscope now has shown that the individual cells maintain their identity and that the characteristic intercalated disks eventually form on these membranes. Thus, the cells are mononucleated at least during early life. However, in dogs within 10 weeks after birth, 85% of the myocytes contained more than one nucleus (Bishop and Hine, 1974). Soon after fusion, the myofibrils develop along the periphery, with Z-disks, I- and A-bands, as in the skeletal variety, except that the nucleus (or nuclei) remains near the center of each cell (Figure 4.9). In the opossum the transverse (T-) tubules, which are a characteristic of the final stages of cardiac muscle cell differentiation, do not complete their development until the animal is over 100 days old (Hirakow and Krause, 1980).

Whether fusion is preceded by a period of proliferation does not seem to have been ascertained, but it is quite likely that such a stage is absent. The chief reason for the latter statement is that the myocardial cells continue to divide after fusion and even after the myofibrils have developed (Manasek, 1968; Hay and Low, 1972; Rumyantsev, 1972; Goldstein et al., 1973; Goode, 1975; Hurle and Lafarga, 1978). Although the cells usually do not undergo division in mature hearts, they have been observed to do so in wounded areas of adult newt hearts (Oberpriller and Oberpriller, 1971). Since the myocardial cells are thus quite different in structure and behavior from corresponding ones of skeletal muscle, it is here proposed that the early cardiac muscle cells prior to myofibril formation be referred to as cardiogens and the later ones as cardiocytes, the terms myogen and myoblast being reserved for the proliferating (mitotic) and postmitotic cells of skeletal muscle, respectively.

Electron micrographs of cardiocytes in longitudinal section reveal a number of unique traits (Myklebust et al., 1980). While the sarcomeres have an appearance strikingly like those of skeletal muscle, a number of distinctions can be noted, such as the H-band being narrow and only indistinctly subdivided by M-lines. Moreover, the I-bands are much less extensive than the A-bands. But the most pronounced differences lie in the breadth of the Z-disks, which in both birds and mammals are broad, rather than linear, and very electron-opaque. Furthermore, there is an irregular row of fine particles at a slight distance from the disk on either side, quite unlike the irregular cloud of dark material that borders Z-disks in skeletal muscle (Peachey, 1965). The nucleus is strongly ovate and elongate and has the inner membrane of the envelope thickly set with dark particles that make it appear much thicker in section than the outer component. In mammals at least, the Z-disks are attached to the plasmalemma, providing that outer covering with a scalloped appearance in transmission electron micrographs, a condition that prevails in teleost fishes also (Leknes, 1980; Midttun, 1980). However, under the scanning electron microscope, quite to the contrary, the Z-disks show as a series of sharp ridges on the surface of the myofibrils, probably as a result of shrinkage during preparation (Myklebust et al., 1980). Use of immunofluorescent techniques has demonstrated that anti-α-actinin stains the Z-disks, antimyosin specifically reacts with the A-bands, and antitropomyosin is specific for the I-bands (Lemanski et al., 1980). One final distinctive feature is provided by the so-called atrial specific granules in the cells of the atrium, the nature of which remains unknown (Saetersdal et al., 1980).

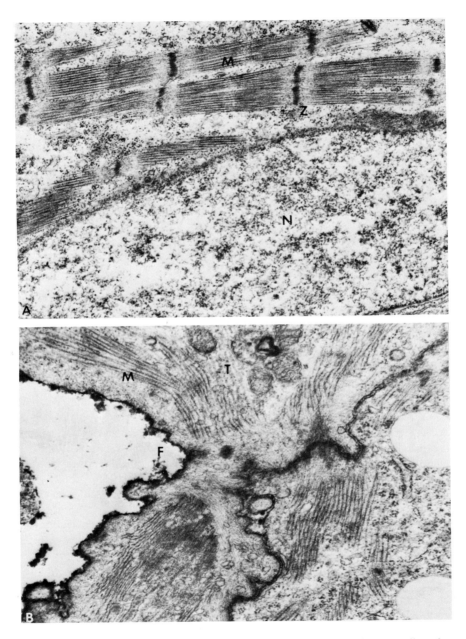

Figure 4.9. Developmental features of cardiocytes. (A) The young cardiocytes have a small number of incomplete myofibrils (M), with very thick Z-disks (Z), especially above the ovate nucleus (N). 21,000×. (B) A cardiocyte undergoing mitotic division. Unlike myogens (of skeletal muscle), cardiocytes frequently undergo mitotic division after myofibrils are present; myofibrils (M) and microtubules (T) may be noted above the cleavage furrow (F). 27,000×. (Both courtesy of Hurle and Lafarga, 1978.)

Further characterizations between the two types of contractile cells become evident during cell division in ultrastructural studies of cardiocytes. Following a well-marked S phase, distinct typical chromosomes were found to form as mitosis began (Rumyantsev, 1972; Goldstein *et al.*, 1973). Up to late prophase, the myofibrils present in these cells remained unchanged, while the nuclear membrane and dictyosomes largely disintegrated (Hay and Low, 1972). Then in prometaphase the majority of the Z-disks began to degenerate, freeing the myofibril bundles and entire sarcomeres to become scattered throughout the cytoplasm. Thick filaments of the latter structures tended to persist, whereas thin ones became indistinct. However, the sarcoplasmic reticulum remained intact, including the typical cisternae that lie beneath the plasmalemma. Following telophase and the restoration of the nucleus, the Z-disks were gradually reformed, thereby reconnecting the isolated sarcomeres while the thin filaments became better defined. Somewhat contrasting to the foregoing report were the results of an investigation on cultured cardiac muscle cells, for it showed that myofibrils were not necessarily disintegrated during mitosis but remained sufficiently intact so that the cells maintained their rhythmic contractions (Kelly and Chacko, 1976; Chacko, 1979).

Cells of Other Types. Within the ventricles of avian and mammalian hearts are two populations of cells, the cardiocytes and Purkinje cells, which are quite similar in structure. Both contain myofibrils, but these bundles tend to be less densely placed in the latter type of cell than in the former, possibly because of their considerably larger diameter of 50 to 70 μm instead of 15 μm. Among ultrastructural differences that may be observed is the contrast in mitochondrial cristae, which in cardiocytes are thin and flat, with lumina scarcely evident, whereas those of Purkinje cells are broad with distended lumina (Osculati *et al.*, 1978; Myklebust *et al.*, 1980). Both types of cells show extensions of the sarcoplasmic reticulum in the form of distinct, single cisternae, but those of cardiocytes are associated with mitochondria and not with the plasmalemma as are those of the other cell type. However, a more reliable identifying characteristic of Purkinje cells is the absence of transverse tubules in the sarcoplasmic reticulum in contrast to their presence in the cardiac muscle proper (Sommer and Johnson, 1968). How the absence of these tubules, which extend along the Z-disks of myofibrils, correlates to function is unknown, but the physiological activities of the opposing types are quite pronounced. The Purkinje cells form fibers which extend as the bundle of His from the atrioventricular node along both surfaces of the intraventricular septum, penetrating thence throughout the muscle tissue. These cells, being conductive, serve in the regulation of the rate at which the cardiocytes contract; thus, their absence is difficult to correlate to the important role of these organelles in excitation–contraction coupling within the cardiocytes themselves. How and when during development these two populations become differentiated has not been established.

In the simple tubular heart of ascidians, the wall is comprised of a single layer of striated cells, which tend to be flat rather than cylindrical (Nunzi *et al.*, 1979). During development, the organ arises as an aggregate of undifferentiated cells enclosed by a basal lamina. After a period of proliferation, the mass undergoes invagination and differentiation into prospective pericardial and myocardial cells. The latter are polarized, in that the nucleus lies beneath the outer surface of the tubelike organ, while the dictyosomes and centrioles occupy the inner region adjacent to the lumen. Subsurface cisternae of rough endoreticulum then form, followed by the appearance of Z-disk precursors and randomly oriented thick and thin filaments. With the passage of time, these parts become assembled into typical myofilaments arranged obliquely to the long axis of the heart adjacent to the lumen. Sometimes secondary myofibrils develop more deeply in the cells at right angles to the first set. These cells reflect their primitiveness in their shape as well as in having the sarcoplasmic reticulum poorly developed.

Other Cellular Events in Heart Development. The development of the embryo involves so much active growth, including the production of new tissues and organs one after the other, that ordinarily one does not associate cell death as an active feature of the processes. Yet it is a common phenomenon during the morphogenesis of many organs and tissues (Glücksmann, 1951; Saunders, 1966). Two steps seem to be involved, the spontaneous death of cells, followed by phagocytosis on the part of neighboring ones or invading macrophages. In the embryogeny of the heart of the chick, cell death has been described as taking place in cardiocytes (Manasek, 1969), mesenchyme, the endocardium (Pexieder, 1972; Ojeda and Hurle, 1975), and more recently, the bulbus (Hurle *et al.*, 1977, 1978). According to the latter reports, during the fourth day of incubation mainly the right side of the bulbus becomes necrotic, so that this entire portion is eventually eliminated, possibly to permit the later transformation of the distal part into proximal regions of the aorta and pulmonary artery. Both adjacent cells and macrophages were found to be active in engulfing the cellular debris. Similar, but less extensive, necrosis has been reported also in the development of the truncus, conus, and aortopulmonary septum, as well as in the semilunar valves (Hurle and Ojeda, 1979).

Inductive influences active during heart morphogenesis have been identified by means of a cardiac mutant in the axolotl. In homozygotes for the "cardiac lethal" gene, the embryonic heart fails to beat, even though initial development appears normal. Subsequently, however, the developing organ becomes distended and remains thin-walled; the mutant larvae survive for about 20 days after the heart would normally have begun to beat, during which time they exhibit swimming movements, suggesting that the mutation does not affect skeletal muscle (Lemanski *et al.*, 1977). However, if the hearts of mutant embryos are cultured with anterior endoderm from wild-type ones, the organs develop normally and contract rhythmically (Lemanski *et al.*, 1979). Still later investigations demonstrated that the mutant cardiocytes were deficient in tro-

pomyosin although they contained near-normal amounts of actin, myosin, and
α-actinin (Lemanski *et al.*, 1980).

Molecular Aspects of Heart Development. Since the heart consists
nearly entirely of muscle tissue, it is not surprising that the majority of investigations on this organ at the macromolecular level have dealt with the contractile proteins (Klotz *et al.*, 1981; Sartore *et al.*, 1981; Woodroofe and Lemanski, 1981); however, a small proportion have been concerned with enzymes,
especially those of cellular respiration. One such protein that has received extensive attention is pyruvic acid kinase. In adult brain and in skeletal and cardiac muscle this protein is represented by type M (Strandholm *et al.*, 1975;
Ibsen *et al.*, 1976), whereas type K is characteristic of the early embryo. Although the two isozymes are cross-reactive in immunological analyses, they
have been reported to be products of separate genes (Harkins *et al.*, 1977) and
both appear to be tetramers like their bovine counterparts (Strandholm *et al.*,
1976). An electrophoretic analysis of various embryonic and posthatching stages
was inconclusive, because the multiple bands might have indicated the presence
of isozymes from tissues other than cardiac, but there was a definite trend away
from type K with the approach of hatching, with possibly hybrid bands pre-
dominating until the second week of the chick (Cardenas *et al.*, 1978).

Whereas dog hearts, for example, gain multiple nuclei in the cardiocytes
with maturity, as already mentioned, the nuclei in a number of other species
become increasingly polyploid. In children up to the age of 7 years, 80% of
the cardiocytes are diploid, whereas in normal adults only 5 to 10% are diploid,
60% being tetraploid and 25% octoploid (Adler and Costabel, 1975). In mice
the cardiocytes may either become tetraploid or binucleate, the latter condition
prevailing in 70% of the cells (Brodsky *et al.*, 1980). Thus, it would appear
that increased DNA content per cell is physiologically advantageous in mature
cells, an increment that can be made by either multiplicity of whole nuclei or
by endoreduplication of the genome. Perhaps this feature serves the purpose of
increasing transcriptive input per unit volume of cytoplasm. How general such
enlarged genomes are throughout the vertebrates as a unit does not appear to
have received investigation.

4.2. DEVELOPMENT OF APPENDAGES

For experimental studies on morphogenesis, the limbs of vertebrates, and
in particular the forelimbs, are outstandingly convenient systems, especially in
view of their having proven to be nearly independent, interacting combinations
of epithelial ectoderm and mesenchyme. Investigations have largely employed
amphibians at the embryonic, larval, and adult stages, but embryonic chicks
and adult rodents have contributed also to the accumulation of knowledge,
through both experimental morphogenetic and regenerative studies. Determi-

nation, induction, competence, and other influences are all seen to be active in the processes, but much still remains enigmatic (Bryant *et al.*, 1981).

4.2.1. Embryonic Aspects of Limb Formation

Among vertebrates in general, one particular inductive influence plays a critical role early in the differentiation of the embryonic skeleton. Epithelial–mesenchymal cells derived from the neural crests in amphibians have been shown to differentiate into cartilage only after they have left the neural crest and during migration have experienced an inductive interaction with endoderm of the pharyngeal region (Holtfreter, 1968; Drews *et al.*, 1972; Epperlein, 1974; Epperlein and Lehmann, 1975). But an even earlier influence is exercised on those cells, for a positional effect is manifest in that only cells that originate in the posterior cranial region of the crest have this capacity, those from other regions of the cranium and trunk having other fates (Detwiler and van Dyke, 1934; Hörstadius, 1950; Johnston, 1966; Le Lièvre, 1974, 1978). However, it has recently been demonstrated that the ability to engage in cartilage formation (chondrogenesis) in birds is established while the cells are still in the neural tube (Hall and Tremaine, 1979). Nevertheless, the main story of differentiation is to be found only after the cells have arrived at their definitive sites on the sides posterior to the gill rudiments.

Limb Development in Embryonic Vertebrates. When the epithelial–mesenchymal cells reach the site of the prospective limb of developing amphibians, the first evidence of their presence is a circular mound of tissue. This area, extending over 3½ somites in diameter, consists of accumulated mesenchyme overlaid by a layer of ectoderm. In the chick, the processes are similar, except that after the wing bud first becomes evident, a ridge forms between it and the leg bud, only to be resorbed later. Otherwise the development of these appendages is remarkably similar in all tetrapod vertebrates. Growth is by rapid proliferation of cells within the bud or disk, rather than by immigration of cells from other parts of the body; however, the limbs are not islands of development but are influenced by other body parts, especially by the mesonephros, quite unexpectedly, as shown in a later section. At the earlier stages of growth a stemlike projection, slightly narrower at the base, is formed, the apical part later expanding into a paddle. Beneath the epidermal covering of the projection, the mesenchyme is more or less uniformly distributed at first but becomes locally condensed in patterns that reflect the species bone characteristics. Later the condensed areas give rise to cartilages from which the bones themselves are developed.

During growth, the mesenchyme plays the major role. If these cells are completely removed from the disk or bud, no limb develops, nor does one form if the ectoderm alone is transplanted to another site. However, one does develop if the mesenchyme is introduced into a new location, as long as it is placed beneath an ectodermal layer. The latter observation makes clear that while mesenchyme is the primary tissue in which the ability of limb formation is localized, it cannot express that potential in the absence of epithelium. Especially in the differentiation of the feet, cell death also is an active process. Necrotic areas appear first in shaping the wrist or ankle and then in removing the interdigital webbing as the digits grow in the chicken, or in ducks along the distal edges of the webbing as it acquires the species characteristics (Saunders and Fallon, 1966).

Results of Experimental Investigations. A number of the earlier experiments on limb morphogenesis were designed primarily to discover when the several polarities of the appendage were established (Harrison, 1921; Slack, 1976). Transplantation of a whole limb bud to another site resulted in normal limbs; however, if the bud were rotated 180° in its new location, its dorsal and ventral orientation was normal relative to the remainder of the body, but its anterioposterior relations were reversed. Thus, the anterior polarities of the limbs were shown to be established earlier in the embryo than the dorsoventral. Later investigations have shown that in the chick the first of these axes is established at the 5-somite stage, the second at the 13-somite, but the limb disks themselves are not distinguishable until the 14-somite stage. However, recent studies on the axolotl have found that reversal of polarities gives rise to supernumerary limbs (Maden and Goodwin, 1980). If half of the limb bud were destroyed, the remaining half gave rise to a complete limb; similarly if the bud were slit vertically into two segments and prevented from fusing by means of an inserted membrane, each part developed into a normal leg. Fusing two limb buds with all axes in normal orientation produced a single large limb that was soon reduced to usual size. Other experiments on late (tail bud) axolotl embryos have yielded comparable results (Figure 4.10; Slack, 1980a), and supernumerary structure production has proven also to depend on the orientation of a graft (Javois and Iten, 1981; Javois *et al.*, 1981).

Additional experiments gave rise to the field concept. When all the limb disks normally involved in producing the limb were removed, a limb still developed after a brief lapse of time, but when another ring of tissue was also removed around the disk, no appendage was formed. Thus, there appeared to be a field, all of which had the full potential for forming the entire structure, even after some major part had been extirpated or added; however, each such field was limited in area. This property can be viewed, as it has been, as a positional effect, but it could also stem from the early inductive influences of the endoderm already pointed out.

Later Influences in Wing Development. While the amphibian limb is more readily available for study, its small size proved a deterrent to further progress in experimental embryogeny, so the larger areas offered by the chick embryo soon replaced the former, after the sophisticated techniques devised by Zwilling (1961) made such studies feasible. As in amphibians the ectoderm has

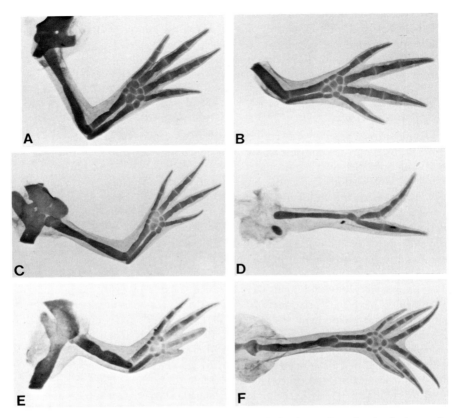

Figure 4.10. Regulation of forelimb development in axolotl embryos. In each pair of micrographs, the left-hand member shows the results of development in place of one half of a given forelimb bud, the right-hand member the other half of the same bud transplanted elsewhere on the embryo. (A) The posterior half developed *in situ*. (B) The anterior half developed after grafting onto the side of the embryo. (C, E) Anterior halves developed *in situ*; (D, F) the corresponding posterior halves developed following grafting onto the head (D) or onto the side (F). (All courtesy of Slack, 1980a.)

proven to be essential for development of the fore appendage and as there induces growth but does not serve in differentiation. However, a contrast has been found in that only the special apical ectoderm that covers the mesoderm is effective. Epidermis from other regions of the embryo fails to influence limb growth, as does also like tissue from earlier embryonic stages (Berrill and Karp, 1976). The apical ectoderm consists of two cell layers, the first of which lies beneath the basement membrane and consists of a plate of tall, irregular columnar cells, loosely associated except at their bases. In turn this is covered by the peridermal layer, comprised of flattened cells. In these layers, as well as in other developing limb tissues, the cells are uniformly polarized, the nucleus of each component being located toward the same end of the cell as that of each neighbor (Holmes and Trelstad, 1977, 1980).

If the apical ectoderm, or apical ridge as it is also called, were removed early in embryogeny, the mesoderm grew and differentiated but only to a limited extent, the proximal portion being produced nearly normally to the elbow, at which point development virtually ceased (Hampé, 1960). When only the cranial half of the apical ridge was excised, the radius and thumb portion failed to develop, and correspondingly when the caudal half was removed, the ulna and most of the phalanges and associated parts were wanting (Saunders, 1948). However, the ridge does not carry specific instructions for differentiation but only permits growth, for replacing it during limb elongation with comparable tissue from either younger or older embryos had no effect (Amprino, 1965).

As the wing develops, the mesoderm undergoes specialization into presumptive regions influenced by positional effects along the proximodistal axis. Apparently from the time of its arrival at the limb bud site, the mesoderm is competent to form the basal region of the wing, as already indicated. At stage 18 of the chick, when the bud is still a low mound, the extreme outer portion develops into the presumptive region for forearm and carpus formation (Figure 4.11). This enlarges along with the basal area until at stage 22 the distal part becomes the prospective metacarpus tissue. Recent investigations have demonstrated that the mesenchymal cells in the central area (core) are more inclined to form cartilage when isolated and cultured than are peripheral ones (Ahrens *et al.*, 1979), but on the other hand, the latter give rise most frequently to myogens (Figure 4.12). Thus, a transverse pattern of determination exists even in these early stages. Commitment to either cartilage or muscle is made by stage 25 in developing chick limbs, an act involving the conversion of NAD into poly(ADP ribose) with the excision of nicotinamide (Harris, 1974; Caplan *et al.*, 1979).

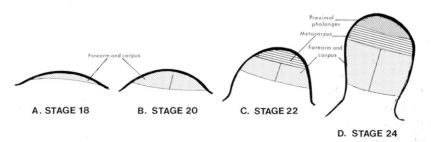

Figure 4.11. Development of the chick wing. As the wing develops from the low initial bud (A), it gives rise to the several presumptive tissues indicated, which increase in size with time. (Based on Amprino, 1965.)

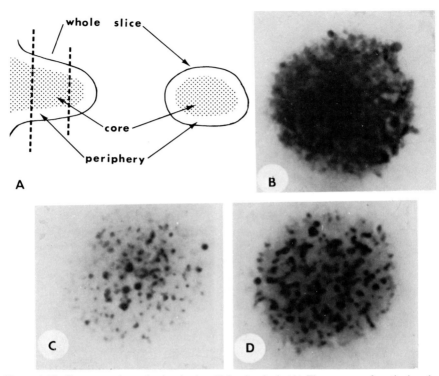

Figure 4.12. Transverse determination in the chick wing bud. (A) The manner of sectioning the wing bud. (B) A 3-day-old culture of cells from the core stained with alcian blue at pH 1.0. The cartilage matrix is darkly stained. (C, D) Similarly prepared cultures of the same age, (C) from cells of the peripheral area and (D) from the whole slice. Cartilage nodules are few in number in the former, relative to those in the latter. B–D, 10×. (All courtesy of Ahrens *et al.*, 1979.)

Increase in mass continues in each of the three portions until stage 24 when a long, stout cylinder represents the forming wing, the distalmost portion being converted to the proximal phalanx tissue (Figure 4.11D; Amprino, 1965). Similar patterns of growth and differentiation also appear to exist during mammalian limb formation, including activities of an apical ridge, which is active also in amphibians. According to Hamilton (1952) all regions of the wing are present from the beginning but occupy differing portions of a gradient, the parts along less steep slopes developing more rapidly. Thus, the proximal limb (stylopod) develops first, the distal limb (zeugopod) next, and the carpus and phalanges (autopod) last. More recently, hand representation, too, has been established as being present in the earliest limb bud by marking with [3H]thymidine-labeled blocks of cells transplanted into various regions of growing limbs (Stark and Searls, 1973; Stocum, 1975a).

Differentiation of Tissues. Just prior to the formation of the autopod, skeletal and muscle differentiation are initiated in the proximal one-third of the limb bud (Stocum, 1975a). The differentiation of bone commences with the synthesis of proteoglycans (Karasawa *et al.*, 1979) and the condensation of the mesenchyme cells into a central core of cartilage precursor; this is followed in turn by the synthesis of chondroitin sulfate in that region, accompanied by a degree of that activity in the remaining tissues (Searls, 1965). However, the differentiation of cartilage is also preceded by changes in the intercellular communication centers at specific sites in the precartilage mesenchyme (Newman and Frisch, 1979; Newman, 1980). Around this early frame, myoblasts align in cords and fuse into myotubules, as already described. These differentiating tissues are consistently separated from the ectodermal ridge by a narrow zone of undifferentiated cells until the autopod begins to develop, when it is lost. Thus, three types of cells are derived from the early mesenchyme, muscle, fibroblasts of the soft connective tissue, and chondroblasts (Newman, 1977), but their precursors still remain problematic.

4.2.2. Limb Regeneration

Additional details of limb formation have been provided by the numerous experiments that have been conducted on the regeneration of limbs, a phenomenon exhibited among postnatal vertebrates only by salamanders, for even the anurans lose the ability by the time of metamorphosis (Forsyth, 1946; Polezhaev, 1972; Scadding, 1977). However, all adult vertebrates can regenerate muscle tissue lost through injury, largely through myogenesis of mononuclear satellite cells (Nag and Foster, 1981). In salamanders, prolactin and thyroxin play important roles in the processes (Hessler and Landesman, 1981).

Essential Stages in Regeneration. When an entire limb is amputated for experimental purposes, the general practice is to leave a short stump of the humerus or femur. After amputation, the muscle, skeletal, and connective tissues just proximal to the sectioned surface have been thought to undergo dedifferentiation into single mesenchymelike cells, whose tissue of origin can no longer be determined (Thornton, 1938; Hay, 1958, 1959; Hay and Fischman, 1961; Lentz, 1969; Schmidt, 1969). This concept, however, has currently been reevaluated and the dedifferentiation of cells, at least those of muscles, no longer is accepted (Mauro, 1961; Moss and Leblond, 1971; Ontell, 1974; Bischoff, 1979; Snow, 1979). All recent evidence points to the muscle satellite cells as the source of new myogens during regeneration, cells that are laid down early in the embryonic development of those organs. In light of this knowledge, it is not unlikely that the connective tissues, too, will prove to contain a population of undifferentiated cells that provides new mesenchymelike cells during regeneration. Nor is the information for regeneration segmentally arranged as in insects, but is organized in a single limb sequence (Pescitelli and Stocum, 1981).

At any rate, while the replacement cells are developing, a wound epidermis grows over the exposed surface to become covered later by an apical epidermal ridge not unlike that of the embryo. After this covering has developed, the new cells from the proximal tissues migrate distally and accumulate into a mass referred to as the blastema. Formation of this mass, however, is dependent upon the presence of a neuron, a requirement that provides the greatest distinction between embryonic and regenerative processes (Harrison, 1907; Hamburger, 1938; Singer, 1952). The blastema elongates into a conical configuration as the cells proliferate rapidly, in general undergoing differentiation much in the fashion of an embryonic appendage.

Originally it was believed that the blastema possessed no capacity of its own for organizing the differentiating tissues but was guided by the adjacent stump tissues, or field, which had given rise to it (Milojević, 1924; Weiss, 1925, 1927; Schotté and Hummel, 1939). However, it has subsequently been established that, in limb regeneration, the field effects which specify the missing parts are actually properties of the blastema itself, because even the youngest of that type of tissue is capable of regenerating complete appendages in the absence of a stump, providing the systemic requirements have been met (Polezhaev, 1936; Trampusch, 1966; Stocum, 1968a, b, 1975b; Dinsmore, 1974; Carlson, 1978).

Nevertheless, changes in determination of the blastema do occur while it becomes increasingly distal in location, as shown by experimentation. When a blastema was transplanted onto a stump shorter than its origin, that is, one that ended proximally to the original level of the transplant, a normal leg was produced under the regulatory influences of stump tissue. In contrast, when one was grafted onto a stump longer than its own, that is, distal to its point of origin, it was capable of producing only the outer parts of the appendage (Stocum, 1975b, 1978; Holder *et al.*, 1980; Krasner and Bryant, 1980). The regenerating blastemas formed over proximal stumps have been found to contain 60% more cells than those of distal origins (Maden, 1976).

Apparently the skin, too, plays an important directive role in limb regeneration. If a half cuff of skin from either the posterior or anterior portion of skin was appropriately grafted to a host limb and the latter then amputated through the graft after it had healed, results were obtained that varied in correlation to the skin source. Limbs with double anterior skin formed normal or slightly reduced replacements, whereas those with double posterior skin produced double posterior regenerates (Slack, 1980b). However, it does not appear that any specific role can be assigned to skin or any other single tissue, if the results of experiments with mirror-image halves in various combinations (double-half limbs) are of significance (Tank, 1978). If double-half forelimbs comprised of symmetrically arranged flexors and extensors were covered by normally arranged skin, they underwent complete regeneration but did not do so when covered by double-half skin (Tank, 1979). On the other hand, limbs with double-half deep tissues and normal skin failed to regenerate normal products.

Irradiation and Regeneration. When given a sufficiently high dose of X rays, regeneration of an amputated urodele limb is inhibited permanently, regardless of whether the irradiation was applied to the whole body or locally (Brunst, 1950; Maden and Wallace, 1976). In adult specimens, irradiated stumps merely healed over, but in young larvae the remnant continued to regress until the entire limb disappeared (Butler, 1933). The loss of regenerative powers has been attributed to the resulting abnormal mitoses (Horn, 1942), blockage of the cell cycle being in either the G_1 or G_2 phase (Maden, 1979a). Although for a while it appeared that grafts of unirradiated tissues, such as skin, muscle, or cartilage, could restore X-irradiated amputated limbs to their normal regenerative capacities (Umanski, 1937; Trampusch, 1951, 1958), it has since been found that the cells for the regenerated parts actually had been derived from the grafted tissue (Umanski, 1938; Maden and Wallace, 1976; Wallace and Maden, 1976). Further experimentation with rotated blastemas has demonstrated that, while incapable of cell division, the irradiated tissue is still capable of providing positional signals (Maden, 1979b, 1980).

4.2.3. Chondrogenesis and Osteogenesis

Since the preceding discussions of limb development and regeneration repeatedly intimated the importance of the skeletal system in those processes, examination of the formation of such elements is an obvious prerequisite to the molecular aspects of the subject. Although in a strict sense the term chondrogenesis refers to the formation of cartilage, here the developmental processes of other connective tissues are given occasional attention, along with the inseparable companion topic of osteogenesis.

As cartilage undergoes development it passes through several well-marked stages: (1) Initially in limb buds the mesenchyme becomes organized in the proximal half as a core of loosely packed cells, interconnected by sparse cellular processes (Jurand, 1965). (2) The core becomes more compact as the cell density and number of interconnections increase to form the so-called cartilage blastema, or bone anlage (Searls, 1973; Thorogood and Hinchliffe, 1975). (3) Secretion of a metachromatic extracellular matrix then begins the expression of the characteristic cartilage phenotype, that is, chondrogenesis proper.

Collagen Formation. In all connective tissues, the one indispensable substance is collagen, the formation of the several types of which has been extensively explored. The precursor to the protein, procollagen, is processed in the endoreticulum (Nist *et al.*, 1975; Olsen *et al.*, 1975) and dictyosomes of fibroblasts, after which it undergoes condensation in the Golgi vesicles, before being secreted into the milieu by exocytosis (Revel and Hay, 1963; Trelstad,

1971; Weinstock, 1972, 1977; Trelstad *et al.*, 1974). After being secreted, the procollagen molecules must have the amino and carboxyl termini removed before they can be assembled into collagen fibrils (Bornstein *et al.*, 1972; Morris *et al.*, 1975). Although the *in vivo* assembly mechanisms by which additions are made to the small initial fibrils have not been established, intermediate aggregates possibly exist as they do in experiments. *In vitro* the aggregates of the short fibrils interact to produce long, linear subunits, to which later terminal and lateral additions gradually form a subfiber (Gross and Kirk, 1958; Veis *et al.*, 1967).

This preliminary outline of the formative processes has recently been extended through an ultrastructural investigation of tendon collagen-fibril synthesis in chick and mouse embryos (Trelstad and Hayashi, 1979). The presence of aggregates of the collagen fibrils within fibroblasts suggested that fibrilogenesis *in vivo* begins by the intracellular formation of subassemblies which are then secreted by exocytosis. Once in the external environment, the subassemblies are added to the ends of fibrils that are contained in deep recesses of the plasma membrane, the additions being made in such a fashion that the fibroblast exercises control over the particular characteristics of the fibril morphology.

The Nature of the Fibroblast. Although it was established many years ago that fibroblasts from different tissues were not identical in behavior, the early observations received attention only recently. Parker (1932a, b) had demonstrated clearly that nine different tissues from a chick embryo gave rise in cell cultures to that same number of contrasting populations of this type of cell, each quite stable and distinguished from one another by several unique characteristics. Among the more currently uncovered distinctions that exist between populations are different morphological traits, concentrations of lysosomal enzymes, reactions to such reagents as trypsin-EDTA and prostaglandin, and types of glycosaminoglycans and interferons synthesized (Milunsky *et al.*, 1972; Beug and Graf, 1977; Conrad *et al.*, 1977a, b; Ko *et al.*, 1977; Colonndo, 1981). Moreover, fibroblasts from chick cornea, heart, and skin have proven to be distinct antigenically, some of the antigens being located on the cell surfaces (Garrett and Conrad, 1979). The glycosaminoglycans from the several cell types also have been shown to be distinct, as were also the properties of the respective hyaluronic acids and chondroitin 6- and 4-sulfates (Conrad *et al.*, 1977b). One type of these cells that has been especially investigated, the myofibroblast, is contractile and contains numerous microtubules; it seems to be active in the contraction of wounds and scars of mammals (Rudolph and Woodward, 1978).

Other Chondrogenetic Molecules. Besides collagen, three classes of substances have been found to be important in chondrogenesis, glycosaminoglycans, chondroitin sulfate, and hyaluronic acid, as pointed out above. In the formation of cartilage, complex interactions between fibronectins, glycosaminoglycans, and collagen occur that result in the formation of cartilage beads or nodules (Ruoslahti and Engvall, 1980), which products then accumulate to form the cartilage proper. A current study focused on the activities of the chondroitin sulfate and hyaluronic acid in the hind limbs of normal and brachypod mouse embryos (Shambaugh and Elmer, 1980) and found that in normal embryos synthesis of the latter substance decreased beginning at 12½ days whereas that of the other increased. Hyaluronidase activity also experienced a sharp rise at the same time, but the increase was transitory. In the brachypodal mutants the changes were similar but occurred a half-day later; most striking was the slower loss of hyaluronic acid, which took place when turnover rate would be expected to be increasing. cAMP has been shown also to increase in abundance during avian limb chondrogenesis (Solursh et al., 1979).

Changes in the fibrose content of the forming cartilage have attracted the attention of a number of investigators recently. In the chick limb bud, type I collagen was reported in the extracellular matrix during stage 2 of chondrogenesis, which occurred in that structure in stage 23 and 24 embryos (Linsenmayer et al., 1973; von der Mark et al., 1976).* Shortly afterwards (chick embryo stages 25 and 26), stage 3 of chondrogenesis commenced, being marked in part by the appearance of type II collagen and the onset of metachromatic staining of the matrix (von der Mark, 1979). By the time the cartilage was mature, type I collagen was no longer present. These results have undergone extension somewhat by a current investigation that employed immunofluorescent techniques with antibodies against fibronectin and the two types of collagen (Dessau et al., 1980). Both fibronectin and type I collagen were present in the extracellular spaces, even during stage 1 of cartilage development, but both substances increased more rapidly in the core than in surrounding mesenchyme as stage 2 proceeded to reach a maximum and stage 3 was initiated. Thereafter the type I protein was gradually replaced by type II, disappearing completely from mature cartilage as noted previously, the loss being accompanied by a similar one on the part of fibronectin.

Influencing Factors. A small number of factors have now been established as influencing growth or maturation of cartilage or other connective tissues, one of which is bone matrix gelatin (Urist et al., 1978). Much of the knowledge of this substance has been garnered from tissue culture and regeneration researches. Normally connective tissue cells derived from muscle do not undergo differentiation into any other form, but when experimentally treated as by transplantation or explantation, they migrate and proliferate, whereas the muscle fibers degenerate. During proliferation, which begins within 24 hr after treatment, the cells synthesize DNA and hyaluronidase at high levels, providing bone matrix gelatin is present. Slightly later, these syntheses are followed by production of large quantities of chondroitin sulfate, addition of which sub-

---

*The nature of the collagen molecule has to be passed by without discussion, as the subject, a highly complex one, is currently in a state of flux. The reader is referred to von der Mark and von der Mark (1979) and Upholt et al. (1979) for insight into the problem.

stance to the medium enhanced the further formation of cartilage, whereas hyaluronic acid depressed it. Consequently, it was made evident that mature muscle tissue exhibits a developmental potential equal to that of embryonic limb mesenchyme, but whether the tissue harbored inactive embryonic cells programmed for cartilage or simply contributed fibroblasts that became dedifferentiated could not be determined. However, the gelatin clearly switched the path of development of such cells from the fibrous connective cells they normally would have become in muscle tissue to chondroblasts.

Dedifferentiation of chondroblasts has been shown to be induced by a basic protein purified from chick embryo extract (Schiltz and Ward, 1980), as did also the impure fraction I of the same material. The former, which had a molecular weight of 72,000, led chick chondroblasts to lose their metachromatic matrix and become motile, assuming a spindle shape like that of fibroblasts in the processes, accompanied by ultrastructural changes (Holtzer et al., 1960; Anderson et al., 1970). They also have been found to synthesize such characteristic substances of fibroblasts as hyaluronic acid and type I collagen (Hamerman et al., 1965; Nameroff and Holtzer, 1967; Schiltz et al., 1973). Purified extracts of the avian substance inhibited chondroblast collagen synthesis at low concentrations, an effect that proved not to be tissue specific. However, it did exhibit some degree of species specificity in not being effective on human fibroblasts (Schiltz and Ward, 1980).

Another factor, either a glyco- or phosphoprotein having a molecular weight of 50,000, has been purified from mouse embryo extract that had an opposite effect (Richmond and Elmer, 1980). This component, when added to the cultures of 11½-day mouse limb mesenchyme, led to a threefold increase of $^{35}SO_4$ incorporation into sulfated glycosaminoglycans, along with an even more pronounced rate of the latter's accumulation. Furthermore, it stimulated type II collagen deposition and the formation of cartilage nodules. The protein was active in both 10- and 13-day embryos but increased in effectiveness in the older examples.

During the embryogeny of the chick and quail, mesenchyme cells from the developing wing were unable to produce cartilage cells until the embryo had attained stage 22 (Hamburger and Hamilton, 1951), and somewhat comparable observations have been made on the mouse (Grüneberg, 1963). However, later studies have refined this point somewhat, by showing that the capability is actually acquired by stage 19 embryos (Solursh and Reiter, 1980). Moreover, the cells form cartilage in cultures only when they are maintained at adequate densities, as in pellets (Karasawa et al., 1979), an observation that has given rise to a concept of a critical cell mass requirement for differentiation (Grobstein, 1955). Thus, it has been supposed that interaction between small groups of cells plays an essential role.

Osteogenesis. The later events in the development of the skeleton have also received detailed attention. In the formation of long bones in vertebrate embryos, the perichondrium that envelops the cartilaginous precursor has been shown to be transformed into the inner layer of the periosteum of the eventual bone, the perichondrial cells being converted into osteoprogenitor cells (Scott-Savage and Hall, 1980). Concurrently, the outer (fibrous) layer was formed from cells of the adjacent connective tissue. The next step in the osteogenetic processes was the deposition around the periphery of osteoid, the unmineralized product of fully differentiated osteoblasts. These subperiosteal activities were revealed to be dependent upon continuous interaction between the osteoblasts and adjacent hypertrophied chondroblasts (Scott-Savage and Hall, 1979). In the chick embryo the timetable of events included the conversion of the perichondrium into the inner periosteum and the presence of outer periosteum at 6½ days, whereas osteoid was present a half-day later. Mineralization of the cartilaginous matrix, the early stage of bone formation, was initiated at 7½ to 8 days (Lufti, 1971; Holder, 1978).

In muscle of adult rat and in cultured neonatal rat muscle (Urist *et al.*, 1968; Nogami and Urist, 1970), bone matrix gel induced the formation of cartilage and bone within 7 to 15 days and lamellar bone and marrow in 20 to 30 days (Urist *et al.*, 1973), supposedly due to a morphogen named bone morphogenetic protein (Urist *et al.*, 1977). The substance, apparently a glycoprotein whose molecules were rapidly diffusible, did not seem to be species specific, because the protein from rabbit induced new bone formation also in rat tissues (Urist *et al.*, 1979).

A number of biochemical changes have been found to precede the actual deposition of calcium phosphate, particularly involving the proteoglycans. Four discrete forms and great heterogeneity characterize the latter class of substances, including aggregated, aggregating, nonaggregating, and intermediate size (Hardingham *et al.*, 1972; Hascall and Heinegård, 1974; Vasan and Lash, 1977, 1979). Shortly before being transformed into bone, the cartilage in the growing zone of the epiphysis, previously avascular, became invaded by capillary sprouts, largely through lysosomal activities. Enzymes from those organelles induced a shift from the large proteoglycan aggregates that previously had occurred there to small aggregates and nonaggregating monomers, thereby creating a new environment favorable to the accretion of calcium phosphate. However, more recently it has been demonstrated that the nature of the proteoglycans synthesized likewise underwent a change during differentiation (DeLuca *et al.*, 1977). At the early wing-bud stage (18), the proteoglycans were small monomers; later these were followed by intermediate-size types and, finally, by aggregated ones, the latter increasing in relative abundance during further differentiation (Ovadia *et al.*, 1980). These observations may be correlated to a point raised in Chapter 3, Section 3.2, which showed that proteoglycans were essential to development beyond the blastula stage.

4.2.4. Controls of Limb Development

Although there can be no doubt that each of the factors active in the formation of the skeletal substances affects limb development to at least a comparable extent, there are others whose effects are of a broader nature. One of these that is especially striking in the production of the vertebrate limb is the presence of neurons, but there are others of a more specific nature that also have become evident. However, the role of nerves has received by far the greater portion of the attention.

Neuronal Influences. Although it has long been established that gross morphogenesis of limbs, but not myogenesis (Sohal and Holt, 1980), can occur quite normally in amphibian embryos in the absence of innervation of that structure (Harrison, 1904, 1907; Hamburger, 1939; Yntema, 1959),* limb regeneration in adults is dependent upon the presence of neural elements (Singer, 1952, 1974; Thornton, 1970). However, reformation of certain other skeletal parts, including the jaw of adults, is completely independent of nervous influences (Finch, 1969). Since the problem is thus one of exceptional complexity, the approaches that have been taken toward its solution have necessarily been greatly diversified.

Denervation Experiments. One of the most frequent techniques employed to that end is that of denervating the growing or regenerating limb, as illustrated by a recent investigation into the mechanisms of developing the individual muscles (Grim and Carlson, 1979). In this study 58 limbs of adult newts were amputated at the middle of the humerus and later denervated when regeneration had progressed to the middle or late bud stage. Those appendages that had the nerves removed at the earlier stage either ceased development or underwent regression, but 62% of those denervated later continued to regenerate and subsequently developed the individual muscle primordia quite normally. Because denervation and X irradiation behave similarly in inhibiting stump regression, a number of newts have been exposed to various levels of X rays prior to amputation of nerve-dependent parts (limb) or nerve-independent (lower jaw) (Wertz and Donaldson, 1979). Unirradiated salamanders and those exposed to only 250 R of X rays regenerated jaws or limbs normally, but those treated with larger dosages failed to do so in all cases. Since both systems gave similar responses, it was concluded that nerves were not involved directly in X-irradiation effects.

Although the mode of action of neural elements in regeneration remains obscure, some progress has been made at the molecular level. Synthesis of protein, RNA, and DNA was reported to decline rapidly after denervation of

---

*A reexamination of this aspect of embryogenetic development makes the supposed distinction less sharp (Sohal and Holt, 1980). Whereas forming muscle paralyzed chemically differentiated nearly normally, the myoblasts and myotubes in developing muscle (that was prevented from becoming innervated) died and degenerated, being replaced by connective tissue.

late-stage regenerating limbs (Dresden, 1969; Morzlock and Stocum, 1972; Bantle and Tassava, 1974), but the major effects of interruption of nerve supply were displayed in the early bud stage. In such denervated parts, synthesis of the various classes of macromolecules dropped off rapidly (Singer and Caston, 1972; Singer and Ilan, 1977). Since all the decreases seemed to point toward a possible change in polysome number, a search was subsequently made to detect and quantify polysome size and quantity through use of [^{35}S]methionine (Bast et al., 1979). The results indicated that 48% less radioactivity was present in denervated regenerating limbs than in the controls; consequently, it was concluded that the nerve-dependent depression of protein synthesis was in part mediated through a diminished number of ribosomes. But since the greater portion of ribosomes consists of proteins, it is more likely that the reduced quantity of those organelles was a result of the decreased protein synthesis, rather than a cause.

If denervation occurs sufficiently late in regeneration, differentiation and morphogenesis are not influenced (Singer and Craven, 1948), although growth is always inhibited by that treatment. The critical point apparently depends on the degree of differentiation that has occurred in the blastema (Dearlove and Stocum, 1974). Because the initiation of differentiation of this mass is marked by deposition of cartilage anlagen, researches have been conducted into the effects of denervation on collagen production (Mailman and Dresden, 1979). Among the results obtained was the demonstration that, in early regenerates, synthesis of collagen was reduced at a rate three times as great as that of other proteins. Differentiation of the blastema is negatively influenced also by the apical ectodermal ridge in embryonic development (Saunders, 1948; Summerbell, 1974). Throughout limb development it maintained, in an undifferentiated condition, those mesenchymal cells that lie within 0.5 mm from it, but if cAMP levels were raised through use of various agents that stimulate its synthesis, they underwent differentiation (Kosher and Savage, 1980).

The question has arisen whether the various types of nerves, sympathetic, motor, and sensory, exercise different kinds of controls. For a time evidence appeared both to favor and to deny the existence of a special influence on the part of catecholaminic (sympathetic) fibers, but the problem unknowingly was complexed by lack of complete recognition of such nerves. Now it has been established by means of histofluorescence techniques that supposed strictly motor or sensory nerves may actually contain a number of catecholaminic fibers, too (Taban et al., 1977), and that fluorescent dendritic cells are present in regenerating limbs (Taban et al., 1978).

Patterns of Innervation. In light of the increasing complexity that is being revealed in neuronal effects on limb development and regeneration, a number of experimental studies have recently focused on the patterns of innervation in appendage formation. One investigation used horseradish peroxidase as a label for identifying cells of the lumbar ventral horn that sends projections into developing hind limbs of *Xenopus* (Lamb, 1976). This horn actually is lateral in location and corresponds to the lateral motor column in birds and mammals; it supplies only the musculature of limbs, including that of the pelvic region, however. During early growth of the limb bud, the first motor axons grew to the mesenchyme closest to the point of entry, but later they appeared to be guided to limb regions more approximate to the site of their cell bodies within the ventral horn. Briefly stated, the pattern of innervation of this appendage included the following generalizations: (1) Cells supplying proximal muscles lay rostrally in the ventral horn; (2) those that extended to distal muscles tended to lie caudally; (3) medial cells (near the central canal) innervated those muscles that were ventral during embryogeny, including knee flexors; and (4) ventrolateral cells (away from the canal) supplied the dorsal muscles (Lamb, 1977). Still later, as a number of the ventral horn cells perished, various abrupt changes in projection patterns brought about the definitive innervation. No mechanism for guidance of the neurons to their particular sites was identified, but it has been suggested to be related to positional information. Previously Weiss (1941) had suggested that the earliest fibers innervating a given region did so in random fashion and that subsequent ones followed the nearest of these pioneer ones. However, in reversed grafts the motor axons did not actively seek out their appropriate targets (Summerbell and Stirling, 1981).

The innervation of supernumerary hind limbs in *Xenopus*, both naturally occurring ones and transplants, intimates that more may be involved than that provided by the foregoing simplistic model. Using grafts and deviating the three normal limb nerves from their usual courses, it has been shown that only the nerve known as S9 could lead to muscular contraction in the grafted leg (Kleinebeckel, 1979). Although the other two, S8 and S10, were involved along with S9 in innervation of normal legs and were capable of providing movement of such parts, they did not do so in grafts. In chick embryos as well as *Xenopus*, artificial supernumerary limbs reduced the total number of nerve cells that died by about 20% (Hollyday and Hamburger, 1976; Hollyday and Mendell, 1976) and naturally occurring supernumerary limbs in the African clawed toad were found to have a comparable effect (Lamb, 1979a).

Neuronal Death. Among the striking features of limb development is the involvement of neuronal death as a normal constituent of the processes. After the transition toward acquisition of the adult pattern of innervating *Xenopus* hind limbs had progressed for a period, there was an abrupt disappearance of the earlier neural projections (Lamb, 1977). Although part of this loss may have stemmed from degeneration of older branches, much of it appeared to derive from the death of the neurons—as many as 75% of the total ventral horn cells that had been produced experienced this fate, the caudal cells generally dying to a greater extent than the rostral ones. While it has been commonly supposed that the caudal neurons of the ventral horn which perish are those that have lost in competing with rostral ones for the limited number of postsynaptic sites present in the limb, other factors seem to be involved as well (Lamb, 1979b). This was effectively demonstrated by experimental removal of the rostral part of the ventral horn, after which the caudal cells perished in large numbers despite the lessened competition.

4.3. LIVER DIFFERENTIATION

Current investigations on the vertebrate liver have more frequently centered on regeneration and carcinogenesis in this organ than on development, but studies on the latter aspect also have been active to a considerable extent. In vertebrates as a whole, the liver arises late in somite formation as a large evagination on the ventral side of the archenteron; the outpocketed appendage then becomes intimately associated with the surrounding mesenchyme, which acts as an inducer. Briefly stated, the inductive influence of the mesenchyme promotes the differentiation of the endothelium to produce the hepatic cells, accompanied by a number of changes at the macromolecular level. It is of interest to note that when larval *Xenopus* liver cells were grown in cultures in which they formed only two-dimensional aggregates, they nevertheless developed bile canaliculi with microvilli and complex junctions between cells and also synthesized liver-specific proteins (Wahli *et al.*, 1978).

Fetal Liver Protein Synthesis. During the fetal stages of mammals, the liver secretes two major proteins into the bloodstream, which, while having 35% homologous primary structures (Innis and Miller, 1980; Gorin *et al.*, 1981), display diametrically opposite life histories. Moreover, the gene structure is identical, consisting of 15 separated sectors in each case (Chapter 8; Kioussis *et al.*, 1981). One of these is albumin, whereas the other is α-fetoprotein (Abelev, 1971), the appearance and subsequent history of each of which has recently been followed in fetal and neonatal pigs (Carlsson and Ingvarsson, 1979). In young fetuses, 2.5 to 9.0 cm in crown-to-rump length, all the hepatocytes were found by immunofluorescence to secrete α-fetoprotein actively, but with increasing age and size, synthesis gradually decreased in quantity, although all cells still participated in its production. Further diminution in quantity continued after birth (Karlsson, 1970; Gitlin, 1975; Nayak and Mital, 1977), but no cells that were not active in this process were detected until the sixth day after parturition. No cells in adult pigs appeared to produce this protein, and investigation into the mRNA and use of a complementary DNA confirmed that in adult rats this protein is virtually absent (Innis and Miller, 1977).

In contrast, almost no liver cells synthesized albumin until the fetus had attained a length of 9 cm, when 50% of the hepatocytes showed a low level of such activity. An increase then continued steadily, 20-cm-long fetuses showing 95% of the cells active in albumin production, and neonatals displayed 100% of the cells very active in its synthesis (Carlsson and Ingvarsson, 1979). While the precise rate of synthesis of this protein was not determined in adults, it has been described as one of the dominant blood proteins during all of postnatal life (Schreiber *et al.*, 1970; Peters, 1975). Three populations of hepatocytes have been recognized during development, one of which secreted α-fetoprotein only, another that secreted albumin as well as the other protein, and a third that produced neither (Valet *et al.*, 1981).

In rat and mouse fetuses, much the same sequence of events has been found to exist, the chief proteins being identified as albumin and α_1-fetoprotein, the latter a glycoprotein with a molecular weight of 72,000 (Watabe, 1974; Watanabe *et al.*, 1975; Hannah *et al.*, 1980; Liao *et al.*, 1980). However, in the rat the yolk sac also proved to be active in secretion of the fetoprotein (Masseyeff *et al.*, 1975). Because antibodies to either of these substances showed strong cross-reactivity with the other one also, it has been suggested that α_1-fetoprotein is chemically related to the albumin and may serve as a fetal type of that protein. In addition to this property, it has been reported to bind estradiol selectively and accordingly has been conjectured to protect the fetus from influences of the maternal endocrine system or perhaps from the maternal immune response through interaction with certain lymphocytes (Keller *et al.*, 1976; McEwen *et al.*, 1976; Murgita *et al.*, 1977).

A large number of liver proteins appear to undergo quantitative or qualitative changes during ontogeny, to judge from the diversity that has so far been reported (Goldsmith, 1981). Among these is a metallothionein, a ubiquitous sulfhydryl-rich heavy-metal binding protein in the adult human, containing 6.7 g atoms of zinc, 0.2 atom of cadmium, and 0.1 g atom of copper (Bühler and Kägi, 1974). In the fetus, however, the protein contained much more of the latter metal, there being 1 or 2 g atoms/mole, but no cadmium was detected (Riordan and Richards, 1980). Another interesting set of studies focused on the changes in serine metabolism in the late fetal and neonatal rat, quantifying activities of four enzymes of the liver that act upon that amino acid (Snell, 1980). Just before birth the *de novo* biosynthesis of serine was demonstrated to be greatly enhanced relative to this activity after birth. Then during the suckling period, serine catabolism in the liver became diminished, at the same time being accompanied by increased gluconeogenesis, with serine acting as the source (Snell, 1974). At weaning when the liver grew rapidly, the serine appeared to serve primarily as a precursor for nucleotides along with its usual role in proteinogenesis.

Changes in Nucleic Acids during Differentiation. Because the liver cells of the bullfrog (*Rana catesbeiana*) do not divide during metamorphosis (VanDenbos and Frieden, 1976), yet secrete a number of new enzymes at that time, it has been hypothesized that changes in the tRNA population might play a role in the regulation of the genes involved (Klee *et al.*, 1978). To investigate this suggestion, the relative amounts and heterogeneity of 10 tRNAs were examined in tadpoles and adults by reversed-phase column chromatography. The profiles of isoaccepting species of seven of these showed no qualitative or quantitative differences, but tRNAs^{Phe} from tadpoles contained a minor species that was absent from adults. Moreover, quantitative differences were observed in several types. In the isoaccepting species of tRNA^{His}, slight contrasts in relative proportions were found between tadpoles and adults, whereas those of tRNA^{Met} displayed marked distinctions, possibly as a result of the higher levels of the initiator species present in the tadpole.

Ultrastructural Changes during Ontogeny. The developmental history of liver cells has been followed under the electron microscope in both the chick and rat embryos (Karrer and Cox, 1960, 1961; Ceico, 1964; Dallner *et al.*, 1965, 1966a,b; Luzzatto, 1981) and in the case of the latter animal into early postnatal life (Chedid and Nair, 1974). In this rodent, the liver primordium appears on day 11 of gestation (Elias, 1955), at which time the cells contain prominent centrioles, multiple large dictyosomes, a few peroxisomes, and numerous free ribosomes. In addition, the irregularly formed nucleus bears several prominent nucleoli, the rather sparse mitochondria are nearly circular and contain small, flat, irregularly arranged cristae, and a rough endoreticulum consiting of one or two single flat cisternae may also be noted in electron micrographs. Two days later, however, the rough endoreticulum had become extremely abundant, occupying much of the cytoplasm with irregular single cisternae, whereas the mitochondria had increased in number, although unchanged in structure. On day 15 of gestation, the rough endoreticular cisternae were so swollen that they appeared to be of the vesicular type, and the mitochondrial cristae were somewhat better organized. However, on day 17, the organelles had begun to acquire more of their definitive characteristics, the rough endoreticulum commencing to form orderly arrays of cisternae and the mitochondria displaying intracristal lumina for the first time. Thus, by day 20, the latter organelle had acquired the elongate-ovate shape and flat transverse cristae that characterize it in the vertebrate tissues as a whole. In addition, a peculiar type of smooth endoreticulum could be noted for the first time. By the time of birth, the nuclei had become rounded, the rough endoreticulum was in the usual multiple arrays typical of vertebrate cells, with small patches of smooth here and there, and well-formed mitochondria and perixisomes were quite abundant. Smooth endoreticulum remained relatively rare even through 5 days following birth, and attempts to induce an increase with phenobarbital proved unsuccessful (Chedid and Nair, 1974; Dillon, 1981, pp. 221, 225).

Studies in Liver Regeneration. The liver of mammals has an unusual ability to replace damaged or removed tissue, but the mechanisms that control these regenerative processes so far have remained elusive (Bucher, 1963). DNA synthesis reaches a greatly enhanced maximum rate within 24 hr of hepatectomy, but chromatin structure is not changed (Simpkins *et al.*, 1981). Although there is a modest increase in the rate of protein synthesis following partial hepatectomy, a greatly decreased rate of degradation also must occur to account for the rapid net increase of protein accumulation. Such a decrease has now been documented through the demonstration that the half lives of proteins become nearly doubled during the first 2 days of regeneration (Scornik and Botbol, 1976; Tauber and Reutter, 1978). Since lysosomes have been shown to be involved in protein degradation, as discussed in earlier sections, the changes in two important lysosomal endopeptidases following partial hepatectomy were the subject of a recent investigation (Suleiman et al., 1980). The two, cathepsins B_1 and D, were compared to changes in total synthesis of proteins, all species of which decreased in parallel for the first 18 hr. However, at 24 hr total liver protein increased rapidly, while the two proteolytic enzymes continued to decrease, cathepsin B_1 falling to a level of 12% of controls at 36 hr at a time when total protein had reached 40% of normal.

Researches into mRNA changes during regeneration have typically also included hepatomas as the experimental subject, as well as normal liver tissues. Development of hepatomas of varying degrees of malignancy typically was accompanied by reduced concentrations or absence of such liver proteins as albumin and α_{2u}-globulin (Schreiber et al., 1969; Sell, 1974; Sippel et al., 1976). As might be expected, the molecular basis for the depressed synthesis has been found to be correlated with decreased mRNA levels (Sippel et al., 1976; Tse et al., 1978; Sala-Trepat et al., 1979). Although 97% of the detectable cytoplasmic and nuclear proteins of Novikoff hepatoma ascites cells and of regenerating and normal liver cells have been demonstrated to be identical and to occur in similar proportions (Hirsch et al., 1978a; Takami and Busch, 1979; Takami et al., 1979), a limited number of mRNAs that were abundant in regenerating liver were shown to be present in greatly reduced quantities in hepatomas (Hirsch et al., 1978b). Using this information, a later study attempted to determine whether posttranscriptional or transcriptional control mechanisms were responsible for the differences by employing cDNA–RNA hybridization analyses, the results of which indicated that the latter was chiefly responsible (Reiners and Busch, 1980).

Some additional light is thrown on such pathological changes in protein content by a study of the chromatin during D-galactosamine-induced liver-cell injury similar to that of viral hepatitis (Keppler et al., 1968; Weiss et al., 1976). During experimental induction of some cell damage, the concentration of uridine triphosphate has been reported to decrease, which loss has been suspected in turn to inhibit synthesis of RNA. This deficiency is generally considered to have to endure for a period of 2½ hr in order to generate hepatitis, but once induced the cell damage is irreversible, as all the injured hepatocytes perish. Since nonhistone proteins are often considered to be active in gene regulation (Elgin and Weintraub, 1975), one group of researchers investigated the chromatin-associated proteins of that class to find whether any changes could be observed. The SDS-gel electrophoretic analyses revealed that a number of such proteins were greatly reduced in quantity during induced hepatitis and in several cases, completely absent (Weiss et al., 1976).

Although liver cells of adult rats divide only rarely under normal circumstances, they regain the ability to proliferate under the influence of stimuli such as removal of part of the liver mass or loss through carbon tetrachloride dosage (Mourelle and Rubalcava, 1981). Such growth, in contrast to neoplastic growth, ceases when the original mass of the organ has been regained. Recently two investigations traced the changes in gene expression that followed partial hepatectomy (Colbert *et al.*, 1977; Scholla *et al.*, 1980). The sequence complexity in the polysomal mRNA ranged up to 20,000 species about 72 hr after the operation, somewhat exceeding the diversity of normal livers at that point but not previously. However, no evidence for regenerating-liver-specific mRNAs could be found. Consequently, quantitative differences, rather than qualitative, were deduced to exist in the mRNAs of this organ during regeneration.

4.4. DIFFERENTIATION OF REPRODUCTIVE ORGANS

As will be recalled in the first chapter it was necessary to outline the early period of gonad development in both sexes in order to understand the beginning stages of gametogenesis. Accordingly the present discussion can be largely confined to the later aspects of the differentiation of the reproductive organs, with mammals and birds receiving the major share of attention. In all higher vertebrates, two pairs of potential reproductive tracts, the Wolffian and Müllerian, develop in the embryo, only one set of which undergoes differentiation into the definitive form, the particular pair that is developed being dependent on the sex of the individual.

Early Differentiation. In males the set of Wolffian ducts, derived from the involuting mesonephri, are the basis for the future sex organs, for from them are formed the vasa efferentia and deferentia, seminal vesicles, ejaculatory tubules, and epididymides. On the other hand, the Müllerian ducts provide the basis for much of the female system, including the oviducts, uteri, and the anterior three-fifths of the vagina (Zuckerman, 1940; Forsberg, 1973; Cunha, 1975). That the testes play the principal role in the early processes has been shown by castration of fetal rabbits (Jost, 1947). Regardless of the sex, in all such individuals the Müllerian ducts differentiated, whereas the Wolffian underwent regression. In contrast, if fetal testes were implanted into castrated fetuses of either sex, the Wolffian ducts developed while the Müllerian set degenerated; however, crystals of testosterone similarly implanted had a like effect on the Wolffian organs but did not induce regression of the second set of ducts. Thus, it was proposed that the fetal testis produces two morphogenetic substances, an androgen and an unknown substance which inhibits Müllerian duct differentiation.

An ultrastructural investigation of these processes found extensive cytolysis in both developing and regressing male and female reproductive organs

(Dyche, 1979). In the involuting Wolffian ducts and differentiating Müllerian ducts of females, the destruction of cells was carried out by intracellular lyso-somal activities and by phagocytosis on the part of neighboring tissues. In males both of these processes were active in the degenerating Müllerian duct, whereas the former type of action alone served in the morphogenesis of the Wolffian. Furthermore, during the loss of the Müllerian duct of males, re-gressed epithelial cells were extruded that appeared to induce the transforma-tion of adjacent mesenchyme into an epitheloid cell cuff, absent during break-down of the Müllerian duct in the other sex.

Influences in Female Tract Differentiation. In avians and also in some reptiles a modified set of events occurs in females, whereas differentia-tion in males, which begins around day 8, is as just described. On day 9 of incubation, the right Müllerian duct of female chick embryos begins to regress in company with both Wolffian ducts, whereas the left one commences to dif-ferentiate, ultimately to become the functional oviduct of the hen. Conse-quently, this system affords unusual opportunities for the study of control mechanisms, that have not gone entirely unnoticed. Early experiments had in-dicated that sex steroid hormones influenced the loss of both Müllerian ducts in male chicks and the right ones in females (Wolff and Wolff, 1947, 1951; Hamilton, 1961; Groenendijk-Huijbers, 1962). [³H]-estradiol showed that sites were present in the cells of the left Müllerian duct that reacted specifically with that hormone, the number of which increased from day 8 to day 12 of incuba-tion, where a plateau was reached (Teng and Teng, 1975a,b). The receptor was proteinaceous and in two forms, one sedimenting with a coefficient of 8 S, the other with 4.5 S. After estradiol had reacted with the receptor, the complex was rapidly transferred to the nucleus (Teng and Teng, 1976), a reaction that has been noted in adult tissues also (Shyamala and Gorski, 1967, 1969).

Comparisons of chromatin changes in the right and left female Müllerian ducts have been fruitful to a degree. In the left organ the nonhistone chromatin protein increased gradually to day 15 and remained level beyond that point until after hatching, whereas that of the right member increased at first but then slowly decreased (Teng and Teng, 1978). Additionally, although no specific information emerged concerning the nature of the changes, antibodies to the histones of newly hatched chicks were found to react only slightly with the chromatin of early embryos and still less with that from the degenerating right duct.

Still another line of investigation has been employed to pursue the ques-tion of how these dissimilarly differentiating ducts and ovaries produced steroid hormones, secretion of which has been reported to be initiated in the embryonic stages (Weniger and Zeis, 1971; Galli and Wasserman, 1973; Guichard *et al.*, 1973; Haffen, 1975). Organ culture techniques applied to embryonic reproduc-tive systems, along with additions of various hormones and other reagents, showed the right ovary to respond more actively than the left in several regards

(Teng and Teng, 1977). Although both ovaries were stimulated by the addition of chorionic gonadotropin to the medium, the right one produced testosterone and cAMP more efficiently, secreting the latter substance at a rate 80% greater than that of its mate. Both responded to the presence of the gonadotropin approximately equally in estrogen production; however, other hormones including thyrotropin, growth hormone, and insulin exhibited no effect.

Influences on Male Tract Differentiation. Since there are no asymmetric reproductive systems in male vertebrates comparable to those of female avians, mammalian fetuses have proven to be more popular than those of avians for developmental studies of this sex. Although secretion of androgens by the fetal testis had been established about a decade ago to play an important role in the differentiating processes (Jost, 1970; Jost *et al.*, 1973), the factors regulating testosterone secretion remained unknown. In the earlier stages of development, chorionic gonadotropin was found to stimulate androgen production, the levels of this hormone being at their maximum when testosterone was first synthesized (Abramovich *et al.*, 1974; Clements *et al.*, 1976; Huhtaniemi *et al.*, 1977). Cultured fetal testes from pigs and radioimmunoassay of steroids from the culture medium have recently been employed in exploring the possible role of the fetal pituitary in early testis function (Raeside and Middleton, 1979). Regardless of the age of the fetuses when the organs were explanted, the addition of chorionic gonadotropin to the medium consistently induced the testes to secrete testosterone; however, the quantities elicited did increase with age. Moreover, secretion of this hormone appeared to commence at a later stage of development than androgen synthesis *in vitro* could be induced by gonadotropin.

Experiments with fetal guinea pigs, while stressing the differentiation of the male reproductive organs, have afforded comparisons with hormonal effects on female systems, too. In individuals of the former sex, the testes became capable of synthesizing androgens between days 24 and 26, at the time when they acquired morphological distinction from the undifferentiated gonad (Block, 1967; Brinkmann, 1977; Rigaudiere, 1977; Sholl and Goy, 1978). Whereas testes retained this ability throughout the remainder of their intrauterine term, ovaries synthesized only minimal amounts of those hormones before day 40. Both types of gonads *in vitro* could also aromatize androstenedione to estrogens, but ovaries were superior in this activity. In developing male guinea pigs, androgens have been shown to be important, not only for the differentiation and maintenance of the reproductive tract, but also for the differentiation of the central nervous system, which during adulthood controlled sexual behavior and the release of gonadotropins (Goy *et al.*, 1964; Price *et al.*, 1967). Possibly the effects on the nervous system were actually induced by estrogens that had been aromatized from those hormones (Naftolin *et al.*, 1971). At least in some mammalian species, the female tract was claimed to be protected against the masculinizing effects of the androgens by the presence of progesterone (Cagnioni *et al.*, 1965); however, in view of the levels of progesterone being the same in fetuses of both sexes throughout prenatal life (Buhl *et al.*, 1979), this is scarcely likely.

4.5. DIFFERENTIATION OF BLOOD CELLS

One further tissue of vertebrates is worthy of space here—the blood; in fact, the genetic basis for differentiation of the red and various white blood cells from a single progenitory stock is sufficient in itself to disclose much of the problem involving control of developmental processes. The embryonic origins of the hematopoietic tissues and their subsequent paths of migration are so complex as still to remain subject to controversy. Current dogma considers their pluriopotential stem cells, along with primary erythroid cell lines, to arise from the mesoderm of the yolk sac, from which locale of origin they are carried in the forming bloodstream to colonize a diversity of hematopoietic sites (Moore and Owen, 1965, 1967a,b; Moore and Metcalf, 1970).

In lymphocytes two differing pathways of development are followed, correlated to the site of origin. Those stem cells that occupy the liver of embryonic mammals or the bursa of Fabricius of birds become the B cell (bursa type) (Moore and Owen, 1966; Owen *et al.*, 1976), whereas those that become established in the thymus epithelial rudiment become T cells (thymus type) (Moore and Owen, 1967b; Owen and Ritter, 1969). However, these differences become more significant in Chapter 7 where they are shown to play important roles in immune reactions. The remaining cell types often share common points of origin, the liver being especially active in the early processes of granulocyte production and secondary erythroid differentiation. Later, the myelopoietic tissues of other regions, including the bone marrow, and still later the spleen and thymus, secondarily are supplied pluripotential stem cells from this organ and become the principal site of hematopoiesis in adults (Moore and Metcalf, 1970; Moore *et al.*, 1970). In larval frogs some differences have been noted in that the erythrocytes are the principal blood cell produced by the liver, the generation of which takes place in discrete foci of the sinusoids. The point of embryonic origin of the frog liver hematopoietic tissues remains in doubt, however, but it may be an extrinsic source located dorsally (Turpen *et al.*, 1979).

Comparative Aspects. In order to provide an overall view of the several aspects of hematopoiesis in vertebrates, Table 4.1 lists the organs or tissues in which the four principal classes of the processes occur. At the lowest levels of the subphylum, the spleen, in which all the types of blood cells are made at first, is not a discrete organ, but in the hagfish consists only of cords of cells in the submucosa of the intestine and in the lamprey of tissues in the intestinal typhlosole. Thus, the erythrocytes, granulocytes, lymphocytes, and megakaryocytes (which give rise to thrombocytes or platelets) may be perceived to have

Table 4.1
Blood-Cell-Producing Areas of Vertebrates [a]

Vertebrate group	Erythropoiesis	Granulopoiesis	Lymphopoiesis	Megakaryopoiesis
Hagfish	Splenic cords (intestinal submucosa)	Splenic cords	Splenic cords	Splenic cords
	Divide in bloodstream	—	—	Divide in bloodstream
Lamprey	Splenic tissue (intestinal typhlosole)	Splenic tissue	Splenic tissue	Splenic tissue
	Intestinal submucosa	Intestinal submucosa	—	—
	Divide in bloodstream	—	—	Divide in bloodstream
Sharks	Spleen	Spleen	Spleen	Spleen
	—	Kidney	Kidney	—
	Divide in bloodstream	Intestinal submucosa	Intestinal submucosa	Divide in bloodstream
Ganoid fishes	Spleen	Gonads	Spleen	Spleen
	—	Kidney	Kidney	—
	Divide in bloodstream	Intestinal submucosa	Intestinal submucosa	Divide in bloodstream
Teleost fishes	Spleen	—	Spleen	Spleen
	Kidney	Kidney	Kidney	Kidney
	—	Intestinal submucosa	Intestinal submucosa	Intestinal submucosa
	Divide in bloodstream	—	—	Divide in bloodstream
Lungfish	Spleen	—	Spleen	Spleen
	Intestinal submucosa	Intestinal submucosa	Intestinal submucosa	—
	Divide in bloodstream	Kidney	Kidney	Divide in bloodstream
Salamanders	Spleen	—	Spleen	Spleen
	—	Intestinal submucosa	Intestinal submucosa	—
	—	Liver	Liver	—
Frogs	Spleen	—	Spleen	—
	Bone marrow[b]	Bone marrow	Bone marrow	Bone marrow
	—	Intestinal submucosa	Intestinal submucosa	Divide in bloodstream
	—	Kidney; pronephros in embryo and tadpole	—	—

(*Continued*)

Table 4.1 (Continued)

Turtle	Spleen	Spleen	Spleen	Spleen
	Bone marrow	Bone marrow	Bone marrow	Bone marrow
	—	Intestinal submucosa	Intestinal submucosa	—
Birds	(Spleen)[c]	—	(Spleen)	(Spleen)
	Bone marrow	Bone marrow	Bone marrow	Bone marrow
	—	Intestinal submucosa	Intestinal submucosa	—
	—	—	Bursa of Fabricius	—
Mouse (adult)	Spleen	Spleen	Spleen	Spleen
	Bone marrow	Bone marrow	Bone marrow	Bone marrow
	—	—	Thymus	—
	—	—	Lymph nodes	—
	—	—	Peyer's patches of intestine	—
	—	—	Appendix	—
Mouse embryo (age in days)	Yolk sac (7–13)	—	—	—
	Liver (10–20)	Liver (8–20)	—	Liver (8–20)
	Spleen (14→)	Spleen (13→)	Thymus (13→)	Spleen (13→)
	Bone marrow (15→)	Bone marrow (15→)	Lymph nodes (16→)	Bone marrow (15→)

[a] Based in part on Metcalf and Moore (1971) and Siegel (1970).
[b] Red blood cells produced here only before metanephros forms and during hibernation.
[c] Only to a limited degree.

had common origins even in adult cyclostomes, that is, they all arise from the same original population of progenitory stock, the stem cells. Although at the somewhat higher phylogenetic level represented by the sharks the spleen has become a separate organ, this early location of hematopoietic tissue in the intestine remains reflected in the continued existence of at least lymphopoietic activity in the submucosa of that organ here and throughout the entire subphylum Vertebrata, including the most advanced classes. Among the less advanced members, the primitive nature of some of the blood cell types may be observed in their undergoing replication in the bloodstream after being released from the hematopoietic tissues. While beyond the level of the lungfish the erythrocytes become too specialized to continue this trait, the megakaryocytes continue to do so to the frog level of evolution. Another particularly noteworthy feature is the relatively late phylogenetic advent of the bone marrow as a blood-producing tissue, which arrives on the scene only with the frogs and other anurans (Table 4.1).

What is difficult to understand from an evolutionary standpoint is the absence of participation in the blood cell production on the part of the liver among the lower classes of vertebrates, since in mammalian embryos that organ is the sole or principal site of activity early in embryonic development. For instance, the pronephros is the only source of granulocytes in embryonic and early larval stages of *R. pipiens* (Carpenter and Turpen, 1979). According to the principle of ontogeny recapitulating phylogeny, it would appear that the liver should be an active site of hematopoiesis in the cyclostomes at least. If in the adult of the hagfish and lampreys that organ does not contain the necessary tissue types, it should surely be expected to be active in this function during the developmental stages.

4.5.1. Erythropoiesis

To avoid unnecessary repetition of needless details in this section on the production of erythrocytes, or erythropoiesis, the processes are examined at only the principal site of synthesis, and a similar practice is followed in the other sections. The chief locale of synthesis of red blood cells in adult mammals is the bone marrow, in which better than 44,000 colony-forming units, or stem cells, out of a total of 51,500 are located in mature mice (Metcalf and Moore, 1971). However, in neonatal mice less than 10% (250) of the total present (3700) are located in the bone marrow, the liver containing about 75%. The stem cells have proven to persist throughout the life of the individual and to be multipotential in that each can produce progeny that lead to the production of any of the major lines of blood cells (Ford *et al.*, 1956; Lajtha, 1970). However, it should be borne in mind that such stem cells do not behave identically throughout the body or even in a given tissue, a number of diverse populations often coexisting at many sites (Playfair and Cole, 1965; Hodgson, 1967; Lajtha *et al.*, 1969). Also it should be remembered that the marrow is an extremely complex tissue (Castro-Malaspina *et al.*, 1980), containing a large variety of cells aside from those involved in blood formation (see Weiss, 1970, for a concise review).

The stem cells that give rise to erythrocytes are of two general types, based on their colony-forming abilities in response to a hormone called erythropoietin to be discussed in more detail in a later paragraph. That variety referred to as CFU-E gives rise to erythroid colonies containing between 8 and 256 erythroblasts, as described in the next section; it responds to low concentrations of the hormone and the colony develops quickly. The second type, BFU, requires high levels of erythropoietin to produce often macroscopic colonies containing up to 1000 erythroblasts requiring several days to mature (Barker, 1980).

Stem-Cell Kinetics. Stem cells exist in two physiological states in blood-forming tissues of all sorts. While a large fraction continues to undergo endless cell divisions with doubling times of 10 to 12 hr (Till *et al.*, 1964; McCulloch, 1970), for extensive periods the remainder is in a resting state, not undergoing mitotic division. As might be expected, these stages are reversible and either cycling or resting cells may be induced to enter the opposite state by unknown triggering factors. In general, the proliferation rate is higher among the larger cells, quite low in the smaller ones, and intermediate in those between the two extremes of size (Yoffey, 1980), an observation which intimates that the reversibility of state may be not so real as has been suspected. However, a point is ultimately reached in a substantial portion of the progeny where the cell becomes a potential target for activating substances to induce its entrance into an irreversible process leading to the formation of definitive blood cells. Thus, a parallel to gametogenesis may be perceived to exist between the early stages of these processes. A difference between the two that sharply sets them apart is that in hematopoiesis, multiple cell divisions occur beyond this point of "decision" in contrast to only the two of meiosis that are characteristic of gamete production.

Erythropoietin. The activating factor in the formation of red blood cells is erythropoietin, a glycoprotein containing hexose, hexosamine, and sialic acid (Gordon and Zanjani, 1970; Lowy, 1970; Erslev *et al.*, 1978). The factor from man, which has a molecular weight between 50,000 and 60,000, appears to be active on other mammals but not on birds or frogs, the converse being equally true (Rosse *et el.*, 1963; Rosse and Waldmann, 1966). Once it was believed that the kidney was the sole and immediate source for this activator, but now it is known that the hormone is produced in the blood serum induced by another chemical (renal erythropoietic factor or REF) which is chiefly of renal origin (Peschle *et al.*, 1967). Although other sources of REF are known to exist, they have not been identified.

The effect of the erythropoietin is to induce certain of the committed cells, those known as erythropoietin-sensitive cells, to differentiate into proerythroblasts, the first morphologically distinguishable precursor of erythrocytes. Secondly, it also appears to stimulate proliferation of such cells (Hodgson, 1970). However, at the macromolecular level its chief action is on transcription of DNA by increasing both RNA polymerase and DNA-template activities (Goldwasser and Inana, 1978). The earlier stages of erythropoiesis are controlled by factors other than erythropoietin (Iscove, 1978).

Developmental Stages. The production and maturation of erythrocytes involve a number of stages, most of which have received detailed ultrastructural analysis, at least in those from mammalian sources (Ackerman *et al.*, 1961; Beams and Kessel, 1966; Bank *et al.*, 1970; Orlic, 1970). Much of the present discussion is based on the text and micrographs contained in the last citation, which deals with the processes in the spleen of the house mouse. The first cell type is, of course, the stem cell, the progenitor of all the varieties of blood cells. It is characterized by the presence of a very irregular nucleus, bearing two or more nucleoli and typically having condensed chromatin around the periphery, which trait continues into the proerythroblast stage. The stem cells of the yolk sac and liver appear to be similar to those from the spleen (Bank *et al.*, 1970), whereas those of the mesonephros in frogs may be distinctive (Broyles *et al.*, 1981; Hågå and Kristiansen, 1981). Another feature of these cells that exists throughout the erythropoietic processes until just before their close is the presence of numerous free ribosomes throughout the cytoplasm. The rather scarce mitochondria are largely rounded in form, with one or two elongate-ovate members also being present as a rule, and contain relatively few swollen but poorly defined tubular cristae. In addition, scattered examples of endoreticulum may be observed, heavily coated with ribosomes; although these organelles are usually described as of the cisternal variety, they appear to be more aptly considered tubular.

The first committed stage, the erythropoietin-sensitive cells, is indistinguishable under the electron microscope from the stem cell, at least at the present time. After this type has been exposed to erythropoietin, however, a small number of structural changes may be noted, especially in the nucleus. Although the undulant configuration of that body persists, the irregularities are somewhat diminished, the chromatin becomes less compactly arranged beneath the nuclear envelope, and the nucleoli appear somewhat more vesicular. In the cytoplasm of these young proerythroblasts, the presence of numerous polysomes may be perceived, and the cristae of the mitochondria seem to begin a transition from the tubular type toward the more familiar flattened saccules of other organs. At least in later populations of proerythroblasts, the Golgi material becomes increasingly abundant, especially in the neighborhood of the centriole.

After an undetermined number of proerythroblast generations, the progeny eventually begin to acquire deposits of ferritin within their cytoplasm and then are marked as early erythroblasts. Generally speaking these iron-containing molecules appear as siderosomes, that is, electron-opaque particulate clusters contained in a vesicle that is not enclosed by a membrane. The presence of these particles ushers in the secretion of hemoglobin by the cell, deposits of which gradually fill the cytoplasm and even the nucleus. The latter body, now almost completely devoid of the irregular contours that characterized earlier stages, undergoes a series of changes in the nature of its chromatin and steadily decreases in size until it is less than half the original diameter. In the very young (or basophilic) erythroblast, the nucleolus (or nucleoli) remains as a prominent feature but gradually loses its identity as the chromatin becomes increasingly more compact and electron-opaque. By the time the second substage (the polychromatophilic erythroblast) has been attained, the chromatin has been compacted into a number of disconnected, irregular bodies placed around the envelope. In the final substage, the orthochromatic erythroblast, those isolated bodies increase in size and interconnect, until near the close of this stage the entire nucleus, now greatly reduced, consists entirely of that material except for scattered patches of hemoglobin-filled nucleoplasm. This stage terminates as the nucleus first assumes an eccentric location and then is expelled from the cell to form the early erythrocyte substage, called a reticulocyte. After this activity is completed, the enucleated cell gradually loses its ribosomal content and other organelles to become the transparent, definitive erythrocyte.

Expulsion of the nucleus from the erythroblast of mammals may be carried out by any one of several procedures, but autophagic destruction, once believed to be a chief mechanism, has been found to be nonexistent in these cells (Awai et al., 1968). In bone marrow, the nucleus may be removed as the cell passes from the compartment in which it has formed into the venal sinus for transport by the bloodstream (Tavassoli and Crosby, 1973). The pores through the partition between the two chambers being too small for passage of the whole cell, the cytoplasm works its way through by means of amoeboid movements, but the nucleus is too rigid and is left behind. In other hematopoietic sites, the aperture appears to be unnecessary in an essentially similar series of steps (Simpson and Kling, 1967; Skutelsky and Danon, 1967).

Ontogenetic Development of Erythrocytes. As shown in Table 4.1, hematopoiesis begins in mesenchyme areas of the yolk sac on day 7 or 8 of mouse fetal life, with the initiation of erythropoiesis (Moore and Metcalf, 1970). On the next day immature erythroblasts enter the bloodstream, where they mature into nucleated erythrocytes (normoblasts) (Craig and Russell, 1964; de la Chapelle et al., 1969; Marks and Rifkind, 1972; Rifkind et al., 1974). At day 11 of gestation, while still in the erythroblast stage having ribosomes, the cells actively synthesize hemoglobin of embryonic types (Kovach et al., 1967) and undergo frequent mitotic divisions in the bloodstream until day 13 (Fantoni et al., 1969). Rounded mitochondria are also present at this stage, albeit in very small numbers (Bank et al., 1970). Later, at days 14 to 15 after the ribosomes disappear in the normoblast stage, the ability to synthesize hemoglobin is, of course, lost along with protein production in general. In the opossum the yolk sac stage is extremely short, for all traces of its activities have been lost by the time of birth, 12½ days after conception (Cutts et al., 1980); this is in contrast to the mouse fetus in which the yolk sac normocytes can be detected until day 14 or 15 of gestation (Fantoni et al., 1969; Rich and Kubanek, 1979).

Between days 10 and 11 of fetal mice, stem cells enter the bloodstream from the yolk sac islands and are carried through the body until they enter the liver, where they undergo proliferation, maintaining red blood cell production thence until just after birth. During the first 5 days of hepatic erythropoiesis, that is, until day 14 or 15, the proerythroblasts are erythropoietin-sensitive and undergo rapid cell divisions, showing doubling times of about 8 hr (Tarbutt and Cole, 1970), after which it is slowed to 48 hr. The erythropoietin-sensitive cells have been found to undergo one or two cell divisions before becoming recognizable proerythroblasts (Cole et al., 1975). In any case, the blood cells produced by the hepatic hematopoietic tissue are enucleated and appear in the bloodstream beginning with day 12. These somewhat smaller products, how-

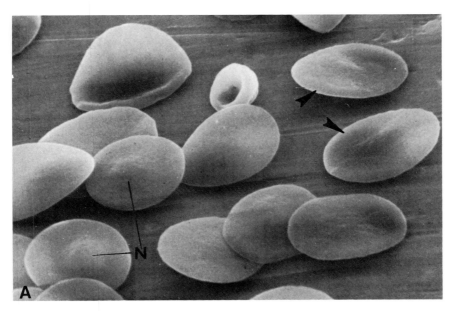

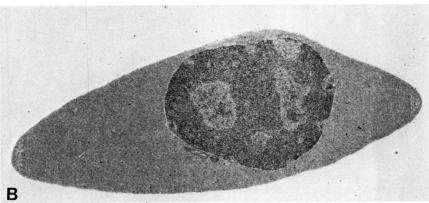

Figure 4.13. Red blood cells of the neonatal opossum. (A) This scanning electron micrograph reveals most of the large red blood cells (megaloblasts) to be ovate and nucleated, the nucleus (N) producing a bulge; in addition some enucleated cells (arrowheads) lacking a central depression are also present, while a small enucleated cell is located near the top. 2700×. (B) These cells are found by transmission electron microscopy to possess few organelles aside from the large nucleus and a few mitochondria. 13,500×. (Both courtesy of Cutts *et al.*, 1980.)

ever, contain ribosomes, at least early in their life cycles, and consequently are able to produce hemoglobin, which is apparently of the adult type (Kovach *et al.*, 1967).

In the neonatal opossum the red blood cells are large erythroblasts of a peculiar form (Figure 4.13), referred to as megaloblasts, being irregularly ovate and nucleated and containing ribosomes and mitochondria (Cutts *et al.*, 1980). These persist for about 3 weeks after birth, gradually becoming increasingly rare as the usual enucleated erythrocyte becomes predominant. In kangaroo pouch young at birth the red blood cells were likewise found to be megaloblasts which predominated in the bloodstream until day 10 postpartum, after which they decreased rapidly in numbers until they disappeared entirely at day 25 (Richardson and Russell, 1969). These were probably early products of the liver tissues, despite the claim that they were of yolk sac origins; normoblasts were their first replacement, which cell type remained abundant during the 200 days of the study. Unlike the opossum, the fetal type of hemoglobin was present after birth until day 7 to 40, depending on the individual, after which only the adult type could be found; thus, no correlation between hemoglobin and cell type was in evidence.

The very beginnings of the blood-cell-forming processes have received only scant attention (Wilt, 1974), but what has been established is highly provocative. In the chick, the first cells already determined for hemoglobin production are found in the newly laid egg embryo in the form of the marginal zone components of the blastoderm. Within 24 hr of oviposition, these cells have become transformed into tight clusters of basophilic cells in the splanchnopleuric mesoderm that soon gives rise to an endothelium, from which hemoglobin-containing erythroblasts are liberated after about 10 to 14 hr. Once these blood islands have thus been formed, X irradiation and antimitotic agents are without effect, nor is erythropoietin effective (Malpoix, 1964; Wilt, 1967). A further study showed that, during the early formation of the blood islands from splanchnopleuric mesoderm, the erythropoietic precursor cells sorted themselves into foci that underwent further differentiation (Miura and Wilt, 1970). If such aggregation was prevented, no blood islands developed and hemoglobin synthesis was nearly inhibited. Both processes also appeared to be dependent on association with endoderm, perhaps for an inductive influence.

Changes in Hemoglobins. The changes in the molecular structure of hemoglobins during development undoubtedly provide the most thoroughly explored example of ontogeny at the macromolecular level. In man, cattle, and goats, but not rodents nor horses, three major categories of this substance may be recognized, embryonic, fetal, and adult, with numerous minor variations and mutant forms (Gratzer and Allison, 1960; Muller, 1961; Bertles, 1970, 1974). Basically four different polypeptide chains are involved, various combinations of which produce the several major and minor types, the definitive molecule being a tetramer. At least in humans two clusters of genes exist, one of which encodes the α-family (α and ζ) and the other the β-family or non-α chains, including β, δ, and γ, and ϵ (Kabat, 1974).

The first hemoglobin to appear in human embryos is the hemoglobin (Hb) Gower 1, which has the tetrameric structure $\zeta_2\epsilon_2$ (Huehns *et al.*, 1961), followed closely by Hb Gower 2, which has the subunit structure $\alpha_2\epsilon_2$. Hence, the α chain is synthesized quite early in embryogenesis. Synthesis of the ϵ chain ceases at the 12th week of pregnancy, but before that event, it seems also to become combined with an additional type of subunit, γ, in the form of $\gamma_2\epsilon_2$ (Kleihauer and Stöffler, 1968). At the close of the third month of gestation, HbF (fetal hemoglobin) becomes the dominant form of the pigment. While this blood protein has the subunit composition $\alpha_2\gamma_2$, two alleles of the second subunit exist, designated as $^A\gamma$ and $^G\gamma$, depending on whether alanine or glycine occupies site 136 of the polypeptide. As a result of recent studies, it has been found that the proportions of these two nonallelic forms change shortly after birth (Schroeder *et al.*, 1971; Vedvick *et al.*, 1980). During late fetal life and in the neonatal, the chains are in a ratio of 75 $^G\gamma$: 25 $^A\gamma$, but this becomes rapidly altered in the first several months of life to the definitive 40 $^G\gamma$: 60 $^A\gamma$. However, the later reference cited was able to demonstrate that the reduction in the glycine-containing component was actually initiated by month 6 of pregnancy.

Then at week 32 of gestation in man, β-chain synthesis is begun, whereas δ-chain formation is initiated just prior to birth. Thus, the umbilical cord of the newborn contains three types of hemoglobin, 75 to 90% of which is HbF, the remainder largely HbA ($\alpha_2\beta_2$) with perhaps 0.2 to 0.4% HbA$_2$ ($\alpha_2\delta_2$) (Kabat, 1974). The α, β, and γ chains have all proven to be coded by multiple cistrons in man and other mammals (Nute, 1974; Rucknagel and Winter, 1974; Schroeder and Huisman, 1974). After birth the production of HbF gradually is reduced, whereas that of HbA is increased, until the former has almost disappeared at about month 9 of age.* How the switch from the γ to the β chain is controlled remains an unresolved problem, but the fetal type may reappear under stress or disease, such as in thalassemias β (Pearson, 1974). Some evidence supports the concept that reprogramming of Hb synthesis occurs in erythroid precursorial cells (Terasawa *et al.*, 1980; Vainchenker *et al.*, 1980), but at least two mechanisms appear to exist in sheep (Barker *et al.*, 1980).

A similar transition from larval to adult types of Hb accompanies metamorphosis in *Plethodon* and *Xenopus* (Flavin *et al.*, 1979; Just *et al.*, 1980). Although larvae were shown to have less than adult Hb in the latter genus, by completion of metamorphosis this amount had increased to 30%, and 2 weeks later the red blood cells of froglets contained 90%, while mature specimens

---

*Between 0.2 and 7.0% of adult human red blood cells are so-called F cells, which contain between 14 and 30% HbF. However, all early erythroid precursors from normal adults produced both HbF and HbA when cultured (Peschle *et al.*, 1980; Dover and Boyer, 1981).

displayed around 99% adult type. The suggestion was advanced that the rapid transition resulted from elimination of larval erythrocytes, while a new line of those cells brought about the increase in adult Hb.

Other Changes. After transcription, the several variants of the α, β, and γ chains may undergo enzymatic modification (Abraham *et al.*, 1979). Among these modifications is acetylation and combination with a hexose molecule (Bunn *et al.*, 1978), but the functional significance of such treatments is still obscure. However, the most important other changes that occur in red blood cells are those that take place on their surfaces (Aizawa *et al.*, 1980). A recently studied example of these alterations is provided by antigens on the chick erythrocyte surface (Miller *et al.*, 1979), which were reacted with a label consisting of hemocyanin complexed with specific antisera. The antigens were detected on the very earliest red blood cells formed in the extraembryonic mesenchyme, even before circulation began, and continued to be present until hatching. At the latter time the antigenic sites completely covered the cell surface, but they gradually diminished with age and no longer could be detected in 7-month-old chickens.

Somewhat comparable studies using double fluorescence staining on differentiating mammalian erythrocytes have yielded parallel results, those accompanying enucleation being especially striking. For instance, an irregular distribution of certain membrane constituents was observed during those processes in rat cells (Skutelsky and Farquhar, 1976). As the nucleus acquired an eccentric location, the density of receptors of the reagent known as concanavalin A became markedly greater in the membrane over the nuclear portion than elsewhere, whereas those membrane components (possibly sialoglycoproteins) that stained with colloidal iron hydroxide were more abundant on the contrasting part. Moreover, with mouse erythroid cells a comparable set of events involving spectrin was observed, the latter protein becoming concentrated in the membrane over the cytoplasmic region, while concanavalin A became restricted to the nuclear section as before (Geiduschek and Singer, 1979).

4.5.2. Granulopoietic Gene Changes

The traditional view of granulopoietic events held that (1) a common granule-bearing precursor, the progranulocyte, gave rise to the three varieties of granulocytes, the neutrophils, eosinophils, and basophils. From this common point of origin, it was conjectured that (2) each type followed a similar pattern of differentiation and granulogenesis, and (3) that the specific granules were derived from the so-called azurophil granules of the progranulocytes, after (4) those granules had undergone partial degradation. Furthermore, it was conceived (5) that the transition from the rounded nucleus of the progranulocyte to the polymorphic ones of the definitive blood cells began at the midpoint of differentiation of the latter and could be used as an index to the age of the later stages.

Evidence from more recent sources, however, has painted a somewhat different picture of the events (Wetzel, 1970a). Perhaps the most drastic change in interpretation is that (1) no common progranulocyte is regarded as existing, because the very earliest granule-bearing cells can be recognized as early stages of either neutrophils, eosinophils, or basophils. Moreover, (2) the "azurophil" granules of each line differ structurally and cytochemically, and (3) in many cases the specific granules are derived from different precursorial particles. In addition (4) each type of granulocyte follows a distinctive pattern of development, especially with regard to the respective granules and the structure of the nucleus, the latter organelle (5) undergoing change to the polymorphic condition at different rates in each case. Thus, the nucleus does not provide a reliable index to the maturity of the cells. To adjust to the newer knowledge it has become necessary to follow Wetzel (1970a,b) in dropping the older terminology for precursorial cells, the term myeloblast alone being retained for the earliest nongranulated precursor (Sainte-Marie and Sin, 1970).

The Myeloblast. The myeloblast of the marrow is characterized first by the large, round nucleus, in which the chromatin is extremely dispersed, and by the absence of leukocytic granules and the paucity of endoreticulum (Capone *et al.*, 1964). Further, the nucleolus is large and finely vesicular, while the cytoplasm contains few mitochondria. Although scarce in normal marrow tissue, cells of this stage are more abundant during myeloblastic leukemia, to the cells of which they are morphologically similar. They also appear to give rise to monocytes (Moore *et al.*, 1976) and macrophages (Williams and Eger, 1978; Hirai *et al.*, 1979) and undergo rapid proliferation, about 40% of a given cultured colony synthesizing DNA at a given time. The products of leukemic marrow and fetal liver tissue, but not normal bone marrow, respond strongly to a substance known as a colony-stimulating factor (Moore *et al.*, 1976), monocytes and macrophages apparently being a principal source of this hormone. Under certain conditions monocytes themselves can give rise to macrophages and epitheloid cells (van der Rhee *et al.*, 1979).

That the earliest myeloblasts undergo a series of stepwise alterations in becoming differentiated toward any one of the three lines of granulocytes has been well established, but the morphological traits, if any, associated with each successive step remain undetermined. Although the degree of chromatin condensation has been suspected to reflect new patterns of genetic control activity, no correlation to overall differentiation has become apparent (Hsu, 1962; Littau *et al.*, 1964). Furthermore, the large nucleoli must undergo reduction during the acquisition of cellular destiny, for they are much reduced in circulating cells, a reduction that does not occur, however, until the late granulocyte stage (Bernhard and Granboulan, 1968). Finally, it remains impossible to distinguish the myeloblast from proerythroblasts or lymphoblasts; consequently all the immediate progenitors may prove to be pluripotential for development into any of the major types of leukocyte.

In frog development, the pronephros rather than the liver has been demonstrated to be the principal site of granulopoiesis (Carpenter and Turpen, 1979; Turpen, 1980), where slight (< 10%) erythropoiesis and almost no lympho-poiesis occur. Although the origin of the stem cells could not be determined, it was not from the yolk sac blood islets but appeared to be from a dorsal source.

  The Neutrophil. The earliest differentiated stage that can be recognized as clearly neutrophil (often called heterophil in nonprimate mammals) contains a sparse number of large electron-opaque granules, most aptly referred to as primary granules. These rounded or oblong-ovate bodies have a mean diameter of 0.4 μm and are produced in dictyosomes. Consequently, the appearance of the granules is preceded in turn by development of an extensive cisternal rough endoreticulum and an abundant Golgi system. Since these and other granules of the granulocyte are largely lysosomes of various types, their description, formation, and enzymes, having been detailed elsewhere (Dillon, 1981, pp. 278–284), need not be repeated here. Later in development of the neutrophil, a second population of granules begins to appear, consisting of bodies less than half the size of the primary, the mean diameter being 0.3 μm. The content of these secondary granules is much finer than that of the primary and is less electron-opaque and often includes crystalloid deposits. After this type of gran-ule has made its appearance, the chromatin begins to condense, the nucleolus becomes less evident, and the outline of the nucleus becomes somewhat irreg-ular in appearance. Later, as the primary granules become quite scarce, tertiary granules develop that resemble the secondary ones in size; in fact, they are morphologically nearly indistinguishable from them after glutaraldehyde fixa-tion. Cytochemically they resemble the primary granules, except in lacking peroxidase and lysozyme activity, and differ from the secondary type in not showing the alkaline phosphatase activity which is unique to that class (Wetzel, 1970a). Following the advent of this third kind of granule, the nucleus becomes increasingly lobate.

  The Eosinophil. The earliest eosinophils are at once distinguished from neutrophils of the same stage by the more abundant and larger primary granules that develop within Golgi vesicles. At first these bodies are spherical and quite electron-opaque, with diameters ranging up to 1.0 μm, but later they become elongate and somewhat angular as crystalloid deposits grow within them. Ap-parently the young eosinophils undergo an increase in diameter, for large cells of this stage are much more frequent in marrow than are smaller ones (Wetzel, 1970a). This increase then is followed by a gradual decrease in diameter, as the granules become increasingly crystalloid, and the nucleus undergoes loba-tion, with accompanying condensation of the chromatin and degeneration of the nucleolus.

  The Basophil. As in the eosinophil only a single type of granule devel-ops in the basophil. Although electron-opaque as those of other granulocytes, they are much smaller, ranging only from 0.15 to 0.5 μm, with a mean diam-eter of 0.33 μm. The supposed early basophil is relatively small, with the rounded nucleus containing prominent nucleoli; granules are scarce, as is the endoreticulum. With additional maturity, the granules increase in number as the chromatin condenses markedly, but the rough endoreticulum never becomes as abundant as it does in neutrophils and eosinophils, mitochondria being as large as those of the latter type of cell. Late in differentiation, the nucleus becomes moderately lobate, the endoreticulum disappears, and the number of ribosomes is greatly reduced. In man at least, mast cells appear to share origins with basophils (Zucker-Franklin, 1980).

Controlling Factors. The mechanisms controlling the formation and release of the granulocytes are complex and poorly known. Eosinophil production is normally far in excess of release; estimates exist of 300 to 400 eosinophils being contained in the marrow to every one present in the circulating blood (Hudson, 1960; Rytömaa, 1960). Release appears to be stimulated by stress-induced histamines and to be inhibited by corticosteroids (Archer, 1970), but until recently little had been demonstrated concerning the nature of a differentiation-stimulus comparable to erythropoietin. At least two opposing factors had been shown to exist, colony-stimulating unit and colony-inhibitory unit (DiPersio *et al.*, 1978). The former substance even was capable of partially overcoming the inhibition of proliferation in myeloblasts induced by X irradiation (Sugavara *et al.*, 1980). It probably corresponds to what has been termed eosinophilopoietin, which now has been established as stimulating eosinophil differentiation both *in vivo* and *in vitro* (Bartelmez *et al.*, 1980).

4.5.3. Lymphopoiesis and Megakaryocytopoiesis

Ontogeny of Lymphocyte Production. The lymphocyte appears to be the sole exception to the rule that blood cells have their origins in the extraembryonic mesenchymal islets, a point clearly established in frog embryogenesis (Turpen *et al.*, 1973). Moreover, at least in large measure, these leukocytes appear to arise from epithelium, rather than mesenchyme (Ackerman, 1962, 1965, 1970; Rugh, 1968). In hamsters as well as chick embryos, a continuous sequence of morphological intermediates has been found between the undifferentiated epithelium of the thymus and the precursorial cell of lymphocytes, the lymphoblast, seemingly under the influence of several thymic factors (Gelfand *et al.*, 1978), one of which is known as T-cell growth factor (Rosenberg *et al.*, 1980). The lymphoblast is a large discoidal cell, much like the myeloblast and proerythroblast in having a large, very irregular nucleus containing prominent nucleoli. However, mitochondria are more abundant than in those cells and display the flat, transverse cristae typical of metazoan cells in general. In rabbits, however, a number of lymphoblasts and lymphocytes have been reported in the capsule and surrounding connective tissue that later invades the thymus (Ackerman, 1970). Thus, the epithelial origins described may be exceptional rather than a general rule.

In lymph nodes, a principal source of these cells in the adult mammal,

these leukocytes appear in the anlage of the organ as intermediate-size lymphocytes along with a few, if any, lymphoblasts (Hostetler and Ackerman, 1966).
Since typical lymphoblasts do not develop in the lymph node until near the end
of term, it is probable that the lymphocytes arise there by transformation of
mesenchymal cells, possibly followed late in neonatal life by a secondary invasion of lymphoblasts, most likely from the thymus. Lymphopoiesis in the
appendix also appears to have dual origins, the initial one by transformation of
reticular or mesenchymal cells, the second by invading cells from the thymus.

Megakaryocytopoiesis. Although the actual origin of the stem cells for
megakaryocytes has not been specifically determined, it is believed to be identical to that of other blood cell lines (Ebbe, 1970). Hence, the bone marrow
sites of megakaryocytopoiesis in postnatal and adult mammals probably are
derivatives of the same progenitory stem cells from which the granulocyte and
erythrocyte stock originated. In neonatal opossums, however, the liver is the
active site of these processes (Paone *et al.*, 1975). As usual, the precursorial
cells proliferate rapidly, some of the progeny ultimately being induced to become committed to megakaryocytopoiesis. After an unknown number of additional mitotic divisions on the part of these committed stem cells, a stage is
entered in which nuclear division is unaccompanied by cytokinesis, resulting
in polyploid precursors having up to $67n$ nuclear DNA content in rabbits and
$32n$ in rats (García, 1964; Odell *et al.*, 1965; Nakeff and Bryan, 1978). The
mean ploidy in human precursors was $8n$ (Levine, 1980).

However, not all these final undifferentiated precursors attain the same
degree of polyploidy, but may begin to differentiate into promegakaryocytes
(also called stage I megakaryocytes) with various degrees of ploidy. In this
stage, the cells have increased somewhat in size through the acquisition of a
greater relative ctyoplasmic content, a process that continues through the remaining two stages (Ebbe, 1970). The cytoplasm originally is homogeneous
and uniformly basophilic, but as the cell enters the next stage, possibly accompanied by mitotic division, the intensity and uniformity of basophilia decrease.
In these stage II cells or promegakaryocytes, azurophilic granules may form a
patch or two in the cytoplasm, but the occurrence of such granules throughout
the cytoplasm characterizes only the megakaryocyte proper or stage III cells.
At first the members of this last class, which arise from the promegakaryocytes
without cytokinesis, may be basophilic, but that trait is lost with maturity as
they become ready for platelet formation. Although knowledge of regulation of
the breakdown of the megakaryocytes into platelets is in a preliminary state,
plasma stimulatory and inhibitory factors seem to be involved (Shreiner *et al.*,
1980).

5

Gene Action Changes during Nonvertebrate Differentiation

Although a large number of gene action changes were made manifest by the several aspects of vertebrate differentiation described in the preceding chapter, a fuller picture of their nature and universality emerges from an examination of various life-history aspects of protistans, especially those of fungi and ciliates. Germination in green plants, too, has much to contribute to a more thorough understanding of the problems associated with such changes, as does also sporulation in prokaryotes. This diversity of topics provides the greater quantity of facts to the present discussion, but a few invertebrates like *Hydra* also have been sufficiently investigated to round out the account still more.

5.1. DIFFERENTIATION IN FUNGI

Differentiation investigations on fungi have been based primarily on two major types, filamentous varieties, such as the members of the genera *Neurospora* and *Aspergillus*, and slime molds like *Physarum polycephalum* and *Dictyostelium discoideum*. These two basic groups share a common trait that makes them particularly favorable for researches on the topic, for while the activities are carried out in widely different ways, both undergo changes in cell types during the course of their life cycles. Although discussion is by no means restricted to those two groups, they do provide the skeletal structure for the account, with additions from other fungal representatives wherever feasible.

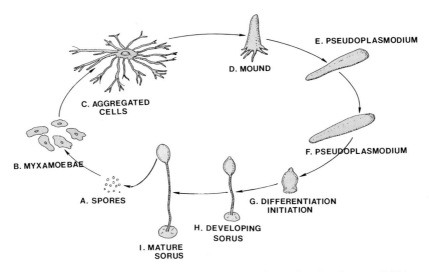

Figure 5.1. Life cycle changes in *Dictyostelium discoideum*. (Based on Bonner, 1957.)

5.1.1. Gene Changes in Slime-Mold Differentiation

Morphogenetic Events in Dictyostelium. When deprived of food, the normal vegetative solitary amoebae of the slime mold *D. discoideum* move into close proximity of one another to form aggregation centers, where they first become arranged as single files of cells.* With the passage of time these eventually condense into spirally arranged streams around a central axis (Clark and Steck, 1979). Further condensation results in mounds, or grexes, each containing up to around 100,000 cells, which then give rise to apical papillae; in this, as in many later stages, amoeboid cells may continue to migrate around the circumference of the multicellular body or in helices over its entire surface. At first the papillae are conical, but they quickly assume a cylindrical form projecting vertically from the surface (Figure 5.1). Each vertical column then drops to the surface to produce a sluglike pseudoplasmodium, which typically undergoes migration, secreting a slimy sheath continually as it does so. Upon reaching a site where high light intensity, low humidity, or other suitable microenvironment prevails, it partially reassumes a vertical orientation, the anterior portion being directed upwards while the remainder expands into a thick base; consequently, the resulting combination is often like a sombrero in conformation. The central cells then develop into a stalk, over which the peripheral cells move to its apex as they become transformed into spores (Figure 5.1); when

---

*This complex behavior is characteristic only of advanced members of this group, for the post-starvation activities of lower forms like *D. minutum* are far simpler (Schaap *et al.*, 1981).

mature, the spores are dispersed, eventually to germinate into amoeboid cells that as a rule live free in the soil.

Thus, the multicellular reproductive body consists of only two major differentiated cell types, spore and stalk cells. Initiation of differentiation involves several events that recall traits of developing zygotes, the chief difference being that, in the present instance, a multicellular body is involved instead of a single cell. Probably the most striking similarity is that, during the spore-producing processes, the tip structure of the forming spore mass specifies a developmental axis; as in fertilized eggs this feature provides positional information which in the present case influences the subsequent differentiation of the associated cells along either a prestalk or prespore pathway (Bonner, 1957; Farnsworth, 1973).

Transitional Changes in Nucleic Acids. When the vegetative amoebae undergo morphogenetic transition into the two types of reproductive cells, the necessary energy and component substances are supplied, at least in part, by the turnover of endogenous proteins, RNAs, and other macromolecules (Bonner, 1967; Loomis, 1975). The rRNA, however, is simply replaced during differentiation, not broken down, the newly formed substance being preferentially incorporated into polysomes, while the undegraded rRNA of the vegetative cells becomes confined to monosomal ribosomes (Cocucci and Sussman, 1970). Although the new rRNAs differ further from the vegetative in having more stable precursors and in a characteristic defect in the 17 S species (Kessin, 1973; Batts-Young et al., 1977), no differences in primary structure of 25 S, 17 S, or 5 S rRNAs could be found by fingerprint comparisons (Batts-Young et al., 1980).

Employment of two different types of RNA excess hybridization reactions permitted insights into the complexity of the poly(A)$^+$ RNAs of growing cells (Blumberg and Lodish, 1980a; Jacquet et al., 1981). The results of both procedures indicated the existence on the polysomes of the cytoplasm of between 4000 and 5000 polyadenylated sequences represented by more than one copy per cell, with an additional 9000 varieties confined to the nucleus. In total these transcripts correspond to the expression of about 53% of the single-copy portion of the genome and indicate a complexity in the mRNA population more than triple that of rapidly growing yeast cells (Hereford and Rosbash, 1977). Similar techniques applied to four different stages of the life cycle demonstrated that transcription of a significant number of new genes occurs in only a single time period of development, about midway in the life cycle (Blumberg and Lodish, 1980b). Whereas 5000 RNA species were found to be present throughout vegetative as well as developing stages, about 3000 new ones appeared just after multicellularity had been achieved but prior to differentiation into stalk and spore cells. During the late aggregation and culmination stages, close to 80% of the single-copy genome was expressed in the total population of poly(A)$^+$ RNA, but here as in the vegetative forms only about one-third of this was expressed as mRNA (Blumberg and Lodish, 1981).

In vegetative cells, some mRNAs were shown to be relatively more abundant in the fractions bearing poly(A) tracts about 112 nucleotides long, while others were equally more abundant in the fraction having segments only 60–65 nucleotides in length (Palatnik *et al.*, 1979). Accordingly, it was suggested that the poly(A) segments might play a regulatory role in cell differentiation, but a later investigation proved this not to be the case (Palatnik *et al.*, 1980). However, qualitative changes in the RNA during the life cycle have been revealed by means of cDNA probes (Jacquet *et al.*, 1981). Species of RNA that were abundant in vegetative cells (2½ hr) were found to fall to low levels of occurrence in aggregation (8 hr) and later stages. Thus, during preculmination (18 hr) 50% of the total RNA population was of species absent in vegetative amoebae, some of which had first appeared during aggregation, while the remainder appeared in postaggregation (12 hr). Moreover, the composition of the polysomal population became markedly altered in the 18-hr cells.

Finally the results of recent studies on a poorly known class of RNAs of this slime mold appear to be pertinent to the present topic, even though they were not directly concerned with developmental changes. The class of nucleic acids is that referred to as small nuclear RNA (snRNA) because of their size of 100 to 250 nucleotides and a sedimentation coefficient of 4.5 S and their being confined to the nucleus. In mammals at least eight species of snRNAs have been categorized, five of which from rodents have had their primary structures established (Ro-Choi and Busch, 1974; Lerner and Steitz, 1979; Lerner *et al.*, 1980; Wise and Weiner, 1981). The three known as U1, U2, and U3 have proven to be metabolically stable, and the first of these is nearly as abundant in the nucleus as rRNAs are in the cytoplasm. U3 has been shown to be confined to the nucleolus, while the others occur as small ribonuclear proteins (Weinberg and Penman, 1968; Zieve and Penman, 1976). The recent studies of *Dictyostelium* just mentioned revealed the presence of these nucleic acids (Wise and Weiner, 1981) and showed that the several species resembled those of mammals but were represented by far fewer copies per cell (Blumberg and Lodish, 1981). That fungal species which was called D2 was demonstrated to be homologous to U3 of the rat and was encoded by a dispersed multigene family (Wise and Weiner, 1980).

Other Factors in Dictyostelium Differentiation. The first step in development of *Dictyostelium* is the production of aggregates of the amoebae after a few hours of nutrient deprivation, followed by differentiation into the precursors of the mature stalk and spores as already described. The act of forming aggregates has been shown to be a vital preliminary step in differentiation and has accordingly received considerable attention. First, as they form the moundlike aggregates, the amoebae secrete a diffusible compound, now known to be cAMP (Konijn, 1974), which serves as a pheromone that attracts others of the population (Bonner, 1947, 1949). As the aggregates enlarge, the cells become increasingly cohesive and develop several new antigens on their surfaces (Beug *et al.*, 1973; Siu *et al.*, 1976; Muller and Gerisch, 1978). These new proteins have been suggested to interact with one another or other membrane constituents and thereby aid in holding the cells together (Loomis, 1979), both of which processes having proven to be of vital importance in the differentiating activities. On one hand elevated intracellular levels of cAMP are necessary for the expression of numerous (all?) genes active in development, and cell contact is specifically prerequisite for entry into the prespore pathway (Kay *et al.*, 1979). In addition, there is a timing mechanism involved in these activities that consists of at least two separate components (Mercer and Soll, 1980).

The surface glycoproteins of the membranes are proving to undergo drastic changes during the course of the life cycle, but the substances have only begun to receive the attention they merit. In one recent study, they were labeled with tritium and then analyzed by gel electrophoresis of the lysate of whole cells (Toda *et al.*, 1980). During the early aggregation period, at least 39 distinct bands were found by one-dimensional analysis, six of which increased in density and four decreased as the stage advanced, while two new ones appeared. By two-dimensional separations, 63 individual spots were obtained, 45 of which underwent marked changes in size during the processes of aggregating. The surface-membrane constituents that provide the essential cohesion during aggregation fall into two major categories on the basis of their reaction to EDTA, those that are resistant to it being collectively referred to as contact sites A, while those that are sensitive are called contact sites B (Beug *et al.*, 1973). Only the latter type is present during the vegetative phase, whereas both are found in aggregating cells. These intercellular interactions have also been demonstrated to be sensitive to the presence of monosaccharides; two types of sites that are specifically reactive to galactose have been identified and are known as discoidin I and II, or CBP-26 and CBP-24, respectively (Rosen *et al.*, 1973; Frazier *et al.*, 1975; Reitherman *et al.*, 1975). Furthermore glucose, but not galactose, inhibits site B-mediated cohesion (Rickenberg *et al.*, 1975; Marin *et al.*, 1980). In other studies, the conditions necessary for full expression of contact sites A were shown to be amino acid starvation for at least 5 hr and high cell density for 3 hr of that period (Marin, 1977).

After the aggregates have achieved a sufficient mass and become transformed into the sluglike pseudoplasmodia, they may either proceed directly into sporulation or undergo migratory activities for a period of time (Newell *et al.*, 1969). Since the cells of the anterior region of migrating pseudoplasmodia give rise to stalk cells, whereas the posterior portion produces spore cells, such bodies have been treated with [^{35}S]methionine to label the newly synthesized proteins (Alton and Brenner, 1979). After being cut into five segments, the proteins of each part were analyzed by gel electrophoresis and visualized by autofluorography. About 10% of the 500 or more polypeptides detected showed regional variation (Figure 5.2). Because the greatest difference was between the anterior fifth and the remainder of the pseudoplasmodium, it was clearly

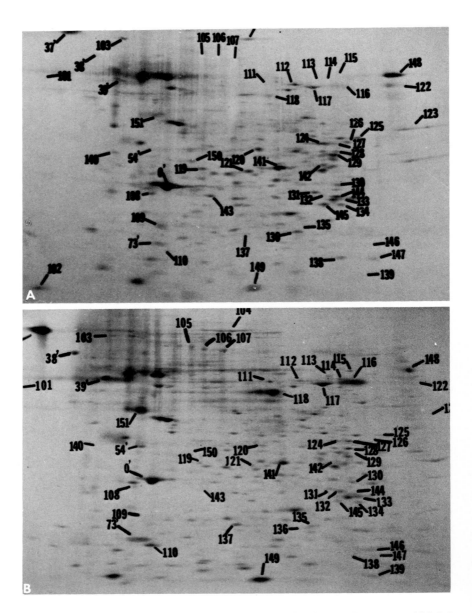

Figure 5.2. Proteins of pseudoplasmodia of *Dictyostelium*. The two autofluorograms of labeled proteins were from contrasting regions of pseudoplasmodia. (A) In the anterior fifth are found six proteins (Nos. 109, 121, 123, 126, 138, and 150) absent from the more posterior portions. (B) In the proteins from the posteriormost fifth, as well as those from the second fifth caudad, several proteins are present that are not found in (A), labeled as 101, 105–107, 110, 113–115, 132, 135, 139, and 146. (Courtesy of Alton and Brenner, 1979.) Thus, the amoeboid cells of the respective regions express a number of different genes.

indicated that differentiation into precursorial stalk and spore cells had already occurred. It is to be observed that these results are not entirely in agreement with those from mRNA studies reported on a preceding page.

Quantitative changes in the synthesis of the mRNAs for actin and two other proteins have been described during differentiation of this slime mold and four phases of actin gene transcription have been observed: (1) An increase up to 13.5-fold occurred during the first 90 min of differentiation, (2) followed by a strong decrease; (3) then after 4 to 8 hr, a second increase took place which raised production to an intermediate level; (4) after 16 hr a final decrease was noted. Unfortunately qualitative differences in the messages or their translocational products were not sought, but the mRNAs were found to have unusually short half lives (Alton and Lodish, 1977; Margolskee and Lodish, 1980). They underwent an abrupt increase (about 8-fold) similar to that of actin synthesis during the first 45 min, and then decreased equally precipitously. Polyacrylamide gel electrophoretic analyses of protein changes during differentiation also have been conducted, the results indicating about 25% of the 400 or more polypeptides detected to undergo changes in rates of synthesis during development (Alton and Lodish, 1977).

The Roles of cAMP in Development. Because of its serving as a pheromone and in other activities in gene expression in *E. coli* and perhaps other organisms, cAMP has received attention from a number of investigations into the development of *Dictyostelium* (Gerisch, 1979; Varnum and Soll, 1981). In the first place, it should be noted that during the service of this substance as an attractant in aggregation, it was produced solely by the central cells and then only intermittently (Konijn, 1972). In addition, similar pulses of cAMP synthesis have been observed to occur during differentiation at 16 hr and again before culmination (Brenner, 1978). Moreover, it has been found to serve during aggregation as an inducer of phosphodiesterase production and later for the syntheses of glycogen phosphorylase and UDP-galactose polysaccharide transferase and for the formation of prespore and stalk cells (Kay, 1979). Ammonia, on the other hand, inhibited each of these activities. Thus, rather than being inducers of specific syntheses, these agents were suggested more likely to be coordinators of the rates of biochemical differentiation of individual cells. However, it is equally possible that at least cAMP serves as a chemical messenger, similar to its role in hormone stimulation in metazoan cells (Wallace and Frazier, 1979; Dillon, 1981, pp. 36, 37).

5.1.2. Differentiation in Other Fungi

In contrast to the obvious relations in *Dictyostelium* between differentiation and nutrient deprivation, factors which lead to sporulation in other fungi tend to be obscure. Many investigations into the induction of this activity in *Aspergillus,* by way of illustration, have failed to find direct relationships between substrate changes and spore formation. Reduction of citric acid content resulted in increased sporulation, but restricted quantities of glucose rarely led to the formation of their characteristic conidiospores, more frequently instead inducing autolysis (Ng *et al.*, 1973).

Filamentous Fungal Differentiation. The filamentous fungi are especially adapted for investigations into cell differentiation, because, in the first place, they can be grown in the laboratory under conditions that permit growth of only vegetative cells. Then at will they can be induced by nutrient deprivation to produce in synchronous fashion large numbers of pigmented asexual spores called conidia. In the genus *Aspergillus*, the spores are formed on special multicellular structures, called conidiophores, comprised of three types of cells. Thus, the organism can be induced to differentiate a total of four cell types, (1) the conidia and the parts of the conidiophore known as (2) the primary and (3) secondary sterigmas and (4) the foot-cell and vesicle combination (Smith *et al.*, 1977), aside from the vegetative hyphal cells.

Differentiation in Aspergillus. The onset of differentiation in *Aspergillus* is marked by the transformation of a vegetative hyphal cell into a foot cell from which a stalklike conidiophore soon emerges. Both the foot and the conidiophore develop a secondary wall within the primary one that is continuous with the single convering of mycelial components (Oliver, 1972). In some cases, including *A. flavus*, the foot cell becomes ornamented with spines, sometimes covered by a fibrillar layer, as in that same species. Within the cytoplasm of the conidiophore are numerous microtubules and microfilaments that run longitudinally and appear to be engaged in the active cytoplasmic streaming which can be observed in these slender cells (Oliver, 1972). After the conidiophore has attained its full length, the apex gradually increases in diameter to form what is known as the vesicle, a structure that provides the conidiophore with a clublike conformation.

The semifinal stage in differentiation begins with the formation of a larger number of synchronously produced spherical elevations over the surface of the vesicle, which represent the primordia of the sterigmata (Tokunaga *et al.*, 1973). Depending on the species, as the primordia elongate, they either become cylindrical in form or develop subdivisions or branches, each part of the sterigma having terms that are unnecessary here. In any case, the apex enlarges into a spherical knob that soon elongates into an ovate spore, or conidium. At this point, the nucleus of the sterigma divides mitotically, one of the daughter nuclei migrating into the young conidium. After the latter has increased to its ultimate size, a septum develops between it and the mother cell. The latter then repeats these processes to form a second conidium, which is cylindrical from its very beginning, not spherical as the first one (Hanlin, 1976; Smith *et al.*, 1977).

Sexual reproduction in the members of this genus appears to take place in darkness, as when the mycelium is buried in the medium (Zonneveld, 1977), and seemingly is initiated by loosely looped hyphae developed from the base of a conidiophore. As differentiation proceeds, the hyphae branch as they elongate to form a clump, the cells of which are thicker than ordinary vegetative ones. Many of the branches anastomose with one another, but others develop swellings subterminally or intercalarily, which enlarge to form subspherical so-called Hülle cells. Within the latter, ascocarps, or cleistothecia, become differentiated, by processes involving the formation of multiple layers of hyphae in which asci arise, each ascus ultimately producing eight ascospores. Although many investigations have been conducted on the energetics of sexual reproduction, only slight progress has been made as to the gene changes that accompany the processes.

Molecular Aspects of Differentiation. The beginnings that have been made at the macromolecular level of this topic include evidence drawn from cDNA-hybridization analyses. The results of such studies demonstrated that during both conidiophore formation and sporulation, many poly(A)$^+$ mRNAs appeared that could not be detected in vegetative cells (Timberlake, 1980). Over 1000 characteristic poly(A)$^+$ mRNA sequences were shown to be present during sporulation that were absent in somatic cells, and 300 different ones that were confined to spores, including some which have been cloned (Zimmermann *et al.*, 1980). In a study on rates of synthesis and turnover of poly(A)$^+$ mRNAs in the related genus *Neurospora*, it was concluded that the synthesis of rRNA established both the ribosomal and the steady-state levels of mRNA (Sturani *et al.*, 1979). However, in view of the storage of mRNAs for long periods in ova and other cells, the latter supposition is subject to doubt.

5.1.3. Gene Changes during Fungal Germination

The changes in proteins that accompany release of the spores and their germination under favorable conditions have been especially well documented in water molds. In these fungi, the spore gives rise to a zoospore, which takes in no nutrients but swims about actively for a prolonged period, using endogenous food reserves, until under certain environmental conditions it is induced to cease movement and transform into a vegetative cell. It then grows, accompanied by repeated mitoses without cell division, so that eventually it forms a large syncytium. During growth of this multinucleated mass, deficiency of nutrients at any stage may trigger the onset of cytokinesis, which processes subdivide it into numerous uninucleated cells, each of which becomes transformed into a zoospore (Lovett, 1975).

Changes in Nucleotide-Associated Activities. In *Blastocladiella emersonii*, cAMP and activities associated with it have captured a major portion of the researches that have been conducted on developmental changes. The activity of the enzyme adenylic acid cyclase was shown to fluctuate widely during the life cycle of this water mold, while its substrate remained fairly uniform in concentration, except for a transient increase during germination (Vale *et al.*, 1976). During the entire period of vegetative growth the enzyme was barely detectable, but when the syncytium underwent cytokinesis, it became 70-fold as abundant as originally (Gomes *et al.*, 1978). This high level then continued throughout the zoospore stage, decreasing only when germination into the germling hyphal cell occurred.

Since certain of the protein kinases of *Blastocladiella* have been found to be cAMP-dependent, a study was made of its enzymes of this class by means of DEAE-cellulose chromatography. The enzyme activity could be resolved into three peaks, only the third of which was dependent on cAMP. This peak III substance acted upon histones, as did also that of peak II, but the latter was independent of cAMP (Juliani and da Costa Maia, 1979). In contrast, the peak I protein acted upon casein and, like peak II, was independent of cAMP. A related investigation later demonstrated that the peak I enzyme remained at a steady state throughout the entire life cycle, whereas the peak III protein appeared only during sporulation (Juliani *et al.*, 1980).

5.1.4. Events during Fungal Spore Germination

That the germination of fungal spores is a particularly favorable system for exploration into the nature of gene expression has not gone completely unnoticed in the literature, for recently a small number of studies have investigated this problem.

Germination in Dictyostelium. In *Dictyostelium,* germination is completed within 3½ hr after activation of dormant spores and may be subdivided into four phases: activation, postactivation lag, swelling, and emergence (Cotter and Raper, 1966, 1968; Cotter *et al.*, 1976; Sussman and Brackenbury, 1976). Since the entire process is dependent on the synthesis of protein, one laboratory labeled activated spores with [^{35}S]methionine at 1-hr intervals from germination until emergence to detect whatever changes might take place (Dowbenko and Ennis, 1980). Analyses by means of two-dimensional polyacrylamide gel electrophoresis disclosed the existence of six classes of proteins, correlated with the times of production. Three included those produced only during hr 1, 2, or 3, respectively; another contained the proteins produced in both hr 1 and 2, but not in hr 3, while a fifth embraced the products made in hr 2 and 3 but not hr 1, and finally those that were synthesized throughout germination. Analysis of the products of mRNAs translated in a wheat-germ system then indicated that the production of the several classes was largely controlled at the level of transcription.

Germination in Other Fungi. In the germination of *Botryodiplodia theobromae* conidiospores, a somewhat different set of macromolecular events has been reported (Brambl and Van Etten, 1970). Here the first activity that could be observed was at the level of translation of stored mRNA, transcription not beginning until 90 min later. Similar requirements of protein synthesis for germination to progress have also been uncovered in members of the genera *Colletotrichum* and *Peronospora* (Holloman, 1969; Furusawa *et al.*, 1977). In the first genus mentioned, preparation for cell division did not take place for more than 2 hr, at which time nuclear and mitochondrial DNA syntheses were initiated simultaneously (Dunkle *et al.*, 1972).

However, in *Collectotrichum*, as a whole the prime focus of investigations has been on cell respiration and the mitochondrion. In dormant spores, no cytochromes could at first be detected in the mitochondria, in spite of oxygen-consumption studies having indicated that a potentially functional aerobic respiratory apparatus must be present (Brambl, 1975; Brambl and Josephson, 1977). The latter investigation, however, demonstrated that cytochromes *b* and *c* were actually present, but not *a*, in those organelles of dormant conidiospores; then after germination had proceeded for 2½ hr of the 4-hr period required for its completion, cytochrome *a* was found to have been actively synthesized (Brambl, 1977). Later, by use of more sensitive techniques, this respiratory protein was revealed to have actually appeared within 30 min after activation of the spore (Brambl, 1980; Josephson and Brambl, 1980). In addition, some attention has been devoted to the nonrespiratory proteins of germinating fungal spores. For example, when comparisons were made of translation products of poly(A)$^+$ RNAs from dormant and various stages of germinating spores, great differences were discovered (Wenzler and Brambl, 1978), the mRNAs of dormant bodies differing qualitatively from those of germinated ones.

Although certainly not identical to germination, the transition between two contrasting stages of fungi like *Histoplasma capsulatum* presents a parallel situation. In such dimorphic species, the organism is in the form of a mycelium as long as it is living in soil, but it becomes transformed into yeastlike cells when it parasitizes the tissues of its host. The transition from the mycelial phase to the yeast has been demonstrated to be accompanied by marked changes in RNA synthesis (Cheung *et al.*, 1974). Accordingly, the RNA polymerases of the two phases have been analyzed, three types proving to be present in each (Kumar *et al.*, 1980). However, when purified further, it became clear that each of the three in the mycelium differed strongly from the corresponding one of the yeast phase with respect to subunit composition, sensitivity to α-amanitin, and enzymatic properties.

5.2. GENE ACTION CHANGES IN BACTERIA

With their rapid rates of proliferation and near absence of specialized cell types, the prokaryotes do not afford many opportunities for investigating the occurrence of changes in gene expression. However, a number of bacterial types do undergo spore formation under controllable conditions, and analyses of these have made evident that even in these minute, seemingly simple organisms, alterations in gene activities do occur. Unlike the fungi, in which the bulk of attention has centered on germination of the spore, here the formation of that dispersive body has been the principal objective. Usually in discussions of prokaryotic functions one is accustomed to having *E. coli* play the leading role, but since that organism does not sporulate, *Bacillus subtilis* has served as the principal model for researches in the present field.

Early Events in Spore Formation. The developmental processes involved in spore formation in *B. subtilis* may be induced by depriving cultures of either glucose or amino acids or by limiting the quantities of phosphate in the medium (Schaeffer *et al.*, 1965; Holmes and Levinson, 1967; MacKechnie and Hanson, 1968). Under one or more such influences, a total of six highly phosphorylated nucleotides appear, collectively referred to as HPNs. Four of these, ppGpp, pppGpp, ppApp (HPN-I), and pppApp (HPN-II), are produced after amino acid deprivation (Rhaese and Groscurth, 1976), whereas the last two, HPN-III and HPN-IV, are synthesized when sporulation commences, especially under either phosphate or glucose deficiency. Although the chemical structure of the first of these is not actually known, it is suspected to be ppUpp, whereas the other is pppAppp.

Induction of spore formation in *Bacillus* also seems to involve a specific factor, called sporogen, which is known to appear only in cells undergoing sporulation (Srinivasan and Halvorson, 1963). Moreover, when the substance was added to a culture in a medium in which the organisms did not normally sporulate, it induced them to do so. In an effort to identify the substance chemically, a series of nucleosides were added to cultures of *B. subtilis* 168 in which sporulation had been inhibited by *m*-aminobenzeneboronic acid (Davis-Mancini *et al.*, 1978; Sekar *et al.*, 1981). Additions of guanosine or adenosine were found to alleviate the inhibition in part and the pyrimidine nucleosides had a lesser effect, whereas xanthosine was totally ineffective. However, inosine completely reversed the inhibition. Moreover, the chemical and physical properties of this latter nucleoside, including its ultraviolet and infrared spectra, were markedly similar to those of the purified sporogen.

Changes in tRNAs during Sporulation. One of the first macromolecular observations that was made regarding sporulation-related changes in tRNA populations of bacteria, loss of the 3'-CCA terminus, subsequently proved to be an aging effect, because it has been found to occur also in nonsporulating mutants of *B. subtilis* (Vold, 1974). However, other analytical studies have succeeded in demonstrating alterations strictly associated with these processes. For instance, it has been shown that in exponentially growing cells the tRNAs did not receive their full quotas of methyl groups, while those in sporulating ones became more completely methylated (Singhal and Vold, 1976). Moreover, chromatographic analyses have indicated that qualitative differences occurred during development, some of which were the result of lack of modification to the hypermodified bases of the postanticodon nucleoside (Vold, 1978). During exponential growth this nucleoside in several species of tRNAs remained N^6-(Δ^2-isopentenyl)adenosine (i^6A or A_1), while in the stationary phase it was modified to 2-methylthio-N^6-(Δ^2-isopentenyl)adenosine (A_s) (Dillon, 1978, pp. 259–262). For example, in vegetative cells, $tRNA_1^{Tyr}$ was by far the most abundant of the isoaccepting species, whereas in stationary phase cells and in spores, $tRNA_2^{Tyr}$ was the predominant form (McMillan and Arceneaux, 1975), the chief difference between the two types being that species 1 had A_i as the postanticodon nucleoside, whereas species 2 had A_s (Keith et al., 1976; Menichi and Heyman, 1976).

Changes in Other Macromolecules. At one time it had been thought that synthesis of rRNA ceased at the onset of sporulation (Hussey et al., 1971), but it was later revealed that the process did actually continue, but at a reduced rate (Testa and Rudner, 1975). Moreover, the latter investigation demonstrated that the several components of rRNA of the vegetative phase were replaced during sporulation by new species. When isolated and tested in cell-free systems, the 30 S subunit from sporulating *B. subtilis* was found to display reduced activity relative to that from vegetative cells (Guha and Szulmajster, 1977). Although not analyzed thoroughly, the rRNAs produced during germination appeared to be similar in composition to those synthesized during vegetative growth (Sloma and Smith, 1979).

The mRNAs made during early and late stages of sporulation and translated in a cell-free system showed a dramatic decrease in protein production to occur, but the autoradiograms also revealed the appearance of a number of new polypeptides, which were demonstrated not to be degradation products of others (Arnaud et al., 1980). Although as a rule bacterial mRNAs are free of poly(A) segments, in *B. polymyxa* poly(A)$^+$ RNA species put in an appearance during sporulation (Kaur and Jayaraman, 1979). Some evidence supports the view also that the RNA polymerase which transcribed the DNA may itself undergo change, possibly through loss of σ function, but the results of experiments have been inconclusive (Murray et al., 1974).

Changes Associated with Spore Germination. Although the formation of the spore has received the greater share of attention, some progress has also been made with regard to those changes that occur during germination. When dormant, *Bacillus* spores carry on no detectable synthesis of either proteins or RNAs; furthermore, they do not appear to engage in energy-related metabolic processes, the level of ATP dropping to less than 1% that of vegetative cells (Church and Halvorson, 1957; Sakakibara et al., 1965; Setlow and Kornberg, 1970a,b). All these activities are quickly resumed when the spore begins to undergo germination, the phosphates and necessary energy being supplied by the ample reserves (Setlow and Kornberg, 1970a). Similarly, during the first 75 min the nucleotides for RNA synthesis are obtained by breakdown of preexisting RNA (Setlow and Kornberg, 1970b).

Protein synthesis changes during germination have also been reported, in this case in *B. megaterium*. During the first 75 min of germination, the necessary amino acids were shown to be derived by proteolysis of the proteins of the dormant spore, the products first being excreted into the medium, after which they were resorbed, often accompanied by metabolism of the amino acids (Setlow and Primus, 1975). By the close of this initial period, the developing bacillus had regained the full capacities of the normal vegetative cells for synthesis of all amino acids, for which activity they required an exogenous source for the necessary nitrogen. Since mRNAs are scarce or perhaps even absent in dormant spores, DNA transcription obviously is also a necessary prelude to these processes. The proteolysis of the proteins began by min 3 of germination and by min 25 had degraded 15 to 20% of the total to amino acids. These processes were selective in that a unique class of low-molecular-weight (6000–12,000) proteins was the major substrate, while enzymes and coat proteins remained untouched (Setlow, 1975). The products of the first 12 min of germination also were degraded rapidly, the rate being 20% per hour; on the other hand, those produced after min 90 of germination were broken down at a rate of only 4% per hour.

Gene Changes in Advanced Bacteria. Although gene changes that occur during certain life cycles of advanced types of bacteria have been investigated to only a limited extent, the results nevertheless contribute significantly to a fuller picture of gene expression alterations in prokaryotic cells. In comparisons between aerobic and anaerobic cultures of the photosynthesizing form (*Rhodopseudomonas spheroides*), variations in isoaccepting species of tRNA[Phe] and tRNA[Trp] were observed (DeJesus and Gray, 1971). Furthermore, similar changes in protein and RNA synthesis under comparable contrasting conditions were reported in the related species, *Rhodospirillum rubrum* (Biedermann *et al.*, 1967; Cost and Gray, 1967; Gray, 1967; Biedermann and Drews, 1968).

Comparable changes under different environmental conditions have been described in a number of other bacteria, including *Pseudomonas putida*. With the ample supplies of oxygen and favorable media needed to induce logarithmic growth, the cytochrome *c* oxidase present was determined to be that known as cytochrome *o*, but under oxygen deficiency or other less favorable conditions that led to a stationary phase, cytochrome *d* was produced instead (Sweet and Peterson, 1978), a change that has also been reported in *Proteus vulgaris, Klebsiella aerogenes, Haemophilus parainfluenzae, E. coli*, and *Achromobacter* strain D (Castor and Chance, 1959; Arima and Oka, 1965; Smith *et al.*, 1970; Pudek and Bragg, 1974; Dillon, 1981, pp. 341, 344). Moreover, in *Pseudomonas*, NADH was sensitive to cyanide and other inhibitors only under rapid growth conditions, thereby indicating that other changes in the respiratory chain had occurred.

The myxobacteria are a group of highly specialized prokaryotes whose life cycles show remarkable parallelisms to those of such slime molds as *Dictyostelium*. Vegetative colonies of these organisms grow on decaying organic matter and on the bark of trees, gliding over surfaces and often preying upon other microorganisms. When nutrients become depleted, the cells aggregate to form mounds, or fruiting bodies, on which the rodlike vegetative cells become converted to spherical or ovate spores (Sudo and Dworkin, 1973). Recently a study was made of the total soluble protein changes that occurred during the sporulation of *Myxococcus xanthus* (Inouye *et al.*, 1979). Both quantitative and qualitative changes were found during the 55-hr period required for spore formation. Protein S, by way of illustration, gradually increased in abundance during the process but became quite scarce in the completed spore. Others, including proteins O, P, and Q, gradually decreased with time; some, like M and R, remained almost at a uniform level; and N increased markedly in abundance at hr 5, as T did at 10, both to remain at high levels until late in the processes. Finally still others, such as U, appeared only late in sporulation (at hr 45), but persisted in the dormant spore. Moreover, the spore being covered by a thick coat, a number of new structural proteins and other ingredients necessarily must have been produced during development that were not studied in the work cited.

Gene Changes during Caulobacter Life Cycle. Among the advanced bacteria whose protein changes have received pertinent investigation are the unusual organisms of the genus *Caulobacter*, forms that certainly merit much additional attention. In these stalked bacteria, cell division is asymmetrical, each resulting in two types of daughters, swarmers, which are flagellated, and immotile stalked cells (Figure 5.3). The former soon attach to the substrate, where they become transformed into the latter type, the free half of each

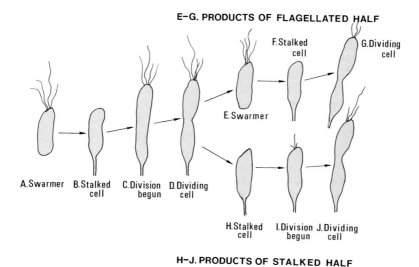

Figure 5.3. Life cycle of *Caulobacter*. (Based on Agabian *et al.*, 1979.)

of which produces a swarmer at every subsequent division. Recently, the protein changes that accompanied the several phases of the life cycle have been particularly thoroughly analyzed, with outstanding results (Agabian *et al.*, 1979). Three separate aspects of the organism were examined, the components of the outer and inner membranes and the soluble proteins of the cytoplasm; only the constituents of the inner membrane and cytoplasm need to be detailed here, however.

The proteins of the inner membranes, besides proving surprisingly complex in composition, showed a large number of life cycle-related changes—examination of the autofluorogram, in fact, suggests that nearly all of the numerous species underwent quantitative changes to at least a slight degree (Figure 5.4B). By way of illustration, W43 can be noted to have increased in abundance by min 10 and then to have decreased only slightly, until at min 150 it became barely perceptible. In contrast, W90 was synthesized at a high rate from the very beginning of the life cycle but decreased to a slight extent during the first hour; at min 60 there was then a distinct drop in quantity, from which point its synthesis appeared to have been maintained on a plateau until min 150, when a second lowering in rate occurred. Others, including 120Kd and 127Kd, reached a maximum near the center of the life cycle, decreasing toward both ends, and still others were most abundant near the termination of the 180-min cycle. In the soluble fraction, comparable patterns were obviously present in the autofluorograms. Some, including W34, were at the maximum rate of production at min 0, or immediately thereafter, as with W29, W24, and the undesignated one just above the latter (Figure 5.4A). Others such as W85, T98, and 130Kd reached a peak within the first 30 min of the cycle, then declined slightly to a lower plateau maintained throughout the remainder of the period. In contrast to the proteins of the inner membrane, few of the soluble ones built up to their maxima near the close of the cycle.

A later study along comparable lines (Milhausen and Agabian, 1981) differed in that two-dimensional electrophoresis was employed, so that the changes which occurred to a large number of species could be followed more precisely. The 37 species that were given numbers for detailed analysis fell into three major categories based on the points of the cycle at which the respective maxima were attained. Protein 1 can be seen in Figure 5.5 to have been moderately abundant at the initiation of the cycle, from which level it dropped off rapidly; thus, at 20–30 min it was scarcely evident, a condition that prevailed through the remainder of the period. Neither protein 22 nor 34 was evident at the onset of development, but the former reached its peak synthetic rate by 20–30 min, maintaining a plateau until 80–90 min, after which it became reduced. Contrastingly, production of protein 34 and M remained at a low rate until 60–70 min, after which they became increasingly abundant to the close of the cycle. Comparable patterns of changes in the proteins of the nucleoid have also been reported for this bacterium (Evinger and Agabian, 1979).

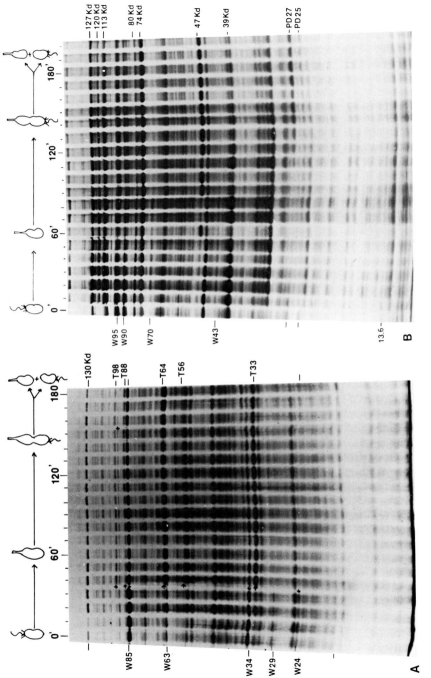

Figure 5.4. Changes in gene action in the life cycle of *Caulobacter*. (A) Autofluorograms of the soluble proteins of the entire bacterium. (B) Autofluorograms of proteins from the inner membrane. See text for discussion. (Courtesy of Agabian *et al.*, 1979.)

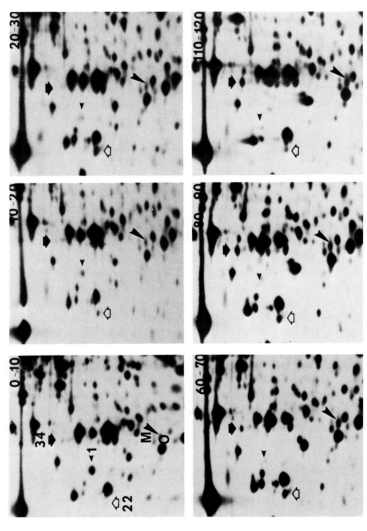

Figure 5.5. Protein changes during life cycle of *Caulobacter*. The two-dimensional autoradiograms were made from synchronized cultures processed at 10-min intervals during the 120-min life cycle. As examples of the changes that many of the proteins exhibit, four are indicated by numbers or letters and distinctive pointers, while the time is denoted by numerals in the upper right-hand corners. That labeled 1 and indicated by a small arrowhead is abundant during the first 10 min but becomes increasingly scarce through the remainder of the cycle; 22 is nearly absent during the initial moments, increases rapidly during the middle 60 min, and then fades out of the picture once more. In contrast, 34 and M increase from nearly nil at first to peaks of abundance near the termination of the cycle. (Courtesy of Milhausen and Agabian, 1981.)

5.3. DEVELOPMENTAL CHANGES IN HIGHER PLANTS

The development and differentiation of the embryo of higher plants represent quite as complex sequences of events as those of many metazoans, but unfortunately they have received far less attention. Since the macroscopic events are not familiar to many biologists, the discussion of protein changes that accompany the processes are prefaced by a brief sketch of differentiation of the maize embryo.

Beyond the level of embryonic development discussed in Chapter 3, Section 3.2.3, ending with the establishment of the plumule–radicle axis, further differentiation begins with the elaboration of the coleoptile primordium into its characteristic sheathlike form (Randolph, 1936). About midway in these processes, the anlagen of the first two leaves gradually are laid down (Figure 5.6), eventually to be followed by the appearance of several others as the plumule approaches the mature embryonic stage. In contrast, very few changes have been taking place at the radicle end, the most marked ones being the formation of a pocket around the tip of that structure, freeing it from the investing tissue as it gradually increases in size, and another, the reduction of the suspensor, which is resorbed until only a vestige remains. Although lysosomal activities

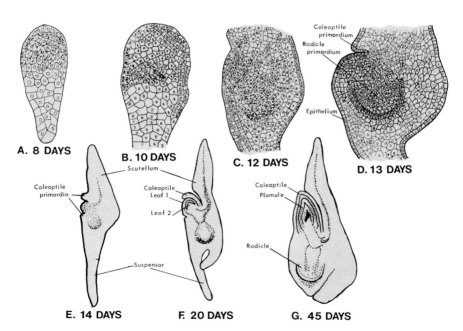

Figure 5.6. Later stages in the development of the maize embryo. The scutellum and coleoptile are absent in the embryos of dicotyledonous plants. (Based on Randolph, 1936.)

may be suspected to play the chief role in the degradation of this structure, the macromolecular events have not been explored to establish the actual steps involved.

5.3.1. Nucleic Acids in Plant Germination

As the seeds of many flowering plants ripen, water is lost and the embryo becomes quiescent, the cells being in the interphase stage and largely dehydrated. Under conditions favorable for germination, the first sign of activity in *Zea mays* occurs at day 2 as the radicle commences growth, followed some hours later by resumption of growth of the plumule and other embryonic parts.

DNA in Germination. When radicle growth begins, DNA replication does too, with mitotic divisions of the cells following within a few hours (Deltour and Jacqmard, 1974). Before these events can occur, however, the nuclei must undergo a remarkable sequence of changes in becoming converted from their resting condition to that of growth (Deltour *et al.*, 1979). In quiescent cells the nucleus contains a strong network of electron-opaque chromatin, which gradually disperses as germination proceeds (Figure 5.7A). During the first 8 hr, a nucleolus organizer region may be noted on one side, associated with the strongly vacuolated nucleolus, which is reduced to about one-fourth its typical mass. The organizer persists until about hr 24, at which time it disappears, as the nucleolar vacuoles diminish in numbers and the nucleolus itself regains its definitive size (Figure 5.7B, C). As the chromatin decondenses, Feulgen-positive material can gradually be detected, at hr 24 becoming evenly dispersed as fine granules throughout the nucleoplasm and to a limited extent within the nucleolus. These granules then commence to clump and by hr 72 have formed small aggregates in the nucleoplasmic matrix (Figure 5.7D).

One of the outstanding differences between plant DNA and that of bacteria and metazoans is the relatively high proportion of cytosines that are methylated, 5-methylcytosine being present to the extent of 5–30 mole% in the former in contrast to the less than 2 mole% in metazoans and nearly zero in bacteria (Vanyushin and Belozerskii, 1959; Dillon, 1978, pp. 70–74). Yet surprisingly little has been learned in plants about the mechanism and timing of the formation of this substance, which is catalyzed by DNA methyltransferases (Hotta and Hecht, 1971; Bayen and Dalmon, 1976). In a recent study of the processes in germinating wheat embryos (Theiss and Follmann, 1980), DNA synthesis was found to increase from near zero in the dormant embryo to a peak at hr 18, after which it decreased until at hr 30 it had been reduced to about 20% of its maximum extent. Contrastingly, the methionine-dependent methyltransferase activity remained nearly nil for about 9 hr before commencing a gradual increment throughout the remainder of the 30-hr study. In soybean germination, a somewhat different pattern emerged in an investigation of the polymerase activity (D'Alesandro *et al.*, 1980). This class of enzymes became detectable as early as 6 hr after the onset of germination. The activity of the soluble

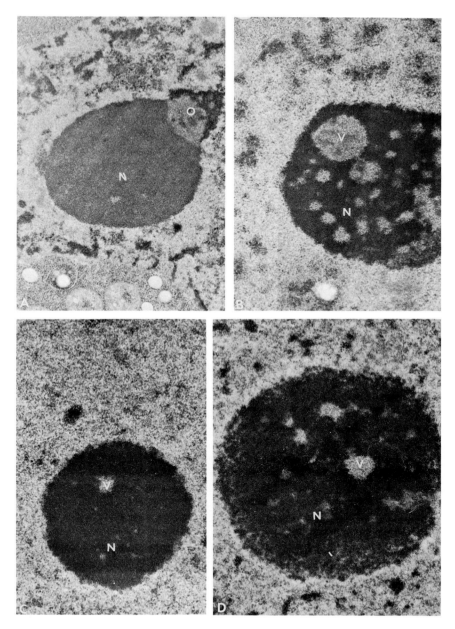

Figure 5.7. Ultrastructural changes in the nucleolus. (A) In quiescent cells, the nucleolus (N) is strongly electron-opaque and contains a distinct organizer region (O). (B) After 8 hr of germination the nucleolus has become filled with vacuoles (V), which decrease in abundance in the 24-hr (C) and 72-hr (D) stages of germination. All 12,000×. (Courtesy of Deltour *et al.*, 1979.)

enzyme, DNA polymerase α, increased rapidly beyond that point, as in other systems undergoing rapid cell division, whereas the chromatin-bound polymerase β remained at relatively unchanged levels.

tRNAs in Germination. During the first half of the past decade, reports on the nature of the first RNAs synthesized during germination presented conflicting evidence. In a number of species, including *Phaseolus vulgaris, Vicia faba, Triticum vulgare*, and *Allium cepa*, the products were predominantly rRNA and tRNA, mRNAs being absent until after hr 24 (Chen *et al.*, 1971; Melera, 1971; Jakob, 1972; Walbot, 1972). To the contrary, in *Z. mays* and *Triticum aestivum* mRNAs appeared between hr 4 and 8 of germination, whereas rRNA and tRNA were not produced until later (Deltour, 1970; Van de Walle, 1971; Rejman and Buchowicz, 1973). A clue to the solution of the problem was later supplied when a study of the synthesis of RNA and DNA during germination of barley showed that two groups of plants existed (Ahmed and Kamra, 1975), which differed in the stage of the genome in the dormant embryo. In the seeds of those species that produced tRNAs and rRNAs early in germination, the genome was demonstrated to be in the pre-DNA replicative stage, whereas in maize and others that synthesized mRNA first, it was found to be in the postreplicative condition.

Comparisons of ungerminated wheat embryos with 48-hr seedlings and similar researches on other species have disclosed a number of quantitative and qualitative changes to occur in the tRNA population (Vold and Sypherd, 1968). One such study examined the changes in the $tRNA^{Phe}$ population during germination and early growth of barley, a total of nine isoaccepting species of which were detected (Hiatt and Snyder, 1973). In the dormant embryo, species 1, 3, and 4 alone were found to be present, the first two of which were in minor proportions; after 24 hr of germination, species 6 characteristic of chloroplasts appeared in minute quantities in the embryos, and species 1 increased in quantity to a degree. At hr 40, species 2 and 5 were detected for the first time, while 6 became more abundant. This distribution pattern remained relatively stable until day 4½, when species 1 could no longer be detected and 7 and 8 began to be actively synthesized; species 7 subsequently became as abundant as 4, which suddenly diminished in importance. Although such differences in isoaccepting tRNAs could not be found in an earlier study on cotton seed germination, the small amounts of minor species that are typically present may have gone undetected (Merrick and Dure, 1972).

In dry lupine seeds, the tRNAs were shown to be aminoacylated to only a small extent and to include numerous defective molecules that had been degraded at the -CCA sequence of the 3′ terminus (Kedzierski and Pawełkiewicz, 1977). Although during germination the level of aminoacylation increased rapidly while defective molecules gradually disappeared, no concomitant rise in tRNA ligase levels could be detected (Dzięgielewski *et al.*, 1979). Since ATP also existed only in small quantities in the dry seeds, it was suggested that that substance possibly was the factor limiting aminoacylation.

Other RNAs in Transcription. Relatively few investigations appear to have explored the mRNAs of germination. In dry wheat embryos an ample complement of poly(A)$^+$ RNAs has been described, containing numerous species (Cuming and Lane, 1978). During the first 3 hr of germination these proved to be a relatively homogeneous fraction of precursorial forms, having high molecular weights and extensive oligo(U) sections (Dobrzanska and Buchowicz, 1976). Similarly in early radish seedlings, two classes of poly(A)$^+$ RNAs were found; the members of the larger group, representing 60% of the total, had half lives of only 30 min, whereas those of the smaller had half lives of 4 to 10 hr or even longer (Aspart *et al.*, 1979). These results are not readily reconcilable with data obtained from developing wheat and rye embryos. The seeds of these monocotyledonous plants were found to contain vast stores of messengers in the form of RNPs synthesized during the last 5 weeks of embryogeny (Ajtkhozhin *et al.*, 1976; Payne, 1976; Delseny *et al.*, 1977; Peumans *et al.*, 1978). Evidence from later experiments, however, supported the view that most of the mRNPs were not requisite for successful germination (Peumans *et al.*, 1979).

A current investigation combined an ultrastructural approach with high-resolution autoradiography and differential staining for nucleoproteins to trace the transcription in the nucleolus (Fakan and Deltour, 1981). Maize embryos from both dry kernels and those germinated for either 6 or 72 hr were labeled with [^{3}H]-5-uridine and the preparations subsequently examined under the electron microscope. In the ungerminated specimens radioactivity in the nucleolus was found to be centered largely in the organizer region, usually located peripherally (Figure 5.8A). The products of this pregermination nucleolar transcription were assumed to be pre-rRNAs that were still unprocessed, whereas the abundant activity shown in the nucleoplasm could represent combinations of this class plus hnRNAs from other centers. Although the organizer region continued to be the sole site of nucleolar transcription in germlings grown for 6 hr, in those that were germinated for 72 hr transcriptional activity was indicated throughout this body (Figure 5.8B). The nature of the nucleolus itself can also be noted to undergo radical change. Whereas that organelle is highly vesicular in ungerminated embryos (Figure 5.8A), the vesicles rapidly disappear upon germination, so that by 72 hr the structure is nearly uniformly particulate (Figure 5.8B).

Finally, researches into the nature of the RNA polymerases active in transcription of the DNA have failed to reveal the existence of any control activities among them. In the first place the quantity of these enzymes present in the dry embryo showed no increase during the first 24 hr of growth, although transcription activity associated with isolated nuclei increased 25-fold (Guilfoyle and Malcolm, 1980). Hence, the amount of RNA polymerase was demonstrated not to be a limiting factor. Only one change in molecular type was noted, in that the polymerase IIA, which alone had been present during the early period of growth, was later in part altered to polymerase IIB, a change that involved the conversion of a subunit from one of 215,000 daltons to 180,000.

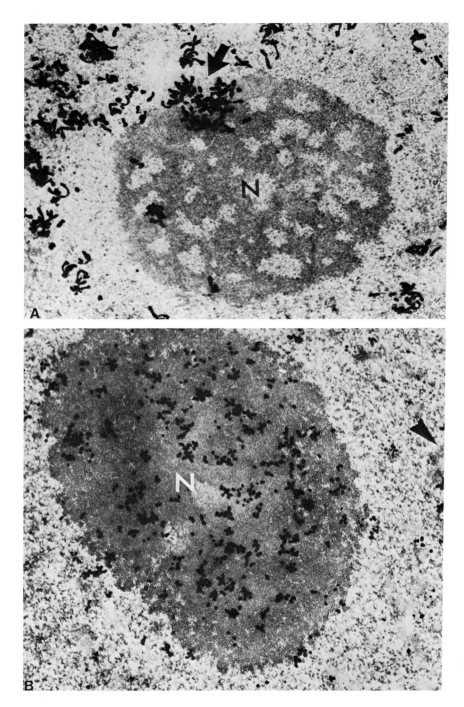

5.3.2. Proteins Synthesized during Germination

Studies of various proteins provide a much clearer view of gene action changes during germination than do those just reported on the several types of nucleic acids. Unfortunately they appear to have been undertaken only in extremely limited numbers.

Overall Patterns of Changes. Probably the most informative account of protein changes is provided by an analysis made by means of one- and two-dimensional electrophoresis of three stages of wheat embryos (Cuming and Lane, 1979), in which newly synthesized polypeptides, identified by [^{35}S]methionine labeling, were examined in dry embryos and in early (0–40 min) and late (5–24 hr) germlings. In the one-dimensional experiments, the autoradiograms showed a previously unsuspected quantity of protein synthesis to occur in the dormant embryos, that resulted in a broad spectrum of species, particularly of low molecular weights. This profile underwent immediate changes in early imbibing embryos, several of the small polypeptides disappearing while a number of heavy ones appeared. Still heavier ones were present at hr 2 to 3, but in limited numbers, whereas at hr 5 to 6 and through the first day, the species increased in diversity and relative size, as well as in abundance.

These patterns of change were shown even more dramatically in the two-dimensional autoradiograms prepared by isoelectric focusing (Figure 5.9A–C). Here, too, the predominance of low-molecular-weight species in dry embryos became apparent, as well as their gradual loss and replacement by high-molecular-weight forms. In addition, the changed properties of the proteins were visualized, since they became increasingly concentrated at the low pH end of the scale. The great numbers of types that were involved in these developmental alterations were especially evident. Thus, when such seeds germinate, many hundreds of proteins must surely be involved in the first 18 hr of the processes, in which period to the unaided eye only the growth of the plumule and radicle appears to occur. In continuation of this investigation the polypeptides of such early and late germlings were examined by two-dimensional electrophoretograms of labeled products of their mRNAs translated in a cell-free system (Thompson and Lane, 1980). As before, a large increase in complexity of species was indicated to occur as germination proceeded (Figure 5.9D, E); also as previously, the enhancement was largely in the more acid end of the pH scale and in those of greater molecular weight.

Changes in Specific Proteins. A few studies have followed the changes

---

Figure 5.8. Transcription in the nucleolus. Embryos from maize were labeled with [^{3}H]-5-uridine both before and during germination and the preparations subsequently studied by electron microscopy. (A) In the embryo of ungerminated grain, radioactivity in the nucleolus (N) was confined to the organizer region, suggestive of the synthesis only of pre-rRNAs. (B) Contrastingly the radioactivity was distributed throughout the nucleolus in embryos germinated for 72 hr. Both 19,300×. (Courtesy of Fakan and Deltour, 1981.)

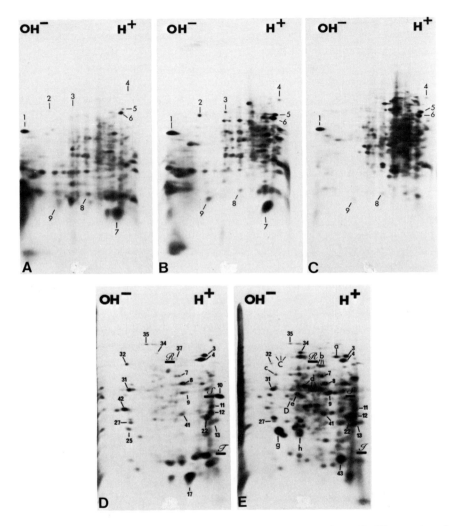

Figure 5.9. Changes in total protein profile during germination of wheat. (A) The proteins of ungerminated wheat embryos. (B) Proteins synthesized by embryos during 0–40 min of imbibition and (C), between 17 and 18 hr postimbibition. (Courtesy of Cuming and Lane, 1979.) (D, E) Polypeptides made in a cell-free system programmed by bulk mRNA from wheat embryos imbibed for 40 min (D) and 24 hr (E). Some that appear only in the later stage are labeled with upper-case letters. Three proteins of known molecular weight were added as markers; these are labeled in round-hand capitals R (bovine serum albumin, $M_r = 68,000$), S (ovalbumin, $M_r = 43,000$), T (soybean trypsin inhibitor, $M_r = 21,000$). (Courtesy of Thompson and Lane, 1980.)

in isozymes of a particular species of protein, representative of which are several investigations into the acid phosphatases in germinating lettuce and peas (Meyer et al., 1971; Johnson et al., 1973). In peas, the report of which is the more extensive, three isozymes were present, designated as I, II, and III, in order of decreasing molecular weight and increasing pH optima. The first of these, acid phosphatase I, was present in the cotyledons of the 24-hr germling, the earliest stage explored, and remained at a constant level of activity through the latest stage observed (14 day). This type was deduced to be located in phytin-containing bodies, a type of lysosome (Varner, 1965; Dillon, 1981, pp. 289–291). On the other hand, acid phosphatase II, which seemed to be cytoplasmic, increased threefold at 3 days, beginning at a level in 24-hr germlings approximating that of the first one; after this initial burst, it continued to become more abundant through the remainder of the period, but at a more moderate rate. Between days 5 and 6, the third isozyme began to appear, but it always provided less than half the level of activity contributed by isozyme II; apparently it was associated with the cell walls, especially those of vascular tissues, where it may have been involved in sugar transport (Sexton et al., 1971; Gilder and Cronshaw, 1973).

In an independent study of phosphatase activity in maize nuclei, the focus was primarily on the source of the high level of inorganic phosphate (P_i) that had been found in the cells of developing embryonic root tips (Deltour et al., 1981). The concentration of P_i was first shown to undergo dramatic increase in the nuclei of such cells during early germination. Nonspecific phosphatase activity was then assayed using three substrates (ATP, pyrophosphate, and β-glycerophosphate) and three levels of pH (4.5, 7.0, and 9.0). Under the most acid conditions phosphatase activity more than doubled with ATP and pyrophosphate as substrates, and more than tripled with β-glycerophosphate between 14 and 72 hr of germination. During the same period, the activity under neutral conditions nearly tripled with ATP and β-glycerophosphate and almost quadrupled with pyrophosphate. In contrast, alkaline phosphatases displayed no significant changes with any substrate, remaining low throughout germination. On the basis of these results, the possibility was raised that a correlation might exist between the high rate of transcription and the levels of acid and neutral phosphatase activities. Nuclear protein phosphorylation has also proven to be at high levels in germinating and in wounded potato tubers, especially if an auxin were added (Schäfer and Kahl, 1982).

Certain seed glycoproteins that are utilized during germination, including phytolectin and cotyledonary reserve protein, contain N-acetylglucosamine as a component of the carbohydrate, which amino sugar is released by proteolytic activities to be employed in the synthesis of new glycoproteins (Li and Li, 1970; Basha and Beevers, 1976; Forsee et al., 1976). Since the proteolytic enzyme that releases the substance should be expected to play a role of unusual importance during germination, an investigation has been conducted to determine the changes that occur during those processes of cotton seed (Yi, 1981). In cotyledons the original level of 0.41 unit at day 0 increased steadily during germination, reaching a total increment of about 250% by day 9. Hypocotyls, while displaying a much lower level of activity, showed a similar net increase, rising from a level of 0.02 unit at day 2 to 0.07 unit on day 9.

Protein Changes in Tuber Development. A differentiation process in plants which is somewhat comparable to the germination of seeds is the sprouting of tubers, those of white potato being especially adaptable to experimental investigation. One recent set of researches was concerned with the changing pattern of nonhistone chromosomal proteins during development, dormancy, and sprouting of these structures (Kahl *et al.*, 1979). Since this class of proteins has been postulated to regulate gene expression in general and to control the transcription of such specific genes as those for histones during the cell cycle, the study cited is of particular pertinence (Kleinsmith, 1975; Stein *et al.*, 1975, 1976; Thompson *et al.*, 1976; Wang *et al.*, 1976; Jansing *et al.*, 1977). But these proteins are in turn subject to such modifications as acetylation and phosphorylation, as became evident in earlier discussions, some of which activities in plants are controlled by hormones, including gibberellic acid (Kish and Kleinsmith, 1974; Trewavas, 1976).

In the study of nonhistone proteins cited (Kahl *et al.*, 1979), attention was confined to the products of the tubers, the sprouts themselves being put aside. Although active tissues have been stated to contain more of these proteins than inactive, the results did not support this view. For example, the electrophoretic pattern from young rapidly growing tubers contained 24 polypeptide bands, including two broad ones of approximate molecular weights of 15,000 and 20,000 and a narrow one that remained near the anode (Figure 5.10A). Later, while the tubers were depositing starch although still undergoing rapid growth, only 16 bands were displayed, none of which was of more than moderate width; in addition, the very light anodal protein had disappeared. Contrastingly, fully ripened tubers, in which growth had ceased, showed 29 bands, several of which were quite wide (Figure 5.10C).

Even after storage for a month at 7°C, the tubers produced more of these proteins than rapidly growing ones, for the electrophoretograms revealed the presence of 31 bands, including three that were quite broad, plus four others of considerable width (Figure 5.10D). Moreover, the very light anodal species, present in the youngest tuber but absent in mature ones, had reappeared, to remain at an even level through the remaining stages. After 2 months of storage at that temperature, however, the number of bands was reduced to 15 as dormancy was finally achieved. Unexpectedly this number of bands increased only to 20 as sprouting began, although the pattern differed greatly from that of dormant tubers and from all others (Figure 5.10F). Comparable changes of protein synthesis were also found when the tubers were wounded by fragmentation of the pith and incubation of the resulting particles; during incubation,

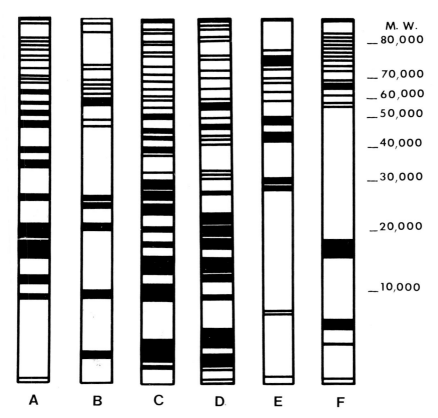

Figure 5.10. Changes in nonhistone chromosomal proteins during tuber development. (A) Nonhistone chromosomal proteins from young, actively growing tubers of white potatoes. (B) From larger tubers, actively depositing starch. (C) From fully ripened tubers. (D) As (C) but after storage for 1 month at 7°C. (E) As (C) but dormant after 2 months' storage at 7°C. (F) From large tubers commencing to sprout. (Courtesy of Kahl *et al.*, 1979.)

gibberellic acid sometimes exercised a stimulatory effect and at others an inhibitory one. However, the hormone did stimulate DNA-dependent RNA-polymerase activity in wounded tubers (Wielgat and Kahl, 1979; Wielgat *et al.*, 1979). It is readily observed in the electrophoretograms that the proteins produced during incubation and the effects of the hormones varied greatly in accordance with the developmental stage and age of the tissues (Figure 5.11).

Ultrastructural Changes. Because cell organelles consist mostly of proteins, fundamental changes in their structure during development and differentiation obviously reflect alterations in the macromolecules that form them and

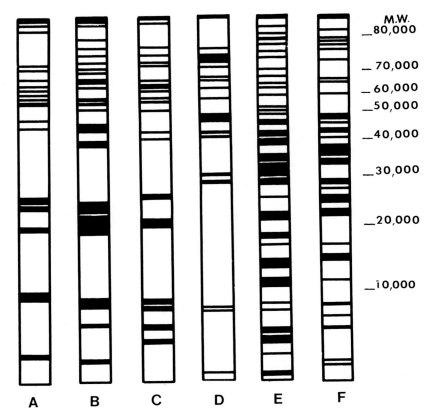

Figure 5.11. Effects of wounding and gibberellic acid on nonhistone chromosomal proteins in white potatoes. (A–C) From actively growing tubers depositing starch. (A) From intact tuber. (B) From wounded tuber tissue, untreated. (C) From wounded tissue treated with gibberellic acid. (D–F) From dormant white potatoes: from intact tubers (D), untreated wounded tissues (E), and wounded tuber tissue treated with gibberellic acid (F). (Courtesy of Kahl *et al.*, 1979.)

thus changes in gene expression. A set of researches into the developing sieve elements of pennycress (*Thlaspi arvense*) makes especially clear this point of view (Hoefert, 1979, 1980).

In these components of the phloem, two types of P-protein (phloem-protein) were present, both of which were absent in the closely associated companion cells that are formed together with the sieve elements by mitotic divisions of mother cells. How soon after division the P-proteins appear in the sieve-element daughter has not been ascertained, but it is evident that gene expression changes either accompany or closely follow cell division in this tissue. Because of the entirely different appearance and behavior of the two P-proteins, they should be considered separate species, not mere variants of a single type. In pennycress, as in cotton (*Gossypium*) and *Passiflora* (Oberhäuser and Kollmann, 1977; Esau, 1978), the commoner species is tubular and is synthesized throughout the life of the cell, even after maturity (Nuske and Eschrich, 1976), whereas the other species is granular and disappears as the cell attains its definitive structure. In order to stress the species level of distinction between the two, it is here proposed that they be designated as Tp-protein and Gp-protein, respectively.

As a rule, the Tp-protein body is of irregular form and appears distinctly fibrous (Figure 5.12A), the actual tubular nature of the apparent fibrils only becoming evident in favorable sections when narrow lumina may be perceptible. Frequently, as the cell approaches maturity, the tubules become less densely arranged and sometimes quite dispersed, a condition referred to as extended (Figure 5.12B). Then after the sieve plate has been completely elaborated, the Tp-protein often becomes loosely congregated on the surface and in the pores of that structure (Figure 5.12C). On the other hand, the Gp-protein is in the form of a compact spherical or ovate body, which is electron-opaque and finely and densely granular; it remains in this condition with no apparent change until the cell has approached maturity, at which point it undergoes dissolution and disappears. Thus, it seems to be merely a storage body that provides amino acids or essential polypeptides for the last stages of maturation.

While the changes in these two protein bodies provide the most distinctive sequence of events in the differentiation of this tissue, a number of other alterations in ultrastructure were to be noted. Even in the earliest stages shown in this study (Hoefert, 1979), the chloroplasts were in the form of advanced proplastids, each containing granular deposits of starch between the four or five photosynthetic lamellae they contained. The latter consisted of a variable number of thylakoids, most of which were short and only rarely stacked to form grana. Later the starch became condensed into rather large grains, followed still later by disintegration of the entire contents of the organelle into sparse, crystalline granules (Figure 5.12C). Mitochondria were relatively uncommon at all stages of development, although they remained constant in structure; the morphology was quite unusual, a point that has not previously been brought out. As among metaphytans in general (Dillon, 1981, pp. 386, 387), the cristae of these organelles were of the microvillose type; in this tissue, however, these parts were greatly swollen, so that instead of being sparingly distributed throughout the stroma of the organelle, they filled the entire interior. Whether or not this condition was natural or an artifact of preparation remains to be established (Dillon, 1981, pp. 377–380). Other organelles were not abundant. Vesicular rough endoreticulum was widespread, and stacks of the cisternal species of this membranous organelle could sometimes be noted; occasional cisternae of smooth endoreticulum and a few dictyosomes appeared late in develop-

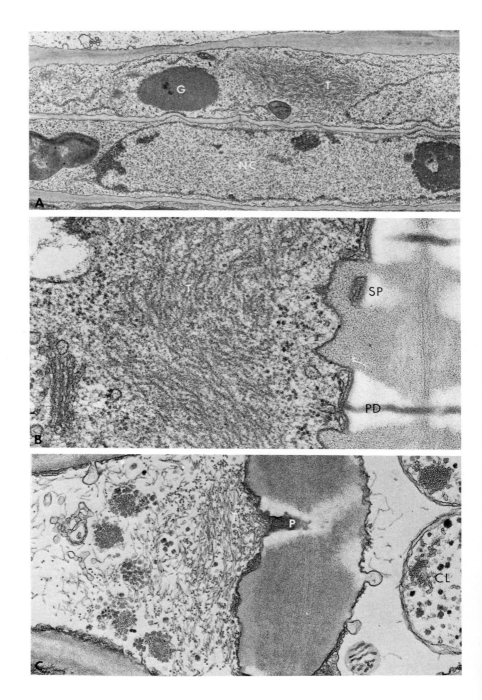

ment, only to disappear entirely as the cell attained maturity. The cytoplasm itself was about equal in electron-opacity to the nucleus in the early stages, but soon became denser than the latter; when the cell underwent further maturation, the opacity decreased as the ribosomes were lost and attained nearly complete transparency at the close of these processes.

5.4. GENE ACTION CHANGES IN DIFFERENTIATING INVERTEBRATES

Despite their ease of culture and diversity of developmental processes, differentiation in invertebrates has received amazingly little attention, especially at the molecular or subcellular level. Two that are exceptional to a degree are the simple coelenterate, *Hydra,* and crustaceans of the genus *Artemia,* the saltwater shrimp. In the first of these experimental models, bud formation had been the principal target of investigations for a long period, but in very recent years a new technique that permitted the growth of specimens having neither nerve cells nor interstitial cells opened additional avenues for research. While time has not permitted any biochemical probings to be conducted on these mutant forms, the very striking results so far obtained promise a bright future for this novel system.

Gene Action Changes during Bud Formation. Although it had long been thoroughly documented that bud cells in *Hydra* arose from parental ones (Tannreuther, 1919; Shostak and Kankel, 1967), the exact pattern of tissue recruitment remained obscure until the investigations of Sanyal (1966) showed that the fate map of the future bud appeared to be in the form of circles about its base. Thus, tissue (both epithelial and gastrothelial) for the growing bud was claimed to be recruited in circular fashion from around its base, those cells that became located near the apex (hypostomal region) of the future offspring being those that had been adjacent to the site of first appearance as a low mound (Figure 5.13; Otto and Campbell, 1977). As the mound gradually developed into a short cylinder, the parental cells that were around the base at this later time were similarly moved outward, and so on in succession as further elongation of the young occurred. While it was not experimentally established,

---

Figure 5.12. Changes in proteins in sieve elements in pennycress. (A) Immature sieve elements of phloem, showing a part of the nucleus (NP) and a Tp body (T) and a Gp body (G), with the nucleus of a companion cell (NC) lying adjacent. 8000×. (B) A more mature sieve element, in which the Tp-protein has become less compact than earlier and lies near the maturing sieve plate (SP) in which plasmodesmata (PD) are evident. 39,000×. (A, B, courtesy of Hoefert, 1979.) (C) Mature sieve element, in which the T-protein has become dispersed and partly fills the pores (P) of the sieve plate. The degenerating chloroplasts (CL) of an adjacent element contain crystalline material. 29,000×. (Courtesy of Hoefert, 1980.)

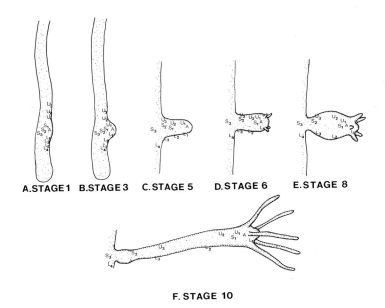

A. STAGE 1   B. STAGE 3   C. STAGE 5   D. STAGE 6   E. STAGE 8

F. STAGE 10

Figure 5.13. Origins of cells in the bud of *Hydra*. As the bud forms and grows, tissue is recruited from the adjacent regions of the parent and distributed more or less in similar sequence in the young. The areas of origin are suggested by the letters (U, upper, S, sides, and L, lower part of parent) and subscript numerals arranged with increasing distance from the developing young. A, apex of early mound and its future location. (Diagrammatic and highly modified from Otto and Campbell, 1977.)

the successive waves of parental cells adjacent to the area must have been continually replaced by mitotic divisions and rapid growth in order to supply the bud; nor is it unlikely that similar mitotic divisions proliferated the parental derivatives after their arrival in the shoot. Recruitment ended after the hypostome of the bud had become partly differentiated and tentacle rudiments began to appear there, so that further growth of the offspring must have been entirely by proliferation of its own cells. Since the young had thus obviously been derived solely from undifferentiated tissue of the parental body, the formation of the tentacles, nematocytes, hypostome, and foot might be attributed to positional effects.

However, in reality morphogenesis in these simple animals is surprisingly complex. Among the complexities is the presence of two regions that assist in regulating the developmental processes, the hypostome and foot (basal disk). For instance, if the former of these is removed from a specimen, young or old, a new hypostome is produced, intimating that the presence of one such structure inhibits the formation of another (Webster, 1971; Wolpert *et al.*, 1971,

1974). The foot, although less thoroughly investigated than the more striking hypostome and its associated tentacles, has also been shown to possess similar properties. Indeed two morphogens (one activator and one inhibitor) have been isolated from this region (Schmidt and Schaller, 1976; Grimmelikhuijzen and Schaller, 1977; Sacks and Davis, 1980) and have proven to be products of the nerve cells, a topic discussed further in the following section.

Morphogenetic Influences in Hydra. As just pointed out, in intact *Hydra* the nervous system has been demonstrated to be the main source of four morphogenetic substances that act either to stimulate or inhibit the formation of the hypostome or foot, depending on their origin (Schaller and Gierer, 1973; Berking, 1977; Grimmelikhuijzen, 1979; Schaller *et al.*, 1979b). However, those techniques mentioned earlier in this section that produced organisms devoid of interstitial cells (Campbell, 1976, 1979; Sugiyama and Fujisawa, 1978; Wanek *et al.*, 1980), and therefore of their derivatives, the nerve cells and nematocytes, have shown that in spite of this absence, the four morphogenetic substances were present in normal or even higher quantities (Schaller *et al.*, 1979a). Moreover, all four types have proved to be chemically identical to those of the normal animal (Berking, 1979). Consequently, it has been made clear that the epithelial cells of normal specimens possessed the potential for producing those substances but simply did not do so when nerves were present (Schaller *et al.*, 1980).

The results of these experiments led to a more detailed investigation of interstitial cells (David and Plotnick, 1980), which actually represent a type of undifferentiated stem cell (Bode and David, 1978). Under typical growth conditions, 60% of the total stem-cell population of normal individuals was shown to divide to produce further stem cells, 30% entered into nematocyte differentiation (Fuijisawa and David, 1981), and the remaining 10% became determined as nerve cell precursors (David and Gierer, 1974; Venugopal and David, 1981a,b). This population grew exponentially, doubling in number every 3½ days, as did the cells of other tissues of the organism. Depletion of the stem cells, however, was found to induce a larger fraction of the population to remain self-renewing, a condition that persisted until the normal density had been recovered (Bode *et al.*, 1976). Other factors also appear to be active in these processes, for only 10% of the stem cells in the hypostome were found to be self-renewing (David and Plotnick, 1980).

RNA Polymerases during Artemia Development. As pointed out earlier (Chapter 3, Section 3.3.1), when the cysts of *Artemia*, containing dormant gastrulae, are immersed in seawater, the embryos emerge and develop into nauplii in a fairly synchronous manner, thereby providing an outstanding system for studies of differentiation at the molecular and subcellular levels. Unfortunately, relatively little advantage has been taken of it for such purposes, and the majority of the few studies that have been made pertain to the nucleic acids. Maximum production of these substances was revealed to occur 30–36 hr after development had been resumed, the rate subsequently undergoing steady decrease until by 72 hr it was less than 10% of peak (McClean and Warner, 1971). In order to understand the basis for the reduction, a series of later researches examined the DNA-dependent RNA polymerases during this period. Whereas in cysts no such polymerase activity could be detected, it was found to appear 1 hr after immersion in seawater (D'Alessio and Bagshaw, 1977). Then at hr 36 polymerase I slightly exceeded polymerase II in quantity, but at hr 72 the latter constituted 80% of the total (Birndorf et al., 1975). However, this change was accompanied by an overall decrease in polymerase activity, part of which resulted from an actual reduction in the quantity of enzyme present on a per nucleus basis—the number of molecules present per nucleus declined from 20,000 at hr 24 to a mere 3500 at hr 72 (Bagshaw et al., 1978). Dormant cysts were discovered to contain a protein S that stimulated transcriptive processes carried out by polymerase II (D'Alessio and Bagshaw, 1979). This protein proved actually to be a complex of several polypeptides, two of which, with molecular weights of 183,000 and 67,000, respectively, were present in a molar ratio of 1 : 2. Its action, which appeared to be species specific, was to enhance the number of RNAs synthesized by *Artemia* RNA polymerase II. During preemergence development and early differentiation after hatching, the protein and its subunits disappeared.

    Other Changes during Artemia Differentiation. In contrast to a number of systems already discussed, the mRNAs of *Artemia* cysts and nauplii have been relatively neglected. Although no protein synthesis proved to be conducted by encysted gastrulae (Hultin and Morris, 1968), assay in an *E. coli* system showed mRNAs were present nevertheless (Nilsson and Hultin, 1974), about 10% of which bore poly(A) segments (Sierra et al., 1976). After development had been initiated and permitted to proceed for 15 hr, total mRNA activity tripled, while that of the poly(A)$^+$ fraction increased sixfold. Moreover, the translation products of the poly(A)$^+$ mRNAs from developed nauplii proved to differ to a degree from those of undeveloped embryos.

    In part the inability of the latter to synthesize proteins was demonstrated to result from the absence of an initiation factor, a protein that was produced in quantity with the advent of development (Filipowicz et al., 1976), but that might not have been the sole deficiency involved. It could also have stemmed from an insufficiency of other enzymes necessary for translation, such as the elongation factor EF-1 (Dillon, 1978, pp. 168–171). This latter type of protein is typically a complex between two interacting factors, even in prokaryotic cells, and it has been described in *Artemia* embryos as consisting of an EF-1α·EF-1β complex. This duality of structure was proposed to serve as a control mechanism through a possible deficiency of one or the other subunit (Slobin and Möller, 1977).

    But the superficiality of this view of control mechanisms is made especially clear by the deficiency of the initiation factor reported above. It is readily comprehensible that absence of such an enzyme would inhibit protein synthesis and that addition of it could permit those processes to occur. What is impossible to perceive is, if it is completely absent as described, how could it ever be produced at any time, since it, like all others, is synthesized by initiation-factor-dependent DNA–RNA–ribosome procedures. Thus, the question is, if the cell cannot initiate protein synthesis, how does it ever acquire the protein-aceous substance needed to do so? The only obvious solution is that protein synthesis in the cyst is not completely inhibited, so that the initiation factor is present but only in minute amounts. Then when development begins, production of that enzyme is increased selectively, thereby permitting an increment in translation to occur. While this proposal appears to solve the problem, actually many additional questions remain unresolved, but discussion of these further aspects is more advantageously held for attention in the closing chapter.

5.5. DIFFERENTIATION CHANGES IN PROTISTA

As Edwards and Lloyd (1980) have pointed out, the growth of unicellular organisms is generally viewed as entirely involving synthesis of new cellular substances, breakdown and replacement of the macromolecules becoming significant only under suboptimal conditions. Hence, it is not an uncommon practice for the synthesis of proteins, RNA, or other biochemicals to be reported as increasing continuously, except perhaps during mitosis (Prescott, 1955; Kessler, 1967; Keiding and Andersen, 1978). But after oscillations in ATP/ADP ratios had been determined and half lives of certain proteins measured, doubts arose as to the validity of this generalization (Chapman and Atkinson, 1977; Bakalkin *et al.*, 1978; Edwards and Lloyd, 1978). Subsequently it was established that proteins, RNA, and other macromolecules were turned over periodically during the cell cycle, even as they are in metazoan and metaphytan cells (Edwards and Lloyd, 1980). Furthermore, there is much evidence which indicates that the nature of the macromolecules undergoes great changes during the cell cycles of unicellular organisms, as well as such less routine activities as encystment. Since the ciliates have received the great bulk of investigation, that taxon alone needs attention here.

Changes in Preconjugant Ciliates. Although the events during and following conjugation in ciliates have long been known to be complex, those which immediately precede that interaction have proven to be little simpler, if at all. When two complementary mating types of a given ciliate species were brought together under the necessary conditions, an interaction was found to be induced that made the cells capable of uniting in bicellular complexes. During this preconjugant stage, individuals of opposite mating types apparently exchanged informational molecules that regulated the processes (Miyake, 1978). One important criterion for the induction of conjugation proved to be the phase of the cell cycle of each cell; mating usually occurred between individuals in macronuclear G_1 (Luporini and Dini, 1975; Dini and Luporini, 1979), but occasional pairing took place with specimens in early S phase of the macronucleus. Once cells had united, macronuclear DNA replication was inhibited, regardless of the cell cycle. According to Verni et al. (1978), there were five stages in the preconjugation processes: (1) The cells contact one another briefly and randomly, during what has often been referred to as a waiting period (Luporini and Dallai, 1980). The cells (2) then congregate. To this point the active cells could be in any phase of the cell cycle, but beginning with (3) the occurrence of clumping or ciliary agglutination, only those in macronuclear G_1 or S phase could participate. The cells (4) then fuse in vis-à-vis fashion, later rotating into (5) a side-by-side union. In at least some cases, it has been reported that when individuals in different stages of the cell cycle unite, their respective nuclei soon become synchronized (Luporini and Giachetti, 1980).

The exchange of informational molecules has been visualized by an unusual technique in which the respective conjugating individuals could be identified; this involved matings between mutants (doublets), which consisted of two cells united, and normal unicellular organisms (singlets) (Dini and Luporini, 1979; Luporini et al., 1979). In the experiments, singlets of one mating type of Euplotes crassus were labeled with [^{3}H]leucine and then mixed with unlabeled doublets of a complementary mating type (Figure 5.14A). Much of the transferal of labeled material into the doublets appeared to occur at stage 3 after fusion of cilia alone had taken place, but the quantity present increased somewhat when bodies of the cells had fused at stage 4. Nevertheless, at earlier stages in which only random contacts had been made, a considerable amount of the labeled product appeared in the doublets (Figure 5.14B).

Changes in Nuclear Macromolecules. One of the striking observations made in recent years was that the nuclear chromatin of ciliates underwent extensive changes in quantity. When the micronucleus of such hypotrichous types as Oxytricha, Stylonychia, and Euplotes developed into a macronucleus, the large molecules of DNA of the former fragmented into relatively small pieces, accompanied by a reduction in size of the genome (Ammermann, 1971; Prescott and Murti, 1973; Ammermann et al., 1974; Lauth et al., 1976). Although similar breakage and reduction is suspected to occur in Tetrahymena and Paramecium, the evidence is not totally clear (Preer and Preer, 1979). Some of this lack of clarity may stem from a second peculiarity of the Tetrahymena macronucleus that has come to light still more recently (Cleffmann, 1980), but first three macronuclear and other traits of ciliates in general must be recalled: (1) The macronucleus is developed from the micronucleus. (2) When the former divides (by a primitive type of mitosis), it does so unequally, so that the daughter nuclei contain different amounts of DNA (Cleffmann, 1968). (3) The macronucleus is able in the absence of micronuclei to sustain all cell

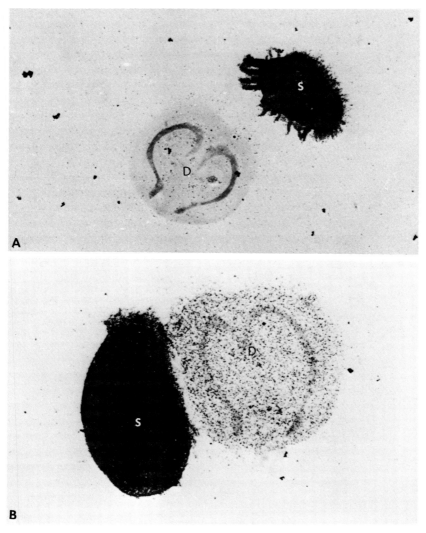

Figure 5.14. Transferal of proteins accompanying conjugation in *Euplotes crassus*. (A) Autoradiogram of a labeled singlet (S) and unlabeled doublet (D) of complementary mating types. That mating reaction has commenced by transfer of labeled protein is evidenced by the presence of that material in the doublet. 200×. (B) The great increase in radioactivity is obvious after cilia fusion (Stage 3) has occurred. 400×. (Courtesy of Luporini *et al.*, 1979.)

functions during vegetative cell multiplication over extended periods of time,* and (4) synthesis of DNA may occur two or more times without cellular division, that is, there may be more than one S phase per cell cycle (Cleffmann, 1975). On the contrary, the S phase may occasionally be omitted during a cycle (Doerder and DeBault, 1978). (5) Finally, chromatin is often eliminated from the nucleus during division (Scherbaum *et al.*, 1958; Shepard, 1965; Murti, 1973; Salamone and Nachtway, 1979).

The extrusion of chromatin from developing macronuclei is a common event that has been found to reduce the DNA of that structure by a mean of around 4% per division (Cleffmann, 1980); in *Tetrahymena*, the chromatin bodies thus formed in the cytoplasm disappear within 20 min. However, the actual amount eliminated at a given time was demonstrated to be highly variable and was clearly not related to the micronuclear (genomic) content nor multiples thereof. In the five cell lines followed for 18 hr, the amount of DNA in the macronuclei fluctuated widely, in one line decreasing by about 25% and in another displaying a threefold difference between the minimum and maximum amounts present.

However, these observations and those from other lines of investigations are difficult to correlate. Both in the present genus and in *Paramecium* the macronucleus in developing from the fused haploid micronuclei following conjugation or autogamy undergoes an increase in ploidy, in the former taxon reaching a level of $50n$ and in the latter one of $840n$—one hypotrich (*Stylonychia mytilus*) has been reported to have a macronuclear ploidy of $4096n$ (Ammermann, 1971; Ammermann *et al.*, 1974; McTavish and Sommerville, 1980). In this hypotrich, the sequence complexity is extremely low, containing only 1.6% of the sequences represented in the micronuclear genome, whereas in *Tetrahymena* its complexity is approximately equal to that of the micronuclear DNA (Yao and Gorovsky, 1974). In spite of the high level of ploidy, the macronuclear DNA of ciliates in general has frequently been found to contain very few repeated sequences and to exist in the form of relatively short fragments produced by specific cleavages of the original macromolecules (Elsevier *et al.*, 1978; Lawn *et al.*, 1978; Lipps and Steinbrück, 1978).

Changes in Histones. The developmental changes in histone species and subtypes that have been described in a number of preceding pages also mark the differentiation of the macronucleus from the micronucleus in ciliates. The former structure contains representatives of all five major classes of histones, all strongly modified by phosphorylation or acetylation (Johmann and Gorovsky, 1976; Gorovsky *et al.*, 1978). Only H2A from this source had been

---

*The micronucleus has been demonstrated recently to play an important, but unknown, role in vegetative growth, for paramecia from which the micronucleus was removed had a greatly elongated cell cycle, imbibed food to a decreased degree, and possessed shortened buccal cavities (Fujishima and Watanabe, 1981). All these characteristics disappeared when a micronucleus was transplanted into the specimens.

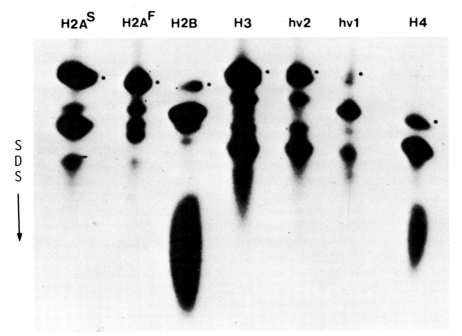

Figure 5.15. Digestion products of the macronuclear histones of *Tetrahymena thermophila*. After digestion of the individual histones with chymotrypsin, the resulting products were analyzed by electrophoresis, followed by fluorography. The large upper spots indicated by dots to their right represent undigested protein. The relationship of hv2 and hv1 to H3 is obvious. (Courtesy of Allis *et al.*, 1980a.)

known earlier to be heterogeneous in primary structure, two subtypes designated as H2A-F (fast) and -S (slow) being present (Johmann and Gorovsky, 1976; Allis *et al.*, 1980a). The latter citation, however, showed the existence of two other histones, called hv1 and hv2, the first of which was tentatively placed as a variant of H3 and the second as an isozyme of H2A. The basis for the latter proposal was not entirely clear, because the electrophoretograms of the digestion products indicated both to be related to H3 (Figure 5.15).

In spite of their progenitory relationship to macronuclei, micronuclei present quite a different profile of histone proteins, as is amply brought out by the two-dimensional electrophoretograms (Figure 5.16). As may be noted there, H2A, H2B, and H4 from both nuclei are similar, but in micronuclei H3 is represented by two subtypes, H3-S and H3-F, not one as in the macronucleus, and both hv1 and hv2 are lacking (Allis *et al.*, 1979, 1980a,b). But the most striking difference is the absence of H1 in micronuclei. In its place are three peptides, referred to as α, β, and γ, which have been reported to be analogs of H1 (Gorovsky and Keevert, 1975; Gorovsky *et al.*, 1978). It should be

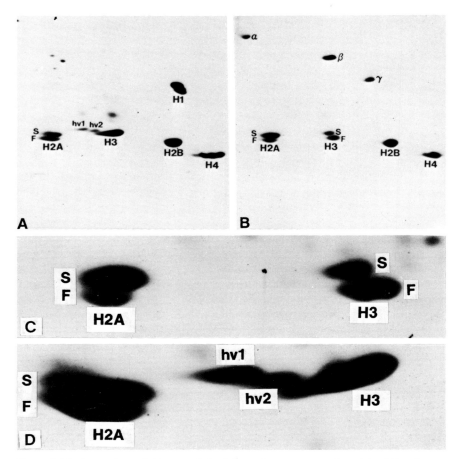

Figure 5.16. Comparison of histones derived from the two types of nuclei of *Tetrahymena thermophila*. When the histones of the macronucleus (A) are compared directly to those of the micronucleus (B), the similarities of H2A, H2B, and H4 from both sources are at once evident. Those of the former differ further from the latter in the presence of hv1 and hv2 and especially in H1; furthermore, α, β, and γ peptides of the latter are absent. (Unpublished autoradiograms, courtesy of C. David Allis.) Individual separations of histones H2A and H3 from the micronucleus (C) and macronucleus (D) clearly reveal the differences between them. (Courtesy of Allis *et al.*, 1980a.)

observed that in the macronucleus, H1 appears to consist of two closely allied isozymes, neither of which are homologs of the three peptides of the micronucleus.

Other Changes in Ciliate Macromolecules. In addition to the several changes in proteins that have been reported (Freiburg, 1981), there are a number of others that must surely occur during the life cycle of these unicellular organisms that so′ far have not been documented at the molecular level. Before cytokinesis occurs, for example, the dorsal and, especially, the ventral ciliature undergoes complex morphogenetic development, particularly in such genera as *Euplotes, Oxytricha,* and *Stylonychia* (Gliddon, 1966; Grim, 1967; Frankel, 1973; Grimes and Adler, 1976; Grimes and L'Hernault, 1978, 1981). The differentiation of these motile organelles involves not only division of the ciliary centrioles (kinetosomes) and production of new cilia, but accurate placement of these structures on the future daughter cell. In addition, lengthening of flagellar stubs occurs and the fusion of the cilia into membranes and cirri, plus many changes in the cortex as well (Grimes, 1972). Furthermore, during encystment of species like *Oxytricha fallax,* a cell coat consisting of four layers is secreted, and both the cytoplasm and nucleus become as altered from the counterpart in the active organisms as in any series of cellular types of metazoans or metaphytans examined in preceding sections. Phagocytotic vesicles abound in such cysts, mitochondria are uniquely structured, the macronucleus becomes almost filled with electron-opaque condensed chromatin, and all the ciliation is resorbed (Grimes, 1973). Hopefully investigations into the protein changes that must accompany such radical morphogenetic alterations will be conducted in the near future. Since other unicellular protistans, such as *Eimeria,* have been shown to undergo radical ultrastructural changes during development (Pittilo *et al.,* 1980), this statement applies to such organisms in general.

6

Gene Expression Changes in Cyclic Functions

Cyclic changes in behavior or activity on the part of eukaryotes in general, correlated to the oscillations in light, temperature, and other variables that characterize the planet on which they live, have become an extremely important area for investigation during the post-1950 period. Circadian and photoperiodic changes related to the day–night pattern have proven especially fertile fields, but infradian (several cycles per day), lunar, and circannual ones have also been productive. A large majority of the investigations have been descriptive of physiological state variations at the organismic level and thus provide only indirect clues that alterations in gene function govern the activities; nevertheless, such studies do serve to reveal the great abundance and wide divergence in character of biorhythms, or chronobiological phenomena, as cyclic behavior has become termed. Nearly all the important life functions have proven to be rhythmic in character, including cell division (Scheving and Pauly, 1973), diapause, energy metabolism, reproduction, sleeping and waking, feeding, types of nutrients consumed, and even the manner of death in man as suicide, coronary disease, and stroke (Kripke, 1974; Reinberg, 1974; Rutledge, 1974; Gorski *et al.*, 1975; Sachsenmaier, 1976; Wever, 1979). But many of lesser importance, such as otolith formation in fish (Barkman, 1978; Dunkelberger *et al.*, 1980; Mugiya *et al.*, 1981), and auditory brain stem response in man (Marshall and Donchin, 1981), also have proven to be rhythmic in occurrence on a daily basis.

Rhythmic behavior can result either as a direct response to a geophysical factor that is itself rhythmic or as an endogenous mechanism of the organism. In the latter case, the periodicity persists under conditions maintained at an invariable level, whereas in the former, the behavior tends to disappear if the

cycling stimulus is removed. Among certain organisms, chronobiological behavior is expressed only under particular environmental influences not related
to the stimulus, the most notorious cases being found among the fungi (Jerebzoff, 1976). In certain *Neurospora* strains, as a case in point, a circadian rhythm
in fructification has been shown to be expressed when either glucose, fructose,
or maltose was present in the medium, but not if sucrose were the sole sugar
(Bianchi, 1964; Jerebzoff, 1976). Similarly in man the circadian rhythm of
ornithine decarboxylase activity in the small intestine is initiated 4 hr after
eating food containing protein (Fujimoto *et al.*, 1978). In analyzing the results
of investigations in this field, the major goals are best achieved by restricting
discussion to those rhythms that appear to be completely endogenous, with
attention devoted wherever possible to systems that reveal changes in gene
action. In addition, a long-term cyclic event in a species' life history, senescence, requires description at the molecular basis to reveal any continuation
that might exist of the series of alterations in gene expression that commences
with the formation of the gametes and extends through growth and maturity.

6.1. CIRCADIAN RHYTHMIC FLUCTUATIONS IN GENE ACTION

Evidence from diverse sources clearly indicates that circadian rhythmic
traits are inherited and therefore are derived from genetic activities, as might
be expected of any endogenous trait. Among the data most convincing of their
hereditability are those provided by the results of breeding experiments of organisms having different rhythmic traits and of those involving the isolation of
mutant strains that display altered circadian rhythms (Bruce, 1976). Additional
support for this conclusion is provided by investigations employing antibiotics
or other reagents to inhibit DNA transcription or RNA translation (Sweeney,
1963; Vanden Driessche, 1975; Mergenhagen, 1976).

6.1.1. Basic Observations

Since circadian rhythms have been shown to be hereditary features, it is
essential that the basic cell processes of DNA replication and transcription and
the translation of messengers into proteins be examined briefly in light of their
possible roles in rhythmic behavior.

DNA Synthesis and the Cell Cycle. Because many cell types of multicellular eukaryotes such as neurons, that do not undergo mitosis, show circadian rhythms nevertheless, it is self-evident that DNA replication is not an
essential component in the cellular mechanism responsible for the recurrence
of functions on a daily basis (Bünning, 1973). Quite to the contrary, the cellular clock mechanism is actually responsible for the rhythmic occurrence of
mitosis and for the synthesis of DNA that precedes it (Burns *et al.*, 1972; Ruby

et al., 1973; Martens and Sargent, 1974). Thus, these aspects of the cycle, along with the one or two growth phases that intervene, are themselves products of an unidentified, independent mechanism. Consequently, in spite of recent statements to the contrary (Edmunds and Adams, 1981), the cell cycle itself is not the clock—rather, to employ a metaphor, its several stages correspond to the hands and the numerals on the face indicating the current time. Although the visible expressions of the rhythm, such as the stages of the cell cycle, may be suppressed, the clockwork continues inexorably, regardless of temperature, most drugs, and even the genome (Brown, 1978).

Attempts have been made to correlate specific enzyme activities to certain aspects of the cycle, particularly to the induction of mitosis. In one such set of investigations, the phosphokinase that phosphorylates histone H1 was studied, because such modifications to that protein enhance its ability to condense DNA (Bradbury *et al.*, 1974; Matthews *et al.*, 1976) and conceivably might thereby lead to the initiation of prophase and chromosome formation. This enzyme, known as growth-associated histone kinase, varied extensively in activity during the cell cycle, increasing 15-fold during the late S and G_2 phases in *Physarum polycephalum* and then declining during M. Furthermore, addition of this substance to the medium in which the fungus was cultured led to early mitosis (Matthews *et al.*, 1976). However, even if it is eventually firmly established that growth-associated histone kinase actually induces mitosis in this organism through its phosphorylating histone H1, it should not be supposed that part of the cellular clockwork has thereby been exposed. For in the first place, in reality this is only the trigger used by that mechanism to induce one event that leads into mitosis, not the whole complex process (Dillon, 1981, pp. 525–556). Furthermore, some unicellular organisms like dinoflagellates have permanently condensed chromosomes, yet undergo mitosis in cyclic fashion. But second and more importantly, the synthesis and activation of the kinase are themselves under the control of the cellular clockwork, as evidenced by the appearance and disappearance of the enzyme at well-defined points in the overall cycle. Thus, the means by which its transcription and translation are controlled and the nature of the cellular clock still remain unexplained. The same conclusions apply equally to other, often unnamed, hypothesized initiators of mitosis (Sachsenmaier, 1976). At one time such mitogens were viewed as being synthesized at a steady rate throughout the cell cycle, attaching to receptor sites on the nucleus as they were produced; then when the required number of sites had been occupied, mitosis was induced. However, this simple model has been shown not to fit experimental evidence and hence is inadequate (Kauffman and Wille, 1976).

One interesting example of the independence of the circadian behavior of the cell and the cell cycle has implications for other aspects of the total problem of gene action changes. In this investigation, uncleaved but fertilized eggs of the Eurasian newt *Cynops pyrrhogaster* were carefully divided into two parts, one nucleated, the other anucleated (Sawai, 1979). The former roughly corresponded to the animal hemisphere, the latter to the vegetal. While the two parts did not always start to divide synchronously, once begun, the rhythm in each had approximately identical time schedules. Both rounded up commencing about 20 min before the first cleavage began to form at the center of the resulting peak; the characteristic furrow then progressed from that pole to the center of the lower surface (Figure 6.1). Nevertheless, it is evident that cleavage and the other behavior patterns displayed were independent of the nucleus and its contained genome and resulted through cytoplasmic control.

Circadian Clock Mutations. Most of the gene mutations that affect endogenous circadian rhythms have been found in *Chlamydomonas, Neurospora,* and *Drosophila,* and in all these organisms they largely influence the length of the repeating cycle (Bruce, 1976). To cite an example of these at the unicellular level, a spontaneous mutation of *Chlamydomonas* has been reported that had a 21-hr cycle of growth and phototaxis, in contrast to the circa 24-hr rhythm of the wild-type organism (Bruce, 1972). Moreover, when mutagenesis was induced in normal colonies by treatment with nitrosoguanidine, one clone gained a mutation which resulted in its having a 27-hr cycle in phototaxis.

The most thoroughly studied day-long rhythms in *Neurospora crassa* are those involving the production of branching hyphae and the formation of conidiospores, but only the latter is truly circadian (Pittendrigh *et al.,* 1959). However, it is expressed solely in those strains that carry the band gene, which affects the activity of the enzyme invertase (Sargent *et al.,* 1966). Using this strain, one laboratory (Feldman and Hoyle, 1973, 1974; Feldman *et al.,* 1973) screened 8000 clones derived from cultures treated with nitrosoguanidine and described three that had a different periodicity from the wild type; one of the two with shorter periods had a cycle of 19 hr and the single mutant with a longer cycle showed a 29-hr rhythm.

Although very little has as yet been learned about inheritable circadian behavior patterns in *Drosophila,* two clock mutants have been cloned by Konopka and Benzer (1971), and two others by Pittendrigh (1974), all induced by ethylmethane sulfonate. The first set of these investigators used gynandromorphs derived from short-period-mutants crossed with wild-type stock, the behavior of which bore out the supposition that the clock mechanism was located in the brain of these flies. Moreover, two systems (or oscillators) seemed to be present, one sensitive to light, the other to temperature.

Rhythm in DNA Content of Nuclei. One circadian rhythm that has been uncovered has proved to be particularly difficult to understand, because it does not fit into current concepts concerning the nature and behavior of DNA. In mature adult rats, the average quantity of DNA per nucleus was demonstrated to increase from the low point attained 3 hr after the initiation of a 12-hr photoperiod to a maximum reached shortly after the beginning of the dark phase (Ruby *et al.,* 1973, 1974). The amount of change was clearly significant statistically, the increment being in the range of 15 to 21%. What was espe-

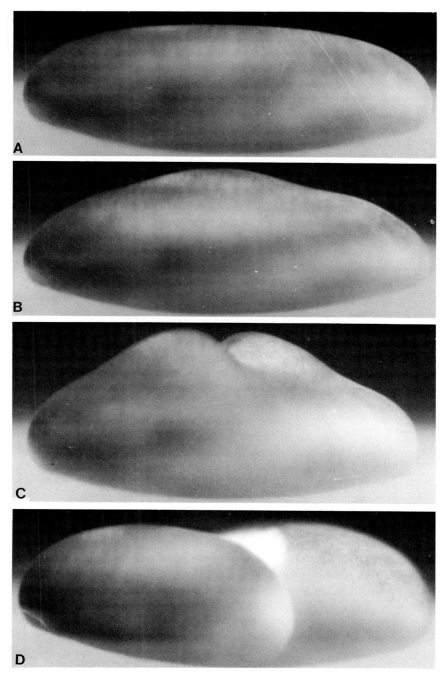

Figure 6.1. Cleavage in the fertilized egg of the Eurasian newt, deprived of the cell coverings. (A) The zygote 60 min prior to cleavage. (B) The same at the initiation of cleavage. (C) The zygote after 20 min of cleavage, and (D), after 60 min. (All courtesy of Sawai, 1979.)

cially confusing was that the increases were not correlated to the rate of [^{3}H]thymidine incorporation, which reached low points at 9 hr after illumination and high peaks at the end of the dark period. Nor was it possible to attribute the observed fluctuation to mitotic divisions, for the mitotic index range was found to be only between 3 and 5 per 10,000 cells (Jackson, 1959).

Rhythmicity in Energy Metabolism. Circadian rhythms have been viewed as an evolutionary adaptation to reap maximum energy harvesting by photosynthetic means through energy conservation and transformation (Pavlidis and Kauzman, 1969; Harold, 1972). As a result of this point of view, it has been thought that the control mechanism involved feedback between compartmentalized sequences of energy transduction, the compartments being constructed of membranes (Wagner, 1976). In support of this hypothesis is a rapidly expanding body of evidence showing the extent of rhythmicity that exists in energy functions (Glick *et al.*, 1961; Sulzman and Edmunds, 1972; Hochberg and Sargent, 1974; Queiroz, 1974), over and above those tied directly to the light reactions of photosynthesis. Perhaps the most thoroughly explored example is provided by growing seedlings of the red goosefoot (*Chenopodium rubrum*), for which approximately 24-hr cycles have been revealed for dark respiration, energy charge, ratio of reduced and oxidized NADP, and changes in activity of adenylate kinase (Dikstein, 1971; Wagner and Frosch, 1974; Wagner *et al.*, 1974). However, a number of related processes showed 12- to 15-hr cycles, such as changes in the activity of malate dehydrogenase, glucose-6-phosphate dehydrogenase, and glyceraldehyde-3-phosphate dehydrogenase (Frosch and Wagner, 1973; Frosch *et al.*, 1973; Deitzner *et al.*, 1974).

Interplay between Hormones. Among multicellular eukaryotes, physiological activities often involve two or more hormones, each of which exhibits an independent circadian rhythm, and in many instances, the effects of one of the substances may depend upon the presence of a second having opposite action. Several especially lucid illustrations of such interplay between two hormones have been provided in amphibians. In the American newt (*Notophthalmus viridescens*), the green aquatic larva undergoes a primary metamorphosis into a red terrestrial immature stage, known as the red eft, under the inductive influence of thyroxine, quite as in anurans. After some time on land, the eft returns to water and undergoes a mild secondary metamorphosis to become the green-bodied aquatic adult, which action is promoted by prolactin (Chadwick, 1940; Grant and Grant, 1958; Grant, 1961). Studies on amphibian late development have led to the generalization that the processes are regulated by antagonistic interactions between prolactin, which favors larval growth, and thyroxine, which induces the first metamorphosis (Etkin and Gona, 1967).

The effects of prolactin, however, have been demonstrated to vary widely in response to a circadian rhythm of the animal itself (Breaux and Meier, 1971; Joseph, 1974). When premetamorphic tadpoles of *Rana pipiens* under long-day photoperiods were injected with prolactin 2 hr after the onset of the light phase, metamorphosis was completely inhibited. In contrast, when the hormone was administered midway or late in the day cycle, no deterrent effect was evidenced. Similarly in red efts, injections of prolactin late in the long-day photoperiod induced migration to the water more frequently than when given early or at the midpoint in the daily cycle (Meier *et al.*, 1971a). Moreover, corticosterone has been found to exert an influence paralleling that of thyroxine, both hormones being effective in the fattening response induced by prolactin in a number of vertebrates from fishes to mammals (Bakke and Lawrence, 1965; Meier and Martin, 1971; Meier *et al.*, 1971b,c; Trobec, 1974). In green anoles (*Anoles carolinensis*) maintained under long-day conditions, it had been shown that treatment with prolactin early in the light phase had no effect, whereas similar injections given midway in the day induced significant increases in stored fat, and those given late led to significant decreases (Meier, 1969a). Later, to determine whether corticosteroids also exercised any influence, experiments were performed on this lizard under continuous light, with daily injections of corticosterone being administered at 6 AM in one group and 6 PM in a second; however, no differing effects could be noted after 9 days (Trobec, 1974). In a further set of experiments with similarly treated lizards, injections of prolactin were given in addition, with the experimental animals arranged in four subgroups injected respectively at 6 AM, 12 noon, 6 PM, and midnight. The animals that received this second hormone together with the corticosterone or 6 hr later showed decrease in fat content, while those treated 18 or 24 hr after receiving the first underwent an increase in fat-body size.

6.1.2. Pineal Gland-Related Rhythms

Since in vertebrates, even in fishes (Kavaliers, 1979, 1981), the pineal gland has often been demonstrated to exercise a regulatory influence over various circadian rhythms (Klein *et al.*, 1981), numerous experiments on chronobiological activities in these animals have focused on this organ. Moreover, these have been conducted at a diversity of levels, including organismic, cellular, ultrastructural, and molecular. Hence, the genetic changes in this aspect of the subject appear to provide an ideal introduction to others that may be less clear-cut. It should first be noted that the gland secretes a hormone, melatonin, in a pattern that is itself circadian in appearance; the substance rapidly increases in abundance after the onset of darkness and then decreases rapidly following the attainment of a peak about midway in the dark phase (Tamarkin *et al.*, 1980).

Ultrastructural Changes in the Pineal Gland. The modern derivative of the former median eye of ancestral terrestrial vertebrates, the pineal gland, has a complex morphology, the ultrastructure of which has been the subject of several reviews (Ito and Matsushima, 1968; Pellegrino de Iraldi, 1969; Matsushima and Reiter, 1975; Korf *et al.*, 1981). Six types of cells are found in the organ: (1) pinealocytes, which make up the bulk of the tissues, (2) Schwann and (3) the associated neuronal elements, (4) glial, (5) epithelial (of capillaries), and (6) pericytes (Kachi, 1979). In mice sampled at 6-hr intervals from populations grown either under 12-hr photoperiod conditions or continuous illumination, several striking ultrastructural changes were observed. Most prominent was the alteration in density/unit area of the granular vesicles of the pinealocytes (Kachi, 1979). Late in the light cycle (7 PM), the vesicles were three times as abundant as they were at their minimal level reached 6 hr later. Glycogen particle numbers showed a parallel course of events, but with a lesser amplitude. The latter pattern had earlier been demonstrated to be eliminated by removal of the superior cervical ganglion and by continuous light, each of which treatment prevented the nocturnal decrease, with a great accumulation of the carbohydrate as a consequence (Kachi and Ito, 1977).

Effects of Pinealectomy. Although scores of investigations into chronobiological effects in vertebrates have employed removal of the pineal gland, a relatively few examples suffice to show the varied reactions to such treatment and the existence of a more fundamental endogenous control mechanism. In the house sparrow (*Passer domesticus*) it had been shown that the circadian rhythm for perching, which persisted even under constant-dark conditions (Binkley, 1974), was lost following pinealectomy (Gaston and Menaker, 1968). Under normal day–night cycles, the body temperature of intact birds also has been shown to drop about 4.5°C in cyclic fashion during the dark phase, a physiological reaction that likewise was lost when the pineal gland was removed (Binkley, 1974). However, if the operated birds were returned to a long-day environment, the rhythmic change became reestablished after 4 or 5 days. A similar drop in body temperature could be induced in intact specimens by injections of the hormone melatonin. Furthermore, when injected with that hormone, comparable temperature decreases resulted in mice (Arutyunyan *et al.*, 1964), and sleeping reactions were obtained in chicks and other vertebrates when the injections were in sufficient quantities (Barchas *et al.*, 1967; Ralph *et al.*, 1967; Hishikawa *et al.*, 1969; Lynch, 1971). Thus, it seems probable that in untreated higher vertebrates, these activities are regulated by the pineal gland, the production of its hormone being reduced during daylight hours and greatly enhanced at night. However, the regaining of normal rhythmic changes in body temperatures by pinealectomized sparrows when placed under standard day–night cycles indicates that some other mechanism exists that is also capable of inducing such cyclic patterns of physiological changes.

In general, results of pinealectomy indicate that the primary effect of removal of this gland is on the control of phase-shift rate rather than on maintenance of the cycle or its entrainment (Quay, 1970a,b). However, generalizations are difficult to draw, because of the species specificity of many circadian rhythms to pineal deficiency. For example, in the rat and white-footed mouse, unlike the sparrow, the 24-hr cycle of running activity remains even after pinealectomy and under normal-day or continuous illumination (Richter, 1964, 1965; Quay, 1968, 1974). Moreover, certain animals that naturally lack a pineal organ, like the alligator, or in which it is poorly developed, as in the Australian possum, nevertheless show comparable circadian rhythms (Kavaliers and Ralph, 1980; Samarasinghe and Delahunt, 1980).

Subcellular Changes in Pinealocytes. Postnatal development of the ultrastructural features of pinealocytes has been observed in a small number of investigations; several of the traits, including numbers of what are called synaptic ribbons and deposits of glycogen, showed circadian rhythmic variations. The synaptic ribbon is an enigmatic structure consistently present in pinealocytes of vertebrates in general, as well as in neuroreceptor cells of sensory organs (Bunt, 1971; Oksche, 1971). Essentially this organelle consists of an electron-opaque rodlet (Figure 6.2A, B), which is surrounded by numerous fine vesicles that recall true synaptic vesicles of neurons in appearance (Vollrath and Huss, 1973; Kurumado and Mori, 1977; King and Dougherty, 1980). Although most synaptic ribbons lie free in the cytoplasm, some are attached to the plasmalemma. The number of them present has been reported to vary in a circadian rhythm (Vollrath and Huss, 1973; Theron *et al.*, 1979), even under constant light or dark (Lues, 1971). During the first 5 days postpartum, however, no rhythmicity was displayed, cells from animals sacrificed at the midpoints of both the light and dark phases of a 12 hr–12 hr cycle increasing in numbers at the same rate (Figure 6.2C). Then for a few days, light-phase cells showed greater concentrations of these organelles than dark-grown ones did, but by day 10 to 12, this situation was reversed, the dark-phase cells having nearly double the numbers of those present during the illuminated period (King and Doughtery, 1980).

A whole series of hormones, enzymes, and other biochemicals have been determined as undergoing daily rhythms of abundance in the rodent pineal. Among these may be listed serotonin and serotonin-*N*-acetyltransferase (Zweig *et al.*, 1966; Illnerová, 1971; Ellison *et al.*, 1972), hydroxyindole-*O*-Methyltransferase (Birks and Ewing, 1981a,b), norepinephrine (Moore and Smith, 1971), and adenylate cyclase (Weiss, 1971), in several of the cycles of which ontogenetic developmental changes were reported. A particularly good example of the changes that occur in biochemicals, both rhythmically and postnatally, is provided by the results of an investigation of the glycogen content of the gland (Kachi *et al.*, 1975). Mice of various known ages between 5 days and 2 years were maintained under a 12 hr light–12 hr dark regimen and samples sacrificed at 1 AM and 1 PM over a period of time to determine the glycogen content of the pineal gland. Five-day-old mice showed a very high glycogen content throughout the day, which decreased rapidly until day 15. However, the first appearance of rhythmic increases during the dark phase did not occur until day 22. The rhythmic changes then became increasingly marked until about day 90, after which there was a gradual falling off in glycogen content

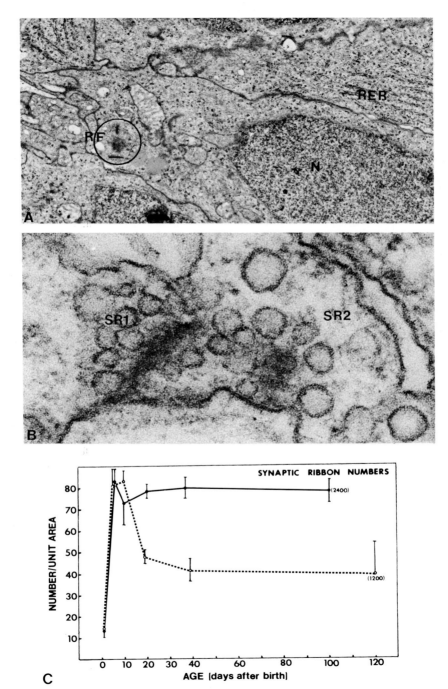

C

to 2 years of age. Although the great majority of researches have studied these organs from rats or mice, similar diurnality and ontogenetic relationships have been revealed in birds—even cultured pineal glands from the chick have been shown to undergo a circadian rhythmic change in N-acetyltransferase activity (Kasal *et al.*, 1979).

This latter enzyme has permitted a demonstration of the intricacies of the rhythmic production of melatonin by this organ (Axelrod and Zatz, 1977; Romero, 1978), and it also is involved in a later discussion of aging effects (Section 6.3.1). The account begins with the release of norepinephrine from sympathetic nerve ends but does not consider the rhythmic behavior of neurons. After its release the hormone binds to pineal cells on β-adrenergic-receptor sites, which display a circadian rhythm in their presence or availability; in broad terms, these receptors more than double in frequency from a low at the beginning of the light phase in a 12 hr light–12 hr dark cycle to a peak reached at the onset of the dark phase, followed by an equally rapid decrease (Romero *et al.*, 1975). When the norepinephrine had bound to the pinealocytes, the synthesis of adenylate cyclase by those cells was stimulated, converting ATP into cAMP; the latter substance in turn stimulated the transcription of a specific gene or genes— and possibly also the processing and translation of the resulting mRNA—to produce N-acetyltransferase. Furthermore, the cAMP was multifunctional for it served also to activate that enzyme and to maintain it in the activated state. When activated, the protein catalyzed the transfer of an acetyl group from acetyl coenzyme A to serotonin to produce an intermediate compound N-acetylserotonin (Figure 6.3). In turn it received a methyl radical from S-adenosylmethionine in the presence of the enzyme hydroxyindole-O-methyltransferase to produce melatonin (Axelrod and Weissbach, 1961; Birks and Ewing, 1981a), which is secreted into the bloodstream. Thus, the cyclic production of this hormone is a consequence of the rhythmic increase in β-adrenergic receptors, perhaps influenced also by the oscillations on the part of the sympathetic neurons. The rhythms in the pituitary production of luteinizing hormone and in the effects of the latter on the gonads are also extensions of the same clockworks located in the pinealocytes and neurons, the nature of which remains unknown. However, it appears evident that the clock is dependent on protein synthesis, for inhibition of those processes with cycloheximide induced phase shifts in sensitive strains of *Neurospora* but not in those that are resistant to the drug (Nakashima *et al.*, 1981).

Figure 6.2. Development of rhythmicity in synaptic ribbons in pinealocytes. (A) Synaptic ribbons in a ribbon field (RF) in a pinealocyte of a 5-day-old rat. Abundant rough endoreticulum (RER) is present near the nucleus (N). 9720×. (B) Greatly enlarged view of a ribbon field containing two synaptic ribbons (SR1 and SR2), lying close to the plasmalemma. 97,200×. (C) The number of synaptic ribbons per unit area is plotted against time in days, the nocturnal counts being indicated by the continuous, the diurnal ones by the broken line. (All courtesy of King and Dougherty, 1980.)

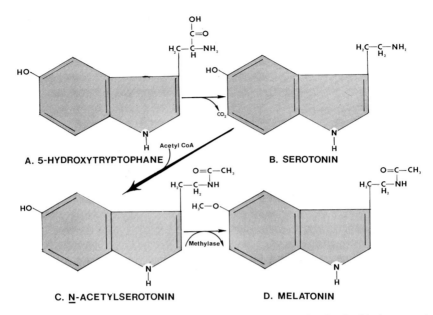

Figure 6.3. The major events in the formation of melatonin. The methylase involved in the conversion of *N*-acetylserotonin to melatonin is hydroxyindole-*O*-methyltransferase.

6.1.3. Other Vertebrate Circadian Rhythmic Functions

Although the pineal gland plays an important role in many circadian rhythmic functions, as has just been seen, a number of others that have been explored show no apparent relationship to that organ (Jacklet, 1981). As in the preceding portion of this chapter, most of the investigations either are at the organismic level or are attempts to find the clock. Others have at least explored the hormones involved in particular cases, and a small fraction have examined the macromolecular changes that accompany the oscillations.

Patterns of Change in Hepatic Enzymes. Systematic studies on the fluctuations in content of various enzymes within the liver have revealed both the presence of numerous independent endogenous rhythms and the complexity of integrative controls. Changes in absolute amounts, as well as in length of the periods and their amplitude, were all uncovered even without varying the composition of the food ingested (Walker and van Potter, 1974). At first laboratory rats were adapted to a regular schedule of feeding, the food being provided for 8 hr early in the 12-hr dark phase and then removed for the remainder of the 24-hr cycle (Potter *et al.*, 1968; Watanabe *et al.*, 1968). One pattern that was displayed, as that shown by ornithine decarboxylase which catalyzed the first step toward the synthesis of polyamines, began with a minimum production rate near zero at the onset of darkness and increased rapidly to the midpoint of feeding. It then decreased with equal rapidity nearly to its original low point by the close of the dark phase. HMG CoA reductase (β-hydroxy-β-methylglutaryl coenzyme A reductase), which is an important inducer of cholesterol production in the liver, showed a similar pattern (Walker and van Potter, 1974), as did tyrosine aminotransferase also.

Somewhat different cycles were found with other hepatic enzymes. One of these was best exemplified by the deposition of glycogen, which rose from its low point at the beginning of feeding as before, but continued to increase throughout the dark phase, even after food was no longer available. With the onset of light, it decreased rapidly in abundance (Watanabe *et al.*, 1968), thus showing a resemblance to the behavior in the pineal gland reported in an earlier paragraph. Glucokinase activity was found to fluctuate in quite a distinctive manner. After the onset of feeding, it decreased markedly for about 2 hr before showing a rapid rate of increment over an equal time span. Then it maintained a much slower increase throughout the feeding period and gradually dropped through the remainder of the dark phase before decreasing rapidly with the onset of light. A number of the enzymatic activities showed effects of the constitution of the diet, glycogen deposition being much greater with low-protein diets than with high, and tyrosine aminotransferase showing the opposite relationship, as might be expected. Furthermore, comparable patterns of change in level of activity have been described for enzymes of liver mitochondria (Philippens, 1974).

Changing Patterns of Metabolic Functions. In a current study several aspects of pyrimidine biosynthesis have been followed in the liver of rats maintained on a 12 hr light–12 hr dark schedule, the light period commencing at 6 AM (Seifert, 1980). In this, as in any study involving the total mass of the liver as a standard of comparison, the circadian variations in size that this organ undergoes must also be kept in mind; in the present case the organ reached its minimal size of about 6 g at noon and its maximal weight of 11–12 g at 8 AM (Figure 6.4), representing a twofold gain over 20 hr and a comparable drop in a 4-hr period. Although differing in scale, the patterns of changes in concentrations were similar for both uridine and cytidine; in parallel with the liver itself, they were at the low point of abundance at 8 AM, but reached their peaks at midnight, after which the quantities present fell off rather steeply (Figure 6.4). However, their rates of synthesis from [2-^{14}C]orotic acid peaked at different points from lows at 8 AM, that of labeled cytosine reaching its high point at 8 PM, four hours ahead of the midnight peak abundance of radioactive uracil.

Changing Patterns of Reproductive Enzymes. Although by far the greater portion of rhythmic alterations in reproductive functions have addressed the problem on a seasonal basis, a relatively few have directed attention to the circadian patterns of the several hormones active in the processes (Stetson,

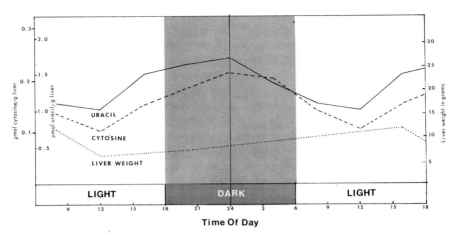

Figure 6.4. Circadian variations in pyrimidine nucleotide synthesis in the liver of rats. The change in liver weight has a rhythm distinct from the two nucleotides. (Modified from Seifert, 1980.)

1978). Among these is a study that focused on the prepubertal development of the blood serum luteinizing and follicle-stimulating hormone levels in hamsters (Smith and Stetson, 1980), beginning with 10-day-old individuals. All were maintained under a 14 hr light–10 hr dark program of illumination. The levels of neither hormone showed any rhythmicity until after day 15, at which time the level of the first of the pair dropped close to the nil point. Beginning on day 16, it began a series of sharp changes in quantity present but in a very irregular fashion; over the next 2 days, the sharp peak that characterized the adult around 5 PM was developed and continued from that period onwards. Similar behavior was observed in the follicle-stimulating hormone levels, except that there was no decrease in concentration at day 15, and rhythmicity could not be noted until day 17. How much of these effects stemmed secondarily from the rhythmic production of melatonin by the pineal gland was not explored.

6.1.4. Circadian Rhythms in Other Organisms

Investigations into circadian fluctuations in organisms other than vertebrates are spottily distributed over the living world, certain fungi and invertebrates like crayfish receiving disporportionately large shares, while others have been totally neglected. Many photoleriod-related functions of the flowering plants are seasonal and accordingly receive attention later; consequently little has been garnered of their actual daily patterns of changes, especially at the macromolecular level.

Circadian Patterns in Unicellular Organisms. Even such simple pro-tistans as the flagellate *Euglena*, the ciliates *Tetrahymena* and *Paramecium*, and the green algae *Acetabularia* and *Chlamydomonas* have long been known to exhibit one or more circadian rhythms (Bruce and Pittendrigh, 1957; Hastings, 1959; McMurry and Hastings, 1972; Edmunds *et al.*, 1974; Schweiger, 1977), and bacteria, but not blue-green algae, appear to show chronobiological prop-erties (Bortels, 1959). One of the more important cyclic functions in unicellular eukaryotes in general is that of cell division, which in many forms occurs once every 24 hr, even in constant darkness (Sweeney and Hastings, 1958; Volm, 1964; Wille and Ehret, 1968; Barnett, 1969; Bruce, 1970). Several enzymes in *Euglena* have now been demonstrated to show daily oscillations in activity independent of those of cell division. One of these, deoxyribonuclease, was found to remain at a constant level for about 5 hr after the onset of the light phase, after which it increased rapidly until the 14-hr dark phase began 5 hr later, when it remained at a plateau (Walther and Edmunds, 1970). Under the same regime of lighting, alanine dehydrogenase reached minimal activity mid-way in the dark phase and peaked late in the light phase, the amplitude amount-ing to about 25% over the low point. Later this same pattern, with still greater amplitude, was revealed to persist for at least 7 days in total darkness (Ed-munds *et al.*, 1974).

At least two circadian rhythms involving photosynthesis in *Euglena* have been brought to light, one related to the cell cycle, the other one not (Laval-Martin *et al.*, 1979). However, both were independent of cell cycle events. A photosynthetic CO_2 fixation rhythm occurred with a period of 24 to 30 hr in either synchronously dividing or in nondividing cultures, grown under either 12 hr light–12 hr dark or $\frac{1}{3}$ hr light–$\frac{1}{3}$ hr dark cycles. Under similar growth conditions, total chlorophyll content showed a comparable oscillation but the maximum followed the CO_2 fixation peak by about 4 to 6 hr.

In the green flagellate *Chlamydomonas reinhardi*, mutations involving the biological clock have been isolated and recombination studies completed (Bruce, 1972, 1974). Among the 24-hr cyclic functions that have been revealed in this organism are responsiveness to light, motility, and growth (Bruce, 1970; Straley and Bruce, 1979). The latter article cited also demonstrated the existence of several other circadian oscillations, including cell division and what was termed "stickiness to glass." This feature really was a reflection of changes in the macromolecules of the cell coat, which is largely pectinaceous. Under a 12 hr light–12 hr dark schedule, the stickiness increased from the low point reached around 7 hr after the light phase began to an abrupt peak at 2 hr into the dark phase. In this form the products of cell division are retained within the cell coat for a period, release of the daughter cells ("hatching") proving also to be a rhythmic activity (Straley and Bruce, 1979).

Still another cyclic function of *Chlamydomonas* has recently been re-ported, one that provides an insight also into the complexity of cellular activities. Tubulin synthesis may be induced by two different mechanisms, one by artificial or accidental loss of the flagella and the second by cell cycle events (Weeks and Collis, 1979). In the first type, tubulin synthesis commenced within 15 min after deflagellation and was found to occur in vegetative, gametic, and early zygotic stages of the organism. During the 1-hr peak rate of production in the latter two stages, the structural component accounted for 15 to 20% of total protein production. However, 1½ hr after initiation of zygote development, neither tubulin synthesis nor flagellum regeneration took place. In the second type, induction occurred 1½ to 2 hr before the onset of cytokinesis. Relatively high rates of tubulin production (ca. 5% of total protein synthesis) resulted and continued throughout the 9-hr period of cell division until just prior to release of fully flagellated daughter cells. Unfortunately, the specific members of the tubulin multispecies complex being produced during the several stages were not determined (Dillon, 1981, pp. 174–176).

   Circadian Rhythms in Fungi. Relatively few circadian rhythms have so far been uncovered in fungi, but undoubtedly exist in numbers as large as those of other eukaryotic organisms. One that has been well established as occurring in *Neurospora crassa* pertains to spore formation. When grown in the dark on solid media, conidiospores were formed with a rhythm that was insensitive to culture temperature and exhibited a periodicity under constant darkness approximating 24 hr (Sargent and Woodward, 1969). Changes in the constitution of the total lipid along the growing edges of the mycelium accompanied this cycle, ranging from a minimum content of 37% unsaturated fatty acids to a maximum of 83%. The high point was correlated to the conidiospore-formative period (Brody and Martins, 1976). One particularly important observation was made recently with regard to a mutation that changed the periodicity of spore formation by 3 hr (Dieckmann and Brody, 1980). This mutant was resistant to oligomycin, a condition that appeared to result from a change in the primary structure of a particular protein of the mitochondria. Consequently, it was contended that the chondriosome might play a vital role in the actual biological clock.

   In addition to the foregoing and those pointed out in Section 6.1.1, one rhythmic cycle of a fungus is of particular interest, because of its relation to development in spite of its being infradian in nature rather than circadian. It will be recalled that during the aggregation stage of *Dictyostelium*, cAMP was released at intervals to serve as a pheromone in guiding the amoeboid cells (Chapter 5, Section 5.1.1). More recent investigations have revealed that the pulses of secretion of this substance occurred at regular intervals of approximately 10 min (Gerisch, 1976). During the interphases between pulses, both the intracellular and extracellular levels of the pheromone were quite low; then when a pulse was begun, there was an extremely sharp rise in the intracellular level, amounting to a 10-fold increment within 2 min, followed by a nearly equally abrupt drop to prepulse levels within 3 min. A similar but less dramatic pulse followed in the external environment with about ½ min delay, the slopes of the peak being similar to those of the intracellular ones but beginning at concentrations close to zero. The decline was shown to result from hydrolytic breakdown of the cyclic nucleotide by phosphodiesterase in the external medium. The synthesis of cAMP was found to be stimulated by its presence extracellularly, possibly mediated by receptors on the plasmalemma of aggregation-competent cells. Thus, the gaining of competence for aggregation in the amoeboid cells involved the new expression of genes for receptor sites, and secretion of cAMP and phosphodiesterase. The changes in the total protein profile of the amoeboid cells during aggregation have not received attention as yet.

Circadian Rhythms in Invertebrates. The majority of the investigations into rhythmic functions of invertebrates at the subcellular level have involved the eye of certain crustaceans and mollusks, while the macromolecular aspects have remained neglected. In crayfish, insects, and mollusks, many of the circadian rhythms at the organismic level are controlled or influenced by those of neurons, so that the latter cells have often served as the primary focal point of investigations (Strumwasser, 1965; Brady, 1969; Jacklet, 1969; Truman and Riddiford, 1970). The optic apparatus of the marine gastropods of the genus *Aplysia* has proven especially valuable for researches, because the eye, together with the optic nerve, can be isolated and maintained in culture media for periods up to a week. Under constant darkness the nerve showed a pulse frequency that was modulated in a 24-hr cycle (Jacklet, 1969, 1974), but the phase of the rhythm could be variously entrained by suitable exposure to light, even in the isolated organ. Gradual excision of parts of the eye from the lens inward showed that the secondary cells provided the compound action potentials to the central nervous system and that populations of cells, rather than single ones, were required to evoke such an action. However, it has been demonstrated more recently that ionizing radiation abolished the circadian rhythmicity of compound action potential generation, without affecting the other functions of the eye (Woolum and Strumwasser, 1980).

The structural changes that take place in the crayfish eye with a daily cycle were described by Eguchi *et al.* (1973). In the cytoplasm of the reticular cells two classes of multivesicular bodies, large and small, were found (Dillon, 1981, pp. 287, 288) along with distinctive organelles referred to as combination and lamellar bodies. The small multivesicular organelles remained fairly constant in numbers throughout the cycle, except for peaks at 30 min of the light phase and again after 6 hr of dark. In contrast, the large class of these particles increased strongly after 1 hr of light and established a plateau of about 4 hr duration before declining in numbers over the remainder of the light phase. More recently the compound and lamellar bodies, which became greatly abundant beginning at hr 1 of the light phase and reached peaks between hr 4 and 6, have been demonstrated probably to represent degradation products of the surface microvilli (Hafner *et al.*, 1980; Stowe, 1980), which break down during illumination.

6.2. SEASONAL AND ANNUAL CYCLIC CHANGES

Since one of the most prominent types of annual and seasonal cycles is that which involves reproductive activity, it is self-evident that its molecular and fine structural aspects have received the majority of attention. But the quasi-semiannual periods of migration, especially in birds (Aschoff, 1955; King and Farner, 1974), and the circannual occurrence of hibernation in mammals (Kayser and Petrovic, 1958; Kolpakov *et al.*, 1974), including changes in hormone secretion (Schulte *et al.*, 1981), have likewise provided the basis for numerous investigations. Although only the surface has been touched in this relatively recent aspect of biology, the responses of organisms to annual changes in light, temperature, and other parameters of the earth have proven extremely diverse, even among tropical forms (Marshall and Williams, 1959; Zimmermann, 1966) and fishes (Kavaliers, 1980, 1981; Kavaliers *et al.*, 1980).

6.2.1. Circannual Changes in Reproductive Processes

In view of the circannual cyclic behavior of the reproductive processes having been more thoroughly investigated than the others, they are reviewed first to provide a basis for comparison for the miscellany that then receives discussion. Later it may be possible to suggest a relationship of these annual oscillations to the circadian rhythms, at least on a causal basis.

Seasonal Cyclic Fluctuations in Avian Sex Hormones. Among birds, the common mallard duck provides an especially appropriate model for investigating circannual changes in reproductive function, because the numerous domestic strains, such as Peking, Rouen, and Khaki Campbell, permit meaningful comparative studies. Pairing of the sexes in ducks, however, endures only to the termination of egg deposition and consequently the pattern of hormonal activity is not typical of those numerous other avian species in which pairing is permanent nor in those in which both parents engage in incubation and posthatching rearing of the young. In spring in all the male and female mallards the gonads increased in size, those of the domestic drakes attaining a greater weight than those of wild ones (Benoit, 1936; Johnson, 1961; Donham, 1979). This growth, which continued into the nesting season, was accompanied by elevated blood plasma levels of luteinizing hormone and testosterone, the peak concentrations of the latter, but not of the former, being higher in domestic than in wild stock (Haase *et al.*, 1975a,b), and follicle-stimulating hormone concentration rose concurrently (Balthazart and Hendrick, 1976). In females the plasma levels of estrogens rose slightly during the nesting season but remained lower than those of testosterone; the peak concentrations of the latter and luteinizing hormone were attained during egg laying, which occurred about 1 month earlier in domesticated stocks than in wild (Donham, 1979). Once incubation began, levels of all these hormones dropped rapidly in all females and wild males, but remained elevated in domestic drakes.

Seasonal Rhythms in Mammalian Reproduction. In many mammals under darkness and short-day conditions, the pineal gland appears to exercise a suppressive effect upon the reproductive system (Pflugfelder, 1956; Quay, 1956; Mogler, 1958). Under those conditions, the ultrastructural changes in the pineal gland that were noted indicated the occurrence of secretory activity, accompanied by reduction in size of the reproductive organs of the animal. In mammals of boreal regions where photoperiods reach especially severe extremes, the pineal gland has been found to be particularly large, the Weddell seal, for example, having a gland 5 to 10 times as massive as that of a dog of equal body size (Cuello and Tramezzani, 1969). Comparable but long-day photoperiod effects have been shown to be active in such rodents as the Syrian hamster which breeds only during the summer, even in the laboratory; by artificially increasing the photoperiod, however, Cusick and Cole (1959) were able to maintain the animals in breeding condition throughout the year. During the annual cycle, the concentrations of melatonin in the pineal underwent dramatic changes (Rollag *et al.*, 1980). Under long-day conditions (14 hr light–10 hr dark) the hormone level rose to a mean maximum of 949 pg/gland in male hamsters 8 hr after the onset of darkness, a change paralleled by that of the *N*-acetyltransferase activity (Rudeen and Reiter, 1979a). Under short-day regimes (8 hr light–16 hr dark), however, they reached mean peaks of 894 pg/gland 13 hr after the onset of darkness.

Consequently, rather than being an endogenous rhythm, the seasonal cycle in these vertebrates appears on the surface to be environmentally induced, but a fuller view of the subject has indicated that such is not completely the case. When hamsters were maintained under extremely short photoperiods of 1 hr light–23 hr dark for 30 weeks, the testes and accessory sex organs degenerated from their average active weight of 3 g to approximately 0.5 g during the first 10 weeks (Reiter, 1971, 1974). Then during the next 20 weeks, these organs increased in size so that by the end of the 30th week, they were fully active in spite of the near-constant darkness.

Other Cyclic Reproductive Activities. The pineal gland is associated with a number of other reproductive functions, especially with certain hormones. In female rats, by way of illustration, removal of that organ has been shown to result in decreased levels of pituitary prolactin (Donofrio and Reiter, 1972; Relkin *et al.*, 1972). In males, similar treatment eliminated the characteristic surge of plasma prolactin that normally occurred each night (Ronnekleiv *et al.*, 1973). But not all such activities are influenced by the pineal. Female rats that have been ovariectomized and given a single injection of polyestradiol phosphate showed a surge of plasma prolactin each afternoon for a period of 3 weeks, after which it diminished in magnitude (Subramanian and Gala, 1976). This circadian surge resembled the elevated plasma prolactin levels that had been reported to occur on the afternoon of proestrus in normal rodents (Pieper and Gala, 1979a) and has been found to be independent of influence by the pineal gland and photoperiod, as well as olfactory stimuli (Pieper and Gala, 1979b).

The range in seasonality of reproductive activities is very broad in scope in harmony with the diversity found among the mammals themselves. For instance, the annual loss and replacement of the antlers in deer is a striking feature of reproductive behavior. However, this trait is induced by lengthening days and thus does not represent an endogenous system (Goss, 1980). Similarly the age at which puberty occurs in many rodents varies with the time of birth (Johnston and Zucker, 1980). Complete spermatogenesis first began in 60-day-old mice grown under long-day (14 hr light–10 hr dark) conditions, whereas it was not manifested until day 140 under short-day (10 hr light–14 hr dark) schedules.

6.2.2. Other Circannual Rhythms

Although numerous seasonal and annual rhythms exist in nature, many are directly related to environmental factors, such as day length or temperature changes. The leafing of trees, flowering of herbs and shrubs, spore production by ferns and mosses, and migrations of birds and certain butterflies all fall into this category—even the blood picture of rodents undergoes annual fluctuations (Berger, 1980, 1981). Often such cycles are highly complex and include a number of subcycles—bird migration, for instance, is one of many associated subcycles, including fat accumulation, molting of feathers, territorial behavior, reproductive activities, and flocking (Farner, 1970; King and Farner, 1974).

Some Factors Involved in Bird Migration. For many years, it appeared that the gonads played a leading role in the seasonal appearance of migratory behavior. Rowan (1925, 1932) very early had proposed that the lengthening photoperiod stimulated growth of the gonads, resulting in the production of gonadal steroid hormones, and that the latter then led to increased food intake and fat deposition, followed by migration. In three species of sparrows of the genus *Zonotrichia,* to cite a specific example, premigratory deposition of fat and the occurrence of nocturnal restlessness (Zugunruhe) were prevented by either castration, ablation of the gonadotropic region of the hypothalamus, or masking the eyes (Weise, 1967; Gwinner *et al.*, 1971; Stetson, 1971; Stetson and Erickson, 1972; Stetson and McMillan, 1974). However, the two responses have proven to be only the terminal effects of a long, complex series of activities. First of all, prolactin appears to play a prominent role, in general having an inhibitory effect on the reproductive organs (Meier and Dusseau, 1968); moreover, in the lesser snow goose it has been shown to undergo changes in abundance correlated to the season (Campbell *et al.*, 1981). Since injections of follicle-stimulating hormone can reverse the inhibitory effect, the action of the prolactin has been thought to be that of suppressing the release of the other hormone (Bates *et al.*, 1937; Nalbandov, 1945).

However, it is now known that in part the reaction involves a temporal element (Meier, 1969b). Although the response of the oviduct to gonadotropins is inhibited by prolactin at any time of the day, that of the ovary is arrested only when prolactin is given early in a 16-hr photoperiod, injections given late having no effect (MacGregor, 1974). On the other hand, administrations of the hormone given in the middle of that period stimulated fattening in the white-throated sparrow but induced loss of fatty tissue when given early (Meier and Davis, 1967). Moreover, this same endocrine product displays comparable time relations with corticosterone (Meier *et al.*, 1965, 1971a). In birds maintained under continuous light, a daily rhythm was entrained by corticosterone in the responses of gonads to prolactin. When injected 8 hr after treatment with that hormone, prolactin inhibited gonadal growth, but when it followed the former by 12 hr it stimulated increase in size, the precise pattern being species specific.

For instance, in the house sparrow, growth of the gonads was stimulated by prolactin if it followed corticosterone by 4 to 8 hr but showed no effects at other times. Under natural conditions the daily peaks in blood plasma of both hormones were revealed to vary according to the season, the two maxima differing by 12 hr during the spring but by only 6 hr in the summer (Meier *et al.*, 1969; Dusseau and Meier, 1971). When birds were injected with prolactin at 12, 8, and 4 hr after treatment with corticosterone, the resulting behavioral and physiological events were typical respectively of those of spring, summer, and fall (Meier and Martin, 1971; Martin, 1974). Further, the specific timing of the level changes in hormones and the resulting behavior has a genetic basis that proved to be population-specific in European warblers (Berthold and Querner, 1981). Thus, in a nonmechanical way, many seasonal activities are really products of circadian rhythms whose timings undergo alteration under the control of changing gene expression influenced by photoperiod characteristics often mediated by the pineal gland, at least in mammals (Rudeen and Reiter, 1979b, 1980; Kennaway *et al.*, 1981).

Circannual Behavior among Invertebrates. A number of invertebrates, especially clams, chitons, other mollusks, and echinoderms, whose life histories span several years, undergo circannual rhythms of behavior, particularly with regard to reproduction. In most Northern hemisphere mollusks and echinoderms that have been studied to date, the mean peak size of the gonads was attained shortly after the vernal equinox (Halberg *et al.*, 1974). The ovaries in the black chiton (*Katharina tunicata*) reached their maxima several days prior to the peak of testicular size, whereas in the sea bat (*Patiria miniata*) the reverse situation prevailed and in the ochre starfish (*Pisaster ochraceus*) both types of gonads peaked on the same day. In such echinoids as the purple sea urchin (*S. purpuratus*), however, the gonads attained their greatest mass shortly before the winter solstice, the male organs preceding the female by several days. Since the hepatic ceca of the starfishes showed their maxima about 180 days after those of the gonads, the existence of several clock mechanisms was disclosed.

In fact the timing mechanisms in these organisms are of great complexity, according to analyses of certain classes of biochemicals (Halberg *et al.*, 1974). The lipid content of the ovaries (percent of dry weight) reached its greatest proportion before the protein of ovaries and testes in both the black chiton and the Pismo clam (*Tivela stultorum*), just preceding maximum size of the organs. However, the carbohydrate content was greatest nearly 180 days after those maxima in both species. Even the plates of the chiton had a separate circannual cycle, their peak protein content occurring in late May. Some of the foregoing changes in reproductive organ biochemical composition of echinoderms may be associated with the fluctuations in sex hormone levels that have recently been described in the starfish *Asterias rubens*. Like the related chordates, these animals synthesize C_{21} steroids from cholesterol and C_{19} ones from progesterone (Schoenmakers, 1977, 1979a, 1980a; Schoenmakers and Voogt, 1980), the ovaries and pyloric ceca alike being active in the processes. Moreover, androstenedione appeared to be metabolized rapidly into other C_{19} steroids, but no estrogens have been found (Schoenmakers, 1979b). Progesterone levels in the ovaries have proven to be high during stage 1 (resting gonads), but decreased during stage 2 (early growth of the organs), remaining low through stages 3 and 4 (late growth and partial maturation, and full maturation, respectively). In the pyloric ceca the profile was only partly parallel, for while it was similarly high in stage 1, it remained at that level through stage 2, decreasing only in stage 3; then just before spawning in the final stage, it regained its original level (Schoenmakers and Dieleman 1981). In contrast, estrone was at a low level both in the ovaries and pyloric ceca, except that during vitellogenesis late in stage 1, it briefly increased in abundance. Further, the activity of an enzyme (3β-hydroxysteroid dehydrogenase) that participates in the conversion of pregnenolone into progesterone has been followed through the annual cycle. During stage 1, this protein was at low levels but began to escalate near the close of that resting period; this increase continued and reached a peak in stage 2. Beyond that point, the enzyme activity decreased rapidly to a low level, where it remained during the rest of stage 3 and the whole of stage 4 (Schoenmakers, 1980b).

Circannual Rhythms of Flowering. Flowering plants have long been known for their responses to seasonal changes in day length—indeed, even the first proposal advocating the existence of an endogenous daily rhythm was based on the flowering of angiosperms (Bünning, 1936). In the laboratory, short-day plants like the red goosefoot (*Chenopodium rubrum*), duckweed (*Lemna perpusilla*), and cocklebur (*Xanthium strumarium*) have proven especially valuable experimental subjects. The first of these has a capacity to flower that oscillates rhythmically in response to a single dark period of a broad range of lengths (King, 1974), whereas the cocklebur is valuable for its extreme sensitivity, just one dark period in excess of 8.3 hr having proven sufficient to trigger flowering (Salisbury and Denney, 1971, 1974).

For the greater part, researches on photoperiod-induced seasonal blooming of plants have focused on the mechanisms involved in the control of expression. Two types have been suggested, endogenous rhythmic ones similar to those of circadian cycles, and hourglass timers (Takimoto and Hamner, 1964). In several genera, including *Pharbitis* and *Chenopodium,* the hourglass type appeared to be represented by phytochrome P_{fr} (far-red) (Evans and King, 1969; King, 1974; Yamamoto and Smith, 1981), for this substance disappeared during the dark periods. Measurements of the period required for its loss in the goosefoot revealed that this pigment increased slightly during hr 1 of the dark phase, then remained on a plateau till about hr 4, at which point it decreased rapidly to nearly a nil level. However, when the dark phase was interrupted at hr 4 by 5-min exposure to red light, the phytochrome content became restored to its earlier high level to decrease to near zero by hr 6, subsequent flowering being greatly inhibited. On the other hand, if the 5-min exposure to red light was given at hr 2, the subsequent patterns of phytochrome loss were unaffected, and flowering was decreased to only a slight degree.

Thus, on the surface it seems that phytochrome P_{fr} serves as an inhibitor of flowering, as its presence is maintained by light; then when darkness induces it to disappear, comparable to the sand running out in an hourglass, flowering is able to be initiated. This view, however, is simplistic in that the pigment is considered merely to disappear in the absence of light. Since its loss is rather rapid, it can scarcely be thought to result from ordinary turnover processes in combination with cessation of synthesis. Consequently, the sharp drop in concentration more likely results from the synthesis or release of an enzyme that converts the phytochrome to a colorless compound, the suddenness of its appearance suggesting it to have lysosomal origins. Therefore, it may not be the disappearance of the pigment that leads to flowering, but the pigment-destroying enzyme or factors associated with it may actually be the active ingredient. Indeed the latter proposal possibly receives support by the known presence of a flower-promoting factor that has been extracted from *Lemna* (Halaban and Hillman, 1974). Because phytochromes have been shown to be associated with the directional transport of ions through the cell (Fondeville *et al.*, 1966; Hendricks and Borthwick, 1967; Satter *et al.*, 1970), those pigments could well prove to be part of the intricate supramolecular genetic mechanism that controls cell activities in general.

The endogenous rhythms, too, have proven to be complex. At least three different circadian rhythms have been demonstrated to be involved in seasonal (photoperiod)-related flowering, along with various hourglass factors. These include (1) an internal rhythm that is triggered by exposure to light (the "light-on" rhythm); (2) another that is activated by the occurrence of darkness (the "light-off" rhythm); and (3) an additional, less well-documented cyclic activity that results from a summation of the first two (Takimoto and Hamner, 1964). Moreover, additional independent timing mechanisms appear to be involved in other plant activities, such as leaf movements and folding and unfolding of leaflets, because no correlation between blooming and the others could be found (Salisbury and Denney, 1974). Comparable seasonality of behavior occurs in gymnosperms, as demonstrated by the extensive changes in ultrastructure of the microsporangiate strobili of Scotch pine that takes place during the winter months (Kupila-Ahvenniemi *et al.*, 1979).

One recent investigation on flower production has provided direct evidence of gene expression changes that accompany those processes. During the transition to flowering in *Sinapis alba* after being transferred from short-day to long-day conditions, a protein referred to as A and found in the meristem of the still-vegetative plants increased in quantity for the first 48 hr in the new environment (Pierard *et al.*, 1980). Until hr 96 it then remained at a constant level, after which it disappeared. Two others, called B and C, that were absent in the apical meristem during vegetative growth, appeared in that of the activated plants between hr 30 and 36 and progressively accumulated in quantity until day 10. These two proteins were said actually to have appeared 8 hr before reversible commitment to flower primordial production by the meristem and 24 hr before the initiation of flower production.

6.3. LIFE-CYCLE-RELATED RHYTHMIC CHANGES

Although all organisms may be considered individually to undergo a life cycle full of changing gene actions, the occurrence of any given major set of events is not duplicated, of course, within a single specimen but only in successive generations. Consequently, the alterations in morphology, physiology, and other aspects of cells and organisms that occur over their life spans, while not cyclic in the same sense as circadian and circannual ones, are rhythmic from a populational or species standpoint. Since the beginning phases of life-cycle-related changes have been documented in the first five chapters, here those of the late phase, senescence or aging (Sacher, 1978), alone remain to be examined. Although the long middle, or adult, phase of the life cycle thus is neglected as a separate topic, many of its aspects, including its most characteristic feature, reproduction, have necessarily received attention in those same five chapters as the basis of comparison with younger stages.

Most, but not all,* multicellular, and probably many unicellular, organisms undergo a period of aging, the changes during which are hereditary. Although in some cases, as in the fungus *Podospora anserina,* the inheritance is by way of extrachromosomal factors (Rizet, 1953; Esser and Kuenen, 1967; Raynal, 1979; Tudzynski and Esser, 1979), this condition appears to be exceptional (Wright and Hayflick, 1975). It is especially noteworthy that even the circadian rhythmic behavior of many functions in rats and other mammals have been demonstrated to undergo changes themselves during the aging processes (Mohan and Radha, 1978). Other gross physiological losses that mark the senescent stage, such as decrease in respiratory capacity, muscular activity, reproductive, heart, and kidney function, and basal metabolic rate (Schneider, 1978; Kanungo, 1980), have been most thoroughly documented in man, where their clinical relevance is self-evident. Important as such reduced organismic functions may be in medical practice, they all stem ultimately from changes in cell and protein structure, as the consequence of gene function alterations, the real theme of this and the other chapters.

6.3.1. Macromolecular Aspects of Aging

The rat and, to a somewhat lesser degree, the white mouse have served as the principal models for experimental and other investigations into the problems of age-related changes at the macromolecular level. Although many studies have been devoted to the problem, the majority of these are only of a broadly quantitative nature or are concerned with functional and behavioral facets. As numerous others address the aging of cells, especially fibroblasts, grown *in vitro*, the macromolecular aspects that best reflect changes in genes have remained relatively neglected in spite of the vast literature in the field.

Alterations in DNA Properties. Although the earliest of current concepts regarding the production of age-related changes was thought to stem from defects in DNA, resulting in loss of information, that simplistic view no longer is tenable (Comfort, 1979; Fry *et al.*, 1981). However, as mammals age, the DNA, together with the associated proteins of chromatin, does undergo a series of changes in properties (Gaubatz *et al.*, 1979). Among the earliest to be studied was the melting temperature (T_m) and hyperchromicity of DNA, both of which increase with senescence (von Hahn and Fritz, 1966; Kurtz and Sinex, 1967; O'Meara and Herrmann, 1972; Kurtz *et al.*, 1974; Dillon, 1978, p. 33). These increments may be related to an increase in the covalent links between

---

*The major exceptions to the generalization are those forms that reproduce sexually only once in their lifetime and perish immediately or very shortly thereafter. Among the exceptional types are lepidopterans and many other insects, such fishes as salmon, the century plant, and most bamboos.

the chromosomal proteins and DNA, for the amount of the former that can be extracted by salt solutions has been shown to decrease in older individuals (O'Meara and Herrmann, 1972). Another trait that increases with age is the occurrence of single-stranded breaks (nicks) in the DNA molecule, as shown by the greater rate of incorporation of [^{3}H]thymidine in material from older individuals (Samis et al., 1964; Price et al., 1971). Furthermore, the presence of additional nicking has been indicated by the increased sensitivity to nuclease S_1 in senescent (20 month) mice relative to that of 1- to 15-month-old examples (Chetsanga et al., 1977).

It is not unlikely that the more abundant nicking results from a decreased repair rate, rather than more rapid damage. In man, with a relatively high body temperature of 37°C, it has been estimated that throughout life about 1000 lesions occur per day per cell as a result of breaks at apurinic sites (Hart and Modak, 1980). Unfortunately, while studies on repair of ultraviolet-induced damage of DNA have been made on a comparative basis among primates and other mammals (Hart and Setlow, 1974; Cleaver, 1977), few appear to have examined changed abilities as a result of aging. However, several reports have indicated that repair of excised regions and single-strand nicks did indeed become defective in terminally differentiating and aging cells (Stockdale, 1971; Karran and Ormerod, 1973; Mattern and Cerutti, 1975; Chan et al., 1976; Milo and Hart, 1976). But to the contrary, a current report on repair DNA found no retardation in aged individuals but proposed that the regulation of that activity was affected (Dell'Orco and Anderson, 1981). If such breaks do actually result from high body temperatures, then one would suspect that dogs, certain other mammals, and birds, whose normal temperatures exceed that of man, would have an even greater rate of nick production, but this condition does not appear to have been investigated as yet.

As just pointed out, experimental researches on this aspect of aging have often been based on observations of cloned cells in culture. Normal human somatic cells have limited replicative life spans in vitro but after a period of proliferation become senescent and incapable of perpetuating themselves (Martin, 1977; Norwood, 1978). A typical pattern of cells subcultured every 3 days would be, first, a period of rapid growth for about 9 days, followed by a long period of constant colony size for around 140 additional days; finally this in turn leads to a stage in which proliferation capacity decreases exponentially, with the colony dying out around 2 months later (Hayflick, 1965). Generally speaking, this lack of longevity in vitro has been found true of cells of most warm-blooded vertebrates, including birds. Moreover, the products of all cultured vertebrate tissues ultimately become a fibroblastlike cell (Hayflick and Moorhead, 1961). In some cases, however, such as mouse tissues, cells tend to undergo spontaneous transformation into abnormal types and often survive for extended periods in cultures (Rothfels et al., 1963). As a rule, it has subsequently been found, cells that remain largely diploid through their limited period of existence in culture have a restricted period of growth and are known as cell strains; on the other hand, cells of tissues that become aneuploid have unlimited potential for growth *in vitro*, and are referred to as cell lines. Other terms were later introduced, including hyperplastoid for strains and neoplastoid for lines; in the latter type, represented by such well-known cell lines as HeLa and mouse L cells, the karyotype usually differs from that of the source organism, and cells have a tendency toward tumor production, whereas the opposite conditions prevail in cell strains (Krooth *et al.*, 1968; Martin and Sprague, 1973).

However, as in most biological subjects, numerous exceptional instances have become known. For instance, mouse teratocarcinoma cells remain diploid *in vivo*, and although displaying slight chromosomal instability, they can be maintained *in vitro* for long periods (Stevens, 1967; Dunn and Stevens, 1970; Kahan and Ephrussi, 1970; Hogan, 1976; McBurney, 1976). Yet when injected into developing blastocysts, they can contribute cells to nearly all the tissues of the growing normal embryo, but, because of their high capacity for producing malignant tumors, they are classed as a neoplastoid type (Norwood, 1978). Furthermore, some evidence has been presented that favors the hypothesis that cells which become established as lines are not present in the primary culture but originate during the *in vitro* processing (Beaupain *et al.*, 1980).

Perhaps more significant are studies of the *in vivo* changes in ploidy that occur in aging mammals. One investigation of this sort employed hepatocytes of male mice of the strain C57BL/6, which had mean and maximum life spans of 24 and 31 months, respectively, under laboratory conditions (Shimo, 1980). In the newborn almost all the hepatocytes had the normal diploid condition, but at 2 months only 40% were diploid, 58% being tetraploid and the remainder having higher degrees of ploidy. After increasing to 60% at 4 months, the frequency of tetraploid cells leveled off until 14 months, after which it gradually decreased to around 20% in 28-month animals. In the meanwhile octoploid cells showed a steady rate of gain in frequency; after amounting to about 6% at 4 months the numbers rose to 20% at 14 months, 40% at 21 months, and about 45% at 28 months. In contrast, $16n$ and $32n$ cells remained nearly constant in relative abundance throughout life, rising only in the oldest animals studied. However, the phenomenon may prove to be strictly confined to mammals, for the same type of cells from the fish *Oryzias latipes*, the medaka, showed no significant differences in ploidy during aging (Shimo, 1980).

Changes in RNA Behavior Associated with Age. To determine whether changes in transcription might provide a possible molecular basis for age-related alterations in biochemical and physiological activities, one study compared the initiation of those processes in two age groups of rats (Miller *et al.*, 1980). When intact nuclei were isolated from the livers of rats grouped at first into two classes, young, ranging from 3 weeks to 9 months, and old, between 12 and 30 months of age, a significant decrease was observed in the

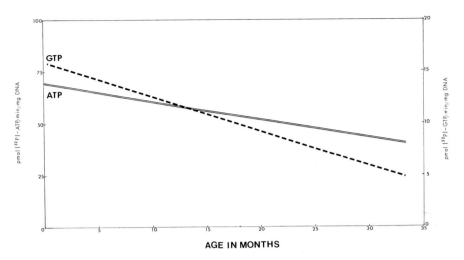

Figure 6.5. Age-associated changes in RNA behavior in maturing rats. (Based upon Miller *et al.*, 1980.)

incorporation of initiating nucleotides (Figure 6.5). Later the animals were arranged into five age groups, with similar results. For example, labeled GTP entered into initiation of RNA synthesis at a rate of 19 pmole/min per mg DNA in the youngest rats (3 weeks to 3 months) to 14 in the next class (4–9 months) and at an irregular rate thence into the oldest rats (30 months). A parallel but more gradual and uniform decrease in initiation was observed with ATP. When rats were hypophysectomized at 12 months and maintained on thyroxine and somatotropin therapy until 22 months, they showed initiation rates at the latter age equal to or exceeding those of the youngest group.

The tRNAs of rat liver appear to undergo a series of changes correlated with age (Singhal *et al.*, 1981). For example, their ability to accept ^{3}H-labeled amino acids was greatly reduced in 24-month-old rats in comparison with 3-month specimens (Mays *et al.*, 1979). The percent decrease was very strong, ranging from a high of 83% with arginine through a 62% drop with phenylalanine to a low of 44% with serine. In some cases the decrease may have resulted from loss of isoaccepting species, lysine tRNA$_5$, for instance, proving to be little more than half as abundant in the aged rats as in the young. Moreover, a defective subfraction of tRNA existed in the 24-month rat class that was absent from the 3-month. The mRNAs, even in fungi (Brown and Hardman, 1980, 1981), also have been demonstrated to undergo age-related changes in properties.

Changes in Cell-Surface Properties with Age. A few investigations have taken advantage of a novel system for "partitioning" cells (separating populations) to show surface-property changes correlated to the age of the organisms. Basically the system consists of two-phase mixtures of aqueous solutions of dextrans and polyethylene glycol, respectively, to which salts such as phosphates are added. As the latter have different affinities for the two phases, an electrostatic potential difference arises between them, with the upper solution bearing the positive charge (Albertsson and Baird, 1962; Johansson, 1970; Reitherman *et al.*, 1973). Through use of radioisotopic labeling, it was found that erythrocytes of young rats accumulated in higher proportions in the positive phase than in the negative and that this ratio decreased in the cells of successively greater ages (Walter and Selby, 1966). When a comparison was later made with human erythrocytes and electrophoretic techniques, it was revealed that the cells from aged rats had a pronouncedly different curve from that of younger ones (Figure 6.6), whereas the two age classes from humans scarcely differed (Walter *et al.*, 1980).

Another feature of the erythrocyte membrane that has received attention recently with regard to cell age-related changes is the insulin receptor (Dons *et al.*, 1981). By use of [^{125}I]insulin, it was demonstrated that the binding to the red blood cells declined quantitatively in exponential fashion as the age of the cells increased. Most of the drop appeared to stem from decreased numbers of the receptors rather than in affinity; however, it should be noted that the change was related to age of the cell, not to that of the donor. Comparable decreases in receptor sites with cell age were described in uterine tissues of rats, in this case in those sensitive to estrogen (Hsueh *et al.*, 1979). Whereas the mean number of estrogen-binding sites on the plasmalemma was 9300 per cell in 4-month rats, the figure dropped to 5200 per cell at 12 months, 3700 at 24 months, and 2200 at 30 months. However, no change was noted in the nuclear estrogen receptors.

Changes in Specific Proteins with Aging. By far the majority of investigations on age-related changes in proteins and other biochemicals have been quantitative in nature. Especially is this the case with sex steroids and gonadotropins, which tend to decrease with advancing years in rats, white-footed mice, and other mammals (Huang *et al.*, 1976a,b; Lu *et al.*, 1979; Steger *et al.*, 1980). The results of two of the few studies on changes in specific proteins in aging cells cast doubts on the validity of identifying alterations in aging cultured cells with the *in vivo* senescent changes. When chondrocytes from the vertebral cartilage of embryonic chicks were grown in culture, the proteoglycan monomeric molecules synthesized between 3 days and 6 weeks decreased in size as the colony aged, along with chain length of the chondroitin sulfate, but the latter chains maintained a relatively constant 6 S/4 S disaccharide ratio near 2.2. Moreover, the keratan sulfate composition remained between 5 and 10% (Pacifici *et al.*, 1981). But when actual cartilage tissues from embryonic, 1-year-old, and 6-year-old chickens were compared, few similarities with the foregoing results could be noted, aside from the decreases in proteo-

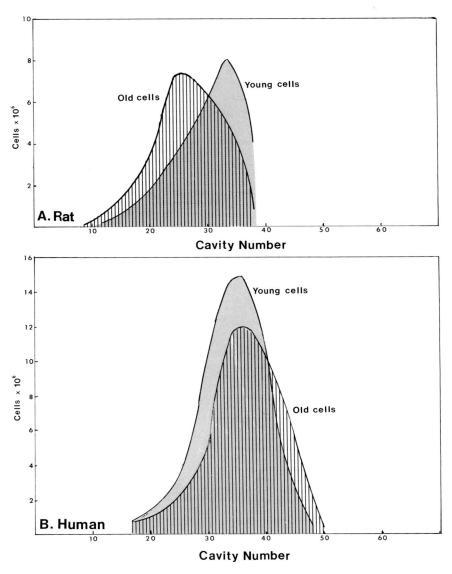

Figure 6.6. Age-related changes in erythrocyte cell-surface properties. The rat (A) and human (B) red blood cells differ vastly in the properties measured. Young cells are shown in stipple, old ones in vertical lines. (Based in part on Walter *et al.*, 1980.)

glycan monomer size and chondroitin sulfate chain length. The 6 S/4 S disaccharide ratio decreased in cartilage taken from old chickens from the 1.7 of the 1-year-old to 0.6, and the keratan sulfate composition rose from 7% in the younger chickens to 40% in the old ones. However, when similar intact cartilages were cultured, instead of dispersed chondrocytes, the changes in the proteoglycans paralleled those of the *in vivo* study (Fellini *et al.*, 1981). Comparable changes in proteoglycan composition from human articular cartilage have also been reported (Bayliss and Ali, 1978).

Perhaps the greatest age-related changes that occur in mammals are those which are associated with the endocrine system, particularly the pituitary–adrenal axis. In culture adrenal glands from old rats released a lesser quantity of corticosterone than those from young individuals (Pritchett *et al.*, 1979), and a subnormal level of Δ^5-3β-hydroxysteroid dehydrogenase activity has been reported to decline with age in female rats and mice (Shapiro and Leathem, 1971; Albrecht *et al.*, 1977). A restudy of the activity of this enzyme made on male rats 4, 5, 12, 18, and 24 months of age obtained parallel results but in addition showed that aging specimens remained equally sensitive as younger ones to stimulation of adrenal function by adrenocorticotropin (Albrecht, 1981). The cyclic fluctuations described earlier in this chapter have also been revealed to undergo alterations in old male rats. For example, the level of progesterone in blood plasma showed a higher peak in old than in young rats and was sustained on a plateau for a longer period (Simpkins *et al.*, 1981). However, the testosterone levels in the plasma of senescent animals failed to show the dramatic rhythms displayed by young ones, whereas dihydroxysterone levels were alike in the two age classes.

Changes in Enzymic Composition during Aging. The changes with age that occur in a number of enzymes that exist as families of isozymes have received considerable attention in the literature, lactate dehydrogenase having been especially well documented. In different rat tissues, five isozymes of this protein family have been reported, each consisting of two subunits in various tetrameric combinations (Wieland and Pfleiderer, 1957). The subunits, designated as H and M, have proven to differ in primary structure and to be encoded by two separate genes (Shaw and Barto, 1963); these were assembled in the five possible tetramers, H_4, H_3M_1, H_2M_2, H_1M_3, and M_4, which occurred in varied proportions from tissue to tissue. In general, H_4 and H_3M_1 tended to be prevalent in aerobic tissues such as the heart and adrenal cortex, while M_4 and H_1M_3 predominated in anaerobic ones like skeletal muscle and liver (Cahn *et al.*, 1962). Investigations into the age-related changes that occur have shown that in all tissues studied in the rat (Figure 6.7), the quantities present of the M subunit increased rapidly from birth to 12 or 30 weeks of age and then declined gradually to 96 weeks (Kanungo and Singh, 1965; Singh and Kanungo, 1968; Kanungo, 1980). Contrastingly, the activity of the H subunit increased strongly postnatally in all tissues until week 12, after which it showed

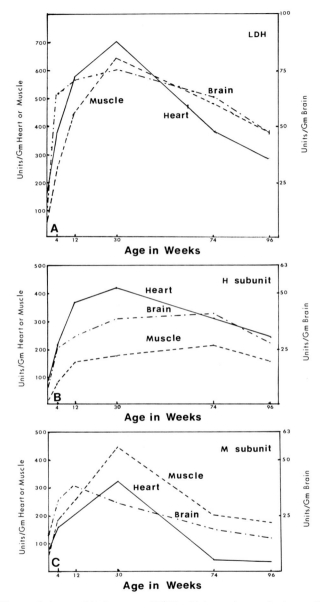

Figure 6.7. Changes in lactate dehydrogenase (LDH) with increasing age in the rat. The total LDH contents of three tissues are compared in (A), while those of subunits H and M are similarly contrasted in (B) and (C), respectively. (Based on Singh and Kanungo, 1968.)

lesser gains until week 74 in both skeletal muscle and the brain, but only to week 30 in the heart; in every case it declined from those peaks at a gradual rate in aged rats (Figure 6.7). As may be seen in those graphs also, total enzyme activity in muscle was more similar in pattern to that of the brain than that of the heart, despite the former being considered aerobic like the latter.

Other Changes in Proteins. Actual alterations, whose precise natures have remained unascertained, in protein structure have been lucidly demonstrated to occur with age in the vinegar eel, *Turbatrix aceti*. Among enzymes that have been established as becoming altered are isocitrate lyase, aldolase, enolase, and phosphoglycerate kinase (Reiss and Rothstein, 1975; Gupta and Rothstein, 1976; Sharma *et al.*, 1976; Reznick and Gershon, 1977; Sharma and Rothstein, 1978). Moreover, similar results have been obtained in enzymes from various tissues of aging rodents, including superoxide dismutase from rat livers and aldolase from heart and skeletal muscles of mice (Reiss and Gershon, 1976; Chetsanga and Liskiwskyi, 1979). In other instances no compositional differences occurred with age and in still others posttranslational modifications took place in the senescent cells that could possibly induce conformational changes. As examples of the former condition in man may be cited creatine kinase of muscles, aldolase in muscles and lymphocytes, and superoxide dismutase of erythrocytes (Steinhagen-Thiessen and Hilz, 1976, 1979; Joenje *et al.*, 1978), while two enzymes of the rat, skeletal muscle phosphoglycerate kinase and liver tyrosine aminotransferase, appear to exemplify the second (Sharma *et al.*, 1980; Weber *et al.*, 1980).

Two functions of a single enzyme (glucose-6-phosphatase) associated with endoreticular membranes from rat liver illustrate the contrasts in striking fashion. The glucose-6-phosphate phosphohydrolase activity of this enzyme, that synthesizes glucose-6-phosphate from inorganic pyrophosphate and glucose, was demonstrated to increase rapidly in abundance from low prenatal levels to a maximum between 2 and 5 days in the neonatal, after which the quantity present showed a steady decrease to adult levels by day 35 (Goldsmith and Stetten, 1979). At first the activity was associated with rough endoreticulum of the hepatocytes but decreased there after day 2, whereas the activity that appeared slightly later in the smooth endoreticular membranes increased to day 10 and maintained a plateau thence to day 70 (Figure 6.8). Thereafter it experienced a slight decrease to 2½ years. On the other hand, the enzyme's pyrophosphate-glucose phosphotransferase activity in rough endoreticulum displayed an extremely high gain from near nil at birth to a high peak at 2 days, before undergoing a threefold decrease to day 35. That of the smooth endoreticulum rose undramatically from zero at birth to a low maximum at day 9, followed by a very slight decrease to day 70, when a plateau was reached that persisted through the remainder of life.

In the vinegar eel, which has a mean life span of 52 days, a strong decline with age was noted in another enzyme of the sugar-metabolizing system, fruc-

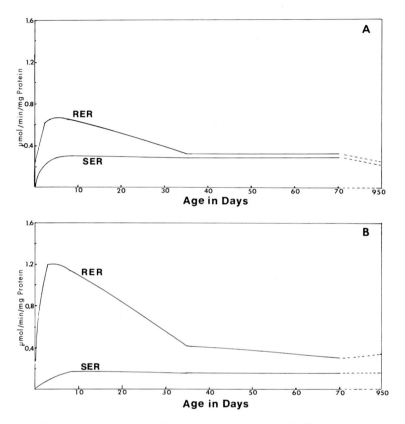

Figure 6.8. Glucose-6-phosphatase activities as a function of age. (A) The enzyme's glucose-6-phosphohydrolase activity of rough endoreticulum (RER) and smooth endoreticulum (SER) is plotted against age in days. (B) The PP_i-glucose phosphotransferase activity associated with these same organelles is similarly plotted. (Based on Goldsmith and Stetten, 1979.)

tose-1,6-diphosphate aldolase (Reiss and Rothstein, 1974; Bolla and Brot, 1975). This enzyme showed a regular curvilinear decrease in specific activity from the time of hatching to 40 days, the oldest stage examined, as did also DNA polymerase. However, two other enzymes that were studied, elongation factor 1 and RNA polymerase, had a somewhat different profile in that sharp increases occurred, to day 5 in the first of these substances and from day 5 to 15 in the second (Bolla and Brot, 1975). Both then declined rapidly over a 5- or 10-day period, after which the decrease was at a more gradual pace.

Total protein synthesis has been shown to decrease in relation to age in cell-free translation systems prepared from rat livers (Moldave *et al.*, 1979). When the source was from 30-month-old animals, synthesis was 30% lower than when it was from 3-month, both in extent and rate. One of the few published studies on age-associated changes in total protein profile comparable to those cited in the earlier chapters on development and differentiation employed the flesh fly *Sarcophaga peregrina*. Heads of adults of this species, which at 27°C has the relatively long life span for an insect of 35 days, provided a convenient uniform source for the comparisons (Utsumi and Natori, 1980). As a whole the picture that emerged was one of decrease in protein content, as is made especially clear by the graph in the cited article. In newly emerged flies the total soluble protein showed a mean of 0.42 mg/head, which amount fell off rapidly to about 0.28 mg/head by day 6. Thereafter the decrease was at a much more gradual pace, so that by day 32 approximately 0.23 mg/head remained. As shown by two-dimensional electrophoresis, the decrease varied among the more than 400 species present in the newly emerged imago (Figure 6.9). Certain types, such as those labeled 6, 10, and 11, underwent almost no change during the life span, while others, such as 4, 7, and 9, decreased very slightly with time. Still others, such as 1, 2, and 3, disappeared very early in adult life, 1 being lost by day 3, and 2 and 3 by day 6. Finally a very few were noted to increase with age, that labeled as 8 being one of the exceptions (Figure 6.9).

While the DNA-replication concept was still widely accepted, another theory regarding the aging of cells and organisms was advanced, known as the error catastrophe concept, which postulated that increased numbers of errors in protein synthesis eventually led to a progressively lessened level of fidelity in the production of these and other biochemicals. Hence, the cells thus ultimately accumulated lethal proportions of aberrant proteins (Orgel, 1963). The similarity of this concept to the DNA replication one is at once apparent, the end results, the infidelity of the protein products, being the same in both views. Recently a system was developed capable of quantitatively assaying error frequency in cultured human fibroblasts (Harley *et al.*, 1980), and the results of studies employing it proved to be in opposition to the error catastrophe hypothesis, for old cells and those from aged donors showed no increase in protein error over those of young cells or from youthful subjects. However, a line of cells transformed by simian virus 40 did exhibit an enhanced error frequency. Still another, more recent theory on the subject has proposed that deterioration of cell membrane function might prove to be a causative factor in loss of reproductivity in cells and ultimately to cell death (Berumen and Macieira-Coelho, 1977; Zs-Nagy, 1979). Thus, in substance, this view, like two earlier ones, visualizes aberrations in proteins or their decreased production, but differs in specifying only those of the membrane. An investigation into D-glucose uptake kinetics of cultured fibroblasts demonstrated no impairment of transport of that carbohydrate in senescent cells still capable of replication (Cremer *et al.*, 1981), but that incapacity set in only after their reproductive powers had been lost, that is, in terminally differentiated cells alone.

sheep red blood cells to stimulate senescent mice than young ones to produce antibody at a maximal rate (Price and Makinodan, 1972a,b). Even then the maximum response of the latter exceeded that of the former 25-fold. The decreases noted are difficult to correlate with other observations. In the first place, the number of B cells in the spleen showed no change with age (Adler *et al.*, 1971; Makinodan and Adler, 1975); neither did the number of those cells decrease in the human bloodstream (Díaz-Jouanen *et al.*, 1975), nor their ability to proliferate (Hung *et al.*, 1975). However, it has recently been demonstrated that certain Ca^{2+}-dependent processes in the activation of lymphocytes became impaired with increasing age (Kennes *et al.*, 1981).

   Autoimmune Diseases and Cancer. As a general principle, there appears to be a decrease in immune function as age increases in man beyond early adulthood, two results of which seem to be higher frequencies of autoimmune diseases and cancer (Burnet, 1970; Teller, 1972; Cunningham, 1976). Both types of disease show an apparent relationship to T lymphocytes, the latter from their decreased numbers, the former from a drop in suppressor T-cell functional ability (Kanungo, 1980). Thus, it may be that the suppressor cells fail to prevent B lymphocytes from reacting against the body's own cells, resulting in the production of antibodies against "self" cells, with autoimmune disease as a consequence. Such diseases include conditions like thyrotoxicosis, rheumatoid arthritis, allergic encephalomyelitis, maturity-onset diabetes mellitus, pernicious anemia, and amyloidosis. While the T-cell-dependent immune response has been reported to decline markedly with age (Makinodan *et al.*, 1971; Kishimoto *et al.*, 1976; Weigle, 1980), experimental data are often conflicting. For instance, the activity of suppressor T cells in certain responses has been reported both to increase (Segre and Segre, 1976) and to decrease (Hirokawa *et al.*, 1978) with age in mice. However, the population of these cells has been shown to become less dense with age in particular breeds of mice, like the New Zealand Black, that are especially susceptible to autoimmune pathologies (Talal and Steinberg, 1974; Kanungo, 1980).

   Undoubtedly the decline is correlated to the changes in composition of the thymus that accompany increasing years (Figure 6.11). In man, the cortex of the gland constitutes 60% of the tissue at birth but commences to diminish in extent thence to old age, falling to 50% at 5 years, 25% at 20, 10% at 35, and around 8% for the remainder of life after 40 (Boyd, 1932). While the medulla increases from the 20% of the whole at birth to 50% at 5 years, it remains fairly constant thereafter until age 20. Subsequently it too declines in extent, to about 13% at age 30 and perhaps 4% after 40. Thus, after age 25, 60% or more of the thymus consists of connective tissue and fat.

   Reduced immune function also appears to be correlated to the occurrence of cancer, at least to a degree, especially when cell-mediated immunity is deficient (Mackay, 1972; Roberts-Thomson *et al.*, 1974). Persons who develop immunodeficiency in childhood have a 10- to 20-fold higher incidence of can-

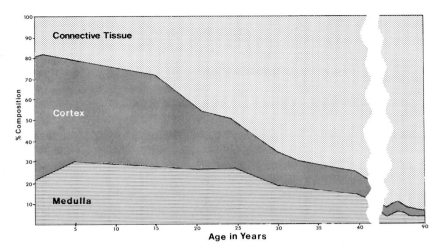

Figure 6.11. Changes in composition of the human thymus. In general the proportions of cortex and medulla in this gland decrease with age, while connective tissues increase. (Based on Boyd, 1932.)

cer, even though their life span is much shorter than normal human beings, a condition paralleled in persons that become immunodeficient during adult life (Southam, 1974). While the cause of this correlation remains unestablished, it is suspected to stem from the decrease in T-cell activity (Burnet, 1970), or oncogenic viruses might be favored by the loss of those cells. But perhaps these and related aspects of aging will become clearer as the gene action changes in general related to immunology and cancer are discussed in the chapter that follows.

7

Gene Action Changes in Immunity

In contrast to the topics of cyclic and aging changes in gene action, in which little progress has been achieved at the molecular level of inquiry, immune reaction investigations have amassed great quantities of pertinent data. One characteristic of this field of research is the great complexity that it embraces, another being the close relationships it bears to tumorous and malignant growths. In approaching this topic, the complicated nature is best breached by viewing, first, the antibodies of the immune reactions, followed by the cellular constituents, and, finally, the interactions of the several component types.

7.1. THE ANTIBODIES

Among vertebrates it is generally accepted that most of the antibodies involved in major immune reactions are secreted by a type of blood cell known as the B lymphocyte, which receives attention later in the chapter. Although all antibodies of vertebrates are a type of glycoprotein referred to as immunoglobulin, this is probably not a condition that prevails in invertebrates and other eukaryotes. However, immune reactions undoubtedly occur widely among living things, as evidenced in green plants by the rejection of grafts in incompatible hosts (Knox and Clarke, 1980), similar reactions in sponges and other lower metazoans (Hildemann and Jokiel, 1979), and by a previous discussion involving pollination (Chapter 1, Section 1.3.3). Even in the vertebrates, there are other classes of substances, such as complement, that are of great importance in the overall picture of immunity, but since they do not react directly with antigens, they do not fit the classical definition of antibodies. Because the molecular aspects of the topic have received adequate exploration only in the vertebrates, and more specifically, the mammals, discussion is devoted almost exclusively to those animals. Even among the mammals, the immunoglobulins from man, and, to a somewhat lesser extent, the mouse, are the only source species adequate for present purposes.

7.1.1. Structure of Immunoglobulins

In man and probably most higher mammals, there are five classes of immunoglobulins (Ig), known as IgA, IgD, IgE, IgG, and IgM, some of which are represented by several subclasses (Roitt, 1974; Nisonoff *et al.*, 1975; Kabat *et al.*, 1979; Sell, 1980). In their simplest forms, all consist of four subunits in the general structural pattern $\alpha_2\beta_2$, but in these substances the contrasting subunits are referred to as light (L) and heavy (H) chains. The light chains are of two kinds, κ and λ, both of which may be present in any of the five major classes; however, under normal conditions, a given immunoglobulin monomeric molecule has either two κ or two λ chains, never one of each kind. While the actual ratio of κ to λ light chains in the total immunoglobulin picture varies from species to species, in man it approximates 3 : 2 in that same sequence (Fahey and Solomon, 1963). The heavy chains differ markedly from one class to another but nevertheless possess several universal traits, as well as a number of amino acid sequence homologies, as shown later.

The Light Chains. As the two types of light chains exhibit about a 40% homology in their primary structures, it is not unlikely that they had a common ancestry; the κ type appears to be closer to the ancestral stock, because preliminary studies of shark immunoglobulins report it to be the only one present in that taxon. In addition, the two types share a number of other traits. Both have molecular weights in the range of 22,000 to 23,000 throughout the Vertebrata, both have two, or occasionally three, intrachain disulfide loops, and a cysteine residue is present at the very end of the κ and in the penultimate site of the λ chain that provides a disulfide bond to the heavy chain (Table 7.1). Since both types occur in the urine in a proportion of patients having myeloma, together they originally were called Bence–Jones proteins, before their true identity was established. That they actually represent the two types of immunoglobulin light chains was discovered by Korngold and Lipari (1956), in whose honor the Greek letter designations were later made (Franklin, 1962; Mannik and Kunkel, 1962). Because only one type usually is present in urine of a given myeloma patient, in such cases the protein is obviously the product of a single clone of cells. With such an abundant supply of uniform material available, it is not surprising that many molecular studies have been made.

The molecules of either light chain contain about 212–214 residues, in both cases containing two contrasting regions that correspond rather closely to half-molecules (Baglioni *et al.*, 1966; Milstein, 1966a,b). The C-terminal half

Table 7.1

Comparisons of Immunoglobulin Light Chains[a,b]

	10 20 30 40 50
Human κ[c]	DIQMTQSPSSLSASVGDRVTITCQA--SQ-DISIFLNWYQQKPGKAPKLLIYDAS
Human λ[d]	ESALTQPPSSASGSPGQSVTISCTGTSSDVGDNKYVSWYQQHPGRAPKLVIFEVS

	60 70 80 90 100 110
Human κ	KLEAGVPSRFSGTGSGTDFTFTISSLQPEDIATYYCQQFDNLPLTF--GGGTKVD
Human λ	QRPSGVPDRFSGSKSDNTASLTVSGLADEDEADYYCSSYVDNNNTFVFGGGTKLT

	120 130 140 150 160
Human κ	FKRTV-AAPSVFIFPPSDGQLKSGTASVVCLLNNFYPREAKVQWKVDNALQSGNS
Human λ	VLRQPKAAPSVTLTLPSSZZLQANKATLVCLISNFYPGVVTVAWKADGSPVKAGV

	170 180 190 L 200 210 220I
Human κ	QESVTEQDSKDSTYSLSSTLTLSKADYEK-HKVYACEVTHQGLSSPVTKSFNRGEC_{COOH}
Human λ	-ETTTPSKQSXXKYAASSYLSLTPZZW-KSHKSYSCQVTHQG--STVZKTVAPTECS_{COOH}
	N R

[a] Based on Hilschmann (1967) and Wikler and Putnam (1970).
[b] Four common mutant sites of the C chain are indicated. The V domain may be considered to extend from site 1 to 110 and the D segment thence to the carboxy end.
[c] Variety Roy.
[d] Variety Bo.

is relatively invariable, with only one or two site differences resulting from minor variations among the multiple alleles. For instance, κ chains of the allotype known as Inv(1) have leucine at site 191, whereas Inv(3) proteins have valine. In contrast to this constant (C) half or domain, the N-terminal half or variable (V) domain exhibits many variations, even in a given class of immunoglobulins from a single normal individual. In part, the specificity of antibodies stems from this V-domain diversity.

Light-Chain Amino Acid Sequences. Since Bence–Jones proteins afford a ready source of high-purity κ or λ chains, the amino acid sequences of many types have become established, representative forms of which are supplied in Table 7.1. Where necessary to maximize homology between the chains as much as is realistically possible, hyphens have been inserted as is the common practice. When a count is made of corresponding pairs of sites, a total of 91 such identities may be found. Although on a theoretical basis one might expect the lion's share of homology to be concentrated in the constant half, surprisingly this proves not to be the case. Instead the V regions may be noted to contain a total of 49 identical sites, equal to a 45% homology, whereas the C portion has only 42 sites or 38%. Thus, the latter domain of the λ chain (or C_λ) may be perceived to have diverged further from its counterpart than the V_λ. Moreover, it should be noted that diversification has involved the entire chains in both cases, for the longest identical segments are only 5 sites in length, the V domains having GGGTK in common at sites 104–108 and the C halves bearing AAPSV (sites 117–121) and VTHQG (sites 204–208). While not infrequently, as in cytochromes and others bearing hemes or similar prosthetic groups, the region adjacent to each bonding residue is frequently fairly invariable, no stability is evidenced around the first cysteine (site 23) in the V regions, and the second (site 91) is preceded by only YY on a consistent basis. Similarly the proximal cysteine (site 140) in the C domain is invariably bordered by a valine residue on one side and a leucine on the other, but no constant residues are immediately associated with the distal cysteine (site 201) and only a glutamic acid residue uniformly neighbors the terminal or subterminal (site 221). One other noteworthy feature is provided by the high frequency of serine in the invariant sites in which it occurs at 14 points, a percentage occupancy of over 15%.

The Nature of the Variability in the κ Chain. The nature of the variability that exists in the inconstant domains of the two major varieties of light chains is most readily perceived by examining a sampling of the numerous amino acid sequences that have been established. In Table 7.2, 15 sequences of the V_κ region are listed, 11 of which are complete, while 4 others (Dav, Fin, Fr4, and Rad) are represented by only the first 50 residues; three subgroups have been recognized, the first of which is subdivided into a and b sections. When these primary structures are scanned beginning with the N-terminal region, both highly variable and invariable sites are immediately evident. Among the constant residues is the isoleucine of site 3, threonine and glutamine (sites 6 and 7), proline (site 9), leucine (site 12), glycine (site 17), cysteine (site 24), serine and glutamine (sites 27 and 28), and so on. These are usually considered to represent major structural or interacting residues, loss or alteration of which renders the protein less fit for its function in the organism—in this case loss or diminution of the ability to bind antigens. In addition there are constant sites within the several subgroups that help to distinguish them from one another. For instance in subgroup I all nine of the examples given have glutamine in site 4, whereas a valine residue occupies that position in the other two subgroups. An even better example is found in site 10, which is occupied by serine in subgroup I, leucine in subgroup II, and glycine in subgroup III. A count of the correspondences between subgroups in this category of homology reveals that subgroups I and II share 7 residues not found in III, I and III share 13 such characteristics, and II and III, 11. Thus, subgroup III is almost equally related to subgroups I and II while I and II are relatively widely disparate. Hence, subgroup III may be considered to be ancestral to the other two, a conclusion that will be found to be reached again from a later consideration.

But further thoughtful comparisons of sites reveal almost none where variation from one representative to another is totally random. Site 32 shows a high level of variability, being occupied by 9 different amino acid residues among the 15 representatives, at site 52 six different ones may be noted among

Table 7.2
The Nature of the Variability of the Human κ-Chain Inconstant Domain (V_κ)[a,b]

Subgroup	Variety					
		10	20	30	40	50
Ia	Roy	-DIQMTQSPSSLSASVGDRVTITCQASQDISI------FLNWYQQKPGKAPKLLI
	Ag	-DIQMTQSPSSLSASVGDRVTITCQASQDINH------YLNWYQQGPKKAPKILI
	Bel	-DIQLTQSPSSLSASVGDRVTITCQASQDISK------FLNWYQQKPGKPPELLI
Ib	Hau	-DIQMTQSPSSLSASVGDRVTITCRASQSISS------YLSWQQQKPGKAPQVLI
	Ou	-DIQMTQSPSSLSASVGDRVTITCRASQTISS------YLNWYQQKPGKAPXLLI
	Eu	-DIQMTQSPSTLSASVGDRVTITCRASQSINT------WLAWYQQKPGKAPKLLM
	Dee	-NIQMTQSPSSLSASVGDRVTITCRAGQSVNK------YLAWYQQKPGKAPKVLI
	Dav	-DIQMTQSPSSLSTVVGDRVTITCDASQDIDS------WLIWYQQYP( )
	Fin	-DIQMTQSPSSLSTVVGDRVTITCDASQDIDS------WLIWYQQYP( )
II	Cum	EDIVMTQTPLSLPVTPGEPASLSCRSSQSLLDSGDGNTYLNWYLQKAGQQPSLLI
	Mil	-DIVLTQSPLSLPVTPGEPASISCRSSQNLLES-DGN-YLDWYLQKPGQSPQLLI
III	Ti	-EIVLTQSPGTLSLSPGERATLSCRASQSVSN------FLAWYQQKPGQAPRLLI
	B6	-ZIVLTQSPGTLSLSPGERAALSCRASQSLSG------YLAWYQQKPGQAPRLLM
	Fr4	-ZIVLTQSPGTLSLSPGERATLSCRASQSVRN------YLAWYQQRPGQAPK( )
	Rad	-EIVLTQSPGTLSLSPGDRATLSCRASQVSRN------YLAWYQQKPGQAPR( )
"Ancestral"		-DIVLTQSPSSLSASPGDRATISCRASQSLSS------YLNWYQQKPGQAPKLLI
		60	70	80	90	100	110
Ia	Roy	YDASKLEAGVPSRFSGTGSGTDFTFISSLQPEDIATYYCQQFDNLPLTFGGGTKVDFKR
	Ag	YDASNLETGVPSRFSGSGFGTDFTFISGLQPEDIATYYCQQYDTLPRTFGGGTKLEIKR
	Del	YDASTLKTGVPSRFSGSGSETHFTLISSLQPDDFATYYCQQYDHFPLTFGGGTZVEVKR
Ib	Hau	YAASSLPSGVPSRFSGSGSGTDFTLISSLQPEDFATYYCQQNYITPTSFGGGTRVEIKR
	Ou	YAASNLHSGVPSRFSGSGSGTDFTFISSLQPEDFATYYCQQSYSSPTTFGQGTRLEIKR
	Eu	YKASSLESGVPSRFIGSGSGTEFTLISSLQPDDFATYYCQQYNSDSKMFGQGTKVEVKG
	Dee	FAASSLKSGVPSRFSGSGSGTDFTLISGLLPEDFATYYCQQSYTTPYTFGPGTKVEMTG
II	Cum	YTLSYRASGVPDRFSGSGSGTDFTLISRVQAEDVGVYYCMQRLEIPYTFGQGTKPEIRR
	Mil	YLGSNRASGVPNRFSGSGSGTDFTLISRVQAEDVGVYYCMQALQTPLTFGGGTNVEIKR
	Ti	YVASSRATGIPDRFSGSGSGTDFTLISRLEPEDFAVVYCQQYGSSPSTFGQGTKVELKR
	B6	YGVSSRATGIPDRFSGSGSGADFTLISRLEPEDFAVVYCQQYGSSPFTFGQGSKLEIKR
"Ancestral"		YDASSRASGVPDRFSGSGSGTDFTLISRLQPEDFAVYYCQQYDSSPLTFGQGTKVEIKR

[a] In large part based on Nisonoff *et al.* (1975).   [b] Areas in parentheses have not been established.

the 13 sequences given there, and at site 60 five are found among the 11 sequences, a count repeated at site 62. Sites 97 and 100 are somewhat more variable, having six different occupants, while 98 again has but five. Probably the most highly variable is site 99, where the 11 sequences contain seven different residues. But in view of there being between 107 and 114 sites in the V_κ domain, a high level of consistency among the representative forms is at once apparent.

The Nature of the Variability in the λ chain. As just shown for the κ chain, the diversity of the amino acid sequences in λ chains also appears to derive from combinations of small variations at a relatively few points. On the basis of homologies among the first 25 or 30 sites in λ Bence–Jones proteins, five subgroups have been recognized, and three serologic subtypes have been identified, resulting from interplay between two types of antigenic markers, ST and 111 (Tischendorf *et al.*, 1970). More recently a third marker has been revealed, referred to as VOR (Rivat-Peran *et al.*, 1980). The presence of ST and VOR and absence of the 111 were shown to be characteristic of subgroup I, whereas subgroup IV lacked ST and 111 but had VOR. Subgroup II lacked all three, whereas subgroup III, and possibly also subgroup V, had only 111.

In Table 7.3 are listed a total of nine primary structures of representative V_λ domains, distributed in the five subgroups. A number of invariable sites are at once apparent near the N terminus, a trio provided by leucine–threonine–glutamine in sites 4 to 6, and a near-constant sector consisting of one serine and two proline residues in the next three positions being especially striking. In fact the entire molecule is so marked by invariant and near-invariant sites that enumeration of them results only in tedium. Both because of the relative stability and the small numbers of representatives known in the various groups, it is difficult to find subgroup characteristics comparable to those obvious ones of the V_κ subgroups. The most evident differences in the majority of cases involve missing sites, rather than distinctive occupants. For example, subgroups III and V lack an occupant in site 1, and there is an additional series of vacancies in sites 28 to 30 in both cases. But subgroup III also has seemingly experienced deletions at sites 98 and 99, which are occupied in subgroup V, whereas I and V alone have site 99 occupied.

A narrow range of variation at any given position is as characteristic of the λ molecule as was in the κ. Among the variable positions is site 3, where five contrasting amino acid residues can be noted among the nine sequences, and a like number is to be found at sites 31, 33, 41, 52, 53, 71, 91, 95, and 97; this quantity is exceeded at only two positions, 32 and 96, at each of which six different residues occur. In contrast, the other variable sites show at most four differences. Although the picture of variability that thus emerges does not seem equal to the task of providing antibodies for the million or more probable antigens that any organism must be prepared to neutralize, it should be remembered that the nine sites listed that contain five variables each could in theory

Table 7.3
The Nature of the Variability of the Human λ-Chain Inconstant Domain
$(V_\lambda)^{a,b}$

Subgroup	Variety	
		10 20 30 40 50
I	New	ESVLTQPPSVSAAPGQKVTISCSGGSTNI-GNNYVSWHQHLPGTAPKLLIYEDNKR
	Ha	ESVLTQPPSVSGTPGQRVTISCSGGSSNGTGNNYVYWYQQLPGTAPKLLIYRDDKR
II	Nei	ESALTQPASVSGSPGQSITISCTGTTSDVGSTNFVSWYQQNPGKAPKLMIYEGNKR
	Vil	HSALTQPASVSGSLGQSITISCTGTSSDVGGTNYVSWFQQHPGTAPKLIISEVRNR
III	Ker	-TALTQPPSVSGSPGQTAVITCSGDNL---EKFTVSWFQQRPGQSPLLVIYHTSER
	X	-TDLTQPPSVSGSPGQTASITCSGDKL---GDKDVCWYQQRPGQSPVLVIYQDNQR
	Bau	-TGLTQPPSLSGSPGQTASITCSGDKL---GEQYVCWYQQKPGQSPVLVIYHDSKR
IV	Bo	ESALTQPPSASGSPGQSVTISCTGTSSDVGDNKYVSWYQQHPGRAPKLVIFEVSQR
V	Sh	-SELTQDPAVSVALGQTVRITCQGDSL---RGYDAAWYQQKPGQAPLLVIYGRNNR
"Ancestral"		ESALTQPPSVSGSPGQTVTISCSGTSSDVGGNNYVSWYQQHPGTAPKLVIYEDNKR
		60 70 80 90 100 110
I	New	PSGIPDRISASKSGTSATLGITGLRTGDEADYYCATWDSSLDAVVFGGGTKVTVLGQ
	Ha	PSGVPDRFSGSKSGTSASLAISGLRSEDEAHYHCAAWDYRLSAVVFGGGTELTVLRQ
II	Nei	PSGVSNRFSGSKSGKTASLTISGLQVEDEADYYCCSYAGNST-RVFGGGTRVTVLSQ
	Vil	PSGVSDRFSGSKSANTASLTISGLQAEDEADYYCSSYTSSNS-VVFGGGTKLTVLGQ
III	Ker	PSEIPERFSGSSSGATATLTISGAQSVDEADYFCQTWDTIT--AIFGGGTKLTVLSQ
	X	SSGIPERFSGSNSGNTATLTISGTQAMDEADYYCQAWDSMS--VVFGGGTRLTVLSQ
	Bau	PSGIPERFSGSNSGTTATLTISGTQAMDEADYYCQAWDSYT--VIFGGGTKLTVLGQ
IV	Bo	PSGVPDRFSGSKSDNTASLTVSGLRAEDEADYYCSSYVDNNN-FVFGGGTKLTVLRQ
V	Sh	PSGIPDRFSGSSSGHTASLTITGAQAEDEADYYCNSRDSSGKHVLFGGGTKLTVLGQ
"Ancestral"		PSGIPDRFSGSKSGNTASLTISGLQAEDEADYYCSSWDSSSSAVVFGGGTKLTVLGQ

[a] Based largely on Nisonoff *et al.* (1975).
[b] Although much of each molecule is occupied by invariable sites (screened), two broad areas of hypervariability can be observed.

together provide for nearly 4,000,000 combinations. Hence, with the more limited variation available at the other sites, this V_λ chain alone could provide a nearly limitless number of peptides. How many of the combinations would be actually efficacious against the various antigens, however, is an unanswerable question.

A Question of Ancestry. In Tables 7.2 and 7.3 are contained also an "ancestral" molecule for the V_κ and V_λ domains, respectively, derived from the other sequences in standard fashion. In each case, invariant and nearly invariant sites have provided a large proportion of the residues for the assumed ancestral form, so that the choice was largely made evident by the consistent presence of a given residue in a majority of the subgroups. That is to say, the total number of occurrences did not necessarily provide the basis, but rather the number of subgroups in which a given amino acid was present. However, a simple majority did provide the basis for an occasional decision, and in those few instances where no type of residue predominated, the base found in subgroup I was arbitrarily selected.

The two resulting sequences appear straightforward enough, but when they are placed adjacent to one another as in Table 7.4, it is at once evident that these supposed ancestral types are highly divergent. For the most obvious points of distinction, the ancestor for V_λ has six sites not represented in that for V_κ and the latter possesses one that is absent in the former. In each of these sequences, sites that are invariable among the representatives of the given chain are italicized, such invariability often being viewed as representing positions of vital importance to the configuration or reaction sites of the molecule. Contrary to expèctations, however, although the chains have similar functions, features that are universal in one peptide are not usually so in the other. Only in 11 cases out of 33 and 37, respectively, for V_κ and V_λ are these invariable sites occupied by identical residues in both of the variable regions, two of which involve the cysteines that provide the disulfide bonds for formation of intrachain loops. At two of these contrasting constant homologous positions, a different amino acid residue is the occupant in the λ chain than in the κ. The first of these is at site 11, where leucine is present in all the representatives of V_κ,

Table 7.4
Comparisons of Ancestral Human Light Chains of Immunoglobulins[a]

		10	20	30	40	50
"Ancestral"	V_κ	DIVLTQSPSSLSASPGDRATISCRASQSLSS---YLNWYQQKPGQAPKLLIYDASSR
"Ancestral"	V_λ	ESALTQPPSVSG-SPGQTVTISCSGTSSDVGGNNYVSWYQQHPGTAPKLVIYEDNKR
"Ancestral"	$V_\kappa V_\lambda$	E?VLTQ?PS???ASPG?RATISCQ?G?S??GGNNY?AWYQQKPGQAPKLLIYGVSNR

		60	70	80	90	100	110
"Ancestral"	V_κ	ASGVPDRFSGSGSG-TDFTLISRLQPEDFAVYYCQQYD--SSPLTFGQGTKVEIKR-
"Ancestral"	V_λ	PSGIPDRFSGSKSGNTASLTISGLQAEDEADYYCSSWDSSSSAVVFGGGTKLTVLGQ
"Ancestral"	$V_\kappa V_\lambda$	PSGVPDRFSGS?SGNT????ISGLQAED?A?YYCQ?YD--SS?R?FGGGTKL?V?RQ

[a]Residues in italic indicate sites that are invariant in the given chain.

whereas serine is universally the occupant in V_λ. The second instance is at site 75, where threonine invariably occurs in V_κ and leucine in the other.

This lack of interchain consistency even at sites of intrachain uniformity exemplifies the difficulty encountered when an attempt is made to derive a model sequence ancestral to both types of chains. In many instances, as at site 2, one chain may have an invariable condition, as isoleucine in the V_κ derived sequence, while none of the individual representatives of the other chain have that residue present, as witness the threonine and serine residues of the V_λ ancestral primary structures. In each such irresolvable position, a question mark has been inserted in the ancestral $V_\kappa V_\lambda$ sequence given (Table 7.4). At site 3, however, where valine and alanine are present in the two ancestral sequences, examination of Table 7.2 shows either valine or glutamine to be the occupant in V_κ representatives, and in Table 7.3 the former of which, but not the latter, is found among the representatives of the V_λ. Thus, it appears that the valine is more probably the residue in the ancestral stock than glutamine. Although it proved not to be possible to assign a residue to a number of sites at the N-terminal region and again at around site 75, objectively made assignments could, surprisingly enough in view of the evolutionary advancement of the source organism, be made in a majority of the sites—only 23 of the 114 remain in doubt. But not until full sequences of the κ chains derived from a number of lower vertebrates have been established can really meaningful estimates be made of the ancestral condition. The present analysis is designed primarily to provide a deeper insight into the nature of the variability, and, consequently, into that of changing expressions of gene functions.

7.1.2. The Classes of Immunoglobulins

By and large the heavy chains of immunoglobulins resemble the light chains structurally, except that they are twice or more their length and are more complex accordingly. A variable domain (V_H) occurs in the N-terminal sector that is similar to the V_L in length and in having an intrachain loop formed by disulfide bonding between two cysteine residues. The C_H portion of the immunoglobulin molecule is comprised of either three or four domains, each approximately equivalent in length, which shows the presence of a disulfide loop and other major structural properties to a C_L domain. Moreover, there is a hinge region located between C_H1 and C_H2, in IgG1 located from site 221 to 223 inclusive; as its name suggests, this short section is located at a bend in the molecule, but in addition it contains several cysteine residues, one of which bonds with the terminal or subterminal cysteine of the light chain. Two or more other cysteine residues interact with those in a second heavy chain to assist in forming the dimeric complete molecule of two heavy and two light chains.

The Classes of Immunoglobulins. The classes are based on combinations of several characteristics, including molecular weight (both of the entire

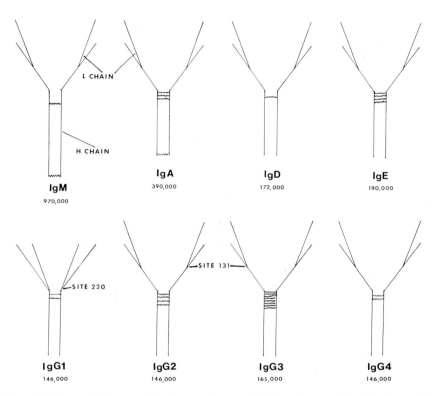

Figure 7.1. The main features of the classes of immunoglobulin molecules. The molecular weight of each class of the secreted substances is given below the figures. In the blood, IgM consists of five of the tetramers shown, plus a J chain which assists in joining them. Similarly in secretions, IgA consists of two tetramers, plus a J chain and a molecule of secretory product, while all the remainder function in the tetrameric form shown. Wavy lines represent disulfide linkages between heavy chains; only a minimal number of such interchain bonds are shown in IgG3, but may range up to as many as 15. Light chains are also joined to heavy ones by disulfide links.

molecule, but especially of the heavy chain), numbers of domains in the latter, percentage of sugar present, and number and location of inter-heavy-chain bonds. The more important of these properties are given in Figure 7.1. While much stress is placed on the numbers of interchain disulfide bonds, they are not the sole interactants responsible for the structural integrity of the molecule, for the several chains do not separate when the disulfide bonds are cleaved. Cleavage of the molecule by means of proteases has become an important procedure in the study of the several classes, papain and pepsin being the usual enzymes. Papain acts on the heavy chains at the hinge region on the N-terminal side of the inter-heavy-chain disulfide bonds, thereby creating three fragments, two of which are identical (Figure 7.2). Since each of the latter consists of a light chain and the NH_2-half of the heavy chain, each contains both the V_L and V_H regions; consequently these have become known as the Fab fragments, the capital letter signifying "fragment" and the two lower-case "antigen-binding." Also present, of course, are the C_L and C_H1 domains. The third fragment, called Fc because of its being crystallizable, is comprised of the remainder of the heavy chains still bound together; that is, each fragment includes the two C_H2 and C_H3 domains and also C_H4 where it is present, plus part of the hinge region.

Pepsin under nonoptimal conditions has a similar action but cleaves the molecule at the hinge region on the C-terminal side of the inter-heavy-chain bonds. Consequently, instead of three nearly equal-sized fragments resulting from the enzymatic treatment, the products include a single bivalent large peptide and a variable number of small ones, depending on conditions. The bivalent particle is distinguished by the designation $F(ab')_2$ or FAB' if the connecting bond becomes broken, while the peptides are poorly known. One larger fragment, however, which roughly corresponds to the dual C_H3 domains, has been denoted as pFc' (Goodman, 1963; Utsumi and Karush, 1965).

Immunoglobulins A and M. The two immunoglobulins that have inter-

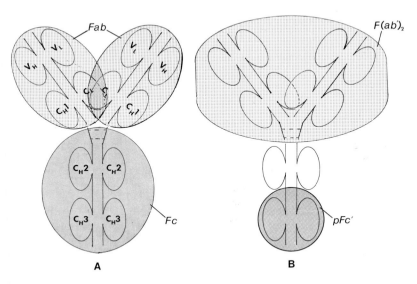

Figure 7.2. Cleavage products of immunoglobulins. The diagram on the left (A) shows the products of cleavage by papain. This enzyme cleaves the molecule on the NH_2 side of the hinge, yielding one Fc and two Fab fragments. In contrast, pepsin breaks the molecule on the COOH side of the hinge, resulting in the production of one $F(ab')_2$ fragment and others, among which may be one called pFc'.

heavy-chain bonds near the C terminus, IgA and IgM, are also the only ones that exist as polymers, the former as a dimer, the latter as a pentamer. However, the dimeric condition of IgA occurs only in secretory products, such as saliva and colostrum, that present in blood serum being monomeric. The two polymers also share a feature called the J (joining) segment, a chain approximating the light chain in molecular weight (ca. 15,000), considered in greater detail in a subsequent section. For the present it is sufficient to point out that it is rich in cysteine, arginine, isoleucine, and aspartic acid and does not resemble the immunoglobulin molecules themselves. In addition, IgA of secretory products (sIgA) contains an additional molecule called the secretory component (SC) that is produced only by epithelial cells of glands. The polymeric immunoglobulins have the highest total molecular weights, that of human IgM being 970,000 and IgA, 380,000 to 390,000; while the heavy chain of IgM, known as μ, has the quite high molecular weight of 72,000, largely as the result of the presence of four C domains in the heavy chain, that of IgA (the α chain) has the relatively low weight of 52,000 to 58,000. In the latter case, the weight is correlated to subclass, α_1 being 52,000 to 56,000 and α_2 between 55,000 and 58,000.

As shown earlier, IgM appears to be the earliest of the five known classes of immunoglobulins, both from phylogenetic and ontogenetic standpoints, for it is the only one universally present among vertebrates (Nisonoff *et al.*, 1975). Although the substance remains poorly characterized in the fishlike classes, considerable progress has been reported in *X. laevis*. In this amphibian the antibody first appeared during development when the larva emerged from the gelatinous coat, at about day 2, whereas the thymus was not recognizable until day 4 (Leverone *et al.*, 1979). Even at that early stage, both pentameric and monomeric forms were present, comprised of heavy and light chains identical in size to those of the adult. The enzyme that is involved in providing this antibody type with one of its most outstanding features, its pentameric structure, has been identified in mouse tissues and proved to be a specific product of B lymphocytes (Roth and Koshland, 1981). Polymerization seemed to be by direct oxidation of monomeric IgM and J-chain sulfhydryl units.

In birds, reptiles, and lower vertebrates including the shark, IgM appears to be the most abundant, and in fishes the only, immunoglobulin present in the plasma. In anurans, IgG has also been reported, but its actual identity in these animals can only be ascertained when sequence analyses become available. That such a complex molecule as IgM should be present in sharks is understandable evolutionarily only if adequate ancestral molecules can be identified in hagfish, lampreys, or lancets, for it is far too large and complex a structure to have arisen suddenly in this single class of vertebrates. Fortunately, some immune activity appears to exist in hagfish and possibly in lampreys, although at low levels (Hildemann and Thoenes, 1969; Thoenes and Hildemann, 1970). However, even in the hagfish, the immunoglobulin, tentatively identified as

IgM, revealed a high molecular weight. Thus, possible ancestral molecules need to be sought in cyclostome larvae and in the cephalochordates in order to establish the origins of the vertebrate's unique immunological system.

IgA is one of two classes of immunoglobulins found predominantly in secretory products, IgE being the second. The former is secreted by local plasma cells as a dimer containing the J chain; then as it passes through the epithelium of the secretory organ it receives the secretory component (Bienenstock and Befus, 1980). From its site of formation, it is transported, presumably in the serum, to the liver where it is selectively moved across the hepatic parenchymal cells into the bile, because ligation of the bile duct results in a pronounced increase in this immunoglobulin in the bloodstream (Lamaître-Coelho et al., 1978). Receptors for the Fc sector of IgA have been reported on the surface of certain populations of T lymphocytes, neutrophils, and macrophages, the former being especially derived from the mesenteric lymph node and thoracic duct. Soon after their formation they are found predominantly in the small intestine and to a much lesser extent in the colon. In these organs, sIgA has been supposed to help protect the mucosal surface against infection and perhaps to interfere with the absorption of antigens from the intestinal tract into the circulatory system. Additionally, this class of antibody has recently been demonstrated to mediate the transport of antigens of foreign proteins from the bloodstream into the bile by means of the Kupffer cells of the liver (Russell et al., 1981). The receptors for IgA on neutrophils appear to be related to the ability of this type of immunoglobin, when in an antigen–antibody complex, to stimulate those leukocytes to release the contents of their granules, a property shared only with IgG. In fact, these two classes of antibodies have been demonstrated to interact synergistically in certain immune activities (Shen and Fanger, 1981). Although sIgA was found not to mediate antibody-dependent cytotoxicity (lysis) by polymorphonuclear leukocytes, monocytes, or lymphocytes, it did enhance the activity of those cells that had been activated by IgG.

Immunoglobulin D. The three remaining classes that lack a C-terminal inter-heavy-chain bond include two of relative rarity, IgD and IgE, which resemble IgM in having four C domains per heavy chain, a characteristic that is inconstant for the former of these, however. But even with this fifth domain in place, the heavy chain of IgD (the δ chain) is lighter than that of the IgE (the ε chain), i.e., 63,000 to 69,000 daltons vs. 72,000 to 76,000 (Leslie and Martin, 1978). The δ chain differs further from the ε in providing for only one inter-heavy-chain bond, instead of four as the latter does. A peculiarity of IgD is its presence on a modest proportion of adult B lymphocytes (about 7%) and a somewhat higher frequency (14%) on those cells from the cord blood of newborn children. About 75% of these cells, both adult and neonatal, also have IgM (Rowe et al., 1973), despite the fact that each lymphocyte had at one time been considered to bear only a single class on its surface. Subsequent examination of B cells from other species of mammals has revealed a similar condition to prevail and probably will prove to be a class characteristic (Knapp *et al.*, 1973; Abney and Parkhouse, 1974; Melcher *et al.*, 1974; Pernis *et al.*, 1975; Gathings *et al.*, 1976; Goding *et al.*, 1977; Mushinski *et al.*, 1980; Burrows *et al.*, 1981). These two immunoglobulins also have the same antigen-binding specificities and probably share the same V_H domain (Pernis *et al.*, 1974; Fu *et al.*, 1975; Goding and Layton, 1976), as all the rest do. Moreover, a variant in a hybrid mouse cell line has been reported which had switched from secretory IgM to IgD (Neuberger and Rajewsky, 1981), that is, from μ-chain synthesis to δ-chain; as judged from the hapten-binding and idiotypic properties, both the original μ and derived δ chains had the same V_H sectors. The δ chains of IgD secreted into the blood plasma have been found to differ somewhat from the type bound to the membrane, having a molecular weight of 61,000 instead of 64,000 as in the latter. The predominant molecular form of the secreted IgD was $\delta_2\lambda_2$. Perhaps the differences in the δ chains resulted from a condition found to prevail in IgM membrane and secreted molecules, which have proven to be encoded by different mRNAs (Alt *et al.*, 1980; Mushinski *et al.*, 1980; Rogers *et al.*, 1980; Singer *et al.*, 1980) derived from the same primary RNA transcript (Early *et al.*, 1980). The gene for both μ and δ have been shown clearly to be located on chromosome 12 in the mouse (Wabl *et al.*, 1980), as those for the other classes may be also.

   Immunoglobulin E. Aside from the relative scarcity in the serum shared by IgD, IgE displays several distinctive characteristics (Katz, 1980a). In the bloodstream, its molecules appear to have a comparatively short half-life and thus must be synthesized nearly continuously at a slow rate. In addition to regional lymph nodes, it is produced by the mucosa of the respiratory and gastrointestinal tracts, where it possibly is particularly active against parasites invading those systems. The carrying out of its function appears to be mainly by action on tissue mast cells and basophils, inducing them to release the contents of their granules, as described in a later section. But its most distinctive feature is the selectivity displayed toward antigens, being particularly reactive to parasitic nematodes and trematodes but not at all to viruses or bacteria. Moreover, IgE production is enhanced by such allergenic agents as ragweed and other pollen, the synthesis of which is by particular B cells that in no way differ from others, except in their specialization for this type of immunoglobulin (Teale *et al.*, 1981a). However, a further unique trait has been revealed recently, to the effect that the synthesis of this type of antibody is influenced by the diurnal rhythm of bloodstream levels of corticosteroids (Bargatze and Katz, 1980).

   Immunoglobulin G. The last class of immunoglobulins, IgG, is both the most abundant and most complex in man (Nisonoff *et al.*, 1975), constituting about 75% of these substances, a condition that appears to prevail among many of the mammals, not IgM as in other vertebrate classes. That the smaller IgG molecule displaced the very large one of IgM among mammals is easily understandable in light of its distinctive properties. All varieties of IgG can cross through the placenta and enter the fetus, thereby providing it with immunological protection, a benefit that is extended to the newborn child until the latter has developed its own immune system. This property is related to the Fc region of the molecule, that is, it derives from the unique primary structure of IgG, and now has been established as being localized in the C_H^2 domain (Johanson *et al.*, 1981). Unlike typical IgM, the present immunoglobulin is capable of passing through capilary walls to enter the extravascular fluids; this characteristic apparently stems from the small size of the molecule, for in the shark, where a monomeric (7 S) form of IgM occurs along with the pentamer (19 S), the former but not the latter is found in the extravascular fluid as well as in the blood. Still another trait of IgG, shared by IgA but not IgM, is a capacity, when in an antigen–antibody complex, to activate neutrophils to liberate the contents of their granules, which are lysosomal enzymes that induce the active inflammatory processes (Henson, 1971). An additional advantage that is presently still tentative may be that the somatic mechanism for V sector diversification is able to produce greater variability in IgG than in IgM antibodies, a condition found in antibodies from hybridomas and myelomas (Gearhart *et al.*, 1981).

The Subclasses of Human IgG. Originally the four subclasses, or isotypes, of IgG in man were defined by immunological procedures (Grey and Kunkel, 1964; Terry and Fahey, 1964), for each possesses two unique antigenic determinants located in two or three of the C_H domains (Franklin and Frangione, 1969). Some of these are found in the Fab fragment and therefore are in the C_H^1 domain; certain types of determinants may be shared by two or three subclasses, but never by all four. Structurally the four may be distinguished on the basis of the interchain bonds (Frangione *et al.*, 1969). First of all in IgG1 the heavy chain (the γ chain) connects to the light chain by means of a cysteine residue located in the hinge region near site 220 (Figure 7.1), whereas in the remaining three subclasses the H–L disulfide bond arises in a cysteine residue situated at position 131, as in all other human immunoglobulins. Second, the remaining classes are then characterized by the number of heavy-chain bonds, γ_2 having 4 such bonds, γ_3 5 to 15, and γ_4 only 2 (Frangione and Milstein, 1968; Michaelsen, 1973). The γ_3 chain is further distinguished by its greater molecular weight, amounting to 60,000, whereas the other three stand at 51,000 (Saluk and Clem, 1971; Damacco *et al.*, 1972). Consequently, it contains about 20% more amino acid residues, that is, about 540 instead of the 450 of γ_1, all the additional ones of which appear to be located in the hinge region.

7.1.3. Primary Structure of Heavy Chains

Now that the V and several C domains of at least a majority of the classes of immunoglobulins have been completely sequenced, it is possible, along with the partial sequences of the others, to obtain a representative view of their likenesses and differences (Kabat *et al.*, 1979). Since the C_H domains have been more thoroughly explored, these are examined before the V_H, in order to lay a firmer groundwork for comparisons of the latter.

Comparisons of the Constant Regions. While only three classes of heavy chains have had the primary structure of their entire constant regions determined, their numbers include the two most disparate types along with a simpler representative (Table 7.5). IgM and IgA will be recalled as the two that have a total of five domains present and also alone possess an inter-heavy-chain bond at the C terminus, features that are well corroborated by sequences of the μ and α_1 chains presented (Putnam *et al.*, 1973; Liu and Putnam, 1979). Thus, these two should be expected to show a large degree of homology, but examination of the various domains reveals great variation in the number of identical sites. For example, in the first 120 sites which together correspond to the C_1 domain, only 17 positions are occupied by the same residue in the two chains, amounting to a homology of only 14.1%. Even the γ_1 sequence (Edelman *et al.*, 1969; Press and Hogg, 1970; Gally and Edelman, 1972) is more closely related structurally to the μ, sharing 38 sites in the same region for a 31.6% homology. But the most striking distinction in this C_1 domain is the evident absence of a loop in the α_1 sequence, for only two cysteine residues are present, one of which, that at site 23, is involved in bonding the light chain. This absence of a cysteine at site 37 is difficult to understand, especially in view of the presence of one being indicated in the diagram of the molecule that accompanies the presentation of the primary structure (Liu and Putnam, 1979). The loop undoubtedly must be present; it simply is not closed by disulfide bonds.

The second constant sector in Table 7.5 is found only in IgM and IgA immunoglobulins. Hence, in order to facilitate later comparisons with members of the other three classes, it is here proposed that this region when present be referred to as the C_X domain to express the concept that it is extra part in these two types. Here a somewhat higher degree of homology exists between the contrasting members of the pair, for 26 sites of the 120 in the C_X region (including the hinge) are identical, a rate of 21.6%. Undoubtedly the most striking difference that occurs is the presence of 15 additional sites in the hinge sector of α_1, a segment characterized by the high percentage of proline residues, interspersed with five serine residues, each of which bears a carbohydrate group. The unusual richness of this sector strongly suggests that it plays a particular role in the unique immune activities of this molecule. Beyond this segment, the sequences, with representatives of all five classes (Shinoda *et al.*, 1981), are better viewed by the homology analysis that follows, except for a note regarding the differing lengths of the molecules. Here μ and α_1 again show their relationships, for they both exceed the γ chain by 18 residues, the ϵ by 17, and the δ by 9—the large amount of homology that exists between these two terminal parts is also noteworthy.

Table 7.5
Primary Structural Relationships between Human Immunoglobulin C_H Domains in Whole or Part[a,b]

```
                       L chain          C₁loop
         10        20          30      40      50        60        70
μ   ----VSSG--SASAPTLFPLVS⌐ENSNPSSTVAVGCLAZDFLPDSITFSWKYⓃXSXKISSTRGFPSVL-R

α₁  EVQLVESGGGVVQAGTSLRL-SⒸTASAPⓃLSDYAMHWVRQAPGKGLZWVALISTGGSKTYYAX--SVRGR

γ₁  ----VSSA--STKGESVFPLAPSSKSTSGGTAALGCLVKDYFPEPVTVSW--ⓃSGALTSGVHTFPAVLQS

         C₁ loop ⌐
         80        90      100       110       120       130       140
μ   GGKYAATSZVLLPSK-DVMQGTDEHVCKWVQHPNGNKQKXVPLPVIAELPPKVSVFVPPRNGFFGXPRKSK

α₁  FTISRXISKXTLYLZMKTLRTEDVYYCAKLIAVAGTRXFWGZGCTLVTVSLASPTSKVFPLSL-STZPXGXV

γ₁  SGLYSLSSVVTVPSSSLGTQTYITA-CN-VNHKPSNT-K-VDKRVEPLSCDK-TH-CPPCPA----------

              ⌐Cₓ loop                                  ⌐ Cₓ loop ⌐
         150       160       170       180       190       200       210
μ   LI-CQATGFSPRQVWSLRECKQVGSGVTTXZVZAZAKZSGPTTYKVTSTILTIKZXDWLGESMFTCRVDH

α₁  VIACLVQGFFPQQPLSVTWS-ESGSGZGVTARXFPPSZXASGXLYTTSSQLTLPATZCLAGKSVTCHVKH

            H chain                                          ⌐C₂ loop
         220          230       240       250       260       270       280
μ   RGLTFQCNASSMĈ---------------VP-DQDTAIRVFAIPPSFASIFLTKSTK-LTĈLVTDLTTYXS

α₁  YTNPSQXVTV-PĈPVPSTPPTPSPSTPPTPSPSCCHPRLSLHRPALZX-LLLGSZANLTCTLTGLRD-AS

γ₁  -------------------------------ELLGGPSVFLFPPKPKDTLMISRTPEVTĈVVLDVSHEDP

ε   SNPRGVSAYLSRPSPFD-LFRKSP-TITĈLVVDLAPSKG

δ   SHTQPLGVYLLTPAVQD-LWLRDKATFTĈFVVG-SDLKD

                                H chain⌐      C₂ loop
         290       300       310       320       330       340       350
μ   -VTISWTREE-NGAVKTHTNISESHPNATF-SAVGEASICEDXDWS-GERFTĈTVTHTDLPSP-LKQTIS

α₁  GVTFTWPSTSGKSAV---ZGPPERXLCGCYSVSSVLPG-C-AEPWXHGKTFTĈTAAYPESKTP-LTATLS

γ₁  QVKFNWYVDG-VQVHNAKTKPREQQYNSTYRVVSVLTVLHQN--WLDGKEYKCRVSNKALPAP-IEKTIS

ε   TVNLTWSRASGK-PVNHSTRKFEKQRNGTLTVTSTLPVGTRD--WIEGLTYQCRVTHPHLPRA-LMRSTT

δ   AH-LTWEVA-GKVPTGGVEEGLERHSNGSQSQHSRLTLPRSL--WNAGTSVTĈTLNHPSLPPQRLMALRE

                                    ⌐C₃ loop
         360       370       380      390       400       410       420
μ   RPKGVALHRPXVYLLPPARZZLNLRESATITĈLVTGFSPADVFVEW-MQRGEPLSPQKYVTSAPMPEPQAPG

α₁  K-SG-NTFRPQVHLLPPPSZZLALXZLVTLTĈLARGFSPKDVLV-WL-QGSQELPREKYLTWASRQEP-SZG

γ₁  KAKGQPRE-PQVVTLPPSRDFLTKNQ-VSLTĈLVKGFYPSDIAV-WESNDGEPEN-YKTTPPVLDSD-GS--

ε   KTSG-PRAAPEVVYAFATPEWP-GSRDKPTLAĈLIQNFMPEDISV-WLHNEVQ-LPDARHSTTQPPKTKGS-G

δ   PA-AQAPVKLSLNLLASS-DPPEAA-SWLL-GEVSGFSPPNILL-WLEDQREV-NTSGFAPARPPPQPGST-⌐

         ⌐C₃ loop ⌐                                             H chain
         430       440       450       460       470       480
μ   RYFAH--SILTVSEEEWNTGQTYTĈVVAHEALPNRVTERTVDKSTGKPTLYNVSLVMSDTAGTĈY COOH

α₁  TTTFAVTSILRVA-EXWKKGDTFSĈMVGHZALPLAFTQKTIDRLAGKPTHVNVSVMAQVDGTĈY COOH

γ₁  FFLY---SKLTVDKSRWQEGNVFSĈSVMHEALHNHYTQKSLSLSPG COOH

ε   FFVF---SRLEVTRAEWQEKDEFIĈRAVHEAASPSQTVRAVSVNPGK COOH

δ   TFWAW--SVLRVPAPPSPQPATYTĈVVSHEDSR--TLLNASSRSLEVSYVTDHGPM COOH
```

---

[a] μ chain from Putnam *et al.* (1973) and Nisonoff *et al.* (1975); α_1 chain from Liu and Putnam (1979) and the δ chain from Shinoda *et al.* (1981); the remaining partial sequences from Nisonoff *et al.* (1975); and the γ_1 from Edelman *et al.* (1969), Press and Hogg (1970), and Gally and Edelman (1972).

[b] Underlined residues are involved in bonding to carbohydrate groups and those four cysteines shown in italic are concerned in providing interchain disulfide bonding.

Evolutionary Relationships of the Five Types. Examination of the 224-site-long region having all five types of immunoglobulins represented (Table 7.5) uncovers a surprising lack of similarity among them, for only 14 positions are occupied by identical residues in all members and only one of these is a sequence of two or more adjacent positions. Of the homologous sites, four are occupied by cysteine residues that are involved in the formation of the closed loops; while thus these conserved sites are structural, their location at corresponding points in the chains is clearly indicative of common ancestry. In just a few cases are two or more sets of invariable sites occupied by the same amino acid residues, three of which have tryptophan and two proline, but no obvious structural or functional basis for the homology can be found. What is striking is the lack of universality among the serine and asparagine residues that serve for attachment of the carbohydrate groups, shown in bold in Table 7.5 wherever their presence has been established. Only at position 307 is universality of an asparagine residue achieved, and at that point the residues are known to bear carbohydrate groups in the μ and γ_1 chains and probably do also in the δ and ϵ ones, too. However, the α_1 sequence here contains a cysteine residue not involved in this function. Because of this absence of consistency, the impression is gained that many of the carbohydrate adjuncts probably are not entirely vital to the functioning of these molecules.

Degree of relationships among these five chains can be analyzed in two ways, one by the usual procedure of counting the numbers of corresponding sites containing identical residues, the other by examining sites where only four of the five given sequences share a common amino acid, the former method being pursued first. In Table 7.6 both the numbers and percentages of correspondences between sites of various pairs of chains are presented on a region-to-region basis, division between which being derived from Table 7.5. As a whole these correspond approximately to the C_2 and C_3 domains, respectively, and are designed to provide both convenience and a deeper insight into the nature of evolutionary changes in structure, that is to say, changes in genes on an evolutionary basis. Since IgM has been shown to be the only immunoglobulin present in lower vertebrates, and thus best represents the progenitory stock, it is listed first to provide the standard of comparison. Both the total sums and the resulting percentages of identical residues at corresponding positions indicate that the sequence of chains followed in Table 7.5 represents their decreasing relationships to the μ chain with increasing distance from it. Further, this conclusion receives support from the results of comparisons of other pairs—in broad terms the lower sequences ϵ and δ are less closely related to the others than either α_1 or γ_1 is to μ. Still further corroboration is provided by the summation of identical sites between one chain and all the others. For instance, the sum of identities of μ with α_1, γ_1, ϵ, and δ amounts to 249, of α_1 with μ, γ_1, ϵ, and δ totals 251, and that of the γ_1 with the other four, 244, as does also the ϵ chain. Thus, these four bear statistically identical relationships to one another. But the δ chain is highly divergent, for it shows a total of only 198

correspondences. It is of interest to note that in the development of B lymphocytes the gene for μ chains appears first, followed by γ and α or perhaps by α
and γ, the picture not being totally clear at present (Lawton et al., 1975).

The second procedure, that of examining the 23 nearly invariant sites in
these C_2 and C_3 domains (Table 7.6), leads to similar conclusions: at site 252,
for a case in point, leucine residues are universally present except in the μ
chain where alanine occurs; thus, at this one site this last chain appears to have
diverged from the ancestral stock after the others had evolved. Similarly, at
three sites, 261, 317, and 381, the μ chain is exceptional, and in like fashion
the α chain is found to diverge at five sites, 273, 308, 341, 342, and 453, one
more than the μ chain. The γ chain is exceptional only at a single site, 346,
the ϵ sequence at three, 366, 387, and 450, whereas the δ diverges at 10 sites,
283, 355, 361, 363, 384, 392, 395, 454, 460, and 469, thus exhibiting twice
as many divergencies as the α and more than the μ, γ, and ϵ chains combined.
Hence, even at these highly conserved sites, the δ chain has become by far the
most divergent type.

The Variable Domain. As in the light chain, the variable domain (V_H)

Table 7.6
Relationships among the C_2 and C_3 Regions of Immunoglobulin Heavy Chains[a]

Contrasting pairs of chains	C_2 domain				C_3 domain				Total (237)	
	Sites 243–281 (39)[b]		Sites 282–351 (70)		Sites 352–423 (72)		Sites 424–469 (46)			
	No.	%	No.	%	No.	%	No.	%	No.	%
μ–α_1	10	25.6	17	24.3	33	45.8	19	41.3	79	33.3
μ–γ_1	9	23.1	16	22.9	24	33.3	16	34.9	65	27.4
μ–ϵ	11	28.2	18	25.7	17	23.6	14	30.4	60	25.3
μ–δ	5	12.8	13	18.6	14	19.4	13	28.2	45	14.8
α_1–γ_1	6	15.4	18	25.7	22	30.5	16	34.9	62	26.1
α_1–ϵ	8	20.5	19	27.1	21	29.1	13	28.2	61	25.7
α_1–δ	10	25.6	17	24.3	12	16.7	10	21.8	49	20.7
γ_1–ϵ	11	28.2	21	30.0	19	26.3	17	36.9	68	28.7
γ_1–δ	9	23.1	12	17.1	18	25.0	10	21.8	49	20.7
ϵ–δ	12	30.7	21	30.0	13	18.1	9	19.6	55	23.2
Mean	8.9	22.8	17.2	24.6	19.3	26.8	13.7	29.8	59.3	25.0

[a] Based on Table 7.5.
[b] Numbers in parentheses indicate number of sites in each region.

Table 7.7
The Variable (V_H) Domain of Immunoglobulin Heavy Chains[a,b]

```
Subclass                             ┌─V loop
                        10        20 │      30        40        50        60
VHI    (Eu)    *VQLVESGAEVKKPGSSVKVS CKASGGTFSRSAII--WVRQAPGQGLEWMGGIVPMFGPP

VHII   (Ou)    *VTLTESGPALVKPKQPLTLTCTFSGFSLSTSRMRVSWIRRPPGKALEWLARIXXXDKFY

VHIII  (Zap)   EVQLVESGAGLVQPGGSLGLSCAASGFTFSTTSRF--WVRQAPGKGLEWVEFRVQGSAIS


                                       V loop─┐
                        70        80        90 │100      110       120
VHI    (Eu)    NYAQKFQGRVTITADESTNTAYMELSSLRSEDTAFYFCAGGYGI--------YSPEEYNGGLVT

VHII   (Ou)    -WSTSLRTRLSISKNDSKNQVVLIMINVNPVDTATYYCARVVNSVMAGYYYYYMDVWGKGTTVT

VHIII  (Zap)   HYADSVQARFTISRNDSKNTLYLQMNTGEAZXTAVYYCARTRPGG-GGY---FSDVWGQGTLVT
```

[a] Based on Putnam *et al.* (1973) and Wang *et al.* (1973).
[b] * = 2-pyrrolidone-5-carboxylic acid.

of heavy chains is the same in each class, a fact especially clearly demonstrated by a myeloma patient (Til) in which both IgM and IgG occurred (Wang *et al.*, 1973), the V_H regions of both of which proved to be identical. In short, V_H is the product of a single "gene,"* that becomes united to those of several that encode for the C_H regions of the various classes. Although the sector is variable, the variations fall into three major subgroups, which are customarily distinguished by Roman numerals. In each subgroup the molecule has a loop of around 80 residues in length formed by disulfide bonding between two cysteine residues located similarly in each case (Table 7.7). Extensive homology can be noted to exist between the single examples of each subgroup shown, but the actual amount, of course, varies widely with the source individuals. In V_HIII, the N terminus usually is not blocked as seems always to be the case in the other two subgroups, but even here the modified residue may occasionally be present, as it is in a representative member called Nie (Capra and Kehoe, 1975).

As was the case with the V_L domain, variability in the V_H region is not uniform throughout the sector but occurs most extensively in several portions, four short sections occurring in the present instance. These hypervariable parts from 12 different varieties are presented in Table 7.8, where the first inconstant zone is seen to be only six sites in length. Examination of the occupants in each corresponding position reveals a situation similar to that of V_L—only a limited number of amino acid residues is found in any given site. The first one, site 30, for example, has only three different occupants, by far the most frequent of which is serine. Slightly greater freedom as to acceptable residues may be noted in sites 31 and 34, where four different amino acids are repre-

---

*A specialized terminology for such complex genetic components is proposed in Section 7.1.5.

sented. In the other three positions, still more latitude occurs, site 35 with 10 different occupants in the 12 cited examples showing almost no restrictions in this regard. Even if the residues actually reported here should ultimately prove to be the only ones that are acceptable in the respective sites—a most likely suggestion—over 40,000 different combinations of amino acids are possible in this short section alone. Similar restrictions, in most cases not exceeding 7 possible residues per site and having a mean close to 5, exist in the other hypervariable sectors.

Restrictions in Amino Acids at Given Sites. A more meaningful analysis of the nature of the variability is provided by examining the particular amino acids present in each given sector and in all the hypervariable regions in combination. In the region embraced by sites 30 and 35, tallies of the residues present at each of the six positions disclose that serine and threonine are disproportionately abundant relative to the others, the first of these amino acids

Table 7.8
Variable Sectors of the V_H Domain[a]

	ST zone	AA zone	M zone	VG zone
	30 35	51 64	84 90	101 109
Eu (γ_1)	SRSAII	GGIVPMFGPPNYAQ	ELSSLRS	GYGI-----
Daw (γ_1)	SGETMC	AWDIL-NDDKY-GA	IMINVNP	VVNSVMAGY
Ou (μ)	STSRMR	AWRIB-NDDKYWST	TMTNMDP	RHPRTL---
He (γ_1)	TTDGVA	AWLLYWNDDRRFSP	TM---DP	ITVIPAPAG
Cor (γ_1)	SSTGMI	AWRIDWDDDKYYXT	SMNTVGP	SCGG-----
Tei (γ_1)	STSAVY	GWRYEGSSLTHYAV	QMLSLEP	VTPAAASLT
Was (γ_1)	STDAM-	AWKYQEASNS-FAD	QMNRLEA	FRQPFVQ--
Jon (γ_3)	STAWMK	VWRVEQVVEKAFAN	QMISVTP	VVVST----
Zaf (α_1)	STTSRF	EFRVQGSAISHYAD	QMNTGEA	TRPGGY---
Tur (α_1)	SRVLSS	SGRNLASSNLNFAV	QMLSLQA	LSVTAV---
Nie (γ_1)	SRYTIH	AVMSYXGXXKHYAD	NMNSLRP	IRDTAM---

[a]Based on Capra and Kehoe (1975).

occurring in 16 of the 69 sites that are both occupied and the occupant fully identified, whereas the latter occurs in 12. Thus, these two substances account for 23.2 and 17.4%, respectively, of the region, in combination totaling in excess of 40%. In contrast, no other amino acids are represented by more than six residues in this sector, most having only between one and three, and five species (asparagine, glutamine, lysine, proline, and histidine) being absent entirely. Because of the great predominance of the two that are indicated, it is proposed that this variable sector be referred to as the ST (serine-threonine) zone.

Similarly the region between sites 51 and 64, inclusive, has two prevailing amino acid residues, in this case alanine, which occupies 12.3% of the sites, and aspartic acid, which fills 9.1% of the 154 known positions. Here cysteine alone of the amino acids is absent, all the remaining species being represented at least twice. It is especially interesting to note the presence of lysine here at eight sites, whereas in the other three zones it is entirely absent. Histidine, too, is found here, at three sites, a substance which occurs only once in the other hypervariable sections. Since alanine and aspartic acid are thus especially characteristic, this region can be referred to as the AA zone, and the third hypervariable portion as the M zone, where methionine, occupying 14.9% of the 81 identified sites, is the only particularly abundant residue there. Three others (serine, leucine, and asparagine) in nine sites each, are next in abundance in this latter region. Actually, this zone is more characterized by the absence of species than by their presence because six of the 20 species are wanting, including histidine, lysine, tyrosine, tryptophan, phenylalanine, and cysteine. In comparable fashion, the fourth hypervariable sector, which extends from site 101 to 109, inclusive, needs to be called the VG zone, for valine in 15% of the sites and glycine in 13.5% are far more abundantly represented than any of the others.

Correlation to Number of Codons. Before leaving these very significant regions, one is compelled to probe the basis for the variability in occurrence of the several amino acid species, and the question immediately arises as to a possible correlation of abundance to the number of codons that specify the several types. In Table 7.9 the absence of randomness in mutations affecting the four zones is evidenced by two sets of data: first, the lack of clear correlation between the abundance of a given amino acid and the number of codons available to it, and second, the unevenness in distribution that characterizes all the types. Although one species, serine, is both the most abundant and is provided with the maximum number of codons (6) available for any species, arginine with a like number ranks only sixth in frequency, and leucine, also encoded by six codons, stands only in 10th place. Those species provided with four codons each are far more consistent in rank, four of the five ranging from second to fifth in relative abundance; however, the fifth one, proline, ranks only 13th in frequency. Among the types represented by only two codons apiece, most fall into the least abundant categories, five of the nine with this number

of codons ranking from 16th to 20th place. However, two of this group, asparagine and aspartic acid, are more frequent than one of those (leucine) that is
provided with six codons. And even more strangely, one of the pair, each of
which is provided with only a single codon (methionine), is nearly as frequent
as one having six (arginine) and greatly exceeds another with that same number
(leucine). Thus, while there is a general trend of increased abundance with
greater number of codons, the correlation is a very loose one indeed. Moreover, only two species, arginine and isoleucine, are fairly uniformly distributed
among all four zones, all the others fluctuating widely from zone to zone (Table
7.9).

Table 7.9
Occurrence of the Amino Acids in the Hypervariable Regions
Correlated to the Number of Codons Specifying Each

Species	Symbol	Codons specifying each	Number of sites occupied (by zones)				Total	
			ST (69)	AA (154)	M (81)	VG (74)	No.	Rank
Arginine	R	6	6	8	4	5	23	6
Leucine	L	6	1	6	9	3	19	10
Serine	S	6	16	12	9	5	42	1
Alanine	A	4	5	19	3	8	35	2
Glycine	G	4	3	10	2	10	25	5
Proline	P	4	0	3	7	6	16	13
Threonine	T	4	12	3	6	8	29	3
Valine	V	4	3	10	4	11	28	4
Isoleucine	I	3	4	6	3	4	17	12
Asparagine	N	2	0	11	9	1	21	8
Aspartate	D	2	2	15	2	1	20	9
Cysteine	C	2	1	0	0	1	2	20
Glutamate	E	2	1	5	4	0	10	16
Glutamine	Q	2	0	4	7	2	13	14
Histidine	H	2	0	3	0	1	4	19
Lysine	K	2	0	8	0	0	8	18
Phenyl-alanine	F	2	2	6	0	2	10	16
Tyrosine	Y	2	2	13	0	3	18	11
Methionine	M	1	6	2	12	2	22	7
Tryptophan	W	1	1	10	0	1	12	15

The Nature of the Carbohydrate Side Chains. The nature of the carbohydrate or glycopeptide side chains found on immunoglobulins has as yet received relatively little attention. One instance where such an analysis has been completed, examined the substance linked to the asparagine residue at site 297 of most types of IgG molecules from the rabbit (Fanger and Smyth, 1972). This prosthetic group was reported to consist of five glucosamine residues that probably were acetylated, five mannose, two galactose, and one each of fucose and sialic acid. Another whose structure has received greater elaboration was located on the asparagine residue at site 475 (563 of the total molecule) of human IgM (Van Halbeek *et al.*, 1981). Although earlier investigations had suggested it to contain only one *N*-acetylglucosamine residue, the later study cited demonstrated that it had two in the core, in addition to mannose. To this central chain were added at least five more mannose residues, arranged in various branched configurations (Figure 7.3A), some variants having one or two additional ones located on those residues labeled A and/or B.

Several carbohydrate units from light chains have been sequenced in recent years, two of which were from a human λ-type immunoglobulin light chain known as protein Smλ (Chandrasekaran *et al.*, 1981; Garver *et al.*, 1981). The first of the pair was *N*-glycosidically linked to asparagine in site 25 of that protein and consisted of a short core with two identical complex branches and a side chain of fucose (Figure 7.3B, C). The second, which was *O*-glycosidically linked to serine 21, was much shorter, being a disialyated tetrasaccharide. Expecially remarkable was the close proximity of this simple muncin-type substance to the long complex component on the asparagine residue.

7.1.4. Other Chains in Immunoglobulins

Two other types of chains present in one or two classes of immunoglobulins require brief attention, the J chain that is involved in polymer formation with IgA and IgM and the S chain that characterizes the former when produced by secretory bodies.

The J Chain. The J chain that aids in joining some of the monomers of IgM and IgA into polymers has a molecular weight of 15,600 (Schrohenloher *et al.*, 1973) and hence is similar in size to the light chains. Only one such chain is present, regardless of the number of monomers in the molecule, attachment to them being by disulfide bonding with the penultimate cysteine of the heavy chains, which elsewhere is involved in inter-heavy-chain bonding (Mestecky *et al.*, 1974). Similar conditions prevail in all vertebrates from sharks to birds and mammals, that is, in all classes that are known to have IgM (Klaus *et al.*, 1971; Weinheimer *et al.*, 1971; Kobayashi *et al.*, 1973; Meinke and

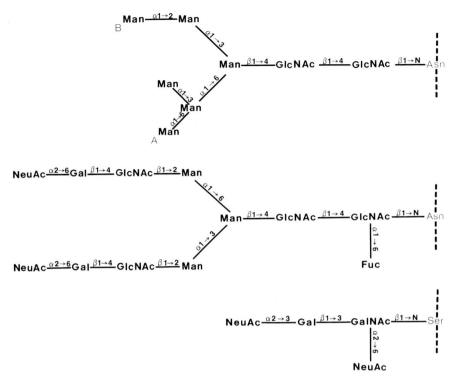

Figure 7.3. Several representative carbohydrate groups of immunoglobulins. The chains, of which many others are also found on immunoglobulin molecules, are often highly complex and variable. Fuc, fucose; Gal, galactose; GalNAc, *N*-acetylgalactosamine; GlcNAc, *N*-acetylglucosamine; Man, mannose; NeuAc, *N*-acetylneuramic acid. Heavy broken lines indicate a portion of the polypeptide chains. (Based on Chandrasekaran *et al.*, 1981, Garver *et al.*, 1981, and Van Halbeek *et al.*, 1981.)

Spiegelberg, 1973). Although involved in polymerization, its specific role in joining the monomers remains unknown, because only one J chain is present in the IgM molecule where it can hold together at most only two of the five units.

The full primary structure of the J chain from man has now been established (Mole *et al.*, 1977a,b) and is reproduced in Table 7.10. Since only a single carbohydrate group is present, attached to an asparagine at site 43, the molecule is at once distinct from the heavy and light chains. Further distinctions are provided by the occurrence of eight cysteines, six of which occur in pairs; the two single ones possibly provide disulfide bonding with the heavy chains of the one or two monomers that bear it, but this point has not been

Table 7.10
The Human J Chain of IgA and IgM[a,b]

```
          10          20          30          40          50
*EDERIVLVDNKCKCARITSRSSEDPNEDEIVRIIVPLDNRENISDPTSP
```

```
          60          70          80          90         100
LRTRFVYHLSDLCKKQCDPTEVELDNQIVTATQCXICDENSASERTYDRN
```

```
         110         120         130
KCYTAVVPLVYGGETKMVZTALTPNACYPX
```

[a] Based on Mole *et al.* (1977b).
[b] * = 2-pyrrolidone-5-carboxylic acid. N indicates the location of a carbohydrate side chain.

established. Nor is it known how many intrachain loops are formed between others of this species of amino acid, but at least a single short one is present, formed by bonding between the cysteines at sites 15 and 17 (Mole *et al.*, 1977b). Although earlier amino acid analyses of the chain had reported unusually high proportions of both aspartic acid and proline, in the neighborhood of 25% (Mestecky *et al.*, 1971), just 8 residues (6.4%) of the latter are to be found in the actual sequence and 11 (8.8%) of the former, a number equaled by the glutamic acid residues. The unequal distribution of the latter two amino acids within the molecule is especially notable, for no aspartic acid and only one of glutamic acid occur in the last 30-odd sites in the C-terminal half. Furthermore, the nonrandom side-by-side association that exists between these two related molecules (Dillon, 1978, pp. 49–54) is also a distinctive feature. Moreover, over half of both these species are concentrated in the N-terminal 50-site region of the molecule, along with half of the proline residues. The presence of dimorphism at site 65 was unexpected, since the polypeptide was from a single patient, but it seemed unlikely that multiple alleles were the basis for the variation (Mole *et al.*, 1977b).

The Secretory Component of IgA. As will be recalled, dimeric IgA in secretory products contains a unit not present in any of the other immunoglobulins, a short chain known as the secretory component (Tomasi *et al.*, 1965; South *et al.*, 1966). It consists of a single polypeptide, with a molecular weight of around 70,000, and contains nearly 9% carbohydrate (Tomasi and Bienenstock, 1968). Unlike the J chain, the secretory component is synthesized only by epithelial cells of the mucosa of such organs as the parotid and submaxillary glands, pancreas, bronchi, stomach, and intestines (Tourville *et al.*, 1969), not by blood cells. The separate origins of the IgA monomers and secretory component are supported also by the fact that persons unable to synthesize IgA nevertheless can produce the secretory component (South *et al.*, 1966). Thus far, its full amino acid sequence does not seem to have been established.

7.1.5. The Genetic Basis of Immunoglobulin Structure

Because of the highly regulated, yet extremely variable nature of immunoglobulin structure, the genetics of antibody production has attracted great numbers of investigations. As was true of the basic morphology, the encoding arrangement for light chains bear many resemblances, as well as differences, from those for heavy chains. Since the genes for the former are of a somewhat less complex nature, they are reviewed before those for the heavy chains. In both instances, the final transcriptional product results from combinations of transcriptional units and/or from recombination events involving the genes themselves, carried out by one or more enzymes referred to as recombinases.

The Organization of Light-Chain Genes. As indicated in the discussion of the light chains themselves, two types, κ and λ, are encoded by separate families of genes, each of which is somewhat comparable in arrangement. In both cases in cells whose immunoglobulin is still unmodified from that of the germ cells (i.e., they possess the germline arrangement of genes), the DNA encoding the V_L sector is separated from that which codes the C_L by many hundreds of base pairs, involving several types of genetic segments. First, there usually are intervening segments which remain untranslated, elsewhere typically called introns but in some studies in this field referred to as I (intervening) segments, with various adjectives like large or small in instances where several occur in the same family. Second are the so-called joining (J) segments of DNA, which are translated and serve to connect the V_L and C_L domains when transcription actually occurs in an antibody-secreting cell. While the use of the word joining and the letter J to indicate the present segment was necessitated to distinguish that type from I segments, some confusion with the J chain of certain immunoglobulins could arise. However, the latter is a polypeptide, whereas the present one is a particular segment of DNA.*

---

*Because of this complex organization of the genome into various size sequences which encode mere fragments of the definitive polypeptide, several new terms are proposed here to alleviate the confusion resulting from use of the term gene for all the various sectors, and are designed for use where complex polypeptides are the encoded products, produced by combination of discrete subdivisions. In other cases the usual terms for translated and untranslated but transcribed parts, respectively called exons and introns, seem to be quite satisfactory. To the smallest segments in complex polypeptide genes such as the DNA sectors encoding the J segments and V and C domains, the name genelet is applied here, and the sectors resulting from combination of such regions are referred to as pregenes. Thus, the term gene is applied solely to the final combination of introns and exons that is actually used in the transcriptive processes of forming the precursorial mRNA.

The Organization of the κ-Chain Genes. A large portion of the κ-chain gene family has recently had its nucleotide sequence determined (Max *et al.*, 1981), a 5500-base-long sector that included the genelets for the several J segments and the C_L domain. This began with a leader section 740 residues long that was transcribed but not translated, followed by a series of five J-segment genelets (J_1 to J_5), separated from one another by introns varying from 267 to 316 bases in length. Each of the genelets was preceded on what was identified as the 5' side by two short sequences, a heptanucleotide that was CACTGTG in two instances (J_1 and J_5), CACTCTG (in J_4), CACTGTA (in J_3), and CAGTGTG (in J_2). Thus, none of these was actually a palindrome as claimed (Boime *et al.*, 1976; Bolivar *et al.*, 1977; Sakano *et al.*, 1981), but those which preceded J_1 and J_5 were concatemers as they displayed complementary ("sticky") ends*; in each instance these sequences were separated from the respective J genelets by one or two sites, which may or may not prove to be equally a part of these supposed signals. The second short sequence in three cases (J_1, J_4, and J_5) was the nonanucleotide GGTTTTTGT, while AGTTTTTGT occurred on J_2 and GGGTTTTGT† on J_3. Perhaps the marked irregularity of composition of the last of these was involved in the failure of J_3 to be transcribed or at least translated, for no polypeptide corresponding in structure to that genelet was detected. Between the heptameric and nonameric sections, there was a sequence typically 23 sites long, but those related to J_3 and J_4 consisted of 21 and 24, respectively. These genelets for joining segments were then followed by an untranslated sequence of 4515 residues in length before the start of that for the C_L domain. Comparisons of the five DNA strands complementary to the genelets for the several J sectors and their translation products (Table 7.11) reveal remarkable consistencies to prevail, even in the DNA where 21 of the 39 sites are seen to be invariant. And when the untranslated J_3 genelet‡ is omitted from these calculations, there are four additional sites, yielding relative universal homology rates of 54% for all five and 64%

---

* As this unnecessary error is appearing in the literature with annoying frequency, it may assist in reducing its occurrence by pointing out that palindromes are words or sentences that read the same in either direction, "radar" being a simple English example of a word and "Madam I'm Adam" a phrase. In contrast, concatemers are objects that can be united in series. Thus, AAGTT-GAA is a palindrome in DNA whereas GAGTTCTC is a concatemer, being capable of forming a loop or a series with identical sequences because of the existence of complementary ends. The DNA of certain bacteriophages (the T-even group) has been suggested to form concatemers during replication (Dillon, 1978, p. 356).

† It should be noted that current practice in the literature, also followed here, is to give the complementary (untranscribed or minus strand) sequence in those cases where the sequence of only a single chain of the actual dual DNA molecule is presented. On the active (transcribed) DNA strand, these heptamers would be placed near the 3' ends of the J-segment genelets and the order of segments would be from J_5 to J_1, not as given.

‡ Technically this may be considered a pseudogene, a sector of DNA that has the structure of related genes or genelets but is not transcribed or at least not translated.

Table 7.11
Base Sequences of the Genes for the
J Sectors of Mouse κ Chains[a]

	Base sequences
J_1	TGGACGTTCGGTGGAGGCACCAAGCTGGAAATCAAACGT
J_2	TACACGTTCGGAGGGGGGACCAAGCTGGAAATAAAACGT
J_4	TTCACGTTCGGGTCGGGGACAAAGTTGGAAATAAAACGT
J_5	CTCACGTTCGGTGCTGGGACCAAGCTGGAGCTGAAACGT
J_3^b	ATCACATTCAGTGATGGGACCAGACTGGAAATAAAACCT

	Gene products
J_1	TrpThrPheGlyGlyGlyThrLysLeuGluIleLysArg
J_2	TyrThrPheGlyGlyGlyThrLysLeuGluIleLysArg
J_4	PheThrPheGlySerGlyThrLysLeuGluIleLysArg
J_5	LeuThrPheGlySerGlyThrLysLeuGluIleLysArg
J_3^b	(IleThrPheSerAsnGlyThrArgLeuGluIleLysPro)

[a] Based on Max *et al.* (1981). [b] Not translated.

for the four active ones. The products encoded by these regions (Table 7.11) are even more constant in structure, differing only in the initial amino acid residue. Were J_3 actually translated, it would differ at four additional sites.

Numerous copies of the V_κ germline genelet had been reported to be present that encode sites 1–95 of the immunoglobulin polypeptide, but the precise number remains undetermined. Moreover, the products of many of the V_κ genelets are not translated into usable polypeptides (Walfield *et al.*, 1980, 1981). During differentiation of the immunoglobulin-secreting lymphocytes, one such genelet becomes attached to that of one for a J segment, possibly through deletion of the intervening DNA between the V_κ and J_κ genelets (Max *et al.*, 1979; Sakano *et al.*, 1979). In addition, creation of the pregene in this manner necessarily also involves deletion of the unused J regions and the long intervening segment separating them from the C_κ genelet. However, what few studies have been made on the actual composition of the nascent mRNA have shown this interpretation to be somewhat simplistic.

Organization of the λ-Chain Genes. The L_λ-chain genes have been investigated in a most interesting manner, in that their sequences were established both before and after the precursorial cells had become mature (Bernard *et al.*, 1978). As a whole, the overall pattern resembled that of the κ-chain genes, except that only a single J genelet was noted. In the case of the most

complete embryonic gene that was cloned, Ig99λ, which most closely corresponded to the λ₀ sequence, the translated leader portion was preceded by an
untranslated segment 92 bases in length; the first active part of the leader, 48
sites in length and coding for 16 amino acids, was followed by a second untranslated and then a translated leader-continuation 90 and 150 base pairs long,
respectively, the latter encoding five amino acids before the actual V_λ gene
began. The later encoded 97 amino acids and ended in a long untranslated
sector of about 260 base pairs. A second germline immunoglobulin gene that
was cloned, referred to as Ig25λ, began with an inactive segment 126 sites in
length that carried the nonanucleotide (GGTTTTTGC) and heptanucleotide
(CACAGTG) sections similar to those of the κ chain, preceding the J sector.
The most notable distinction was that these two segments were separated by
only 11 sites, instead of the 21–24 that characterize the other light chain. As
intimated, these preceded the J genelet that encoded a 13-amino-acid polypeptide, which differed from the product of the J_1 genelet of the κ chain at five
sites. At site 2 valine instead of threonine was present, the latter in place of
glycine at site 10, followed by valine, tyrosine, and glycine in place of glutamic acid, isoleucine, lysine, and arginine in the same order. Beyond the J
genelet was a 1250-base-pair sector that was untranslated, followed by the
genelets for the constant region.

A myeloma (H2020) from the same basic source (BALB/c mice) yielded
an immunoglobulin called Ig303λ. In this type from differentiated cells, the
translated and untranslated leader segments were identical to those of Ig99λ, a
situation that prevailed throughout the V_λ-domain gene, even in the hypervariable regions, with just two exceptions. In the amino acid sequences of the
peptide products, site 25 contained a serine in 99λ in contrast to threonine in
303λ due to a mutation from AGT to ACT, and at site 32 a change of AGT to
GGT in the DNA resulted in a difference between a serine in the first and a
glycine in the second. Beyond this point, the 303λ gene continued directly into
the J genelet found in Ig35λ and had the same long intervening sequence,
followed by the genelets for the constant region. Thus, it appears that during
maturation of immunoglobulin-secreting cells, the only recombination event involves the V and J segments, the remaining beginning and intervening untranslated sequences being retained intact.

The Organization of Heavy-Chain Genes. In the first place, heavy-
chain genes form a family containing a V_H sequence plus at least eight C_H-
domain genelet complexes, μ, δ, γ_3, γ_1, γ_{2b}, γ_{2a}, ϵ, and α (Moore *et al.*,
1981; Nishida *et al.*, 1981). These form a tightly linked cluster joined to V_H-
domain markers (Mage *et al.*, 1973; Cohn *et al.*, 1977). As described more
fully later under B-lymphocyte differentiation, a V_H genelet is first brought
together with one for C_μ, leading to the synthesis of IgM (Early *et al.*, 1979).
Later during further differentiation, other recombination events lead to the production of another class of these immunoglobulins.

Table 7.12
Comparisons of the J_H Gene Signals and Products[a]

	cDNA signals[b]	Translated products	Next codon
J_{H1}	AGTTTTAGTA(22)ACTGTG-C	YWYFDVWGAGTTVTVSS	GGT
J_{H2}	GGTTTTTGTA(23)AGTGTGAC	-----YWGQGTTLTVSS	GGT
J_{H3}	ATTTATTGTC(23)AATGTGCC	-W-FAYWGQGTLVTVSA	GGT
J_{H4}	GGTTTTTGTC(22)ATTGTGAT	YYAMDYWGQGTSVTVSS	GGT
$J_{H\psi}$	GAATCTTGTC(16)CTTGTGAG	[c]	GGT

[a]Based on Gough and Bernard (1981).
[b]Numbers in parentheses indicate number of intervening sites.
[c]This pseudogene is not translated.

But as in the production of the differentiated gene for light chains, the mature pregene for the V_H domain involves the assembly of several fragmental segments by elimination of the intervening sectors. However, in this case assembly is of three separate genelets, the V_H sequence encoding the first 101 amino acids, followed by a short genelet for what is referred to as a D sector that codes for six sites, and several for a J_H portion that encodes for sites 107 to 123 (Early et al., 1980). At least four such J_H genelets have been identified, the amino acid sequences and signals of which are presented in Table 7.12 (Bernard and Gough, 1980; Gough and Bernard, 1981). As in the light chains, during maturation of the secretory cell, the V_H genelet is combined to one of these for a J_H sector to make an uninterrupted V_H pregene, presumably by somatic excision of the intervening sections—but here again knowledge of the precursorial mRNA is incomplete (Figure 7.4). The combined portion is then transcribed, along with all the noncoding portions that separate the J_H sectors from the C_H genelet, as well as the latter and possibly a leader segment, and seemingly in the cases of C_μ and C_α, an additional (M) genelet employed in membrane-associated types as described earlier (Moore et al., 1981). The extraneous parts are then removed from the resulting precursorial mRNA by enzymatic trimming to form the definitive mRNA.

It should be noted that two recombinational events are thus associated with the production of heavy-chain immunoglobulin genes (Sakano et al., 1980), the first of which selects among the four J_H genelets to complete the V_H pregene (Figure 7.4). Then during the course of maturation, the gene that results from union with the C_μ pregene can undergo a second recombinational event when antigen stimulates a switch to a different class of antibody. Thus, the intact V_H complex becomes combined to another pregene, perhaps that for $C_{\gamma 2b}$ or C_α (Pernis et al., 1971, 1976; Davis et al., 1980). The existence of certain signals for the enzymes inducing the switch has been proposed, but since these

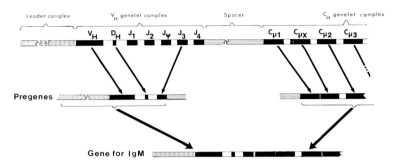

Figure 7.4. Dynamics of forming an IgM gene. The coding regions, or genelets, for the various segments and their introns are diagrammatic and only suggest relative lengths. In the first recombinational event of producing an immunoglobulin molecule, the V_H genelet is combined, together with the D_H genelet, to one of the four J_H genelets to form the pregene for the V_H domain, while similar events prepare the pregene for the $C_{H\mu}$ pregene. When the two pregenes are joined by partial (or complete?) elimination of the spaces, the gene for an IgM molecule has been readied for transcription. The product of transcription presumably requires processing into the definitive mRNA. Another recombinational event, not shown, selects for type of IgM produced, that is, membrane or serum (p. 345).

appear to be part of the coding μ genelet (Sakano *et al.*, 1980), their use in this capacity is subject to doubt. Also questionable is the suggestion that the spacer between genelets for the last J_H sector and C_μ and those that separate the genelets for the other classes of immunoglobulins are degenerate remnants of the single primordial repeating sequence $(AGTCTG)_3GGGTG$ (Ohno, 1981), although the first portion of the suggested repeat admittedly is of frequent occurrence.

The Messengers Transcribed from Immunoglobulin Genes. Relatively little attention has been devoted to the nature of the mRNAs transcribed from immunoglobulin genes, but what has been learned from several recent investigations into this aspect of the genetic processes reveals a compelling need for additional researches along this line. In one report, it was shown that two quite different mRNAs can be produced from a single μ gene by alternative paths of processing the transcript (Early *et al.*, 1981). It will be recalled that IgM exists in two forms, the monomeric type of membranes (mIgM) and the pentameric (sIgM) that is secreted into the bloodstream, the first variety appearing on the surface of lymphocytes prior to the appearance of the latter in the blood serum. Structurally the two types of μ-chain polypeptides appear to differ primarily at the segment preceding the C terminus. In the formation of the mRNA for sIgM, the last 187 residues are transcribed from DNA contiguous to the 3' end encoding the $C_{\mu4}$ domain, whereas this part is not employed in the formation of the mRNA of μ_m. Instead 392 residues are encoded by two exons located 1850 base pairs beyond the genelet for the $C_{\mu4}$ domain; the two genelets are separated by a spacer 118 base pairs in length. A similar situation has also been reported for the formation of membrane and secreted varieties of IgD (Moore *et al.*, 1981); the λ_1-mRNA has proven to be translated into two major immunoglobulins (Near and Storb, 1981). Thus, developmental changes in the synthesis of at least several classes of these antibodies involve differences in reading programs, not recombinations as suggested by studies of the genes.

However, transcriptional program alterations are not the only new method of providing gene changes, for in plasmacytoma cells of mice a multiplicity of light-chain mRNAs were found (Schwartz *et al.*, 1981). In this rodent two types of λ chains have long been known, λ_1 occurring in about 4% of the murine immunoglobulins and λ_2 in about 1%, the κ chain providing the greatest bulk. While a third even rarer type (λ_3) has recently been discovered (Azuma *et al.*, 1981), its recognition has been made too recently to enter into the present discussion. An investigation of the mRNAs for λ_1 chains demonstrated that in plasmacytomas producing λ_1 chains, mRNAs for λ_2 of normal size were also produced. However, only the first of these appeared to be translated and the product employed in antibody snythesis. While thus some of the variability of immunoglobulin idiotypes results from differing recombination events, much still stems from somatic mutation in the V_H and V_L chains (Bothwell *et al.*, 1981).

7.2. THE CELLULAR COMPONENTS OF THE IMMUNE SYSTEM

Now that the complexities of the antibodies themselves have been examine, the next logical step in scrutinizing the nature of gene action changes in immune reactions is to focus on the cellular components. The picture that emerges is obscured to some extent, both by the complicated nature of the components themselves and by the persistence of unknown factors, despite the large number of investigations that are completed annually in this field. Among the types of cells involved in the system are monocytes, macrophages, mast cells, and lymphocytes, the last of which being by far the most important. As pointed out earlier (Chapter 4, Section 4.5), lymphocytes fall into two major populations, the B and T cells, depending upon their origins, and are discussed in the two following sections in that same sequence.

7.2.1. The B Lymphocytes

According to the view now prevalent among immunologists (Roitt, 1974), all lymphocytes are produced in adult mammals by bone marrow cells, one population then going to the structures equivalent to the avian bursa of Fabricius to become the B lymphocytes, or simply B cells, the other to the thymus, where they are processed into T lymphocytes or T cells. The presence of an antigen induces both types to proliferate, some of the products of which then undergo morphological changes; thus, B cells become converted to large so-called plasma cells that actively secrete immunoglobulins, and T cells develop into what are known as lymphoblasts, cells that directly carry out a number of immune functions detailed in the next section. Although therefore T lymphocytes are not supposed to secrete immunoglobulins into the bloodstream, removal of the thymus does decrease the production of antibody (Cooper *et al.*, 1966), and other evidence presented later indicates the presence of the same activity. A third class, null cells (N cells), lacks certain traits of both T and B cells, but their ontogenetic development has not yet been followed.

Origin and Properties of B Cells. The origin of B cells remains controversial to a degree, especially in mammals. In the first place, the organs or tissues that are actually equivalent to the bursa of Fabricius of birds have not been fully defined, but they appear to include a miscellany of structures, notably the tonsils, vermiform appendix, Peyer's patches, and certain regions of the lymphoid follicles. For example, when an antibody known to be independent of interaction with the thymus, such as the polysaccharide produced by the bacterium *Paracoccus*, the cortical, but not the paracortical, cells of the lymphoid follicles are induced to undergo rapid mitoses, the resulting plasma cells reportedly migrating to the bone marrow medullary cords (Roitt, 1974).* Other evidence suggests that the liver may also be an active site of B-cell differentiation, in addition to those tissues already cited (Melchers *et al.*, 1975; Abney *et al.*, 1978). The latter organ has been definitely established as the earliest site of differentiation of this type of lymphocyte, progenitory cells appearing there in mouse embryos between 12 and 14 days of gestation and definitive cells at 16 to 17 days (Nossal and Pike, 1973; Owen *et al.*, 1974).

The pre-B cells in the liver and bone marrow of the early fetus did not occur in the thymus or lymph nodes (Owen *et al.*, 1977). Such relatively large cells as these progenitors have also been recognized in *Xenopus*, rabbit, and man (Gathings *et al.*, 1977; Hayward *et al.*, 1977; Zettergren *et al.*, 1977). However, the cells from different species were not entirely identical, for differences in surface markers have been detected (McElroy *et al.*, 1981). The capacity for forming a diversity of antibody-producing cells is not gained until sometime after birth, when a differentiation event of unknown nature takes place (Sherr *et al.*, 1981). In birds the development of early B lymphocytes from the stem cells is confined to the bursa of Fabricius, as is their differentia-

---

*It should be noted that development into a full-fledged plasma cell is at least often a two-stage process. On first contact, a given antigen apparently induces a B cell to become specialized to a degree for action against it. Upon second contact, the same antigen then leads these so-called "memory cells" to develop into full-fledged plasma cells, that appear to be inactive against all other foreign substances.

tion into populations that secrete different classes of immunoglobulins (Lawton *et al.*, 1975).

A current study demonstrated that a number of contrasting populations of B cells were formed during the course of differentiation in the bone marrow of mammals (Deslauriers-Boisvert *et al.*, 1980). The chief distinctions among the up to six populations were in their respective cell sizes, susceptibility to various mitogens, and kinetics of subsequent maturation into immunoglobulin-secreting cells. Maturation, both of B and T cells, also occurs within the spleen, although the precise role of the organ still is not completely understood. However, it has proven to be the major site of antibody production in rats, rabbits, and human beings (Rowley, 1950a,b; Draper and Süssdorf, 1957); moreover, this role is supported by the observation that B cells accumulated in smaller numbers in the peripheral bloodstream in splenectomized mammals (Ron *et al.*, 1981).

In gross morphology, there are almost no differences to be noted between definitive B and T lymphocytes; however, a number of ultrastructural distinctions may be detected, largely on the cell surface by use of the scanning electron microscope, rather than internally with the aid of the transmission type. The entire surface of B cells is rather densely covered with microvillous projections (Figure 7.5), whereas only a few are borne on the others (Reyes *et al.*, 1975). But the two classes are more readily distinguished by several cytochemical and physiological tests. In one standard procedure, fluorescein-labeled anti-immunoglobulin light-chain serum or similarly treated anti-immunoglobulin monomer serum, shows the presence of immunoglobulins on the surface of B cells but not on most T lymphocytes. However, a small proportion of the latter class may react with such sera, as a result of the presence of immune complexes bound to receptors for the Fc segments, but this occurs only when these cells have been activated. Another technique involves the addition of sheep red blood cells to the lymphocytes, the B showing no reaction, whereas T cells become covered with a number of the erythrocytes to form what is termed rosettes. It should be noted that when the red cells are treated with IgG or other immune-related substances, B lymphocytes, too, form rosettes with them, but only under such special conditions.

Ultrastructural Features. As stated above, ultrastructural features with the transmission electron microscope show only slight differences from the T type. In typical small B lymphocytes, the ovate, broadly emarginate or sometimes deeply incised nucleus fills most of the cell and consists of about equal parts of electron-opaque heterochromatin and granular-appearing euchromatin (Figure 7.6A, B; Poulsen and Claësson, 1980; Vos *et al.*, 1980). The scant cytoplasm is free of organelles, except in the broader region provided by the nuclear emargination or incision, where a number of mitochondria and several Golgi bodies occur. The former, which appear to be of the microvillose type

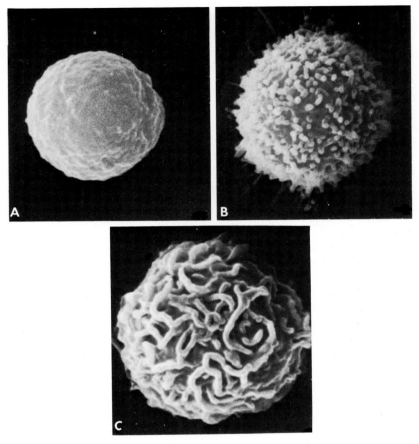

Figure 7.5. Surface features of blood cells. (A) In members of the T class of lymphocytes, the surface is nearly smooth, with just an occasional short microvillus. (B) In contrast, the surface of a B lymphocyte is densely covered with short microvillar projections. (C) The surface of phagocytotic leukocytes is heavily covered with thick microvilli, often appressed against the plasmalemma, as here. All 10,000×. (Courtesy of Vos *et al.*, 1980.)

(Dillon, 1981, pp. 380–392), are circular in outline, while the latter organelles have strongly swollen cisternae that give rise to large, rounded vacuoles.

After contact with an antigen, a mitogen, or certain other substances, the B lymphocytes become activated and commence to differentiate into immuno-globulin-secreting cells known as plasma cells, which transformation processes involve many radical changes including an intermediate stage referred to as plasmablasts. The most notable alteration is the development of the greatly enhanced quantity of cytoplasm, the diameter of the cell becoming virtually

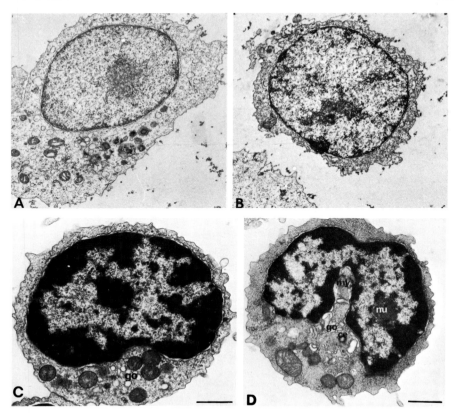

Figure 7.6. Ultrastructure of B-lymphocyte development. (A) Pre-B lymphocyte (or lymphoblast) grown in culture. 6375×. (Courtesy of P. B. Paulsen, unpublished.) (B) Mature B cell, with reduced cytoplasm and few organelles. 6375×. (Courtesy of Paulsen and Claesson, 1980.) (C) Slightly activated B lymphocyte, showing the presence of Golgi bodies (go) along with six mitochondria. 9720×. (D) A larger activated cell at a somewhat later stage with deeply lobed nucleus containing a nucleolus (nu), myelin figures (my) within the nuclear cleft, Golgi bodies (go), and a centriole (ce). 9180×. (C and D, courtesy of Vos *et al.*, 1980.)

doubled. In plasma cells the now nearly rounded nucleus contains a large nucleolus and perhaps a greater quantity of euchromatin than heterochromatin (Figure 7.6C, D). In the cytoplasm, the mitochondria have greatly increased in size, are elongate-ovate, and are either microvillose or cristate. More striking is the presence of an abundant rough endoreticulum, consisting of single tubules or swollen cisternae, including an extensive region around the nuclear membrane (Figure 7.7). The dictyosomes have also increased in size and produce vesicles of prodigious proportions; these bodies, together with the endo-

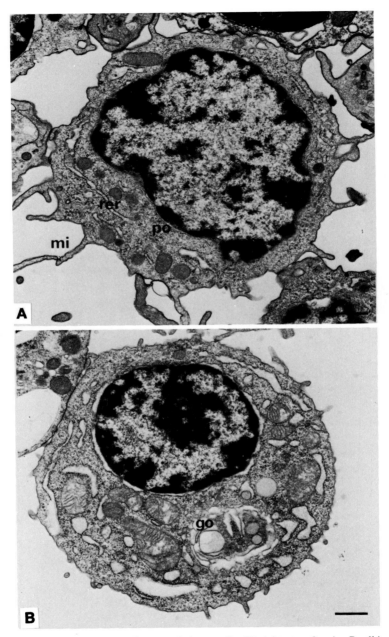

Figure 7.7. Late stages in the development of plasma cells. (A) A late transforming B cell in which the cytoplasmic content is increasing and rough endoreticulum (rer) and polyribosomes (po) are beginning to appear, as are microvilli on the surface. 15,300×. (B) This immature plasma cell has still more greatly enhanced cytoplasm, and extensive vesicular and cisternal rough endoreticulum, and Golgi vesicles (go) that ramify throughout much of the cell, giving it a vesicular appearance. 9900×. (Courtesy of Vos *et al.*, 1980.)

reticulum, give the entire cytoplasm a vesicular appearance and undoubtedly is a reflection of the strong secretory activities of the cells.

Surface Immunoglobulins of B Cells. The B lymphocytes appear to function against antigens in two ways: (1) by secreting immunoglobulins into the blood plasma after they have become transformed into plasma cells, and (2) by immunoglobulins and/or other substances borne on their surface that interact with the antigen or foreign particle directly. As a result of this second important functional property, much attention has been devoted in the literature to the nature of the surface components; however, because of their complexity, controversy still persists, especially pertaining to the manner in which the surface substances undergo specialization for interaction with the particular antigen that happens to be present. Here those surface features which are unique to, or at least, characteristic of, B cells are enumerated, those that are shared equally with other classes of blood cells being discussed where most appropriate in later sections. For instance, the surface antibodies involved in what is known as the major histocompatibility complex are held for attention in that portion that deals with the latter topic.

The best known of the surface reactants, the immunoglobulins, vary with the developmental stage and degree of activation (Shortman *et al.*, 1981). The youngest B cells, like those from fetal mouse liver and cases of chronic lymphocytic leukemia, have only monomeric IgM on their surfaces (Raff, 1977; Vitetta *et al.*, 1977; Scher *et al.*, 1980; Stevenson *et al.*, 1980). As already mentioned, prior to the appearance of this surface immunoglobulin in precursorial B cells of fetal bone marrow, IgM monomers are detectable in their cytoplasm (Raff *et al.*, 1976) and similarly leukemic cells of comparable nature predominantly display a like condition (Vogler *et al.*, 1981). Thus, the acquisition of this type of antibody undergoes a sequential series of changes in the location and form, for, after activation, IgM is secreted into the blood plasma only in the pentameric form $(L_2H_2)_5$, while the early cytoplasmic and surface forms are the monomer, L_2H_2, aside from the structural differences already pointed out (Parkhouse *et al.*, 1977). In the 1-week postnatal mammal, B cells bearing IgD in addition to IgM first appear in low numbers, but these cells with dual isotypes increase substantially during the next 3-week period (Raff *et al.*, 1975; Sidman and Unanue, 1975). However, in contrast to the M isotype, IgD is quite scarce in the blood serum (Parkhouse *et al.*, 1977).

IgD is not the only isotype of immunoglobulin to put in a first appearance in week-old mice, for IgG and IgA are to be found on B-cell surfaces at the same time. They are presently considered to develop directly from IgM-bearing precursors (Lawton *et al.*, 1975), because some cells bear either IgG or IgA along with IgM but never with IgD. Nevertheless, B lymphocytes possessing only IgD on their surface can switch to IgG when activated by antigen (Parkhouse *et al.*, 1977); and those bearing IgM can do likewise upon comparable stimulation. The IgA-bearing B cells are a special case, for in the rabbit and probably other mammals as well, they appear to be developed primarily in

Peyer's patches; the appendix and bronchial follicles are the only important secondary sources of that type of lymphocyte (Cebra *et al.*, 1977; Stafford and Fanger, 1980).

A current study has summarized the ontogenetic events in a particularly lucid fashion (Teale *et al.*, 1981b), after analyzing clones derived from primary and secondary B cells separated according to surface isotypes. First, aside from those that bear IgA, it was found that virtually all mature primary B cells bear IgM on their surfaces; thus, none bear only IgG there, as had been thought. Second, the majority of these cells have the potential for producing multiple classes of immunoglobulins in the presence of helper T cells. After first contact of these cells with antigen, the resulting memory cells include a substantial fraction still bearing IgM on their surface. As those that lack that isotype are unable to produce clones which secrete IgM, they apparently have lost the μ gene, as predicted by Honjo and Kataoka (1978). Finally, most memory cells have the potential for production of multiple classes of immunoglobulins. As might be expected, in mice the mRNA for the heavy chain and the κ light chain are the first to put in their appearance, the former preceding the latter event. At least four different μ-chain mRNAs have been reported in a murine cell line, but whether this heterogeneity resulted from the participation of more than one C_μ allele or from processing could not be established (Perry and Kelley, 1979). More likely, some of the differences reflected the presence of secretory and membrane messengers, the respective types arising by a pretranslational mechanism (Sidman, 1981).

Other Surface Traits. Since many of the activities of B cells are dependent upon the diversity of molecules carried on the surface membrane, it is inevitable that any enumeration of the surface features should cut across an equally broad spectrum of specialized topics that remain to be taken up in later sections. Although the nature of several components thus becomes clear only in subsequent discussions, a list including them nevertheless must be made in order to provide a better understanding of the B lymphocyte and its highly complex organization into a large number of disparate populations.

Many of the surface components are members of what is referred to as the major histocompatibility complex and are arranged into two important classes, the Ia (immune-associated) and the HLA-A, -B, and -C antigens, respectively. The latter classes have been well defined, both serologically and biochemically, and have been established as consisting of polymorphic glycosylated polypeptide chains, with a molecular weight of 43,000, and a substance called β_2-microglobulin (Bridgen *et al.*, 1976; Terhorst *et al.*, 1976). Essentially the members of these groups occur on the surface of all cells except erythrocytes. In contrast, those in the HLA-D category are specific B-cell alloantigens and contain polypeptides of 23,000 and 30,000 daltons (Springer *et al.*, 1977). Like the latter, members of the Ia class of antigens are especially characteristic of B lymphocytes and have a dual chain construction of glycosylated polypeptides, one component having a molecular weight of 28,000, the other 34,000 (Bridgen *et al.*, 1976; Barnstable *et al.*, 1977; Snary *et al.*, 1977). Two members of the class, referred to as L203 and L227, have been identified on human B lymphocytes (Lampson and Levy, 1980), but quite a diversity of populations appears to exist (Greenstein *et al.*, 1981).

An interesting process has been revealed by a late study of another class of surface structures, the receptors for the activated third component of what is referred to as complement. This substance, called C3, occurs as a number of varieties designated by lower-case or capital letters, and these in turn as a series of subvarieties. In the investigation in question (Gormus *et al.*, 1980), the ability of lymphocytes from mouse spleen and human peripheral blood to bind to a complex consisting of bacteria, antibody, and C3 was examined, together with red blood cells. The results indicated that the normal human lymphocytes in the presence of this complex were able to form rosettes with lymphoblastoid red blood cells, which carry the variety C3dR, but not to those of normal subjects, which carry C3bR. On reacted lymphocytes incubated at 37°C, the bound complexes moved from sites scattered over the entire surface to a small area, a process referred to as capping, the significance of which remains unknown (Gormus *et al.*, 1974).

Another series of B-cell-specific alloantigens has only recently been brought to light and thus far consists of only two known members, B1 and B2 (Stashenko *et al.*, 1980; Nadler *et al.*, 1981). These substances were demonstrated to be distinct from other B-lymphocyte-surface markers, including immunoglobulins, Ia-like antigens, and Fc and C3 receptors. Moreover, the two members differ from one another both biochemically and in their distribution on normal and malignant B cells; thus, these surface components serve further in distinguishing subpopulations of this class of lymphocytes.

Although the basis for the differences remains undetermined in each case, an abundance of other cell reactions than those enumerated have been uncovered which indicate the existence of numerous populations. A number of types have been reported, distinguished by their undergoing mitotic division preferentially to different mitogens (Prager and Baechtel, 1973; Galili *et al.*, 1978; Klein and Naor, 1979; Yowell *et al.*, 1979; Klein *et al.*, 1981a,b), and others that responded to thymus-dependent or -independent forms of the same types of antigens (Gahrton *et al.*, 1980; Klein *et al.*, 1980). Still others exhibited different growth characteristics on agar (Brunner *et al.*, 1968; Haas, 1974; Cerottini and Brunner, 1974) or in culture (Wetzel and Kettman, 1981), and additional ones were specific for certain haptens (Boswell *et al.*, 1980; Pillai and Scott, 1981). Thus, the ability of these cells to provide the organism with antibodies against almost any of the innumerable possible foreign substances or invaders does not derive solely from the varieties of expression of the several immunoglobulins but from a whole series of complexly interacting surface and secretory components. The complexity is further enhanced by the circadian rhythm that has recently been shown to exist in lymphocyte number in man. The concentration of cells reached its ebb in the morning from which point it gradually increased during the afternoon to reach a peak at midnight, dropping abruptly thence till morning (Abo *et al.*, 1981). The T and B cell numbers appeared to change in concert, under the influence of a cortiocosteroid (Kawate *et al.*, 1981), but whether there were subpopulational differences remains for the future.

7.2.2. The T Lymphocytes

As pointed out elsewhere, the T lymphocytes are developed in the thymus. In the immunological account, prolymphocytes derived from precursorial cells produced in the bone marrow and spleen are released into the bloodstream to be carried to the thymus where they develop into T lymphocytes (Everett and Tyler, 1967; Miller and Osoba, 1967). The precursors in the bone marrow have had a long ontogenetic history prior to their advent, as described earlier (Chapter 4, Section 4.5; Weissman *et al.*, 1976). From the thymus certain subpopulations of the T cells migrate thence to particular regions of peripheral lymphoid tissue, such as that around the splenic arterioles and the paracortical areas of the lymph nodes (Roitt, 1974), for these areas have been ascertained to become depleted of lymphocytes if thymectomy is performed on a neonatal mammal. However, some evidence exists which intimates that in addition certain mononuclear cells of the bloodstream (T-colony-forming cells) can develop into T lymphocytes without direct association with the thymus (Triebel *et al.*, 1981).

Ultrastructure and Further Development of T cells. The small T cells differ only in the lack of the microvillous projections found on the surface of their B counterparts (Figure 7.5A), but once they have been activated by certain mitogens, they increase greatly in size as they become transformed into a type called lymphoblasts, or more usually, blast cells. Several mitogens are known thus to stimulate T cells specifically, including concanavalin A (Con A), while others, like bacterial lipopolysaccharide (LPS), influence only B cells. From the product of the latter class, the plasma cell, lymphoblasts differ in having a greater volume of cytoplasm relative to the nuclear size, and the nucleus, which is deeply incised at several points, consists largely of granular euchromatin (Al-Hamdani *et al.*, 1981). In the cytoplasm are numerous mitochondria, that recall those of the transforming B cell in being rounded and largely of the microvillose variety. Beyond these organelles, the cytoplasm lacks large structural features, save for a very meager vesicular rough endoreticulum and perhaps a dictyosome or two, the remainder of the region being uniformly filled only with ribosomes.

At least three major classes of T cells are generally recognized, helper, suppressor, and killer (Paul and Benacerraf, 1977), but when and where the respective specializations develop have not been fully elaborated as yet (Klein *et al.*, 1981b). However, there appears to be an unspecialized intermediate stage in their ontogeny, referred to as the recognition cell. The members of the suppressor type (T_S), as well as the helper (T_H), act upon certain other T cells, augmenting or suppressing activated members, but most of their activity appears to be directed toward B cells. The third principal type is the killer cell (T_K) that lyses or ingests foreign or antigen-bearing cells, but in addition, a fourth population (T_D) usually is recognized, which functions in the delayed hypersensitivity response *in vivo*, a reaction involving specific antigens and the secreting of substances called lymphokines (Golub, 1977; Katz, 1977; Rocklin *et al.*, 1978, 1980). However, such secretions are released also by several other types of blood cells, especially by macrophages (DeWeck *et al.*, 1980).

Surface Characteristics. As was seen to be the case with B cells, receptors and antigens on the cell surface largely provide the major features that differentiate the several populations. While the nature of these traits had remained controversial for some time, the basis for the differing opinions is proving to have resulted from their nature, for current knowledge indicates them to be quite as complex as those of the B class. Among the more important types are three Ly alloantigens, often also referred to as Lyt antigens (Lanier *et al.*, 1981). For instance, the T_D and T_H populations have been found to bear Ly-1, but not Ly-2 or Ly-3 (Kisielow *et al.*, 1975; Huber *et al.*, 1976), whereas the T_S and T_K types lack the first of these but have the other two (Shiku *et al.*, 1975; Cantor *et al.*, 1976). Those that bear all three are considered to be precursors (recognition cells?), but in some cases they have cytotoxic properties, that is, they are killer cells (Beverley *et al.*, 1976; Chen *et al.*, 1981). The last paper cited also demonstrated that the Ly-3-bearing cells did not bind bacteria, but those that had Ly-1, with or without Ly-2, did do so. However, the behavior of the cells is not always so precisely related to these factors as the foregoing discussion might suggest, but apparently it arises through the interplay of several contrasting sets, most of which remain unknown. For instance, cultured cell lines of T_D lymphocytes have been reported to be of the typical Ly-1^+ phenotype (Huber *et al.*, 1976; Smith and Miller, 1979; Weiss and Dennert, 1981), but others bear the Ly-2^+ or Ly-3^+ phenotype, that is, they are lacking Ly-1 (Smith and Miller, 1978). Moreover, the T_S and T_K populations have also been demonstrated to carry Ly-1, albeit in small quantities, in addition to a more abundant supply of Ly-2 and Ly-3 (Lanier *et al.*, 1981).

Another highly distinctive surface marker is one known as Thy-l, which occurs also on brain cells (Cohen *et al.*, 1981), but this antigen serves only to distinguish prothymocytes from T cells (Silverstone *et al.*, 1978). When precursors leave the bone marrow or spleen, they lack this trait; then within the thymus they are induced by the polypeptide hormone of that organ, thymopoietin, to express it and another characteristic known as TL (thymus-leukemia antigen) (Basch and Goldstein, 1974; Goldstein *et al.*, 1975; Slomski and Cohen,

1980; Tokuyama and Tanigaki, 1981). Thy-1 has proven to have a primary structure related to that of immunoglobulin, at least in part (Cohen *et al.*, 1981). In addition, another trait, an internal one, however, served toward distinguishing precursorial and mature T cells, but in the opposite direction. A template-independent DNA polymerase, called terminal deoxyribonucleotidyl transferase, was reported present in prothymocytes that later became lost during maturation in the thymus (Cayre *et al.*, 1981). Besides thus serving as a distinction between many prothymocytes and T cells, it also distinguished between precursors that had originated in the bone marrow and those from the spleen, for the latter population lacked the enzyme.

High-molecular-weight glycoproteins in addition to Thy-1 form another class of surface antigens, details of a few of which have become known (Trowbridge *et al.*, 1975; Dunlap *et al.*, 1978; Hoessli and Vassali, 1980). Two groups have been recognized, one of which, termed T170, had a molecular weight of 170,000 and occurred only on thymocytes and T cells from the peripheral blood (Sunderland *et al.*, 1979). The second varied in molecular weight with the source, being present on the surface of thymocytes as a single molecular form weighing 180,000, whereas on peripheral T lymphocytes two forms were represented, having molecular weights in the range of 180,000 and 190,000. Further on B cells, it again occurred in a single molecular species, but in this case weighing 210,000. Still another glycoprotein, one of low molecular weight (11,000), has also been detected on activated T cells (Gately and Martz, 1981).

Although many other surface components have been described and numerous additional ones will probably become known in the near future, only one more needs to be described here to make clear the complexity of gene expression that exists in this class of lymphocytes. A series of surface antigens has been defined by a set of monoclonal immunoglobulins belonging to the IgG2 subclass; since one of the latter, OKT3, reacted with all T lymphocytes, these cells were shown to share a common antigen (Kung *et al.*, 1979; Van Wauwe and Goossens, 1981). Contrastingly, a second representative, OKT4, was specific for only the inducer-helper class, and a third, OKT8, reacted solely with T_S and T_K types (Reinherz *et al.*, 1979a,b, 1980; Friedman *et al.*, 1981; Triebel *et al.*, 1981). Some of these and other factors that are distinctive of the several classes have recently been the subject of a review (Taussig, 1980).

Immunoglobulin on T Cells. For many years it was accepted that one major distinction between T and B lymphocytes was in the former lacking the ability to produce immunoglobulin as the latter type did. Then later this supposed distinction gradually began to fall out of favor as an increasing number of laboratories explored the question and found receptors for the Fc fragment present on T-cell plasmalemma (Warner, 1974; Marchalonis, 1975; Vitetta and Uhr, 1975). A number of investigations reported the κ chain present on T cells and others detected the mRNA for that sequence in the cytoplasm (Putnam *et al.*, 1977; Storb *et al.*, 1977). Moreover, the presence of both the α heavy chain and its mRNA has been established (Marcu *et al.*, 1978; Near and Storb, 1979), and now two functionally distinct populations have been defined on their ability to bind either IgG or IgM, the latter being distinctive of T_H and the former T_S cells (Grossi *et al.*, 1978). The type of immunoglobulin borne on the surface has been demonstrated to be correlated to the source of the population; on T cells in the spleen the γ chain was more prevalent than the μ (Ricardo, 1980), occurring on 32 to 35% of those lymphocytes against 15 to 18% having IgM. Moreover, in the lymph nodes and blood, the proportion of cells bearing γ was far lower than it was in the spleen. In tests with various viral antigens, only T cells bearing the γ chains were found to respond (McFarland *et al.*, 1980).

7.2.3. Other Cellular Constituents

Since most, if not all, cells of the various body tissues produce antibodies and/or antigens on their surfaces or elsewhere, the enumeration of cellular constituents involved in immune reactions could be a nearly endless occupation. Consequently, here only those that are consistently involved in immunity-associated processes through interplay with the various types of lymphocytes are considered worthy of discussion. In addition to the two varieties that now receive detailed attention, occasional mention must also be made of several familiar types, such as the various polymorphonuclear leukocytes.

The Monocyte-Macrophage Series. In current contributions to the field of immunology, no differentiation often is made between the monocyte and macrophage, so that those terms must be employed loosely here, too, with macrophage given some preference. In addition, some investigators distinguish the macrophages of tissues as histocytes, reserving the former term for slightly smaller ones of the blood (Sell, 1980), and on other occasions the cells from the latter tissue are designated as accessory (or A) cells, with the name macrophage confined to those of other tissues. Apparently the monocytes and macrophages bear some sort of ancestor–progeny relationship, the former, which has somewhat less abundant cytoplasm, probably representing the forebear. Both are amoeboid and have the peculiar ability to adhere to smooth surfaces such as glass; furthermore, they are actively phagocytotic, but the ingestion of foreign, dead, and atypical cells is only one of the ways they enter into immunological reactions.

The monocyte-macrophage line consists of large cells, each having a single, large, incised nucleus, which varies between kidney shape to bilobed in conformation. Within it may be seen a conspicuous nucleolus and extensive electron-opaque heterochromatin around the periphery; much of the interior, however, is granular-appearing euchromatin. If monocytes do actually represent either a separate class or stage, they might be distinguishable by their less extensive cytoplasm, the presence of a number of opaque vesicles, and a greater content of mitochondria, which are of the typical cristate type. Although vesicular rough endoreticulum is abundant, little if any of the stacked cisternal variety can be noted (Roitt, 1974). In typical macrophages, on the other hand, the broader cytoplasmic mass contains only a few cristate mitochondria, a very extensive cisternal rough endoreticulum, a number of dictoysomes, and quite numerous heterosomes containing remnants of phagocytosed cells (Dillon, 1981, pp. 274–285).

Phagocytotic Properties. The phagocytotic properties of these cells are indeed remarkable, for those that remain in the sinusoids of the liver are able completely to remove gelatin-stabilized carbon particles injected into the bloodstream during a few passages through that organ (Stuart, 1970). Similarly when dust or carbon particles are inhaled into the lungs, the macrophages of the pulmonary alveolae ingest them. Phagocytosis is in part carried out by the lamellipod pseudopodia that characterize these amoeboid cells, but these organelles enter also into other activities, their great breadth being maintained and activated by an extensive network of actin fibers (Trotter, 1981). During the ensuing intracellular digestion of ingested material, oxygen consumption is greatly increased, which respiratory enhancement does not result from increased mitochondrial activity but involves a cytochrome b_{245} of the cell membrane (Segal *et al.*, 1981). Moreover, similar processes are involved in the initiation of immunogenesis—the first step appears to be the phagocytotic uptake of antigen by macrophages, which process the material. Such antigens are not recognized further in these cells but are treated nonspecifically before contact is made with lymphocytes for their actual recognition and subsequent antibody formation (Nelson, 1976). In addition, macrophages are active in the inflammatory response, for they migrate from blood and tissues in large numbers to sites of inflammation. The basis for this chemotactic response has not been ascertained, but it appears to be induced by the release from specialized lymphocytes of a substance called macrophage-aggregating factor (Badenoch-Jones *et al.*, 1981). Moreover, *in vitro,* activated macrophages demonstrate marked regulatory activities upon tumor cells by restricting their growth (Keller, 1976; Normann *et al.*, 1980). Such suppressor cells are of frequent occurrence in the spleen of rats and other mammals (Veit, 1981).

The phagocytosis of antigen is followed after its nonspecific treatment by what is known as "antigen presentation," involving contact between antigen-bearing macrophages and lymphocytes. These processes are poorly understood but appear to be of great significance to the immune reaction. For example, *in vitro* studies have shown that the normal secreting of antibody by B cells in the presence of antigen and T cells was largely abrogated when macrophages were removed from the culture. Additionally, such antigens as bovine serum albumin evoke a far stronger antibody response *in vivo* when they are injected together with macrophages than when administered alone. More current studies have shown that at least two populations of macrophages exist, only one of which is efficient in presenting antigen (Tzehoval *et al.*, 1981). As among other types of blood cells on the basis of other characteristics, including surface markers and behavior, numerous populations of macrophages have similarly become recognized (Humphrey and Grennan, 1981; Lee *et al.*, 1981).

Other Activities of Macrophages. As among other classes of immune-active blood cells, the functions of macrophages are made complex by the existence of the multiple populations just mentioned, a point made especially clear by a recent study on mouse cells (Lee and Wong, 1980). Macrophages derived from bone marrow precursors were cultured in two contrasting media, one that was conditioned with mouse L cells and the other with lung cells. When the macrophages grew exponentially in the L-cell medium, they reacted to a number of antigens dependent on Ia factors, including tuberculin purified protein derivative and bacterial flagellin, but only to a lower level than that of normal macrophages from the spleen or peritoneal cavity. Then as cell growth reached the stationary phase, this activity declined. Contrastingly the bone marrow-derived cells cultured in lung-cell-activated medium developed a higher activity that did not decline after the stationary phase. In other aspects, however, both populations resembled normal macrophages in antigen uptake, phagocytosis, and other activities.

Another function of macrophages is that of lysing such cells as erythrocytes and tumor-cell lines that have been sensitized to antibody (Shaw *et al.*, 1978; Horwilz *et al.*, 1979; Norris *et al.*, 1979; Randazzo *et al.*, 1979; Pace and Russell, 1981). The mechanism of this antibody-dependent cytotoxicity is not understood, but the binding of antibody-sensitized target cells by Fc-receptor-bearing effector cells is essential to the initiation of the event. Examples of similar behavior include the lysis of sensitized tumor cells by neutrophils and macrophages (Hafeman and Lucas, 1979; Nathan *et al.*, 1979). More recently, however, it has been shown that two independent mechanisms existed, one of which was O_2 dependent, whereas the second was not (Klassen and Sagone, 1980). Perhaps the observation that various prostaglandins have differing effects upon the cytotoxic activities of the cells may form part of the overall picture (McCarthy and Zwilling, 1981).

Still another factor that is sometimes active in the functioning of macrophages is the presence of lymphokines (including interferons), secretions of antigen- or mitogen-stimulated spleen cells (Nacy and Meltzer, 1979; Neta, 1981; Stanwick *et al.*, 1981). The particular lymphokine that was effective in a given case varied with the nature of the antigen, and appeared to vary as to whether tumoricidal or suppressor populations were generated (Taramelli *et al.*, 1981). That which elicited macrophage cytotoxicity against tumor cells proved to be a single protein, with a molecular weight around 45,000, whereas the reagent active against *Rickettsia tsutsugamushi* was complex, consisting of three substances with molecular weights respectively of 10,000, between 35,000 and 45,000, and around 115,000 to 125,000 (Nacy *et al.*, 1981).

Surface Markers of Macrophages. The functions of macrophages as a whole are under extensive genetic control, both the processing of antigens and their presentation by these cells being highly restricted (Rosenthal and Shevach, 1973; Erb and Feldmann, 1975; Rosenthal, 1978; Treves, 1978). Their ability to secrete antigen-specific and -nonspecific mediating substances likewise is controlled in comparable fashion (Gery and Waksman, 1972; Calderon *et al.*, 1975; Rosenwasser and Rosenthal, 1978). During the course of development of monocytes into macrophages, determinants defined by the *I* region of the genome, that is, *Ia* determinants, revealed the development of distinct subpopulations during the course of maturation. To cite a specific example, only a minor group of relatively immature macrophages from the spleen and peritoneum that reacted to antisera against specific *Ia* determinants were found capable of presenting antigen that stimulated antigen-specific T-cell proliferation (Rosenthal *et al.*, 1976; Yamashita and Shevach, 1977; Lee *et al.*, 1979; Louis *et al.*, 1981). One such reaction was the recognition of *Leishmania tropica* by macrophages, an activity that had been demonstrated to be strictly dependent on *Ia*-related factors (Louis *et al.*, 1981).

Among the important classes of surface markers on macrophages are receptors for Fc fragments of various immunoglobulins. In cultures of human monocytes, addition of Fc fragments of IgG was found to decrease the secretion by these cells of C2 and lysosomal enzymes but increased the synthesis of prostaglandin E (Passwell *et al.*, 1980). Another investigation used mouse peritoneal exudate macrophages and eight different varieties of IgG antibodies, all of which activated the cells to lyse and phagocytose erythrocytes (Ralph *et al.*, 1980). However, the varieties of antibodies called IgG2a and IgG2b were more effective than the others in inducing the reactions, whereas similar antibodies for IgM were completely ineffective. Additional populations of these cells both from rat and human sources have proven to have Fc receptors for IgE and to lack those for IgG (Anderson and Spiegelberg, 1981; Boltz-Nitulescu and Spiegelberg, 1981); similar Fc receptors for IgE have also been reported to be present on eosinophils from rat and human tissues (Capron *et al.*, 1981).

Mast Cells. The mast cell receives only occasional mention in investigations of the immune reaction, but it probably will prove to merit more attention as knowledge of this most complicated of body activities increases in subsequent years. Like the macrophage, this type of cell is large, with extensive cytoplasm that contains coarse basophilic granules, and has a rounded nucleus; typically the members of this class are present in blood and in other connective tissues and are especially abundant in the circulatory systems of leukemic individuals. Except for the granules, the cytoplasm usually stains very lightly, providing the cells with a characteristic indefinite, almost ghostlike appearance. Like most other types found in the blood, the mast cell appears to have multiple origins, precursors having been reported from bone marrow, spleen, fetal liver, and peripheral blood of mice (Kitamura *et al.*, 1977, 1979a,b). Most of those in noncirculatory tissues, however, appear to be developed in the spleen (Kitamura *et al.*, 1981).

Very few studies have been conducted on the immune-related functional aspects of this type of cell. Like basophils they carry a glycoprotein on their surface, which specifically binds the Fc region of IgE (Metzger, 1978). When this receptor was activated by antibodies to that immunoglobulin fragment or by interaction of the bound IgE and a multivalent antigen, exocytotic activities on the part of the cells were stimulated. Recently the surface glycoprotein was demonstrated to have a molecular weight of 50,000 and to be monomeric; however, it was found to be associated in a 1 : 1 ratio with a polypeptide of molecular weight of 30,000 (Kanellopoulos *et al.*, 1980). Series of C3 receptors have been uncovered that induce rat peritoneal mast cells to engulf blood cells phagocytotically, so that the suggested role in immunogenesis appears to hold much substance (Vranian *et al.*, 1981).

The exocytotic release mentioned above ranks among the most important activities of the mast cell and involves the basophilic granules, which are actually members of the class of lysosomes known as exophagosomes (Dillon, 1981, pp. 273, 280). Among the proteins known to be contained in these organelles are heparin, histamine, serotonin, bradykinin, "slow-reacting substances," and a varied set of hydrolytic enzymes. Release of these agents as by inducement of a substance called anaphylatoxin has a marked contractile effect on such smooth muscles as those of arterioles and endothelial cells, thereby inducing greater permeability of capillaries. Thus, such effects of atopic reactions like asthma, hay fever, allergic rhinitis, and food allergy and anaphylaxis, including hives, edema, and shock, are induced by this class of cells. However, eosinophils have also been implicated in such reactions, and the blood platelets seem also to be carriers of the active agents. Since IgE is chiefly involved in the activation of mast cells, it is often referred to as atopic reagent, in reference to its reactions in the skin (Ellis, 1969).

7.3. NONCELLULAR COMPONENTS OF IMMUNE REACTIONS

The noncellular components of immune reactions include several of major importance, such as the coagulation, fibrinolytic, and kinin systems, and what is known as complement. In turn, these classes of substances together with such cellular elements as mast cells, polymorphonuclear leukocytes, and some activities of macrophages, are often grouped together under the term accessory systems (Sell, 1980). Consequently, all the noncellular parts are viewed as accessory to the main events, but as the discussion proceeds, it becomes evident they are not to be viewed as incidental or of minor importance. Here the principal purpose of the present study is best served by centering on only two of these systems, complement and the kinins, plus another unit, the major histocompatibility complex.

7.3.1. Complement

Complement should be viewed as one of the mechanisms active in amplifying the effects of immune reactions and as a result, it is often responsible for the tissue lesions that frequently accompany the antibody–antigen precipitations. Basically it consists of a single major series of interacting substances, together referred to as the classical pathway, but the earlier steps are often replaced in part by a so-called alternative pathway. Both sets of reactions occur on the surfaces of cells, during which multimolecular complexes having biological activity are produced (Müller-Eberhard, 1969; Johnson, 1977).

The Classical Pathway. The classical pathway is provided with a backbone series of nine major polypeptides referred to as C1 to C9 which are cleaved and recombined in an intricate series of steps (Figure 7.8). In simplified terms, C1 functions principally as the recognition unit, C2 to C4 are involved with activation, and C5 to C9 attack membranes. In greater detail, only one 400,000-dalton portion of C1 known as C1q (Yonemasu and Sasaki, 1981) actually is concerned with recognition, while the two remaining parts, C1r with a molecular weight of 160,000, and C1s (80,000) in union cleave C2 and C4. After the activation of complement has begun with C1 being fragmented into its several components, the C1q unit becomes bound with antibody that has been altered in its Fc region through reaction with antigen, only that portion of IgM or IgG being effective. The two types of antibody sectors differ in that only one pentameric IgM molecule is needed to activate C1, whereas two of IgG are requisite and these must lie adjacent. Although proximity presents no problems when the antibody is dissolved in blood serum, it does become so when carried on a cell or fragment. For a case in point, if the foreign or transformed cell carrying the antibody is an erythrocyte, only a single IgM molecule would be needed, whereas on the average about 600 molecules of IgG would be required to provide two adjacent molecules (Humphrey and Dourmashkin, 1969).

The Cascade of Complement Reactions. Broadly speaking, the various components of the classical pathway interact like a multiple cascade (Figure 7.8), but in a highly complex fashion. When an antibody–antigen complex fragments C1, one fragment, C1q, is split off; the other two subunits, C1r and C1s, remain combined and become activated. This dual molecule serves as an enzyme that splits two others of the series, C2 and C4, into two subunits each, as stated before. Of the four parts resulting from this cleavage, C2a and C4b, which unite to produce "C3 convertase," are the only two that continue the cascade; C4a has no known further function but C2b interacts with plasmin to produce a substance called "C2b kinin," which increases the permeability of

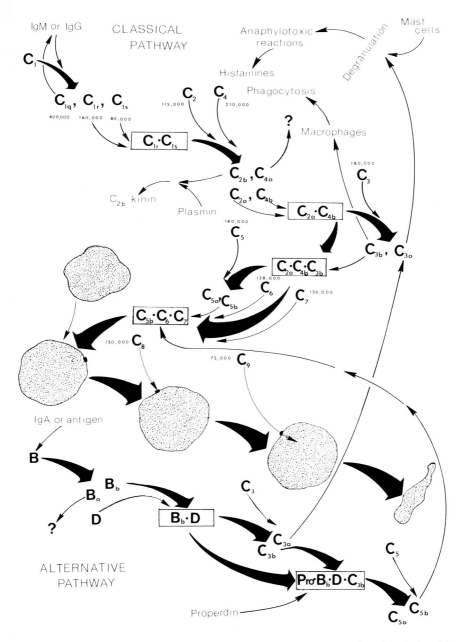

Figure 7.8. The two pathways of complement activity. The classical pathway is activated when C1 reacts with either IgM or IgG, as described in the text; the alternative route is activated by IgA or certain antigens.

capillaries. In similar fashion, the C3 convertase cleaves C3 into two portions, the b subunit of which combines with the C3 convertase to produce the trimeric molecule C2a·C4b·C3b, known as "C5 convertase." Since each molecule of activated C1 and C3 convertase can cleave many molecules of their individual substrates, these steps serve to amplify the whole complement reaction. That same fragment can also react as an opsonin with macrophages, which bear special receptors for the purpose, inducing them to great phagocytotic activity against antibody-coated particles (Figure 7.8). The second part, C3a, interacts with mast cells, inducing the latter to undergo exocytotic release of the basophilic granule contents, thereby initiating anaphylatoxic reactions.

As in the other steps of the cascade, C5 convertase acts upon its substrate (Kinoshita et al., 1981) to produce two fragments, C5a, which reacts with neutrophils and leads to inflammatory responses, and C5b, which joins with C6 and C7 to carry on the cascading steps still further (Figure 7.8). This trimolecular combination binds onto the surface of the cell and affords a means of entry for C8 into the lipid part of the plasmalemma. The final component of complement, C9, then interacts with C8 to induce lysis of the cell.

The Alternative Pathway. Consisting of only three factors plus a series of the members of the classical pathway, the alternate route is somewhat simpler than the corresponding stages of the foregoing. First, it must be activated either by IgA or by such substances as bacterial lipopolysaccharide (endotoxin) or yeast zymosan, resulting in the cleavage of the factor B. However, this series of interactions is highly specific as to the nature of the agents that can activate it (Gadd and Reid, 1981; McConnell et al., 1981a,b). One of the products, Bb, interacts with factor D to form the dual molecule, Bb + D, that serves as a second type of C3 convertase. The C3b portion of this reaction with C3 joins the dual molecule to produce a triplex component of Bb + D + C3b, which serves as a C5 convertase, but only after it has become stabilized by interaction with an additional part of the alternative pathway called properdin. Beyond that point the reactions are those of the classical pathway. Here as before the C3 and C5 convertases, being capable of acting upon many molecules, serve to amplify the subsequent cascading reactions.

7.3.2. Kinins and the Major Histocompatibility Complex

Because it has already been seen that fragments like C3a and C5a of complement enter into sets of reactions other than those of that system proper, it is readily perceived that the various compartmentalizations of immune and immune-related bodily functions are only man-made devices for simplification. This observation receives reinforcement as the discussion of a second noncellular system proceeds.

The Kinin System. The major mechanism that initiates kinin system activity is by way of blood factor VII (Hageman factor) which also initiates blood clot formation. In the latter processes it converts prothrombin to thrombin, which enters into a cascade of reactions similar in many ways to that of complement to produce blood clots, beginning with the formation of fibrin from fibrinogen. At the same time, prothrombin interacts with plasminogen to form plasmin, a substance that destroys fibrin, thereby providing a feedback control mechanism. However, this plasmin also cleaves blood factor VII to produce subunits that activate a substance called prekallikrein, which then becomes converted into kallikrein. This latter substance acts together with plasmin upon kininogen to produce kinin. As pointed out earlier, kinin induces contraction of certain endothelial cells, thus leading to greater permeability of capillaries. Still further interdigitations between the several noncellular systems are provided by plasmin, first in interacting with the C2b fragment of complement to form C2b kinin (Figure 7.8), and second in activating the classical pathway of complement.

The Major Histocompatibility Complex. The major histocompatibility complex (MHC) refers to a portion of the genome in which genetic control of a number of immune responses and antigens for allograft recognition is maintained (Dausset, 1981). While most investigations in this area have centered on the mouse, in which it has been localized to the *H-2* gene complex of chromosome 12, and on the human being, where it was localized in the *HLA* complex of chromosome 6, many other vertebrates, including the chicken, have also been extensively studied (Götze, 1977; Hildemann and Jokiel, 1979; Longenecker and Mosmann, 1981a,b). Since different terminology has been necessary for each source species (Lee and Nordskog, 1981), discussion centers largely on the murine complex, with comparisons with the human system as warranted (Charmot *et al.*, 1981). Probably the most important region of the *H-2* complex insofar as immunological reactions are concerned is the *I* sector, which is composed of a cluster of loci. Among these are the immune response (*Ir*) loci that have the capacity for generating immune reactions. For example, their products determine whether a mouse strain can exhibit a strong or weak immune response to a given antigen or whether it will develop leukemia if injected with certain viruses (Uhr *et al.*, 1979). Other loci (*Is*), the immune suppression genes, are involved with factors that may suppress such resistance to foreign antigens, and still others, the *Ia* loci, that are responsible for antigens of all surfaces, a number of their encoded products having already been described. These functional subdivisions are distributed irregularly between five structural segments of the chromosome designated in sequence as *I-A*, *I-B*, *I-J*, *I-E*, and *I-C*. In general, however, *Ir* genes appear to be located in the *I-A* sector, supplemented, and often augmented, from additional ones situated in *I-C*. Still others of this functional class that respond to IgG allotypes occur in *I-B* (Katz *et al.*, 1973, 1976; McDevitt, 1978). *Is* genes seem to be confined primarily to the *I-J* and *I-E* sectors, those in the former part encoding suppressor factors for IgG responses, those in the latter having similar functions for IgE reactions.

On maps of the MHC region of mice, the *H-2* complex is shown to be interrupted by several others (Sell, 1980). The *H-2K* sector is followed by the *I* and *S* regions in turn, the latter being involved in the control of the serum concentration of complement factor C4. After a series of unrelated genes, the *H-2G* and *H-2D* regions are to be found, followed at some distance by *T-1a*. *H-2K* and *H-2D* products are active in providing the recognition of allografts, those of *H-2G* are erythrocytic alloantigens, and the *T-1a* sector encodes the antigens of thymus leukemia.

Although thus the *H-2* genes are concerned largely with self–/nonself-interactions, the actual interrelationships between different sectors are proving to be far more complicated. One pertinent illustration is provided by an autoimmune response in mice to F antigen (Silver and Lane, 1981), a protein, having a molecular weight of 40,000, that is present in the liver of many mammals (Lane and Silver, 1976). In spite of T thymocytes having been considered to be largely involved in self tolerance, their ability to respond to a given antigen varies with the strain, which is under complex *Ir* gene control (Silver and Lane, 1979). First, there is an absolute requirement for a *k* allele located either in the *H-2K* or *I-A* region, strains bearing other alleles being unable to respond; in addition, the degree of response is under the control of two or more genes located elsewhere in the region (Silver and Lane, 1981). Furthermore, the requirement for T cells was demonstrated by removal of the thymus; low-level responders (that is, self-tolerant mice) became high responders to the antigen after 3 months.

Similar multigenic control of immune responses involving *I* region products has also come to light. For instance, it has been demonstrated that suppression of response against certain antigens in the serum involves the interaction between products, both of *I-S2* and *I-S1* loci (Benacerraf and Dorf, 1977). Further, the Ae polypeptide chain encoded by an *I-A* gene appeared only on the surface of the cells when influenced by a product of a locus in the *I-E* region (Jones *et al.*, 1978). Likewise, the Ea chain polypeptide of another antigen, in this case encoded in the *I-E* sector, was expressed on cells under the influence of a gene seemingly located in the *I-A* or possibly the *I-B* region (Murphy *et al.*, 1980). However, not all T-cell responses are dependent upon multiple gene interactions, as shown by mice immunized with 2,4,6-trinitrophenyl conjugated to mouse serum albumin, but even here dual systems were present nevertheless. High responsiveness was demonstrated by different strains, both by factors encoded in either the *H-2D* or *H-2B* region on one hand and by those either in the *H-2K* or *I-A* sector (Wicker and Hildemann, 1981). When the phenotype resulted from the first locus, it was recessive, whereas it was dominant when controlled by the second.

7.4. CELL INTERACTIONS IN IMMUNE RESPONSES

Few, if any, immune reactions are carried out completely by one type of cell or immune-active substance; virtually all require interplay between several cell types and differing antigens, antibodies, and their respective receptors. Thus, insofar as the genetic activities of any given cell type, or better, cell population type, are concerned, exogenous influences are essential in the activation—or sometimes creation—of the necessary phenotype, whether involving behavior or the production of antibody or antigen.

7.4.1. Cytotoxic and Killer Cell Activities

In previous sections, mention was made of killer T lymphocytes (T_K) and other cells that are actively phagocytotic, including the monocyte-macrophage lineage. However, discussion of their many activities has necessarily been held to this point, because of their dependency upon such factors as the products of the MHC. In addition, a new class of killer cells has recently come to light, that is not directly kin to the others of similar properties.

Natural Killer Cells. The recently discovered class, referred to as natural killer (NK) cells, are present even in nonsensitized normal individuals, but they were not recognized for many years, their activities being considered merely as background (Henney, 1973; Hellström and Hellström, 1974; Herberman *et al.*, 1975; Pross and Baines, 1977; Herberman and Ortaldo, 1981). Since they are lymphocytes that lack markers for both the T and B classes, they actually represent a population of null cells; they occur in normal blood as a number of distinct subpopulations, each one of which is specific for the lysis of a different class of target cells. Most of their targets appear to be derived from tumors, but not all types of the latter are susceptible to NK cell activity. The cytolytic properties have been shown to differ strongly from those carried out by macrophages and T lymphocytes, which, for example, were blocked by low temperatures, whereas those of the present type were not (Roder *et al.*, 1980). Further, while the macrophage and T_K-cell-mediated target–effector interactions in the mutant strain of mice known as beige were normal, the NK ones were absent. In addition, NK cells proved to be inactive in pathogen-free mice and expressed their lytic function only after exposure to pathogens or other agents (Clark *et al.*, 1979), including viruses, tumor cells, or even interferon (Quinnan and Manischewitz, 1979; Senik *et al.*, 1979). Also the NK types have been found capable of lysing such normal, nonmalignant cells as thymocytes, peritoneal macrophages, and fetal fibroblasts (Hansson *et al.*, 1979a; Welsh *et al.*, 1979; Kiessling and Welsh, 1980), and they have been demonstrated possibly to play an important role in regulating normal hemopoietic stem cells in both adults and fetuses (Hansson *et al.*, 1979b, 1981). Not all their natural functions are readily comprehensible, for *in vivo* they lysed normal bone marrow cells of mice and thus may also be concerned with control of normal growth processes (Riccardi *et al.*, 1981).

Although the members of this class have been discovered too recently to have had their surface properties thoroughly determined, several such markers have been demonstrated. For several years receptors for the Fc segment of immunoglobulin have been known to be present (Herberman *et al.*, 1975; Pross and Baines, 1977), and now an alloantibody has been found that proved to be specific for a cell-surface antigen designated as NK-1 (Glimcher *et al.*, 1977), an allelic form of which or an entirely new antigen, NK-1.2, also has been demonstrated (Burton and Winn, 1981). Moreover, a number of alloantigens, such as those related to *H-2K* or *H-2D* products that activate T cells have exhibited similar effects on this type (Clark and Holly, 1981), and interleukin 2 and interferon have proven to have synergistic stimulatory effects on the production of these cells (Kuribayashi *et al.*, 1981).

Killer T Lymphocytes. As pointed out previously, one major population of T lymphocytes is specialized for killing other cells by attaching to them and inducing lysis, much in the same fashion as the foregoing NK type. In much current literature, the members of this class are referred to as cytotoxic T lymphocytes (CTL), but the simpler term killer cells (T_K) is preferred here. The differentiation of these cells *in vitro* has been shown to be associated with collaboration between several T-lymphocyte subpopulations, from which soluble substances called amplifying factors seemed to play important roles (Cantor and Boyse, 1975; Plate, 1976; Finke *et al.*, 1977; Pilarski, 1977; Okada *et al.*, 1979). Experimental production of these amplifiers was induced in cultures by alloantigens encoded variously in either the *K*, *D*, or *I* region of the MHC, so none of these factors was uniquely involved (Kano *et al.*, 1980; Okada and Henney, 1980). However, the respective influence of each class was highly dependent on the phenotype of the T lymphocytes. In order for *I*-region-encoded substances to be effective, Lyt-1$^+$ T cells were necessary for amplifier production, but not Lyt-2$^+$, whereas *K*- or *D*-region-encoded antigens required the presence of Lyt-2$^+$ T lymphocytes, but not Lyt-1$^+$ (Figure 7.9).

Quite a different set of reactions in these T_K cells was obtained in a study of thymocytes employing peanut agglutinin to distinguish populations (Kruisbeek *et al.*, 1980). Those cells that were able to become agglutinated in the presence of this substance were unable to display any cytotoxic reactions to allogeneic cells until a substance called T-cell growth factor was added, when their cytotoxic activities were elicited and subsequently maintained at a constant level. In contrast, T cells not agglutinated by the peanut-derived reagent did not gain killer activity when treated with that growth factor, but rather seemed to secrete the latter substance, an activity shared with spleen cells, especially those of the epithelial covering of the latter organ. As a result of these observations, it was concluded that the agglutinated thymocytes represented a population of T_K-precursor cells that could be activated by suitable

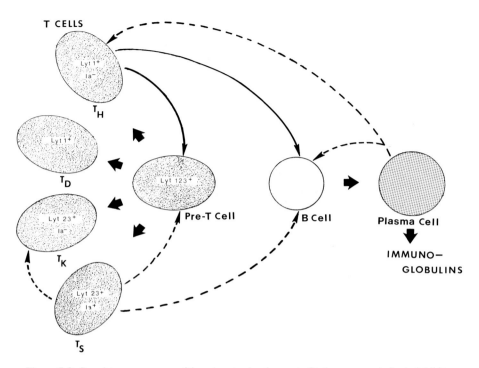

Figure 7.9. Regulatory processes of lymphocyte development. Broken arrows indicate inhibitory actions and solid arrows, accelerating actions. The pre-T cells generate all four classes of T lymphocytes, a process stimulated by members of the helper (T_H) class and inhibited by those of the suppressor (T_S) category. The former also stimulate and the latter retard the development of B lymphocytes into plasma cells. In turn, the plasma cell inhibits both the transformation of additional B and T_H cells by way of its antibodies, the immunoglobulins.

antigens, whereas the nonagglutinated ones were T_H cells, whose presence or whose product, the growth factor, was also essential to the process. This factor has proven to be identical to another reagent with similar activity, interleukin 2, which receives mention on several subsequent occasions (Liepins et al., 1978; Mizel and Farrar, 1979).

Actually it would appear that at least three soluble factors are involved in the activation of T_K precursors (Farrar et al., 1981). The first of these, interleukin 1, with a molecular weight of 15,000, was produced by macrophages, because removal of this type of cell from cultures prevented the induction of T_K lymphocytes (J. J. Farrar et al., 1980; W. L Farrar et al., 1980). The second factor, interleukin 2, was produced by T_H cells as just shown; it could be replaced in the induction of cytotoxic activity by interleukin 1, however (Larsson et al., 1980). In addition to this property, interleukin 2 has proven to stimulate proliferation of T lymphocytes in general and, as mentioned in the preceding paragraph, also to enhance the differentiation of T_S and T_K cells (Simon et al., 1979; J. J. Farrar et al.., 1980). The third factor, immune interferon, was demonstrated to play an especially significant role in the cytotoxic activation of T cells, an activity regulated by interaction between such cells on a one-to-one basis. Moreover, some evidence has indicated that interleukin 2 serves as a signal mechanism for immune interferon production (Farrar et al., 1981), and in turn, the inductive influence of the interleukin may be dependent upon the synthesis of the interferon.

To the present it has not been possible to correlate the results of the foregoing investigations into soluble factors to those that focus on the Lyt-1, -2, and -3 surface features, many of the latter having been concerned with the nature of the precursors, rather than the specific inductive influences. Although it had been established that T lymphocytes that bore all three surface factors (indicated as Lyt-123 cells) were the major source of T_K precursors, it had not been determined clearly what roles those that bore just the last two of the surface features (that is, had a Lyt-23 phenotype) or only the first (Lyt-1) played in generating T_K cells (Simon and Abenhardt, 1980; Simon and Eichmann, 1980). But just recently it has been found that both Lyt-1 and Lyt-23 and/or Lyt-123 must be present to induce H-2-restricted and anti-H-2 killer cells (Simon et al., 1981). Whether or not interleukin 2 could serve in place of Lyt-1 cells has not been explored.

Activities of T_K Lymphocytes. Many of the experimentally established activities of T_K cells have employed tumor cells as the antigens. Allogeneic tumor cells have long been known to induce a strong cytotoxic response on the part of T_K lymphocytes which almost invariably destroyed them *in vivo*; in contrast, syngeneic ones led to only a weak reactivity in the T_K cells and usually resulted in fatal malignancies (Fishelson and Berke, 1981). Through *in vitro* investigations into the basis of the differences in reactions, it was found that, while the lysing of the target cells was identical regardless of the genetic composition, very few T_K lymphocytes capable of binding to and lysing the syngeneic cells were induced by the antigens. Moreover, the intensity of the reaction between individual T_K and tumor cells was decreased when the latter were of syngeneic composition, possibly as a result of the low immunogenicity of the cells with a host of similar genetic properties. However, this point of view may be simplistic as discussed shortly.

A number of tumors are induced through transformation of cells by various viruses, one instance of which is the lymphoblastoid type that results from infection with Epstein–Barr virus. In the presence of cultured lymphoblastoid cells transformed by that organism, peripheral blood lymphocytes of healthy adult persons underwent cell division rapidly, proliferation being similar regardless of the donor's serological status to the virus (Tanaka et al., 1980). However, T_K cells from those persons positive to the viral serum were active against the lymphoblastoid cells, whereas those from seronegative individuals showed little lytic activity. While reports of other laboratories had been conflicting, because cytotoxicity for the Epstein–Barr-virus-infected lymphocytes has not always been observed (Svedmyr *et al.*, 1974, 1975; Viallat *et al.*, 1978), results similar to the foregoing have been obtained elsewhere (Tsoukas *et al.*, 1981). Additional observations also were made in the later study to the effect that lysis by T_K cells was specific against B cells infected by the virus and was controlled by products of the *HLA* complex. Furthermore, a number of cloned lines of these cytotoxic cells have been established that act specifically against the influenza virus (Braciale *et al.*, 1981).

For obvious reasons, T_K lymphocytes must be able to distinguish self (autologous) from foreign (heterologous) cells, an ability provided by substances encoded by the MHC. Thus, in the mouse, T_K lymphocyte activity is restricted by *H-2K*, *-2D*, *-2L*, and *2I* encoded products. Although neither antibodies nor killer cells effective against autologous MHC products are generally demonstrable, they have been found to exist through hybridization studies of mouse strains having contrasting *H-2* genotypes (Nakano *et al.*, 1981). The F_1 generation whose cells were heterozygous for the gene-sets produced T_K lymphocytes specifically sensitized against *H-2* molecules. Whereas they were capable of binding to target cells bearing the products of appropriate *H-2* genes regardless of whether they were of heterozygous genotypes, they could actually lyse only parental-type (homozygous) cells.

7.4.2. Activities of Suppressor Cells

The lysis of target cells by T_K lymphocytes and possibly also by NK cells is in part controlled by the T_S class of lymphocytes briefly discussed earlier in this chapter. Their action, however, is not solely against lysis-inducing components but is much broader in scope, for the cells appear also to exercise regulatory effects on the transformation of lymphocytes in general under the influence of mitogens and allogeneic cells and even on the synthesis of immunoglobulins by plasmablasts (Shou *et al.*, 1976; Haynes and Fauci, 1977; Rice *et al.*, 1979; Golub, 1981).

Origins of Suppressor Lymphocytes. The origins of T lymphocytes having suppressor function have been studied to a degree in primary mixed lymphocyte cultures, one such investigation employing spleen cells from mice of the CBA strain with antigenic factors from mice of the BALB/c strain (Al-Adra *et al.*, 1980). By day 3 of culture when both T_H and T_S cells had become differentiated, the former were found to bear Ly-1.1 antigens on their surface, but not Ly-2.1, whereas the later had both types. However, by day 5, the T_S lymphocytes had developed phenotypes of Ly-1.1$^-$ and Ly-2.1$^+$, but whether the members of this class had undergone further differentiation or the new type had originated from a different set of precursors could not be established. Neither T_H nor T_K cells underwent further changes, the latter showing a phenotype of Ly-1.1$^+$, Ly-2.1$^+$ continually. Substantial evidence has been presented which indicates that in the peripheral blood of normal human individuals, programmed T_S cells are a constant feature (Nadler and Hodes, 1977), their generation apparently influenced by the presence of prostaglandin E_1 (Fulton and Levy, 1981), but they become much more active when appropriate stimulating factors are present.

The mechanism through which T_S lymphocytes exercise their immunoregulatory influences has not been fully elucidated. In some cases the observations indicate that they act directly upon T_K cells by cell-to-cell contact (Figure 7.9; Reinherz and Schlossman, 1979), but the results of other researchers intimate that their activities are wrought by way of their secreting soluble factors (Williams and Korsmeyer, 1978). Experimental data that support the latter concept have now been advanced (Shou *et al.*, 1980). Media in which normal human peripheral blood lymphocytes had been cultured were found to contain a soluble factor that exhibited suppressive activity, because when the supernatant from such colonies was added to mixed lymphocyte cultures, antigen-induced proliferation of the lymphocytes was suppressed and the secretion of IgG and IgM was inhibited. Moreover, similar soluble factors have been shown also to be present in a bovine system (Smith *et al.*, 1981), for neither cell-to-cell contact nor macrophages appeared to be necessary for generation of suppression. In fact, the absence of those phagocytotic cells appears to be a requirement of T_S-cell production, at least in some systems (Feldmann and Kotianinen, 1976; Ishizaka and Adachi, 1976; Pierres and Germain, 1978).

Functions of T_S Lymphocytes. Among the frequent investigations exploring T_S function are a number that have employed as antigens different forms of the same protein. One research of this nature used native and urea-denatured ovalbumin, substances that had been shown not to be cross-reactive serologically (Endres and Grey, 1980); however, the two forms exhibited a high level of cross-reactivity in the proliferation of antigen-induced T cells. Injections into mice of either the normal or the denatured ovalbumin induced the production of T_S cells, but those that had received injections of the former proved to be effective in suppresssing response of recipients immunized with that same substance, but not those exposed to the denatured form. Moreover, a comparable but opposite state of specificity resulted in those T_S cells in animals treated with the denatured ovalbumin. Thus, it was suggested that T_S cells, like the B variety, recognize conformational aspects of antigens, one of the few properties that would differ between the native and denatured proteins. In man, comparable experiments also demonstrated that the concentration of these types of antigens is also an important factor in T_S-cell generation, being correlated in a direct manner (Keystone *et al.*, 1980).

In like fashion, nucleic acids and nucleotides can induce T_S-lymphocyte generation. Although numerous approaches to this area of research have been utilized, conjugation of the various common nucleosides to spleen cells has proven particularly effective in generating suppressor activity. T_S cells induced by spleen cells that had been conjugated to guanosine proved to be especially active, being capable of suppressor immune response to such cells bearing any of the four common types of nucleosides (A, G, C, and T) (Borel and Young, 1980). However, only guanosine and thymine were capable of actually eliciting the suppressive reactivity, but the latter nucleoside could similarly cross-suppress all four common varieties (Rups et al., 1981).

Tumor cells themselves or cell-surface antigens from various virus-induced tumors or malignancies also have been demonstrated to activate T_S-cell generation. In rare cases, by way of illustration, the Epstein–Barr virus, the causative agent of infectious mononucleosis, may lead to malignant B-cell (lymphoblastoid) disorders (Broder et al., 1975); both autologous and allogeneic lymphoblastoid cell lines have been found equally effective in generating increased suppressor activity. The net effect of the increment was to decrease immunoglobulin synthesis by B cells and thus lessened the control of the malignancy (Tsukuda et al., 1981). In mice, sarcoma virus-induced and Moloney, Friend, or Rauscher virus-induced lymphomas bear one identical major cell-surface antigen (Lévy and Leclerc, 1977). Studies on mice both with and without virus-infected blood showed that specific T_S cells present in the spleen of Moloney tumor-bearing mice were capable of enhancing the growth of the sarcoma in vivo by suppressing T_K cells specific for the antigen (Plater et al., 1981).

T_S-lymphocyte production can be stimulated by a number of substances, including mitogens and histamines, but in some cases when the former are the inducers, generation is dependent upon other factors. For example, with Con A both the time of treatment and the presence of monocytes proved to be critical (Mizerski and Cajl-Peczalska, 1981; Mizerski et al., 1981), no T_S cells being produced in the absence of the latter cell type. Histamines have been demonstrated to inhibit antigen-induced lymphocyte proliferation, as well as production of antibody and T_K cells (Plaut et al., 1973; Melmon et al., 1974; Rocklin, 1976, 1977). Apparently the inhibition arose through specific interaction between that substance and a certain population of lymphocytes that bore receptors for it (Plaut et al., 1975). Although at first it appeared that the histamines interacted directly with the lymphocytes to lead to an increase in cAMP, more recently it has been determined that the histamine actually induced the production of a specific set of T_S cells that secreted the cyclic nucleotide (Thomas et al., 1981). Those cells also could suppress delayed hypersensitivity responses as well as the cutaneous sensitivity type. In such reactions, at least three classes of T_S cells proved to be essential (Sunday et al., 1981).

To a degree the specificity of reaction on the part of these suppressor cells may be derived from the presence of sectors of immunoglobulins, according to current studies. While heavy-chain variable-region and idiotype markers have been reported on the surface of these cells (Binz and Wigzell, 1975; Eichmann, 1978; Lonai *et al.*, 1978; Rubin *et al.*, 1979), no C_L or C_H regions have been found. Thus, it was intimated that certain T_S-cell receptors may consist of a heavy-chain variable region plus either a T_S-cell-specific constant region or some other type of protein. The recent chromosome mapping of a gene (Tsu^d) that encodes an idiotypic alloantigen linked to the immunoglobulin heavy-chain gene cluster appears to add substance to this proposal (Owen *et al.*, 1981).

7.4.3. Helper Cell Activities

Since the prime function of helper T lymphocytes, that of acting on B cells to induce antibody specificity (Claman *et al.*, 1966; Miller and Mitchell, 1967), has already received mention, here the main focus is concentrated on such topics as the ontogeny of these T_H cells and the genetic basis for their specializations. Then a brief section enumerates in more detail the manner in which they interact with B cells, for more than these two types of interacting bodies are involved in those processes.

Properties and Origins of T_H Lymphocytes. Ordinarily the T lymphocytes of all potential types are concentrated into recirculating pools, loosely confined to larger bodies of lymph, such as that of the thoracic lymph duct. When antigen is introduced into the system, a percentage of cells, those that bear a suitable phenotype, are conducted out of the pools to become sequestered into such sites of antigen concentration as the spleen. Here they remain for 1 or 2 days, developing antigen-specificity and proliferating extensively. To cite a concrete example, purified T cells, after being exposed to antigen in the form of sheep erythrocytes and then introduced into irradiated mice, were not detectable in the thoracic duct lymph for about 2 days (Sprent, 1978), after which period they occurred in large numbers in the lymph as activated T_H cells. There is some question as to whether the antigen itself induced the T-lymphocyte generation and specialization, or whether the antigen reacted with B cells to stimulate the production of immunoglobulin, which then activated the T cells. An induction of this class of protein synthesis against IgM antibodies has been observed that appeared to be mediated by antibody-specific T_H cells (Forni *et al.*, 1980). Hence, it was suggested that the enhancement of anti-IgM immunoglobulins required T_H cells that possessed specificity for the antigen (Coutinho and Forni, 1981).

The basis for such specificity has recently been tested *in vitro* by use of two related haptens, NP (4-hydroxy-3-nitrophenyl acetyl) and NIP (4-hydroxy-5-iodo-3-nitrophenyl acetyl) (Martinez-Alonso *et al.*, 1981). When helper cells specific for either antigen were cocultured with syngeneic spleen cells and then grown in the presence of homologous hapten coupled to cells, the T_H lymphocytes responded by rapid proliferation, activating large numbers of B cells to do likewise, thereby inducing them to secrete antibody. In each case only homologous antigen-coupled cells influenced such activities.

In general, the activation of B cells by T_H lymphocytes is a three-step process. In the first step, which requires direct contact between the two types of cells, the helper class upon recognizing the antigen on the B-cell surface (L'Age-Stehr, 1981) rapidly leads the latter to become reactive to soluble growth factors (Weinberger *et al.*, 1981). Second, they induce these stimulated B lymphocytes to grow into memory cells (Figure 7.9), followed by proliferation, by means of factors which they secrete into the bloodstream (Martinez-Alonso and Coutinho, 1981; Tse *et al.*, 1981). Since at least certain of the factors exercise their influence within a quarter of a day, they have been referred to as "six-hour factors" (Lee and Paraskevas, 1981; Paraskevas and Lee, 1981). Third, the newly proliferated cells then became differentiated into antibody-secreting plasma cells. Whether identical T_H cells performed all functions or whether several different populations were involved remains an unresolved issue, but it could be that during the cell-to-cell contact in step 1, the B type activates the contacting member of the T class to begin its secretory activities at the same time the latter stimulates the former to grow and proliferate.

At least under certain conditions the interaction of the T cells may also regulate the type of immunoglobulin produced by the B lymphocytes. For illustration, B cells from B-lymphoblastoid cell lines derived from patients with lymphoproliferative disorders secrete IgM as long as T lymphocytes are absent, but when the latter type is added to the cultures, IgG is secreted instead (Kishimoto *et al.*, 1978), and the opposite change from IgG to IgM is mediated in other cases (Kempner *et al.*, 1980). However, it appears that the latter immunoglobulin really was secreted by previously resting cells after they were activated by the addition of the T cells, no class-switch from IgG to IgM actually being involved.

Genetic Control of T_H-Cell Function. The MHC has become thoroughly documented as playing key roles in T_H-cell functions in mammals and birds, as well as in amphibians (Bernard *et al.*, 1981). Earlier studies had demonstrated that selection of purified homozygous T lymphocytes respondent to sheep erythrocytes in irradiated mice required that both the donor of the T cells and the host shared specific *H-2* determinants (Sprent, 1978). On the basis of these observations, it was proposed that *in vivo* T cells do not respond to free antigen but only to that associated with certain *H-2* determinants on the radioresistant macrophages of the host. Further investigation later brought out more specifically that the *I* region of the *H-2* complex was involved in this control and that efficient immune reactions were provided solely when the host and donor had like phenotypes related to both the *I-A* and *I-E* subregions (Sprent and Alpert, 1981).

The majority of the soluble factors which T cells secrete are not under the control of this genetic complex; however, those that act upon other classes of T lymphocytes are governed by its products. In one case a carrier-specific enhancing solute was shown to be associated with control of the *I-A* region and required Thy-1-bearing cells for its effect (Tada *et al.*, 1976). Several experimental investigations on culture media could demonstrate the presence of either a single specific soluble helper factor for B cells (Delovitch and Sohn, 1979), or one for T_K cells (Plate, 1980, 1981), after the T lymphocytes had been removed. In the first instance, an *I-J*-region-encoded product was found and in the second an *I-A*. However, more recent research has indicated that the soluble factor active in Step 2 of B-cell activation may be influenced by a product of the MHC (Tse *et al.*, 1981).

Complex Interplay between Cell Types. In the processes of converting resting B lymphocytes into immunoglobulin-secreting cells, the assistance of macrophages is required along with antigen and T_H cells (Katz, 1980b). At least some of the supportive role of macrophages is exercised by release of interleukin 1 (Hoffmann and Dutton, 1971; Calderon *et al.*, 1975; Wood *et al.*, 1976; Aadeen *et al.*, 1979), which also may be secreted by T_H cells (Hoffmann and Watson, 1979; Hoffmann, 1980). However, the identities of the secretions from these two contrasting sources have not been clearly established, for the results from different laboratories are often conflicting. In general, interleukin 1 activates precursor B cells to acquire such early surface markers as Ia and surface immunoglobulin. Then late in development T_H cells or their secretory product, TRF (T-cell replacement factor), induces the development of complement receptor (CR) and IgD as surface markers on B cells (Dutton *et al.*, 1971; Schimpl and Wecker, 1972; Hoffmann *et al.*, 1976). That the latter two substances were not identical was indicated by adding them to antigen-treated B-cell cultures. When interleukin 1 was added to new colonies early in their development, followed 20 to 40 hr later by TRF, a pronounced synergistic effect was noted (Hoffman, 1980). Thus, it would seem that the early events of differentiation and proliferation were controlled by interleukin 1 and later development into antibody-secreting cells by TRF.

Helper cells seem also to be involved in the generation of T_K cells (Figure 7.9). T lymphocytes can be maintained in culture on a long-term basis in the presence of TRF (Morgan *et al.*, 1976; Ruscetti *et al.*, 1977), which is produced by lymphoid cells that have been treated with T-cell mitogen. Using murine lymphoblast lines successively propagated from mixed lymphocyte cultures stimulated with alloantigens and grown in the presence of this growth factor, it was possible to generate antigen-specific T_K cells from thymocytes added periodically throughout the culture's existence (Narimatsu and Saito, 1981). Moreover, the thymocytes could be induced to proliferate in the presence of T-cell mitogen. However, in order to maintain these abilities for periods in excess of 1 month, it was necessary to add the specific alloantigens at frequent intervals. Similar cooperation between these three classes of cells has been shown to exist in cultures of chicken cells activated by the histocompatibility complex antigens expressed on chicken erythrocytes (Shiozawa *et al.*, 1980). In this case the TRF extracted from T_H-cell cultures was shown to contain Ia antigen and reacted with unprimed B cells in an allogenetically restricted

fashion (Shiozawa *et al.*, 1977, 1979). As before, the presence of either macrophages (adherent cells) or their secretory products (including interleukin 1)
was essential, plus T_H cells or TRF.

Experiments conducted to ascertain the specific effects of surface immunoglobulin have yielded a few results relevant to a discussion of B-cell activation. Although anti-immunoglobulin has been reported to stimulate proliferation
of B lymphocytes from rabbits (Sell and Gell, 1965), activation of immunoglobulin synthesis by those cells did not occur (Parker *et al.*, 1979). However,
secretion of the immunoglobulin was achieved by the addition of either T cells
or TRF, apparently by way of surface IgD (Primi *et al.*, 1980). Furthermore,
if the antisera were prepared against particular idiotypes, the immunoglobulin-
receptor activation proved to be strictly specific for those antigens.

7.5. AGE-RELATED CHANGES IN IMMUNE REACTIONS

In Chapter 6 a statement was made to the effect that many age-related
changes in immune reactions could be presented in a comprehensible fashion
only after the immune responses themselves had been described. Now that the
main features of that subject have been presented, a continuation of the earlier
topic thus becomes feasible. In general terms, the efficacy of the immune system decreases rapidly with advancing years in man (Benner *et al.*, 1981), as
well as in many other vertebrates, a point made especially clear by the frequent
failure of immune responses in older persons to act successfully against tumors,
particularly malignant ones. In England the probability of an individual at the
age of 25 years developing cancer within the next 5 years was 1 : 700, whereas
at 65 years the probability was increased to 1 : 14 (Doll *et al.*, 1970). In great
part the decline in immunity is related to the decrease in thymus size detailed
in an earlier discussion and additionally by the deficiency of coenzyme Q that
prevails (Bliznakov, 1980).

Changes in T-Cell Populations. In a recent study of age-related changes
in T-lymphocyte populations in the peripheral blood of man, the ones (T_M) that
bore receptor sites for the Fc portion of the IgM molecule were demonstrated
to differ from those (T_G) whose receptor sites were for the corresponding region
of IgG. The former type proved to be involved in the mitogen-induced transformation of B cells into plasma cells, while the latter were of the T_S type
(Cobleigh *et al.*, 1980). Although no significant changes could be noted in T_G-
cell numbers with advancing years, the T_M populations decreased markedly.
The peak number of these cells (977 per mm^3) was attained in persons in the
40- to 49-year age range, but that frequency dropped to 629 in people that were
between 50 and 69 years and decreased further to 560 in those who had reached
ages between 70 and 90.

Opposite trends with age were uncovered in T_K-cell populations that were active against self B-plasma cells. Normal human T lymphocytes were cultured with autologous blood cells enriched in B lymphocytes and were activated with irradiated non-T cells in the presence of 20% inactivated autologous plasma (Fournier and Charreire, 1981). The resulting proliferation of cells that formed rosettes with erythrocytes from the same source was related both to the sex and age of the individual, being higher in females of all ages than in males, and underwent increases with age in both sexes.

Changes in Other Cell Types. Somewhat comparable divergences in number with increasing age have been noted in other immune-associated cell types, including B lymphocytes, but owing to the former difficulty in firmly identifying this class of leukocytes, dissonant results of experiments have characterized the earlier literature. In recent years, however, greater reliability has been attained through the use of F(ab′)$_2$ fragments, with results that strongly support the view that the relative numbers of these cells decrease significantly in older individuals (Cobleigh *et al.*, 1980).

The enhanced frequency of tumors with senescence reported in the preceding chapter may result in part from a greater abundance of cells, in this case of macrophages. The class of secretions called prostaglandins produced by this cell type has been found to occur in large quantities in various murine tumor lines, as well as in the plasma of man and rats having one of several types of tumors (Levine *et al.*, 1972; Jaffe *et al.*, 1973). As a rule, the large quantities of prostaglandins destroy the ability of spleen cells to display plaque-forming activity, but treatment with indomethacin *in vivo* reduced the plasma levels of that secretion to nearly normal and restored the plaque-forming abilities of the spleen cells. Other studies have shown that the tumor-related increase in prostaglandins stemmed from a correlated increase in the macrophage population, but whether such an elevated number of these cells is characteristic of older mammals or only tumor-bearing ones has not been determined (Strausser and Rosenstein, 1980). While other investigations have shown that the phagocytotic populations of macrophages also increased in numbers in the presence of tumors or malignancies (Herberman *et al.*, 1980; Moore and Moore, 1980), no attempt has been made to discern age-related effects.

8

The Nature of the Genetic Mechanism

Now that the preceding chapters have viewed the actions of the molecular genetic mechanism through the development, differentiation, and functioning of mature organisms, several observations concerning the nature of the actual genetic processes become obvious that remained obscure or completely concealed when only the macromolecular (Dillon, 1978a) and cellular levels (Dillon, 1981) had been examined. But, as becomes evident in the following discussion, even at those lower levels of biological organization, some important features had actually been disclosed in those analyses but in too intangible form to be expressed in words. In a sense, then, this closing chapter of the present study is designed to serve as a summary for the entire trilogy.

8.1. THE NONMECHANISTIC NATURE OF THE GENETIC MECHANISM

In proposing that the genetic processes do not behave in a manner interpretable in simple chemical or physical terms, as has been the practice on several occasions, no suggestion is made for a return to a vitalistic point of view nor to other philosophies that invoke mysterious forces. Life basically results from physicochemical interactions, and living things are constructed of molecules built from atoms united by ordinary bonding processes, and to that extent it is strictly mechanistic in nature. But the synthesis of macromolecules in live cells from the smaller, mechanistic units is not conducted by ordinary chemical steps, nor do the interactions between various types of the biochemicals *in vivo* resemble those of inorganic substances. All reactions in the metabolism of the cell are at once made far more complex by one of the most fundamental characteristics of life, that of passing down sets of interacting molecules from one generation of cells to another. Any modification of those interactions is subjected to another process unheard of in ordinary chemical laboratories, its elimination, resulting from loss of reproductivity on the part of the possessor of the unfavorable alterations. As a consequence, only the modifications that do not induce actual or virtual death can be passed along to future products of the living system. Thus, there is an inherent evolutionary requirement innate to biological objects that is totally absent from the familiar ones of the chemist. It is because of this influence, perpetuated in organisms by way of the genetic mechanism and limited by the need for survival, that a modified philosophy of life, called biomechanism, was advocated following the analysis of its macromolecular organization (Dillon, 1978a, pp. 426, 427).

8.1.1. The Contrasting Points of View

Examples that could contrast the effects of application of the strictly mechanistic concept of life and the biomechanistic are rampant in the literature, but several illustrations suffice to bring out the differing consequences. The few that are presented are chosen solely for the sake of convenience and clarity, but when first proposed almost all recent and current explanations of cellular activities provide the same glaring discrepancies between concept and ultimate actuality, including the "central dogma" of biology itself.

A Supposed Origin for Catalase. Many hypotheses regarding the possible origins of various important biochemicals were advanced during the early decade following Miller's (1953) synthesis of amino acids under assumed primitive earth conditions, but none is more lucid than Calvin's (1956, 1969, 1975) exposition of a possible autocatalytic development of the complex heme enzyme called catalase. Since the major steps in the suggested processes of forming this biologically significant substance have been summarized earlier (Dillon, 1978a, pp. 56–58), it is not necessary to repeat those details here. The demonstration that porphyrin could be produced by electric discharges in an appropriate mixture of gases (Hodgson and Ponnamperuma, 1968) certainly held validity for the problem of life's origin and early evolution, as might also Calvin's conjecture of its synthesis in the presence of ferric ions in the primitive seas. Even the suggested spontaneous creation of a heme from the porphyrin and iron appears to be acceptable. But beyond that point, the addition to this combination of a peptide, which would necessarily have had to possess a reasonably constant primary structure, could only have occurred within living organisms possessing a genetic mechanism sufficiently complex to enable it consistently to build such an enzyme (Dillon, 1978a, p. 63). A strictly mechanistic approach, such as that just alluded to, can propose reasonable solutions to problems concerned with the origins of the simpler precursorial molecules, like the porphyrin and perhaps the heme, but beyond that point the problem depends more upon biolgoical considerations than chemical.

One method of applying a biomechanistic approach to the problem would be by first referring to the primitive biological objects themselves, preferably when arranged in a logical sequence of increasing complexity, including those schemes advocated elsewhere (Dillon, 1962, 1963, 1978a, pp. 410–426; 1981, pp. 559–565). When suitable systematic lists are examined, it is perceived that simpler organisms like *Beggiatoa*, rickettsias, chlamydids, and viruses do not employ porphyrins as far as is currently known, and that hemes probably did not arise until just prior to the advent of the blue-green algae, at least according to data provided by the tricarboxylic acid cycle and its precursors (Dillon, 1981, pp. 364–374). Thus, it becomes evident that the origins of heme-containing compounds, including catalase, have no real bearing on the problem of life's advent and consequently lack validity in regard to protobiontic evolution. Nevertheless, this topic needs thorough exploration in context with the phylogenetic development of later cellular life, where it could hold great significance.

Origins of the Genetic Mechanism. Probably nowhere else in the studies on the origins of life is the failure of a strict mechanistic point of view so manifest as in experiments on the possible beginnings of the genetic apparatus. Since the molecular apparatus includes several types of nucleic acids, whereas the focal products are polypeptides and proteins, most such investigations have endeavored to disclose direct interactions between polynucleotides and amino acids. All such attempts to find physicochemical relationships between a given amino acid and polynucleotides or oligonucleotides that might correspond to either its codons or anticodons have failed completely (Dillon, 1978a, pp. 215, 216). As shown in the reference cited, this lack of relationship between the two classes of biochemicals should have been anticipated, for nowhere among the living things of today do they display direct interactions of any sort.

From a biomechanistic standpoint, a much more realistic experimental approach could be taken towards solution of the problem. First, examination of living things discloses that the one universal feature of the tRNAs, with which amino acids must be united in order to be processed into proteins, is the -CCA terminus, and that this is the only combination of nucleotides with which amino acids interact. Moreover, it would be found that the interaction takes place only in the presence of a tRNA ligase (Dillon, 1978a, pp. 344–348). Thus, experiments concerned with the beginnings of the coded genetic system could be designed to employ a simple common amino acid, such as glycine, and the trinucleotide -CCA, together with a simple enzyme system to attempt to uncover the elementary requirements for charging such a primitive tRNA. Obviously the success of this approach depends upon finding a suitable enzyme whose molecular structure is sufficiently simple to be convincing in context with the primordial nature of the organisms in which these first steps must have arisen.

Self-Assembly of Macromolecules. Almost invariably in the recent past, it has been the practice when a new ubiquitous type of structural biochemical has been isolated and analyzed, to suggest that the substance assembles itself spontaneously into polymers within the cell as it often can be made to do *in vitro*. Such mechanistic proposals have also invariably proved to be simplistic, totally out of keeping with the actual processes that are eventually found to occur in the cell. Undoubtedly, the most notorious example of this misconception was the describing of DNA as a "self-replicating molecule," a notion that still reappears far too frequently in current literature, especially in that pertaining to life's origins. Such proposals overlook the fact that *by itself* DNA is undoubtedly the most useless macromolecule an organism possesses, for it requires a minimum of 189 proteins in prokaryotes and 279 in eukaryotes for its replication, transcription, and translation into usable products (Dillon, 1978a, pp. 204–210).

A more lucid example is provided by tubulin which was originally suggested to polymerize into microtubules spontaneously under "dynamic equilibrium" between the soluble subunits and the microtubules (Inoué, 1953; Dillon, 1981, pp. 81–90). The results of subsequent investigations have shown that that purely mechanistic point of view is invalid, because the processes have proven to be of great complexity involving a multiplicity of reactants. However, a more realistic view of the nature of the cell would have negated the concept before it was ever presented. Were this substance capable of self-assembly as proposed, the α and β subunits of which tubulin consists would be expected to form dimers almost immediately upon contact after their synthesis on ribosomes. As soon as they had been generated, these dimers would, according to the theory, tend to polymerize in the region of their origin, because of the obvious lack of equilibrium resulting from the absence of microtubules in the locality. Hence, microtubules would form in random fashion, scattered in disarray throughout the cell, rather than in the highly ordered manner that actually exists even in the mitotic spindle, the object first studied in this connection.

Application of a biomechanistic approach would have suggested that the fibers interconnecting the chromosomes and polar caps would have to be formed with great precision and under careful control to permit the vital processes of nuclear division to be carried out successfully. The later findings of microtubular involvement in numerous other important functions of the cell, such as in flagellar movement and fertilization, serve to emphasize a need for pinpoint control over the formation of microtubules, as well as over all the other constituents that comprise these exceedingly complex structural elements. Such control measures would incude (1) regulation of transcription and processing;

(2) translation of the mature transcripts; (3) posttranslational modification of primary structure and development of the correct secondary and tertiary morphologies; (4) conduction of the completed polypeptide to a site where formation of a microtubule is requisite; (5) orientation of those molecules in the required direction; (6) polymerization by enzymes which likewise had to be brought to the same site after themselves experiencing the same five prior steps; (7) polymerization of the α and β subunits, together with incorporation of microtubule-associated proteins (MAPs) and others, each of which likewise had to pass through steps 1 to 5; (8) degeneration of the microtubule when it was no longer needed; and (9) disposal of the resulting by-products. In view of this fuller—but doubtlessly still incomplete—picture, the inadequacies of self-assemblage and similar proposals become more fully evident, not only in regard to microtubules but to myosin, actin, and all other fibers and filamentous structures.

   Origins of Steric Properties of Biochemicals. In the opening statements of this section, it was conceded that a stringent mechanistic philosophy was validly applicable to the chemical elements of living things, the nature of their chemical bonds, and the origins of the simpler molecules of protoplasm. But even the last portion of that concession requires restriction. Obviously, the amino acids which constituted the first interacting proteinoids that can be considered protobionts were formed on the primeval earth spontaneously, and equally by their own properties they united to form these proteinoids (Fox, 1980; Fox and Nakashima, 1980); however, the monomeric units were not consistently identical in structure to the amino acids of modern organisms. Although a large percentage probably were of the α type that alone occurs in living things today, the rest were doubtlessly β, γ, or other varieties. Insofar as the optical properties of the molecules were concerned, dextro- and levorotatory ones likely occurred in unequal quantities, whereas those of modern cells are almost invariably of the latter configuration, aside from glycine which is neutral in this property—even the occasional exceptions that occur are derived enzymatically from the levo-enantiomorph (Dillon, 1973, 1978a, pp. 66, 67, 218–233). Thus, the amino acids clearly demonstrate themselves to be homologous in structure, both in their being α-isomers and in their steric properties. Obviously, for the 20 species of amino acids that make up almost every single protein molecule of all extant organisms to be homologs in regard to two of their most basic structural aspects, they, like all other homologies known to biology, need to be interpreted as having had origins from a common ancestral molecule. These origins by evolutionary processes must have occurred within primitive organisms in the Archean seas of the young earth. Furthermore, analysis of the genetic code presented in those same two references obviously supported the identical conclusion. Contrastingly, none of the numerous experimental or philosophical investigations into the origins of either the homologies of the amino acids or the possible origins of the genetic code (for example, Weber and Miller, 1981) have succeeded in finding even one consistent set of observations to support their mechanistic proposals.

In comparable fashion, the various species of simple sugars, all of which are homologous in structure and in their steric configurations, also show evidence of having shared a common ancestry. Unfortunately, the members of this class of biochemicals have not been thoroughly studied in viruses and other primitive living things in sufficient depth to permit an evolutionary scheme to be proposed. However, the point being made here is not the validity of the phylogenetic scheme that has been advanced in relation to the amino acids (Dillon, 1973, 1978a, pp. 218–273), for other schemes may eventually be forthcoming that are equally or even more acceptable. What is being stressed is that the amino acids and sugars show several features whose homologous nature can be understood only in light of a biomechanistic point of view.

8.1.2. Organizational Aspects of the Genome

Since the analysis of the molecular genetic apparatus was published and its nonmechanical behavior pointed out (Dillon, 1978a), many additional details of its structure and behavior have been revealed that cannot be explained in light of rigid mechanistic philosophy. Some of these unexpected features have already received attention in the preceding chapter in relation to the structure of immunoglobulin genes (Chapter 7, Section 7.1.5). There it was shown that each gene, whether for the light or heavy chains, was comprised of a series of segments, separated by nontranslated regions, the introns. In addition, there were often leaders, parts of which were transcribed—or even translated—whereas the rest were not, including cap structure, trains, and sites of polyadenylation. Thus, instead of a single continuous section of the genomic DNA encoding a polypeptide, as postulated in the mechanistic concept, a number of separate parts are actually encoded that need to be assembled, in part during transcription or afterwards, and extraneous sections require removal. Although enzymatic cleavage has been implicated in the trimming of unnecessary translated sequences from precursorial molecules, the mechanism involved in pretranslational assembly remains unknown. Moreover, extensive pretranscriptional control was manifested also in the selection of the particular class of immunoglobulin to be transcribed. Early in the ontogeny of the B lymphocytes, the μ chain was almost always transcribed, an action that required the universal V_H domain to be combined to the series of genelets or pregenes for the several domains of the μ class, either prior to or during transcription. Then later a switch was made, with the V_H domain becoming attached, transcriptionally speaking, to the several C domains of the γ or other class of heavy chains.

Although no other instance of such great complexity in transcriptional control has as yet come to light, a segmental structure like that of immunoglobulin genes is proving to be of frequent occurrence. The gene for hemoglobin β in mice, for example, contains two introns, one 116 base pairs in length, the second one 646, while the actual coding exons themselves total only 432 base pairs in length (Konkel *et al.*, 1978). Others have been shown to include 20 intervening sections and the α-collagen gene, 51 (Lewin, 1981b). The genes encoding mitochondrial products also may embrace multiple noncoding segments, as shown by that for cytochrome b, which consists of five short segments separated by four noncoding regions (Lewin, 1980). In fact, most of the genes of eukaryotes and many of certain viruses are segmented, whereas those of prokaryotes do not appear to be (Lewin, 1981a). As in the immunoglobulins, the introns are removed enzymatically during processing, the splicing of the remaining segments apparently requiring a GT base pair at the 5' end of the intron and AG at the 3' (Breathnach *et al.*, 1978; Catterall *et al.*, 1978; Ohno, 1980; Rogers and Wall, 1980). Quite frequently, again as in those antibodies, the GT signal in the first intron involves the last nucleotide of the final codon in the preceding coding regions, as in the actin gene of yeast (Gallwitz and Sures, 1980). The nonmechanistic behavior of such signals is indicated by the demonstration that certain mutations which alter the splice junctions nevertheless are correctly processed *in vivo* (Colby *et al.*, 1981). Moreover, in several known instances, the introns are not inert segments to be removed and destroyed but encode proteins, some of which are actually involved in the splicing activities (Lewin, 1980; Schmelzer *et al.*, 1981).

Genes for Nontranslated Transcripts. Since the transcripts of genes for certain molecular types of RNA, such as those for tRNA and rRNA, are not translated into proteins but are employed as ribonucleic acids themselves, they need merely to be processed to a slight degree prior to use. Hence, the family of genes that encode the tRNAs appears to provide an ideal device for introducing the complex subject of gene organization. In only a few viruses has the structure of the pertinent section of the genome been determined, that of bacteriophage T4 being the most thoroughly investigated. The eight species of tRNAs of this organism have recently been shown to be arranged in clusters together with two other RNAs, referred to as C and D, whose functions have not been discovered (Mazzara *et al.*, 1981). The first cluster encodes seven of the tRNAs, the species for glutamine lying toward the 5' end, followed by those for leucine, glycine, proline, serine, threonine, and isoleucine in that order toward the 3' terminus. The second region, separated from the first by a spacer 500 base pairs in length, provides the coding region for tRNA^{Arg} and RNAs D and C. In each case the genes are separated by one, two, or a few residues and in at least one instance by none at all. Apparently each cluster is transcribed as a unit, so the pairs of precursors reported earlier (Barrell *et al.*, 1974; Dillon, 1978a, pp. 199–201) probably represent products of early enzymatic processing of an originally much longer nascent transcript. The short leaders, spacers, and trains, where they exist, are then removed and certain of the bases undergo modification, an activity that proceeds by several steps. In some cases the terminal -CCA sequence is encoded in the DNA, but sometimes it is added during processing by the enzyme known as nucleotidyl transferase. Since no intron is present in any of these RNA genes nor are any of the spacers, where present, of any length, at least 90–95% of the DNA in these clusters consists of active coding regions.

The situation in bacteria regarding stable RNA genes seems to differ little from that just described. Many of the genes appear to be dispersed widely throughout the genome in these organisms, as represented by *Salmonella typhimurium* and *E. coli* (Sanderson, 1967; Gorini, 1970); in the latter at least, however, some of the 60 tRNA genes present are arranged in clusters (Squires *et al.*, 1973). Multiple copies of the same gene may occur, tRNA^{Gly} being an example; of the three for tRNA^{Tyr} present in *E. coli*, two are adjacent and are transcribed as a unit (Ghysen and Celis, 1974), whereas the third copy is entirely separate (Landy *et al.*, 1974). On the average, the immediate products of transcription were reported to be 200 nucleotides in length, which were first trimmed to 120-base lengths before being reduced to definitive size. Thus, the precursors were processed in two steps, whereas trimming in viruses was accomplished in a single stage. Further, in *E. coli* 18 tRNA genes were reported to be interspersed among those for rRNA, forming clusters (called operons) that are transcribed as a unit (Duester *et al.*, 1981). Three identically arranged operons, those referred to as *rrnA* and *rrnD*, plus an unmapped one, have been reported to include a gene for 16 S rRNA, followed in sequence by ones for tRNA$_1^{Ile}$, tRNA$_{1B}^{Ala}$, 23 S rRNA, and 5 S rRNA (Morgan *et al.*, 1977; Sekiya and Nishimura, 1979). Among the details of structure that were ascertained was the presence of a spacer segment 68 base pairs in length between the 16 S rRNA and the tRNA$_1^{Ile}$ genes. The tRNA$_{1B}^{Ala}$ and 23 S rRNA genes also appeared to be separated by a spacer of modest length, but how closely the second tRNA gene followed the first was not reported.

In other investigations the coding region for tRNA^{Tyr} has been demonstrated to be preceded on the 5′ end by a sequence at least 60 base pairs in length that contains a recognition signal (or promoter) for the initiation of transcription (Sekiya *et al.*, 1976). Recently the structure of another operon has been analyzed more fully. In this short cluster identified as either *rrnF* or *rrnG* were the coding regions of 23 S rRNA, 5 S rRNA, and tRNA$_1^{Asp}$, arranged in that order from the 5′ end. A spacer 93 base pairs in length separated the two rRNA genes and another 52 base pairs long lay between those for the 5 S rRNA and tRNA (Sekiya *et al.*, 1980). Moreover, the latter was followed by a spacer of 165 base pairs that included an assumed termination signal for the entire operon, as well as those for binding and ribosome-binding of the transcript. Why rRNA and tRNA transcripts were thought to become bound to ribosomes was not made clear. In no case was the gene for a tRNA interrupted by an intron and the -CCA terminal seemed to be consistently encoded in the DNA.

As might be expected, the eukaryotic genes for this class of substances are far more complexly arranged, their specific disposition varying from taxon to taxon but almost always consisting of multiple copies. In yeast two repeated tRNA^{Phe} genes lie adjacent, whereas those for tRNA^{Tyr} are dispersed through the genome, a condition that seemingly prevails for many of the 360 tRNA genes present in this organism (Schweizer et al., 1969; Olson et al., 1977; Valenzuela et al., 1978). Among the higher eukaryotes, the tRNA genes are characteristically arranged into small clusters interspersed among single-copy DNA sequences; in Drosophila, for a specific example, the genes respectively for tRNA^{Lys} and tRNA^{Val} are clustered (Grigliatti et al., 1974; Delaney et al., 1976). Great redundancy often prevails, 7800 genes for 43 different tRNA sequences being present in Xenopus and about 13,000 being estimated to occur in rat liver cells (Quincey and Wilson, 1969; Clarkson et al., 1973). On the other hand, in the slime mold D. discoideum, only six copies, all identical, have been found of the gene for tRNA^{Trp} (Peffley and Sogin, 1981). A fragment of DNA containing one cluster (or partial cluster) of these genes in the rat genome has recently been sequenced, which contained the cistrons for tRNAs for aspartic acid, glycine, and glutamic acid, in that order (Sekiya et al., 1981). The first and second were separated by a spacer 464 base pairs in length, while the last was removed from the middle one by a spacer–leader combination of 429 base pairs and had a train of at least 700 paired residues. No introns were present in any of these three, nor was the -CCA-terminal triplet encoded in the DNA. Many other members of this gene family also lack introns, including two that code for tRNA$_2^{Lys}$ in Drosophila (De Franco et al., 1980).

Although absent in the three rat tRNAs and others just discussed, a frequent feature of the eukaryotic genes for these nucleic acids is the occurrence of introns. In many cases the single intervening sequence consists of around 13 nucleotides, that seem to form a hairpin on the side of the anticodon loop (arm III) when arranged into the familiar cloverleaf pattern, like those of tRNA^{Trp} from Dictyostelium (Peffley and Sogin, 1981). A number of sequences of tRNAs in yeast have proven to include such an intron (Figure 8.1), among them those of tRNA^{Tyr}, tRNA^{Phe}, tRNA^{Leu}, and tRNA^{Ser} (Knapp et al., 1978; O'Farrell et al., 1978; Valenzuela et al., 1978; Etcheverry et al., 1979; Johnson et al., 1980), while others, like the rest that code for tRNA^{Ser}, apparently are not thus interrupted. The introns that are excised in the yeast species are no longer than those of Drosophila but all are situated in like fashion. Processing of the nascent transcript involves two steps, at each of which ATP is required. The first reaction cleaves the precursor into three parts, consisting of the intervening sequence and the two half-tRNAs, while the second splices the latter to form the complete molecule (Knapp et al., 1979; Peebles et al., 1979). In addition in Drosophila, there is a leader sequence of at least 117 residues and a train of 113 at the 3' end, both of which appear to be transcribed and then removed enzymatically.

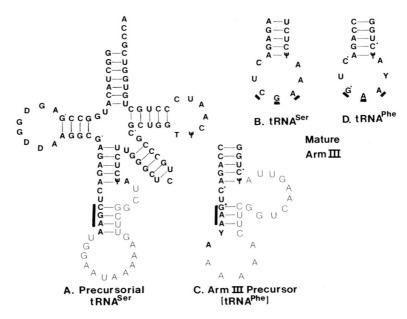

Figure 8.1. Precursorial transcripts of tRNAs of yeast. In the nascent transcript for the yeast minor species of tRNA[Ser] (A) and tRNA[Phe] (D), an intervening sequence is present (shown in light-face type). In all known cases where such introns exist in tRNAs they are similarly placed. The heavy bars indicate the anticodons. During processing the intervening sequence is removed and the resulting two half-molecules are spliced, producing the normal anticodon arms (Arms III) shown in (B) and (C). (Based on Etcheverry et al., 1979, and Valenzuela et al., 1978.)

Phylogeny of tRNA Genes. As the tRNAs are the only specific class of actively functional macromolecules shared by viruses, prokaryotes, and eukaryotes, a possible phylogenetic sequence of gene organization may be derived. In the viral tRNA genes, intervening sequences were seen to be absent and spacers between members of a cluster were either wanting or consisted of only a few base pairs. It is conceivable, too, that in more elementary viruses than bacteriophage T4, the source of the transcripts described earlier, all tRNA genes will be found to lack leaders and trains or to have them virtually absent. In bacteria the genes for tRNAs were similar in lacking introns, but members of a given cluster were separated by spacers of greater length, perhaps in the neighborhood of 50 to 70 base pairs. None have been reported whose -CCA terminus was not encoded in the DNA, at least not in those highly advanced bacterial species that have been studied. A distinct possibility remains, however, that in *Beggiatoa* and other primitive types, and possibly even in the blue-green algae, this feature may be lacking in some cases, and their spacing sequences probably will prove to be shorter than those just described, that is, they will be closer to the viral condition.

Finally, in the eukaryotes, introns are of frequent occurrence and long leaders and trains are the rule. Thus, the overall trend is from the simplest arrangement to the most complex—the fragmenting of genes is an evolutionary advancement, the advantage of which in terms of survival is not apparent. But it seems improbable, as has been suggested (Ohno, 1980), that genes for complex polypeptides, such as immunoglobulins, are the result of fusion of transcripts for smaller chains; fragmentation through the gradual introduction of introns appears to be the more likely event, according to the evidence of the tRNA genes and consideration of the principle of reverse evolution.

No phylogeny of this sort would be fully relevant were the chloroplasts and mitochondria of eukaryotes not included. In each of these types of organelles, both prokaryotic and eukaryotic traits are present. For instance, chloroplast tRNAs of spinach and maize are located in a repetitive section of DNA between genes for rRNAs (Bohnert et al., 1979; Koch et al., 1981; Schwarz et al., 1981), much as in bacteria except that in the present case the sequences include a gene for a type absent from prokaryotes, 4.5 S rRNA, located between the 23 S and 5 S. The region coding for tRNA^{Val} has been found to precede that for the 16 S species, whereas those for tRNA^{Ile} and tRNA^{Ala} lies between the latter and the gene for 23 S rRNA (Koch et al., 1981; Schwarz et al., 1981). Although the former was not interrupted by an intron, the second set was, tRNA^{Ile} having an intervening segment 949 base pairs in length and tNRA^{Ala}, one of 806. Thus, these genes are eukaryotic in being subdivided, but differ in having introns of much greater lengths.

A comparable intermediate arrangement prevails also in the genes for tRNAs in the mitochondrion, a condition that likewise characterizes the 5 S rRNAs of those organelles (Gray and Spencer, 1981; Spencer et al., 1981). While the base sequence of the entire DNA molecules from mitochondria of the mouse displays the utmost economy in gene structure and organization, some genes for proteins do contain introns (Bibb et al., 1981), as is the case also for the yeast organelle (Bechmann et al., 1981). However, the tRNA genes lack intervening segments and are interspersed between those for rRNAs, as in the chloroplast and prokaryotes. Several especially striking features were reported, chief among which was the employment of any combination of AU- with a standard nucleotide to serve as the translation initiation codon, not only AUG as elsewhere. Moreover, UAA (ochre) alone served as the termination signal for translation. Comparable unique coding patterns have also been demonstrated in the mitochondrial tRNAs of *Neurospora,* in that anticodons containing U in the first position were able to read all four codons of a given family, whereas those having a modified U in the corresponding site reacted only with those terminating in purines (Heckman et al., 1980). TGA in these organelles of this fungus appeared to serve for tryptophan, rather than termination as elsewhere; in contrast, this codon does not occur in this organelle of *Z. mays*, but CGG (as well as TGG) codes trytophan, not arginine as typical (Fox and Leaver, 1981). Thus, while the tRNA and other genes of mitochondria shed little light on their origins, they do accentuate the nonmechanistic behavior of the genetic apparatus in all organisms.

8.1.3. The Nature of the α-Globin Genes

Among the sets of genes which have been most thoroughly studied at the molecular levels by the highly sophisticated procedures now available are the two families that encode the subunits for the various hemoglobins, amino acid sequences of certain of which are given in Table 8.1. The first of these contains the α-like globins that form a closely linked group of four functional genes, located in mankind on chromosome 16 (Diesseroth *et al.*, 1977); the second one, containing five β-like genes, is found in this same mammal on chromosome 11. The genes actually encode only subunits, and, as indicated in an earlier section (Chapter 4, Section 4.5.1), the definitive hemoglobin molecules are tetramers, consisting of two identical representatives from each family, such as $\alpha_2\beta_2$, the typical hemoglobin A (HbA) of adult persons. As a general rule, the nascent transcripts from any of the α-like globin genes reportedly are the simpler, having molecular weights of 280,000 compared to the 600,000 for those of the β-like family; after processing, the mature mRNAs of either type are reduced to a weight of 200,000 (Ross and Knecht, 1978).

The α-Globin Gene Family. Both families of genes, although included in different chromosomes, are grouped into closely linked clusters and are arranged in the sequence of their expression during ontogeny (see Chapter 4, Section 4.5.1). Hence, because of their close linkage, transcription of a subunit in each group is concerned with a specific region of one particular strand of DNA. In addition to the active genes, each family also embraces one or more pseudogenes, typically indicated by the symbol ψ. Thus, the full sequence of this family of globins in man is ζ_2, ζ_1, $\psi\alpha_1$, α_2, α_1 (Lauer *et al.*, 1980), reading in the direction in which transcription occurs ($5' \rightarrow 3'$ in reference to the transcript). Since the two ζ globins occur only in the embryo, the macromolecular characteristics of their genes remain relatively unknown, but much attention has been given to the three of the α subgroup, especially in man and mouse (Nute, 1974; Földi *et al.*, 1980; Liebhaber *et al.*, 1981). Contrastingly in a macaque (*Macaca nemestrina*), three active α cistrons but no pseudogenes exist (Nute, 1981). In man the peptide products encoded by the two active loci proved to be identical, whereas each of those of the three of the macaque diverged at two sites (Földi *et al.*, 1980; Liebhaber *et al.*, 1981). However, the actual base sequences of this sector of human DNA have demonstrated the presence of differences between α_2 and α_1 in two sites, the former having CAA at site 54 and GCT at site 123, in contrast to CAG and GCC at the corresponding points in α_1. But since the mutations still encode the same amino acids (glutamine at site 54 and alanine at the other location), the peptide products are identical. In contrast, the pseudogene $\psi\alpha_1$ in man has been found only 73% homologous to its neighbor α_2 (Proudfoot and Maniatis, 1980); while single mutations are scattered throughout the sequence, the most extensive difference between the pair is a deletion of a 20-base sector that has removed the codons for amino acids 38–45 from the pseudogene. Moreover, the defect also results in a trans-

Table 8.1
Amino Acid Sequences of Various Globins

	Exon 1	Exon 2
Ambystoma α^a	FKLSGEDKANVKAVWDHVKGH-EDAFGHEALGR	MFTGIEQTHTYFPDK-DLNE
Mouse α^b	V-LSGEDKSNIKAAWGKIGGH-GAEYGAEALER	MFASFPTTKTYFPHF-DVSH
Human $\alpha_{1,2}{}^c$	V-LSPADKTNVKAAWGKVGAH-AGGYGAGALGR	MFLSFPTTKTYFPHF-DLSH
Human ζ^d	S-LTKTERTIIVSMWAKISTQ-ADTIGTETLER	LPLSHPQTLTYFPHF-DLHP
Mouse β^e	VHLTEADKAAVSCLWGKVNSEDVGG---DALGR	LLVVYPWTERWFESFGELSS
Human δ^f	VHLTPEEKTAVNALWGKVNVDAVGG---EALGR	LLVVYPWTQRFFESFGDLSS
Human $^A\gamma^g$	GHFTEEDKATITSLWGKVNEEDAGG---ETLGR	LLVVYPWTQRFFDSFGNLSS
Human ϵ^h	VHFTAEEKAAVTSLWSKMNVEEAGG---EALGR	LLVVYPWTQRFFDSFGNLSS
Chick ρ^i	VHWSAEEKQLITSVWSKVNVEECGA---EALAR	LLIVYPWTQRFFDNFGNLSS
Rana β^j	G--S--D---LVSGFWGKVDAHKIGG---EALAR	LLVVYPWTQRYFTTFGNLGS
Soybean^k	GAFT--DKQEALVSSSFEAFKTNIPQYSVVFYT	SILEKAFAVKDLFSFLANGV
Ambystoma α^a	GSFA----ALHSHGKKVMGALSNAVAHIDDLEATLVKLSDKHAHDLMVDP	
Mouse α^b	GSA-----QVKGHGKKVADALAS AAGHLDDLPGALSALSDLHAHKLRVDP	
Human $\alpha_{1,2}{}^c$	GSA-----QVKGHGKKVADALTNAVAHVDDMPNALSALSDLHAHKLRVDP	
Human ζ^d	GSA-----QLRAHGSKVVAAVGDAVKSIDDIGGALSKLSELHAYILRVDP	
Mouse β^e	ASAIMGNAKVKAHGKKYITAFNEGLNHLESLKGTFASLSELHCEKLHVEP	
Human δ^f	PDAVMGNPKVKAHGKKVLGAFSDGLAHLDNLKGTFSQLSELHCDKLHVDP	
Human $^A\gamma^g$	ASAIMGNPKVKAHGKKVLTSLGDAIKHLDDLKGTFAQLSELHCDKLHVDP	
Human ϵ^h	PSAILGNPKVKAHGKKVLTSFGDAIKNMDNLKPAFAKLSELHCDKLHVDP	
Chick ρ^i	PTAIIGNPKVRAHGKKVLSSFGEAVKNLDNIKNTYAKLSELHCEKLHVDP	
Rana β^j	ADAICHNAKVLAHGQKVLAAIGEGLKHPENLKAHYAKLSEYHSAKLHVDP	
Soybean^k	VNPTNPKLTGHAGKLFGLVRDSAGQLKATVVADAASGSIHAQKAITNPEF	

(Continued)

Table 8.1 (Continued)

		Exon 3
Ambystoma α[a]	AEFP	RLAEDILVV–LGFHLPAKFTYAVQCSIDKFLHVTMRLCISKYR
Mouse α[b]	VNFK	LLSHCLLVT–LASHHPADFTPAVHASLDKFLASVSTVLTSKYR
Human $α_{1,2}$[c]	VNFK	LLSHCLLVT–LAAHLPAEFTPAVHASLDKFLASVSTVLTSKYR
Human ζ[d]	VNFK	LLSHCLLVT–LAARFDADFTAEAHAAWDKFLSVVSSVLTEKYR
Mouse β[e]	DNFQ	LLGNM–IVIVLGHHLGKEFTPAAQAAFGKVVAGVATALAHKYH
Human δ[f]	ENFR	LLGNV–LVCVLARNFGKEFTPQMQAAYQKVVAGVANALAHKYH
Human $^{A}γ$[g]	ENFK	LLGNV–LVTVLAIHFGKEFTPEVQASWQKMVTAVASALSSRYH
Human ε[h]	ENFK	LLGNV–MVIILATHFGKEFTPEVQAAWQKLVSAVAIALAHKYH
Chick ρ[i]	ENFR	LLGNI---IVLAAHPTKDFTPECQAAWQKLVSVVAKALARKYH
Rana β[j]	ANFR	LLGNV–FITVLARHFQHEFTPELQHALEAHFCAVGDALAKAYH
Soybean[k]	VV–K	EALLK-----TIKEAVGDKWSDELSSAWEVAYDELAAAIKKAF

[a] Boissel *et al.* (1980).
[b] Nishioka and Leder (1979).
[c] Földi *et al.* (1980), Michelson and Orkin (1980), Proudfoot and Maniatis (1980).
[d] Clegg and Gagnon (1981).
[e] van Ooyen *et al.* (1979).
[f] Spritz *et al.* (1980).
[g] Slightom *et al.* (1980).
[h] Baralle *et al.* (1980).
[i] Chapman *et al.* (1981).
[j] Chauvet and Archer (1972).
[k] Hurrell and Leach (1977).

lational reading-frame shift that produced three premature UGA termination codons. The standard initiation signal (ATG) has likewise undergone alteration to GTG.

The Nature of the 3′ Flanking Region. In the literature, the region of the gene on the 3′ side of the messengerlike strand frequently is variously referred to as the 3′ flanking region or 3′ untranslated region. Here for convenience of discussion it is considered to be divided into two portions, the train, which extends from the termination signal to the point where the poly(A) tail is added, while the remainder is merely the intergenic spacer. Table 8.2 supplies the whole of this flanking region of the mouse α-globin gene (Nishioka and Leder, 1979), which extends from site 1087 of that gene sequence to 1441,* along with the trains of the genes for human $α_1$ and $α_2$ globins (Michelson and Orkin, 1980; Proudfoot and Maniatis, 1980), plus that of the mRNA transcribed from the latter (Wilson *et al.*, 1980). Unfortunately, because at the time

*The numbering in the table refers to the base pairs of this sequence only.

Table 8.2
The 3' Untranslated Regions of Globin Genes (Trains)

```
                      1090
Mouse α[a]            -TAAGCTGCCTTCTGCGGGGCTTGCCTTCTGGCCATGCCCTTCTTCTCTCCCTTGCACCTGTACCTC

Human α-mRNA[b]       -UAAGCUGGAGCCUCGGUAGCAGUUCCUCCUGCCAGAUGGGCCUCCCAACGGGCCCUCCUCCCCUCC

Human α2[c]           -TAAGCTGGAGCCTCGGTAGCCGTTCCTCCTGCCCGCTGGGCCTCCCAACGGGCCCTCCTCCCCTCC

Human α1[d]           -TAAGCTGGAGCCTCGGTGGCCATGCTTCTTGCCCCTTGGGCCTCCC--------------------

Mouse β[e]            -TAAACCCCCTTTCCTGCT-CTTGCCTGTGAACAATGGTTAATTGTTCCCAAGAGAGCATCTGTCAG

Human δ[f]            -TGAGATCCTGGACTGTTTCCTGATAACCATTAGAAGACC-CTATTTCCCTAGATTCTATTTTCTGA

Human Aγ[g]           -TGAGCCTCTTGCCCATGATTCAGAGCTTTCAAGGATAGG-CTTTATTCTGGAAGCAATA-------

Human ε[h]            -GTGAGTTCAGGTGCTGGTGA-TGTGATTTTTTGGCTTTATATTTTGAC------------------

Mouse α               -----------------------------------

Human α-mRNA          CAACGCGCCCUCCUCCCCUCCUUCACCGGCCCUUUC

Human α2              --------------------TTGCACCGGCCTTTC

Human α1              CCCAGCCCCTCCTCCCCTTCCTGCACCCGTACCCCC

Mouse β               TTGTTGGCAAAATGATAGACATTTGAAAATCTG---

Human δ               ACCTGGGAACACAATGCCTACTTCAAGGGTATGGCT

Human Aγ              -----------------------------------

Human ε               -----------------------------------
                                             1190      1200      1210
Mouse α               TTGGTCTTTGAATAAAGCCTGAGTAGGAAGAAGCCTGCATGCCTGGTTCTCTGCGTCTGCA

Human α-mRNA          CUGGUCUUUGAAUAAAGUCUGAGUGGGCGGCA*

Human α2              CTGGTCTTTGAATAAAGTCTGAGTGGGCGGCA*

Human α1              GTGGTCTTTGAATAAAGTCTGAGTGGGCGGCA*

Mouse β               TCTTCTGACAAATAAAAAGCATTTATGTTCACTGCA*

Human δ               TCTGCCTAATAAAGAAATGTTCAGCTCAACTTC--CT*

Human Aγ              -----CAAATAATAAATCTATTCTGCTGAGATCA*

Human ε               -------ATTAATTGAGCTCATAATCTTATTGGAAAGACCA*
                          1220      1230      1240      1250      1260      1270
Mouse α               AAGGTGTCATGTTTAGTGTGGGGATGCCGCAGCTCATTTGCCATGGGGCAGTAAAGACAAGG

                          1280      1290      1300      1310      1320      1330
Mouse α               TTCAGAGCAAAAAGCATAATTGGATGCCTACACACACACACATATGTCTTCTGAGTCTGGG

                          1340      1350      1360      1370
Mouse α               AAGATCGTCTTTGGAGGGTCCTTATCACAGGACCTCTGAGGG

                          1380      1390      1400      1410      1420      1430      1440
Mouse α               CAGCAGTCCCTCCCAAGCCCTCCACTGACAGCCATGTGTCTTCTCCTCGAGCCAAAGAAGCCA
```

[a] Nishioka and Leder (1979).   [f] Spritz *et al.* (1980).
[b] Wilson *et al.* (1980).   [g] Slightom *et al.* (1980).
[c] Proudfoot and Maniatis (1980).   [h] Baralle *et al.* (1980).
[d] Michelson and Orkin (1980).   * Indicates presence of poly(A) tract.
[e] Konkel *et al.* (1978).

when the analysis of the messenger sequence was made, it was believed that the two human α genes were virtually identical, some misinterpretations of the peptide fragment arrangements became introduced into the structure; not until later was it shown that the 3' untranslated region of the two were really quite divergent (Wilson *et al.*, 1977; Michelson and Orkin, 1980). Thus, as may be perceived in the table, sectors from both the α_1- and α_2-globin sequences were combined in the transcript.

In general the three molecular structures from human sources show extensive homologies (with uridine in the mRNA being considered identical to the thymidine of DNA), especially directly following the termination signal, T(U)AA or TGA. However, the α gene from the mouse shows little homology after the fourth residue in the subsequent region and lacks a section 15 base pairs in length. If the virtual identity between the two human α-globin genes has been maintained within a given species by homologous but unequal (i.e., offset) crossing over between the pair, as has been suggested (Liebhaber *et al.*, 1981), it would have had to occur almost strictly within the coding regions, otherwise the nontranslated flanks would not be so divergent. Moreover, one must wonder why the pseudogene of this family has not been similarly maintained as a homolog as it has been in the macaque. All four α sequences are identical for nine residues preceding the AATAAA signal and nearly so for 11 sites which follow. On a strictly mechanistic basis, it is not clear why in the mouse molecule 20 base pairs lie between that signal and the GC doublet that serves as the site of attachment of the poly(A) tail, whereas in those from man only 13 base pairs are present. It is of interest to note that the differences in structure that exist between the two human α-globin genes have permitted comparisons of their respective frequencies of transcription (Orkin and Goff, 1981), the analysis of which indicated that the α_2 was transcribed more frequently than the α_1 in a ratio of 60 : 40. Thus, the transcription even of two virtually identical genes that lie adjacent in the genome is under cellular control.

The Introns of the α *Globins.* Even a superficial comparison of the two introns of the three representative α-globin genes shown in Table 8.3 reveals little homology to exist between those of the mouse and the two from man. This lack of correspondence is so marked that no attempt has been made to correlate those from the two differing source species, except near the 5' and 3' ends. Closer examination does reveal several short sequences to be present that suggest conserved regions of homology, however; for example, in intron 1 of the mouse the pentanucleotide GGACC extending from site 46 to 50 is identical to that of sites 45 to 49 in the two human species, but insertion of a hyphen to align the three series fails to expose further likenesses. Similarly between sites 40 and 50 in intron 2, there are suggestions of homology between the murine species and human α_2, but these similarities become less evident in the α_1 sequence. These differences are brought out still more prominently when the proportions of the various nucleoside residues are examined. In the first 60

Table 8.3
Comparisons of Introns of Globin Genes

Intron 1

Mouse α^a	GTGAGAA–CAGGACCTTGATCTGT–AAGGATCACAGGATCCAATATGGACCTGGCACTCGC–
Human $\alpha_2{}^b$	GTGAGGC–CCCTCCCCTGCTCCGA–CCCGGG–TCCTCGCCCGCC–GGACCCAGAGCCCACC–
Human $\alpha_1{}^c$	GTGAGGCTCCCTCCCCTGCTCCGA–CCCGGGCTCCTCGCCCGCCCGGACCCACAGGCCACC–
Mouse β^d	GTTGGTATCCAGGTTACAAGGCAG–CTCACAAGAAGAAGTTGGGTGCTTGGAGACAGAGGT–
Human δ^e	GTTGGTATCAAGGTTATAAGAGAGGCTCAAGCAGGCAAATGGAAACTGGGGCATGTGTAGAC
Human $^A\gamma^f$	GTAGGCTCTGGTGACCAGGACAAGGGAGGGAAGGAAGGACCCTGTGCCTGGCAAAAGTCCAG
Human ϵ^g	GTAAGCATTGGTTCTCAATGCATGGGAATGTGAAGGGTGAATATTACCCTAGCAAGTTGATT
Mouse α	–TCAGTGGGCACGCCTTCTAACTATGCTTTTCTGTGACCTCAACTTCTCTTCTCT––CCTTCTCCCAGG
Human α_2	–TCAACCGTCCTG–CCCCGGGAACCAAACCCCACCCCTCACTCTGGTTCTCCCCG––––––––––CAGG
Human α_1	–TCAACCGTCCTGGCCCCGGGACCCAAACCCCACCCCTCACTCTGCTTCTCCCCG––––––––––CAGG
Mouse β	–CTGCTTTCCAGCAGACACTAACTTTCAGTGTCCCCTGTCTATGTTTC–––CCTTTT––––––––TAGG
Human δ	–AGAGAAGACTCTTGGGTTTCTGATAGGCACTGACTCTCTGTCCCTTGGGCTGTTTTCCTACCCTCAGA
Human $^A\gamma$	–GTCGCTTC–TC–AGGATTTGTG–GTGGCACCTTCTGACTGTC–AAACTGTTCTTGTCAATCTCACAG–
Human ϵ	GGGAAAGTCCTCAAGATTTTTTGCATCTCTAATTTTGTATCTG–ATA–TGGTGT–––CA–TTTCATAGA

Intron 2

Mouse α	GTATGCGCTGGGACCTGGCAGGCGGCATCTGGGACCCCTAGGAAGGGCTTGGGGGGTCCTC
Human α_2	GTGAGCGCCGGG–CCGGGAGCGATCTGGGTCGAGGGC––AGATGGCCTTCCTCTCAGGGC
Human α_1	GTGAGCGGCGGG–CCGGGAGCGATCTGGGTCGAGGGGCGAGATG––CTGCCTTCCTCGCA
Mouse β	GTGAGTCTGATGGGCACCTCCTGG–––––––––––––––––––––––––––––––––––––
Human δ	GTGAGTCCAGGAGATGCTTCACTT–––––––––––––––––––––––––––––––––––––
Human $^A\gamma$	GTGAGTCCAGGAGATGTTTCAGCA–––––––––––––––––––––––––––––––––––––
Human ϵ	GTGAGTTCAGGTGCTGGTGATGTG–––––––––––––––––––––––––––––––––––––
Mouse α	GTGCCCAAGGCAGGGAACATAGTGGTCCCAGGAAGGGGAGCAGAGGCACTAGGGTGTCC––––––
Human α_2	AGAGGATCACGCGGGTTGCGGGAGGTGTAGCGCAGGCGGCGGCGCGGCTTGG–––––––––––––
Human α_1	GGGCAGAGGATCACGCGGGTTGCGGGAGGTGTAGCGCAGGCGGCGCGGCTGCGGACCTGGGCCCTCG
Mouse β	–––––––––––––––––––––––602 base pairs––––––––––––––––––––––––
Human δ	–––––––––––––––––––––––845 base pairs––––––––––––––––––––––––
Human $^A\gamma$	–––––––––––––––––––––––545 base pairs––––––––––––––––––––––––
Human ϵ	–––––––––––––––––––––––810 base pairs––––––––––––––––––––––––

(Continued)

Table 8.3 (Continued)

Mouse α	---------AC--TTT-GTCTCCGCAG
Human α_2	GCG-CACTG----TCT-CTCTGCACAG
Human α_1	GCCCCACTGACCCTCTTCTCTGCACAG
Mouse β	------GTTCTTCCATATTCCCACACG
Human δ	-------TGGGGATCAGTTTTGTGCAG
Human $^A\gamma$	------TGTCTCCTTTCATCTCAACAG
Human ε	------TTTGTC-TTTT-GCCTAACAG

[a]Nishioka and Leder (1979).   [e]Spritz et al. (1980).
[b]Proudfoot and Maniatis (1980).   [f]Slightom et al. (1980).
[c]Michelson and Orkin (1980).   [g]Baralle et al. (1980).
[d]Konkel et al. (1978), van Ooyen et al. (1979).

sites in intron 1 of the mouse, the frequencies of the four types are remarkably uniform, the range being from a low of 20% for thymidine to a high of 30% for adenosine, with cytidine providing 23% and guanosine 27%. On the other hand, in those of the two human α species, which have frequencies nearly identical to one another, cytidine occupies 50% or more of the sequence, and guanosine accounts for 25%, with the remaining sites divided equally between the other two types. The second halves of introns 1 differ slightly less markedly, for the distribution of frequencies becomes greatly altered in the mouse, with guanosine falling to 18% and thymidine rising to 40%. Cytidine likewise becomes more abundant (37%) and adenosine decreases greatly (15%).

In the first 60-site regions of the introns 2, the frequencies of the four nucleosides show less contrast between those from the mouse and man, but they contrast sharply with those of introns 1. Guanosine is the most abundant in all three sequences, providing 41–43% of the totals, with cytidine next in frequency (24–26%); adenosine is the rarest with 11–13%, and thymidine scarcely exceeds it with 15–17%. In the remaining 73 to 92 sites, one of the most notable changes in ratios is an exchange of rank between adenosine and thymidine, the latter becoming the rarest and the former assuming third place. Both of these nucleoside types increase slightly in abundance in the two human species, largely at the expense of guanosine, while in human α_1 the proportion of cytidine becomes greatly enhanced, largely through its presence in sites that are unoccupied in the other sequences.

Closer examination of the terminal regions of the two sets of introns discloses that the 5' ends of introns 1 are identical in the three species for a distance of only five sites, whereas those of the introns 2 are highly homologous for about 20. Thus, the latter display a higher degree of evolutionary conservation than do those of introns 1. The 3' termini show a comparable difference between the two introns, the first having only the last four sites homologous, and the second having the last nine. Another difference of interest is that the 5' initial guanosines of the introns 1 are derived from what would be the last site in the final codons of the first exons, whereas those of introns 2 follow the terminal codons of exons 2. This arrangement also characterizes a number of other proteins whose genes have been sequenced, including certain of the immunoglobulins. During trimming of the nascent transcript, the final G of the 3' end of introns 1 becomes the last nucleoside in the final codon of exons 1. Thus, in these instances the third site of that codon assumes a greater functional importance than the other two in the triplet, reversing the more usual situation.

The Leader Section of the α Globins. As much of a leader sector is really a transcribed portion of an intergenic spacer, only the last 80 or 90 nucleoside residues are shown in Table 8.4. Immediately it is clear that here a condition comparable to those of other untranslated regions prevails, in that the two sequences from human sources are largely homologous, while that of the mouse is highly divergent. As elsewhere, similarities in murine sectors close to corresponding sites of the human sequences can occasionally be noted, such as the TTCTG in sites −50 to −44 and −42 to −38 of the mouse and −45 to −41 of the two from man; however, aligning either of the murine pentanucleotides with the latter through insertion of hyphens fails to reveal further homologies in subsequent sites. Nevertheless, toward the 3' terminus regions of identities and similarities do exist, beginning around site −24 (Nishioka and Leder, 1979). The two leaders from human sources interestingly are strongly divergent only at this terminal region, being identical elsewhere (Michelson and Orkin, 1980; Proudfoot and Maniatis, 1980).

A section of DNA about 40 base pairs in length has been shown to be protected by RNA polymerase B (or II) against digestion by DNase 1, a sequence beginning at about site 17 in those given in Table 8.4 where the pentameric nucleotides TATAA or CATAA are found. This portion is frequently referred to variously as the Hogness, Goldberg–Hogness, or TATA "box," but none of these terms is appropriate. In the first place, Pribnow (1975) had described the region several years before Goldberg and Hogness, so it should be referred to as the Pribnow box, as it occasionally is. Secondly, the term TATA is often inaccurate, because for instance, in two of the three α-globin genes given in that table the sequence is CATA, and other combinations are found from protein family to protein family. Consequently, it should be referred to as the promoter signal, a term in use by bacteriologists for many years before the actual primary structure of such sequences was revealed. Experiments involving excision of a 21-base-pair section of DNA including the TATAA series and its subsequent insertion into various foreign nucleotide sequences have supplied data supporting the view that this signal is both essential and sufficient for initiation of transcription by RNA polymerase B (Sassone-

Corsi *et al.*, 1981). It works together with a "cap site," an -AC doublet that receives one or more modified bases (Dillon, 1978a, p. 132); distance of this site from the promoter signal appears to vary with the protein and organism, but it frequently is in the range of 21 to 27 base pairs. Its distance from the origin of translation also varies extensively, but of course the RNA polymerase is not concerned with that aspect of protein synthesis, only with the production of RNA. However, the cap site proved not to be essential to transcription in a study on β globin, initiation occurring about 30 nucleotides on the $3'$ side of the promoter regardless of the nature of the primary structure in the region (Grosveld *et al.*, 1981). However, caution must be exercised with use of these or other signals, for it has now been clearly demonstrated that the promoters of transcription for tRNAs are actually internal parts of the genes, being those sectors that encode much of arms II and V (Sharp *et al.*, 1981). Consequently, the TATAA and other combinations may prove not to be of real significance in initiation, at least in particular instances.

8.1.4. The Nature of the β-Globin Genes

The β-Globin Family of Genes. The β-globin family of genes in man, arranged on the short arm of chromosome 11, consists of five members arranged in the sequence (beginning from the $5'$ terminus) ϵ, $^G\gamma$, $^A\gamma$, δ, and β (Flavell *et al.*, 1978; Efstratiadis *et al.*, 1980; Spritz *et al.*, 1980), but the number varies with the species. In the mouse the family includes six components, whereas in the rabbit only four are present, and one of these is a pseudogene (Lacy and Maniatis, 1980; Leder *et al.*, 1980; Shen and Maniatis, 1980). Since the latter number is found also in chickens (Dolan *et al.*, 1981; Villeponteau and Martinson, 1981), it seems to represent the total in the common ancestral reptilian stock, or perhaps even that of earlier forms. Hence, the presence of two γ-globin genes in the human family is probably the result of a duplication, as is obviously evidenced by their near-identity of structure. In each case the sequence of appearance during development follows the chromosomal arrangement, beginning at the $5'$ member, ϵ in the case of human beings.

The $3'$ Untranslated Region. It is unfortunate that the primary structure of the ζ-globin gene of man has not been determined to permit more meaningful comparisons of the respective globin gene families. However, even the highly variable trains of these genes indicate a closer kinship between ϵ globin and the α globins than between the former and most other β globins (Table 8.2). In the first place, this train is much shorter in the ϵ locus than in those of the γ and β globins. Hence, it appears self-evident that evolutionary advancement involves the lengthening of this gene sector, the two adult members (δ and β) being nearly identically longer than the others, while the two γ genes are intermediate. Comparison of the primary structures of the respective proteins (Table 8.1) also supports these conclusions of closest relations between the embryonic genes (ϵ, ζ, and γ) and greater kinship distance between the α and β families in adult components, as shown later in more detail.

One marked feature of the ϵ-globin train is the departure from the others at its extreme 5' end, where a guanosine is present before the translation termination signal that is lacking in the rest (Table 8.2). Moreover, the signal involved in termination of transcription differs greatly from the others, the hexanucleotide ending in TGA in place of the AAA consistently present in the remainder (Baralle et al., 1980). Quite unpredictably, this signal is divergent also in the γ-globin primary structure, a guanosine replacing the thymidine that uniformly marks the rest. Another unusual trait characterizes this latter type, for polyadenylation apparently occurs on a -CT dinucleotide, not on -CA as elsewhere. Here then in these signals is additional evidence of the nonmechanical nature of life.

The Nature of the Introns of β-Globin Genes. One of the features of the globin genes that intimates the common ancestry of the α and β families is the presence of two introns in closely corresponding positions (Figure 8.2). However, in all the β globins the first intron lies between the codons for amino acids 30 and 31, whereas in the α globins, it is placed between 31 and 32. Similarly, the second intron of β globins interrupts the coding sequence at codon 104, not at 99 as in the α series (Proudfoot et al., 1980); moreover, it is always much longer in the former type than in the latter, ranging in the

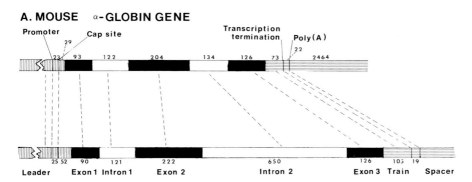

A. MOUSE α-GLOBIN GENE

B. MOUSE β-GLOBIN GENE

Figure 8.2. Structures of the globin gene in the mouse. In this as in other mammals, the genes for each of the α-globin (A) and β-globin (B) families consist of three exons (shown in black), separated by two introns (light stipple); the members of each family differ approximately as indicated, corresponding parts being connected by broken lines. In addition, the genes also bear a leader (vertical ruling) including promoter and cap-site signals, and a train (horizontal ruling) containing transcription-termination and poly(A)-site signals. The portion that follows the latter is here considered part of the intergenic spacer. (Based in part on Nishioka and Leder, 1979, and van Ooyen et al., 1979.)

human genes from about 600 base pairs to nearly 900 in contrast to around 150 in the α (Table 8.3).

As already pointed out, a second intimation of the kinship between the two families is provided by the source of the first nucleotide residue in all the sequences in which this trait was adequately observed (Michelson and Orkin, 1980; Slightom *et al.*, 1980). The final nucleotide in the last codon in the first exon seems consistently to be employed as the first residue in this intron, joining with a thymidine in serving as one end of a future splicing site. Since in most cases the last nucleotide in the intron is also a guanidine, no change occurs after this sector is removed enzymatically and the exons are spliced, but in the human δ and ϵ genes, the adenosine residue that is located here (Table 8.3) would effect a change in the codon but not in the amino acid that is encoded. Although the sequences in that table have been maximized for homology in the usual fashion, correspondences within introns 1 of the β family are scarce, being most frequent between the ϵ and $^A\gamma$ genes and decreasing toward the β unit proper, which shows few relationships to the others. Similarly this sector of the β gene displays kinship only to that of α_1 of man or the murine α, whereas the corresponding region of the ϵ-globin gene has a greater number of homologies with the latter, albeit frequently on a neighborhood basis rather than point to point.

Much the same observations can be made with the intron-2 nucleotide sequences. However, as already seen, the initial G never is derived from the last preceding codon as is uniformly the case in introns 1 (Table 8.3). Because of the great interfamily differences in length of these introns, provision of full sequences of the β-family members would be futile, for beyond the first 24 sites almost no homologies with the α family can be observed until the region near the 3' terminus is attained. But even in the latter sector it is easy to overdo efforts at homologization of the few sequences that have been established. What is needed before reasonable conclusions can be drawn are the primary structures of many more globin genes, especially from marsupials and monotremes and from reptilian, amphibian, and piscine sources. Here, as before, relationships are more readily perceptible between the ϵ and $^A\gamma$ sequences than between the remainder of the β series, as well as between the former and the α_1.

The Leader Sequences of β-Globin Genes. As in the foregoing sectors, the leader sequences suggest a close kinship to exist between the embryonic (ϵ) and fetal ($^A\gamma$) β genes and diminishing ones between the adult genes and the α-family members (Table 8.4). But, also as before, a quick and easy solution to the problem of the probable phylogeny is not provided by these few sequences. Nonetheless, while a convincing evolutionary history must await the primary structures of genes from both embryonic and adult fish and prochordates, some interesting points of correspondence can be noted even at this advanced level of phylogenetic development. The first concern is the promoter signal, in which various modifications of the embryonic and fetal heptanucleo-

Table 8.4
Comparisons of Leader Sequences of Globin Genes

```
              -100       -90        -80        -70        -60        -50
Mouse α[a]    -CAGCCCTTGGAGG--GCATATAAG-TGCTACTTGCGCAGGTCCAAGACACTT

Human α₂[b]   TGCCCCCGCGCCCCAAGCATAAA---CCCTGGCGCGCTCGCGGCCCGGCACT-

Human α₁[c]   TGCCCCCGCGCCCCAAGCATAAA---CCCTGGCGCGCTCGCGGCCCGGCACT-

Mouse β[d]    CAGGA-GCCAGGCAGAGCATATAAGGTGAGTAGGATCAGTTGCTCCTCACATT

Human δ[e]    CAGGAGGACAGGACCAGCATAAAAGGCAGGGCAGAGTCGACTGTTGCTTACAC

Human ᴬγ[f]   GCTGGCTAGGGATGAAGAATAAAAGGAAGCACCCTTCAGCAGTTCCACACACT

Human ε[g]    GAACTTCGGCAGTAAAGAATAAAAGGCCAGACAGAGAGGCAGCAGCACATATC

              -40        -30        -20        -10        -1
Mouse α       --CTGATTCTGACAGACTCA----GACTCAGGAAGAA--------ACCATG

Human α₂      --CTTCTGGTCCC---CACA----GACTCAGAGAGAACCC-----ACCATG

Human α₁      --CTTCTGGTCCC---CACA----G------AGAGAACCC-----ACCATG

Mouse β       ---TGCTTCTGACATAGTTGTGTTGACTCAC--AGA-C-------ATCATG

Human δ       --TTTCTTCTGACATAACAGTGTTCACTAGCAACCTCAAACAGACACCATG

Human ᴬγ      CGCTTCTGGAACGTCTGAGATTATCAATAAGCTCCTAGTCCAGACGCCATG

Human ε       TGCTTCCGACACAGCTGCAATCACTAGCAAGCTCTCAGGCCTGGCATCATG
```

[a]Nishioka and Leder (1979).
[b]Proudfoot and Maniatis (1980).
[c]Michelson and Orkin (1980).
[d]Konkel et al. (1978), van Ooyen et al. (1979).
[e]Spritz et al. (1980).
[f]Slightom et al. (1980).
[g]Baralle et al. (1980).

tide AATAAAA occur; in the adult human types of both families this has become CATAAAA, except that in the two α genes the final adenosine has been lost along with the post-signal guanosine. These two residues are retained in both murine adult sequences in which the signal has been altered to CATATAA. Thus, the adult signals are identical in each mammal but differ from those of embryonic and fetal types. The significance of a guanosine consistently preceding the promotor is not known, but merits attention.

In the 3' half of the leader, a trend toward diminution of sequence length becomes a marked trait in adult sequences, for beginning after site 50, an increasing number of hyphens have been inserted to bring out the homologies of structure, including the near-universal initiation sequence ATG. The ε and ᴬγ chains are longest, the δ is decreased by two base pairs, and the mouse β and all the α-globin leaders are much shorter. Thus, it is apparent that the origins of these genes by duplication or other mechanism must also have involved this leader sequence to some extent in order to have brought about and maintained the correspondences that obviously exist.

The Pseudogenes of the Globins. Since much of pseudogene structure in the α-globin gene family has already received mention, the principal focus now is upon those of the β family, with a few pertinent details pertaining to the former added at times. In the rabbit, four β-like genes have been cloned and their structure and arrangement on the chromosome determined (Hardison *et al.*, 1979; Lacy *et al.*, 1979), numbered from 4 to 1 in descending order in the $5' \rightarrow 3'$ orientation. Recently the one that had been known as β_2 has had its primary structure analyzed and was shown to be a pseudogene, now to be referred to as $\psi\beta_2$. It is obvious that this nomenclature differs from that employed in the human α-globin family, in which the pseudogenes were numbered separately from active ones, a practice followed also with the human β-globin family (Lewin, 1981c).* In the rabbit genome, a number of mutations have occured, so that $\psi\beta_2$ differs greatly from β_1 in its base sequence—even their $5'$ flanking regions have proven to be only 71% homologous (Lacy and Maniatis, 1980). Among the most deleterious defects in the $\psi\beta_2$ that interfere with either its transcription or translation is the occurrence of a translation-initiation codon (ATG) at the usual cap site in the leader, as well as one at its typical location. Even more serious is an apparent deletion involving the last nucleotide of codon 20 that results in a frame shift leading to premature termination. Moreover, the $3'$ ends of both intervening segments have been altered in such a fashion that the splicing clues have been lost, so that even if the sequence were transcribed, the processing of the nascent precursor might not be feasible. Similar alterations in the GA/TA excision signals in intron 1 have resulted in two β pseudogenes in the goat (Cleary *et al.*, 1981), but a later discussion indicates such changes do not always have such an effect.

The seven cloned members of the β-globin gene family in the mouse have been named in still different fashion, the numbering ascending in the $5' \rightarrow 3'$ direction, not descending as the rabbit and mankind, so that the gene sequence given was ϵY_3, βH_0, βH_1, βH_3, β major, β minor (Jahn *et al.*, 1980). The major and minor species differ by nine amino acids, for a homology rate of 95.1% (Konkel *et al.*, 1979). βH_3 proved to be defective in the $5'$ half preceding codon 75, and a frame-shift mutation at codon 90 likewise interferred with the translation of the sequence. Hence, this segment of DNA was recognized as a pseudogene but was not renamed. It should be noted that two additional embryonic genes exist, ϵY_1 and ϵY_2, which were not present in the cloned segment. That the pseudogenes in the respective globin families represent separate evolutionary events is made clear by the description in the mouse

*As the latter procedure allows greater flexibility in naming the pseudogenes as they are discovered, it appears to be preferable to the murine system, but the adoption of some uniform scheme that would facilitate comparative studies is imperative.

α-globin gene family of a pseudogene (α_3) that has lost both introns and has become inactivated (Nishioka *et al.*, 1980). Because the mouse pseudogene was claimed to be otherwise largely homologous to the α_1 gene (despite the presence of several significant regions of deletions and additions), it was proposed that the clean loss of the introns was mediated either through the involvement of the mRNA or its complementary DNA. However, the loss of the introns in this case really may have been secondary to the effects of the deletions and additions, for a recombinant rat preproinsulin gene proved to be normally active without the single intron usually present (Gruss *et al.*, 1981).

Investigations into the human family of β-globin genes have likewise demonstrated independent origins of pseudogenes (Lewin, 1981c). The $\psi\beta_2$ and $\psi\beta_1$ genes of man have been reported to be absent in the gorilla and baboon, but it is quite possible that they were overlooked, for the gene arrangements in those primates have been shown to be otherwise identical to the human series. These two pseudogenes likewise obviously share independent origins, for $\psi\beta_2$ is located to the 5' side of the ϵ gene and $\psi\beta_1$ is placed between the $^A\gamma$ and δ sequences, slightly closer to the former than to the latter (Efstratiadis *et al.*, 1980; Fritsch *et al.*, 1980). The baboon's β-gene family differs further from those of the man and gorilla in that the δ gene is not expressed. At lower levels among primates, the fetal γ gene is not duplicated as in the hominoids, and in the most primitive forms, such as various lemurs, only three functional genes plus a pseudogene comprise the β family. These are set much more closely together than at higher levels, the intergenic spacers being shorter even than those of the rabbit. The pseudogene ($\psi\beta$) of these prosimians apparently represents the remnants of a former active δ gene. Since the genome is identical in the two species of lemurs that have been investigated, it would appear that the primordial ancestral stock of this mammalian order had four genes representing this family, including an active δ sequence that underwent degenerative mutation early in the lemur branch. The general presence of the δ gene in the evolving forebears of the various orders is indicated by the location of a pseudogene ($\psi\beta_2$) at a corresponding position in the rabbit (Efstratiadis *et al.*, 1980; Lewin, 1981c). Thus, the primitive structure of the β-globin families probably embraced four genes, closely set on a single chromosome in the sequence ϵ, γ, δ, and β.

8.1.5. Evolutionary Changes in Globin Genes

That the globin gene families of mammals provide an ideal basis for analyses of evolutionary histories at the molecular level has certainly not gone unnoticed in the literature (Konkel *et al.*, 1979; Nishioka and Leder, 1979; Efstratiadis *et al.*, 1980; Leder *et al.*, 1980; Proudfoot and Maniatis, 1980; Slightom *et al.*, 1980; Lewin, 1981c; Liebhaber *et al.*, 1981). However, most of these accounts have viewed the problem on a limited basis, sometimes being

restricted to a single family of these genes or to those of a particular mammalian taxon, or even to a single pair of sequences. However, what has now been
learned of the two globin families offers an unusual opporunity to examine
evolutionary processes at the gene level from a much broader point of view.

A Basic Principle in Erecting Phylogenies. One of the principles that
must be applied during an analysis of this extent is the so-called biogenetic
law, which is often succinctly expressed as "ontogeny recapitulates phylogeny." Although this principle in its original form has been capably shown to
be biologically untenable (Gould, 1980), the developmental changes undergone
by vertebrate embryos would become meaningless in the absence of the light
cast by a looser interpretation. Further, invertebrate zoology would be deprived
of one of its main guideposts to relationships among the metazoan phyla, if
ontogeny may no longer be considered to reflect phylogenetic history. Just as
few biologists follow Darwin's theory of speciation in its original form, whereas
most still accept it in the modified framework of neo-Darwinism, a less stringent statement of the present principle appears a biological necessity. Thus, the
biogenetic law here is to be phrased: *The developmental stages of higher organisms often reflect past events in phylogeny.* The word "often" is employed
because of an occasional lack of a reflection of such influences; for example,
earthworms develop directly into the adult form, whereas clam worms have
marked developmental stages, including a trochophore larva.

From this point of view then, if all globin genes are at least distantly
related, as appears to be the case, the ζ and ϵ globins should be considered
most like the ancestral stock since they are from the embryo, and the α and β
globins of adults the most highly derived ones. The final decision as to which
of the two developmental ones most probably reflects the single actual precursorial sequence must await the determination of the globin genes of prevertebrate chordates, particularly those from embryonic or larval sources, but a preliminary choice is made later. In theory, one would suspect that the primordial
functional globin molecule consisted of four identical subunits, but only two
could have been present at the very earliest stages of its origin. While it has
been speculated that the globin molecule may have been derived from some
ancient heme-containing protein, such as certain cytochromes, no firm evidence
exists to support that view. The β sequence from frogs of the genus *Rana*
(Table 8.1) implies that the primordial gene was slightly shorter than those of
mammals and birds, but its abbreviated length could equally be a reflection of
independent mutation among the Salientia branch of the Amphibia.

Evolution by Gene Duplication. It is generally accepted that gene duplication plays a fundamental role in the evolution of gene families, a principle
well supported by the evidence presented by the two globin gene clusters.
Moreover, as was already shown in a previous section, many genes of a great
diversity of types likewise occur in proximity on segments of the same chromosome. For instance, the cuticle genes of *Drosophila* consisting of five im-

munologically related members expressed in different ratios during development are grouped in a 36-kilobase sector of DNA (Snyder *et al.*, 1981). In like fashion the histone genes in newts are first grouped into clusters containing coding sequences for all types of those protein; then these clusters are tandemly repeated up to 800 times per haploid genome, each repeat unit being separated by a long spacer (Stephenson *et al.*, 1981). In contrast, in man the histone genes are clustered but are not tandemly repeated (Heintz *et al.*, 1981).

Origins of the Globin Genes. Since the globin genes have been so thoroughly explored at the molecular level, at least in mammals, they can be employed to suggest a possible phylogeny of a gene family, or better, of two closely related gene families. Obviously serious flaws exist in this analysis, as they must in any other that is similarly based on the structure of genes from mammals or comparably highly evolved organisms. Only when the full complement of gene structure of the embryonic, larval, and adult forms of these substances from the primitive members of the phylum have been established will a true picture of the phylogeny emerge. Thus, the present account should be taken merely as a guide to the deductive processes that should be employed when the necessary information finally is available.

As a basis for the present account, the primary structures of the translational products are used (Table 8.1), those of the human being and mouse providing the main foundation, as they are the only ones fully determined. Along with these are also given the embryonic member (ρ) of the chick β-globin family and one representative each of the α and β genes from amphibians to indicate the relations of the mammalian forms with those of lower levels. In addition, the amino acid sequence of leghemoglobin C_2 from soybean is included (Hurrell and Leach, 1977), because it has entered into some related discussions in recent years. One striking feature that becomes immediately apparent upon examining the sequences is that exon 1 of the murine β sequence corresponds quite closely to that of the human δ throughout its length, whereas the murine and human α chains differ much more widely. Another prominent trait of this exon is the extensive homology* that exists at the 3' end throughout the spectrum presented in Table 8.1, whereas to the contrary, many fewer identities can be found at the 5'-terminal region. Probably the first condition may be correlated to the marked folding that exists in that region of the tertiary structure (Gō, 1981).

It is strange, though, that a similar constancy of structure does not prevail in the 5'-terminal sector of exon 2, a region involved with others of this exon in attachment of the heme prosthetic unit (Gō, 1981). The members of the

---

*The homology is furthered if it is noted that alanine, aspartic and glutamic acids, glycine, and threonine are virtual equivalents and appear to be freely substituted for one another during phylogenetic events, despite the differences that obviously exist in their acidity and other physicochemical properties.

β-gene family are remarkably uniform here in the first 11 positions, even including the *Rana* gene, strongly suggesting a functional relationship of vital importance. In the α-gene family, to the contrary, only rare homologies with the β family are in evidence, except for the proline and threonine in the sixth and eighth positions of the exon, respectively. Furthermore, the former of these is absent from the *Ambystoma* peptide. Such occasional harmonies between the α and β series characterize the entire exon, despite the region's serving as the principal support for the heme unit in both families. An additional point of attachment to the prosthetic group is provided in exon 3 by the occupant of the penultimate site in which tyrosine is universally present. The 5' end of this portion is still more constant, the presence of leucylleucine in all sequences save that of *Ambystoma* being especially outstanding. In all the mammalian members of the α series, this pair of amino acids is followed by the nonapeptide sequence SHCLLVTLA, whereas in those of the β series only a pair of amino acid residues (GN) is consistent. When the members of both series are scanned, such contrasts in constancies between the α and β sets are seen to be frequent characteristics of this sector of the molecules.

Two other points need to be made before actually proposing a phylogeny for this class of proteins, the first of which pertains to the nature of the exons. Despite the claim to the contrary (Gō, 1981), a clear correlation between exon subdivisions and function is definitely lacking. It is obvious that both exons 2 and 3 are required to support the heme group; hence, each cannot be a distinct structural domain, and, since this is the case, it is extremely unlikely that exon 2 represents a fusion of two former exons, as that reference also proposed. But what should be stressed even more is that the exons are present only in the DNA and precursorial transcripts; they are in no way evident in the final translational products—the gaps between exons shown in the table are artifacts, introduced only for the purpose of convenience in the discussion. As it is these translational products that are acted upon by natural selection, favored genes and gene structures are perpetuated only indirectly through selective conservation of their products. What advantage the introduction of introns into gene makeup provides has not been demonstrated, but so far as is evident to this point, it perhaps represents an improved method for protein synthesis evolved in the eukaryotes, as shown in a previous discussion.

The second major point is that leghemoglobins of legumes show no correspondence to those of vertebrates above the 5% homology level provided by random chance. It is peculiar that the gene consists of parts, two of which fall at points similar to those of the vertebrate series (Jensen *et al.*, 1981), and it may be that a gene was introduced via a transforming virus into an ancestral legume, perhaps from an invertebrate (Lewin, 1981a)—it certainly was not from a vertebrate nor an insect! But until the primary structures of the hemoglobins and their genes have been determined from one of the relatively few invertebrate metazoans that possess such proteins, that possibility must remain sheer speculation.* The confinement of leghemoglobins to the bacteria-containing nodules which are subterranean structures, makes the suggestion of vectorial transmission of the gene even less palatable.

8.1.6. The Evolution of Globin Genes

Although the concept that genes undergo changes in structure by evolutionary processes is a nearly universally accepted biological principle, only the recent advances in knowledge provided by the relative ease of determining the actual structure of genes (Gilbert, 1981) have begun to make feasible the opening of vistas into the processes that bring about such alterations. The broadest such insight that thus far has been gained is provided by current knowledge of the hemoglobins, so that here the foregoing discussion may be continued into a speculative account of the steps that seem to have been followed in the development of the two families of genes.

The First Globin Gene. To begin the search for a logical phylogenetic history of the globin genes, it is first essential to determine the type most likely to be kin to the original ancestral form. Here the factual basis for the search is a summary of the homologies that exist between pairs of genes, arranged to show relationships by both the several exons and the total counts (Table 8.5). The latter given for any particular type results from summarizing all five combinations, so that the total (423) given for ϵ globin is arrived at by adding those of α–ϵ, ζ–ϵ, β–ϵ, δ–ϵ, and γ–ϵ. All except the β globin, which is murine, represent human proteins, and each is based on the sequences in Table 8.1.

From examination of the percentages given under the total column, it is immediately apparent that the two members of the α family (α and ζ) show homology relationships only near the 40% level, whereas all the members of the β family display levels higher than 50%. Since there are four members of the latter family in these comparisons and only two in the former, it is tempting to view the inequity of kinship ratios as a result of this bias. However, further analysis shows this not to be entirely the case. First it is obvious that α and ζ display about the same degree of similarity between themselves as α does with the β-family members, with the exception of ζ. The same statement is true for ϵ globin, but here the ratio of homology is greater with several β-like sequences, β globin itself being exceptionally low in this instance. Thus, the β family is much more homogeneous than the α, and the contrasting adult genes

---

*The detrimental effect of unfounded speculation in the scientific literature is that it removes attention from the important issue to a trivial one. The really significant aspect of the leghemoglobin gene is its origin in relative isolation among seed plants, but thoughtful examination of the problem would have revealed comparable isolated instances of hemoglobin genes in three genera of unrelated insects and certain other invertebrates. The origin of that protein in each of these instances is the fundamental problem requiring investigation, not a supposed vectorial horizontal introduction of a gene from one species to another.

of the two families are more closely related to one another than they are with the embryonic member of the opposite family; that is, α is more closely akin to β and δ than it is to ϵ, and β resembles α to a greater degree than it does ζ. But the same condition does not prevail for δ, the other adult β-like gene, for there is only one site difference between the comparing sets, 62 for δ with α, and 63 for δ with ζ.

On the basis of these figures, along with the ontogenetic principle, the conclusion is unavoidable that either the ζ- or ϵ-globin gene arose first, and the fact that the latter has more numerous descendants than the former makes it more probable that ϵ is most like the progenitory stock. Thus, the very first prochordate globin likely will prove to have a subunit structure similar to ϵ_4, or even more probably ϵ_2. The relatively high level of relationship between ζ and ϵ, too, suggests that the former arose from the latter by gene duplication early in chordate history and that the two evolved largely in parallel throughout vertebrate evolution. The fact that γ and ϵ display the highest rate of homology (76%) of any contrasting pair of sequences intimates that the γ gene also arose early by duplication of the ϵ gene, so a γ-like globin should be expected to occur in some of the more advanced prevertebrate chordates. The similarity between ζ and δ also implies this close relationship between both embryonic and early fetal genes.

The subsequent origins of the δ and β genes by additional duplications (probably of γ) are more or less routine; what does present a perplexing problem is the origin of the α gene. Since the main difficulty stems from the α and β families being located on separate chromosomes, the more acceptable proposal appears to be that the ζ arose by duplication on the 5' side of the ϵ, whereas the members of the β family arose on the 3' side, as they are now arranged in the higher vertebrates, an observation nicely supported by the decreasing relationship displayed by the β-like family members with increasing distance from ϵ. Then later the segment containing the ζ-like gene became translocated onto a separate chromosome. After this transposition had taken place, the ζ gene diverged evolutionarily from its ϵ forebear for a time sufficient to lengthen the first exon by one residue, shorten the second intron, and gain the other major characteristics of the α-globin family. Only after these steps had been consummated did a gene duplication establish the basis for the origin of the α-globin gene proper. On each chromosome other duplications occurred as the vertebrates evolved further, but most of these transpired at the level of class or order, as in the α_1, α_2, and $\psi\alpha_1$ genes of man.

Evolutionary Changes in Exon Structure. Although only the definitive globin molecule would appear to be subject to natural selective influences, some features of the individual exons are difficult to account for in other terms. Both the amino acid sequences (Table 8.1) and the counts of homologous sites (Table 8.5) indicate that exon 1, whose product does not support the heme unit, has undergone the most frequent mutation and shows a mean count of

Table 8.5
Comparisons of Human Globin Primary Structures by Exons

	Exon 1 (33)^a	Exon 2 (74)	Exon 3 (43)	Total (150)
α–ζ	8	26	29	63
α–β	18	26	17	61
α–δ	16	31	15	62
α–γ	15	32	17	64
α–ε	12	27	13	52
Total α	69 (41%)	142 (38%)	91 (42%)	302 (40%)
ζ–β	6	32	14	52
ζ–δ	10	37	16	63
ζ–γ	10	44	19	73
ζ–ε	8	43	18	69
Total ζ	42 (25%)	182 (50%)	96 (45%)	320 (43%)
β–δ	16	53	30	99
β–γ	16	52	24	92
β–ε	14	48	28	90
Total β	70 (42%)	211 (57%)	113 (53%)	394 (52%)
δ–γ	12	58	28	98
δ–ε	14	56	30	100
Total δ	68 (41%)	235 (64%)	119 (54%)	422 (56%)
γ–ε	16	65	31	114
Total γ	69 (41%)	251 (68%)	119 (55%)	439 (60%)
Total ε	64 (39%)	239 (64%)	120 (56%)	423 (56%)
Total for exon	191	630	329	1152
Mean for exon	13 (39%)	42 (57%)	22 (57%)	77 (51%)

^{a}Number of sites per unit.

only 13 invariable sites in the sequences out of the possible 33, for a homology rate of 39%. In the other two exons, the mean homology rate stands above 50% as does the total of the whole (Table 8.5). Despite this low overall constancy, the five residues before the termination of exon 1 show remarkable uniformity, for even the *Rana* β and chick ρ sequences have -EALAR, while the mammalian genes differ at one or two sites. It is also interesting that the α gene of *Ambystoma* is more closely related in this sector to the β family of genes of mammals than to the α-family members from the same taxon as expected.

At the very beginning of the second exon, a 10-site sequence is found that is remarkably uniform among all the β-family members but is rather variable among those of the α group. Indeed, this is followed by an additional 10- or 12-site-long region that displays much the same characteristics, that is, uniformity in the β family and variability in the other. At a short distance beyond these areas are five residues in the β-globin-like sequences that are missing in all the rest. Hence, the ζ gene must have experienced a deletion in this region shortly after it was translocated, so that its α-duplication has the same basic characteristics here as elsewhere.

Changes in Intron Structure. When the full gene structure of many more globin genes have been determined from a wide variety of source animals, then the intron sequences doubtlessly will prove capable of enriching the account of the evolutionary history of these heme proteins. At the present time, the sparsity of available information (Table 8.3) permits little more than the conclusion arrived at by numerous other investigators, to the effect that the structure of introns is not subject to as severe constraints as that of the exons and therefore has become greatly varied. Only the 5' and 3' termini appear to hold much survival value, in that they are involved in the splicing of the transcripts. Because the introns of the two human α genes are so largely homologous, it is at once evident that the duplication of these genes occurred recently. And since they differ widely from that of the mouse, the duplication must have occurred on the hominoid line, an observation supported by their being present also in the great ape genomes (Zimmer *et al.*, 1980). But a sufficient number of differences occurs between pairs to make unacceptable the concept that the near-identity of these or other gene pairs is maintained by exchange of genetic information (Slightom *et al.*, 1980). To maintain the sequence integrity of exons without affecting intron structure in like fashion is presently inconceivable. The loss of corresponding sections in the members of the human α-gene pair is indicative of its having occurred independently; a similar absent segment in the mouse β gene cannot represent relationships to those two genes, because it is also present in the murine α sequence.

In view of intron 2 being much longer in all components of the β-globin family than in those of the α, it is quite likely that the primordial ζ gene underwent a deletion in this region prior to its giving rise to the α gene, as suggested earlier. The unevenness in length of this intervening segment among the embryonic, fetal, and adult members of the β family probably represents independent reductions in each case through deletions from a primitive form in which more than 845 residues intervened between the terminal sectors shown in Table 8.3. But at the same time the persistence of additional length of this intron over that of the corresponding sector of α genes compels the inference that the length of segment has considerable survival value in the β family that is not evident in the other.

In summary, the phylogenetic events proposed here are (1) the origin of the ϵ gene in a primitive prochordate; (2) the occurrence of two gene duplication events, one on the 3' side, the other on the 5' side of ϵ; (3) the latter ultimately led to the evolution of a precursorial δ gene, whereas the former became translocated to another chromosome; (4) the translocated duplicated gene was subjected to modification to become the forebear of the ζ gene, after which another duplication event provided the basis for that of α globin; (5) in the meanwhile the γ gene underwent successive duplications that evolved into the δ and β genes. Later at higher levels of vertebrate phylogeny, separate and independent duplications of various genes occurred (often followed by degeneration into pseudogenes) that characterize various orders or families of these organisms.

8.1.7. Effect on Evolutionary Concepts

If the foregoing phylogeny is reconsidered in light of current evolutionary thought, certain of the problems in that discipline become clarified to a degree. Chief among these is the apparent absence of survival value of the differing isozyme patterns between tissues or the changes in type of a given protein that occur during ontogeny. Here a proposal is formulated that provides a regimen for future deductions on this aspect of evolutionary change.

The Nature of Embryonic and Fetal Genes. In the first place, it is evident that the genes of early embryos are to be considered as reflections of the primordial gene in each family of proteins or RNAs. Since this would be the case with all the genes that have undergone phylogenetic changes, the cells themselves in early development are to be viewed as primitive, as is also the fertilized egg from which they are derived. This suggestion obviously is only an extension of the recapitulation theory to the macromolecular level of organization. The degree of gametic and embryonic primitiveness probably varies with the taxon. Thus, the ovum and sperm of a coelenterate, for example, would be expected to be less highly diverged from the ancestral metazoan stock than those of mammals, birds, or insects. Consequently, gametes are not an expression of the most distant forebears but only of more immediate ancestors of a given taxonomic unit. Otherwise the gametes of all animals would be identical in protein composition, a condition that would imply that sperm from any source could effectively fertilize the egg of any other animal.

The maintenance of a degree of primitiveness is a function of gametogenesis. In some taxa, such as the vertebrates, the gametes are derived from primordial germ cells set aside early in embryogeny (Chapter 1, Section 1.1.2), so that for all practical purposes their protoplasm is virtually identical to that of the parental egg. However, even in such cases, some of the macromolecules of germ cells have experienced changes that must undergo modification to the zygotic condition during subsequent gametogenesis, thus accounting for the differences in ultrastructure and protein patterns displayed by the successive stadia of gamete formation. Consequently, in those organisms that give rise to gametes from differentiated tissues, reversion of gene expression from an advanced to a more primitive condition must accompany the formation of the sex cells. Because in the majority of the thoroughly studied metazoans, no or little transcription occurs in the zygote, early gene expression is almost exclusively that of the mRNAs supplied to it during egg formation.

Only after the commencement of differentiation do the embryonic cells begin to express their characteristic genes. Although the full complement appears to be present in the genome at that time, those sequences alone that are characteristic of the embryo (including some continued into more advanced stages; for example, Tanksley et al., 1981) are expressed, mainly those that are to be considered more primordial. Thus, the primitive nature of these early cells is maintained by selective reading of the genes—in other words, the primitive cytosol and nucleoplasm (together referred to as the soma of the cell) direct the reading of only the relatively primitive genes during the earliest stages of development. Then as embryogenesis proceeds, environmental influences, including positional effects, induce slight alterations in the programming of the cell soma, so that genes for less primitive members of one or several protein families become transcribed. The resulting products of these transcripts lead to further program changes in the soma of these cells, which then read additional genes of a less primitive nature in other protein gene sets. As the environmental influences differ in the various regions of the early embryo, the extent and kind of effect they exercise would also result in localized differing programming changes, both of a quantitative and qualitative nature. Hence, as development continues, contrasting layers (ectoderm, endoderm, and mesoderm in metazoans) become differentiated, both as to their later fates in the embryo and their present protein contents, as shown in Chapter 3, Sections 3.1.2 and 3.3.2. Another way in which the concept might be expressed is that, as the embryo becomes less primitive in structure, its cells express successively more advanced genes. These processes continue through the juvenile stages into adulthood and, in many instances, even into senescence; although a number of the characteristics of aged individuals undoubtedly represent degenerative effects, these, too, are under the control of the same mechanism.

The Nature of Ontogenetic Changes. Currently it is the vogue to view the characteristic features of the developmental stages of one taxon as reflections of those of other related taxa; that is to say, the various fetal manifestations of mammals resemble the larval stages of fish or amphibians and the like, not former adults. But this concept views only one aspect of the whole picture, in that the origins of the fish or amphibian larval stadia are in turn not considered. If the fish developmental stages are similarly explained on the same basis and those precursors in succession into more and more remote past events, the conclusion ultimately must be reached that even the most primordial forms had larvae similar to those of fish and therefore to mammalian fetuses! This is totally absurd, because somewhere, somehow, the early larval types had to have an origin of a more meaningful nature. Consequently, one is compelled to consider the embryonic and fetal characteristics as reflections of past ancestral adults, but highly modified, of course.

The word that is important here is "reflections," and those seen darkly. Developmental stages are not precise copies of an ancestral form, nor even models, for their function is not that of providing biologists with phylogenetic information, but only that of developing into juveniles that can grow and differentiate into the adult form. And only when that stage has been attained do the gonads develop and become functional, even though the ancestral stock which the embryos mirror must have had active reproductive organs. Similarly other organs of the developmental stages have undergone great modification in becoming adapted for the more immediate needs.

As was seen earlier in the discussion of the phylogeny of hemoglobins, this view is testable and will be tested when the gene structure and amino acid sequences of globins from appropriate prochordates and larval cyclostomes are established. And, beyond that in the future, further detailed analyses of gene families in a wide spectrum of types, whether vertebrate, arthropod, annelid, gymnosperm, or other, will test this point of view and either establish its soundness or expose its frailities. But at the present time, it appears to be the only premise that explains the available data.

8.2. THE SUPRAMOLECULAR GENETIC MECHANISM

A second new concept, advanced under the term "cellular genetic mechanism," was necessitated by the complexities of organization of the macromolecules and ultrastructural features of the cell (Dillon, 1981, pp. 175, 176, 313–316, 556–558). There this apparatus, now referred to by the more descriptive term "supramolecular genetic mechanism," was revealed as an organized unit within the cytosol and nucleoplasm in eukaryotes that was responsible for directing the processing, distribution, and assembly of the products synthesized in crude form by the familiar DNA–RNA–protein system. As a result of the present study at the organismic level, this view must be extended to include genetic functions in a stricter sense, the behavior of immunologic components being especially compelling in this matter, as shown later in this discussion.

Implications of Developmental Changes in Gene Expression. One of the problems of developmental biology that was addressed in the preceding section was the nature of the innumerable changes in gene expression that occur during embryogenesis and differentiation. Such sequential alterations in the transcription of the genome were shown to characterize the life cycles of almost all organisms, including prokaryotes, protistans such as the ciliates, and higher eukaryotes, including fungi, seed plants and their relatives, and invertebrates, as well as vertebrates. Thus, their universality of occurrence, above the viral level at least, has been thoroughly documented.* What requires attention beyond their mere existence is how such changes are consummated. The present proposal, being of necessity entirely speculative, needs to be tested by appropriate experimental analyses.

In former years it was widely believed that the selective reading of particular gene sets was governed by positioning of either the histones or, later, the nonhistone nuclear proteins upon the DNA. Genes to be transcribed were exposed by relocating these substances to areas that were to be inactivated. Although this device appeared to be logical, no mechanism was indicated for providing the movements of the proteins nor for the precise selection of the genes that were to be activated or concealed. Further, this concept has been demonstrated to be untenable by the results of ultrastructural studies of active and quiescent regions of DNA, including those reported in Chapter 1 (Figures 1.11 to 1.17). In each of those electron micrographs, it is obvious that regions of the chromosome loops not undergoing transcription in no way differ in diameter or appearance from those that are, and the nucleosomes are similarly spaced in all regions.

In seeking a mechanism that can induce, control, or carry out such changing gene activities, the most obvious one, the nature of the DNA, deserves the earliest attention. The single type of change that this gigantic macromolecule can effect is in its configuration, for as discussed in a previous section in all other processes it is the most inert of all cellular organic substances (Dillon, 1978a, p. 121). Thus, it is conceivable that the DNA molecule might be in a more tightly coiled configuration in transcriptionally inactive sectors that would unravel slightly when the developmental state was attained in which the particular sector was then needed. Since changes in pH or ionic content can modify the configuration of DNA, the concept appears to be sound—unless one attempts to determine how the requisite localized ionic or pH modulations are themselves induced. Then it becomes evident that an additional mechanism is required to govern the variations in the chemical properties from one section of the genome to another. Hence, the loosening or tightening of the molecular structure would itself not be a control mechanism but merely an effect of another less obvious one. Additionally this view is invalidated by those electron

*The absence of ontogenetic changes in viruses may be more apparent than real, for at the highest level of viral organization represented by the vaccinia group (Dillon, 1978a, pp. 378, 379, 421, 424), it is possible that modified duplicated genes may be differentially expressed during the life cycle. Little would be expected at lower levels because reproduction largely involves direct growth into the mature form.

micrographs just cited and by numerous others of a similar nature. For it is readily apparent, as just pointed out, that the distance between nucleosomes is comparable in both the transcriptionally active and inactive regions, as would not be the case if unfolding of the DNA backbone were involved. These same observations apply in like fashion to other methods of gene control that have been advocated, such as changes in degree of methylation in active genes (for example, Naveh-Many and Cedar, 1981). Any such alteration does not represent the definitive mechanism, only an intermediate stage.

Consequently, the sole ultimate source of control must lie in the soma of the cell, that is, in the supramolecular genetic apparatus, as no other possible mechanism is in evidence. Phrased in different terms, the soma contains an organized system of proteinaceous, and perhaps other, substances that is somehow programmed to carry out selective reading of particular portions of the genome. The programming must be viewed not as a static arrangement but as sensitive to changes in the immediate environment of the cell and continually subject to modification by some of the products of the genes that are read. In brief, a feedback mechanism exists. At the earliest stages of embryogeny in which transcription occurs, the program is set to read a certain number of genes, especially the more ancestral types, including one group that can be called protein set Q. The components of this set are not to be thought to be concentrated into one region of a certain chromosome but as a diversity of types from families of genes scattered throughout the genome. When the transcripts for this set have been translated, along with the others characteristic of this stage, the products effect a slight change in certain parts of the program, inducing the supramolecular genetic mechanism to read some new genes. The latter would not only encode more advanced replacements for previously synthesized substances, including protein set R, but would also code for additional products. The members of set R whose genes likewise would be scattered about the genome, would lead to another set of program changes, inducing the synthesis of protein set S, and so on throughout development.

Concurrently with this feedback arrangement, environmental factors would also play a role in influencing the programmed activities. Among these influences are those discussed in preceding pages, such as the pH and ionic constitution of the medium, position within the growing embryonic mass, pressure, hormones of various types, especially in mammals, inductive secretions of neighboring cells or tissues, and many others. As a consequence, beginning immediately after the first cleavage of the zygote, the supramolecular genetic mechanism in each individual cell is acted upon by a different spectrum of parameters than its congeners. In some cases the differences between small adjacent areas are too slight to influence distinctive features in the program, so that as multicellularity increases, groups of similar cells are produced that differentiate in chorus, but by and large the programming in each region, including those of early stages comprised of only one or several cells, normally would be subjected to a number of contrasting factors and ultimately would become greatly differentiated along their individual paths.

Reverse Differentiation. Under normal conditions, most cells do not undergo extensive dedifferentiation, and those of higher vertebrates as a rule are unable to do so, possibly as a consequence of their being too complexly specialized. In other words, the genetic programming has diverged so widely from more elementary stages that a step-by-step reversal of the differentiating processes is not feasible. Possibly in part this condition results from the absence of the essential external influences; that is to say, the inductive secretions of neighboring tissues, which changed in successive stages during differentiation, would have to be present in reverse sequence, along with the specific other factors that accompanied each stage. Consequently, as was seen earlier, the muscle fibers of regenerating limbs are unable to degrade into myotubes, and those into myogens. Instead new myogens develop from generalized satellite cells and progress through the respective stages into new muscle tissue, as do the forebears of other types through their particular developmental stadia. Since the various tissues of adult mammals and birds are still more highly differentiated than those of their fetuses, regeneration is largely restricted to replacement of small sectors lost through injury, or it is lacking entirely—for instance, scar tissue is often formed in place of the original epithelium. Liver cells are exceptional, in that they can regenerate the complete organ, as reported in a previous discussion (Chapter 4, Section 4.3), but they lack the high degree of specialization that characterizes the remaining types.

Contrastingly, in many complex organisms, reverse differentiation can occur, as in the formation of gametes from somatic cells and in the seed plants of embryoids from differentiated tissues. One can visualize that the processes involved in these instances require reprogramming the supramolecular genetic apparatus by feedback mechanisms as during development, but in this case they proceed in the opposite direction. Perhaps they originate through synthesis of a more primitive species of proteins under instigation of that mechanism after exposure to inductive influences from external stimuli. Those newly secreted substances then influence the reprogramming of the mechanism to a still less advanced level, which leads to the reading of successively more primitive genes and on and on until the basic level of that taxon is attained with the production of gametes, embryoids, or the like.

Functions in Rhythmic Activities. If the supramolecular genetic apparatus can undergo developmental changes in programming and those alterations are reversible to a degree, it is readily understood how cyclic patterns of gene expression may occur on circadian, circannual, or other biorhythmic basis. In such cases, the modifications in transcription would be produced in repetitious oscillating fashion, under the influence of a clock mechanism perhaps. But it is not unlikely that the rate of change in programming itself provides a part of the clock mechanism, which can be modulated in response to factors in the cell's external environment—including effects of various hormones in vertebrates, seed plants, and other complex organisms. As was seen in Chapter 6, light intensity and duration of photoperiod and temperature are also important parameters in the induction of circadian reprogramming events, but how those influences are asserted needs to be given thorough investigation.

Functions in Regulating Genomic Size and Composition. In Chapter 5, Section 5.5, it was shown that the genome of euciliate macronuclei underwent drastic changes in size and composition as they developed from micronuclei following conjugation. In addition to the expression of new types of histones, macronuclear differentiation was described as including loss of up to one-third of the DNA present in the precursorial micronucleus. Since the macronucleus encodes for the vegetative activities, it is obvious that the extrusion of chromatin that occurs must be selective; both this selectivity and the occurrence of genomic changes have now been demonstrated in *Tetrahymena* (Yao and Yao, 1981; Yao et al., 1981; Yao, 1982). Thus, some control mechanism must exist to regulate which segments of DNA are extruded and which retained, and also to induce the reported changes in genome structure. Similar expulsion of portions of the genome has been described in fungi and certain protists, while the ejection of the entire set of paternal chromosomes characterizes meiosis in a number of dipterans. Obviously, then, there is ample evidence that the cell is able to recognize differing sequences in its chromatin and to distinguish individual chromosomes and even the individual genes. The latter observation also is supported by the selective expression of X chromosomes in many mammals, as well as others, as demonstrated by the widespread occurrence of allelic exclusion. Chromosomes themselves are incapable of any activity; their movements, diakinesis, and other behavioral features are all conducted by the extrachromatin matter, and here are ascribed to functions of the supramolecular genetic apparatus.

It is evident therefore that the opposite type of change, increases in genomic size, also must be ultimately derived from the control of this same mechanism. Multiplication of ploidy in the euciliates during macronucleus formation also was noted previously (Chapter 5, Section 5.5), in one case attaining a level of over $4000n$, while the sequence complexity was reduced to less than 2% that of the micronucleus. In other words, there was extensive, highly selective amplification of small regions of the DNA along with chromatin extrusion, again revealing the effects of a carefully organized control device. Similar selective multiplication of histone genes in amphibians and most other vertebrates is too familiar a phenomenon to require more than mention (Dillon, 1978a, pp. 94, 95), but those processes must likewise be carried out through this same governing mechanism. Related to this activity are the qualitative changes in DNA during development of an amphibian that have recently received attention (Lohmann and Schubert, 1980), in which melting and density gradient patterns became markedly altered during gastrulation. It should be noted that such synthesis of DNA during differentiation characteristically is independent of mitosis (Smith and Vonderhaar, 1981).

One aspect of amplification that is of greater importance to evolutionary than to ontogenetic origins is the presence of highly repetitive noncoding but transcribed DNA elements in the genomes of many eukaryotes, including sea urchins, *Xenopus*, and man (Spohr *et al.*, 1981). Two types of such segments are recognized, satellite DNA and interspersed repetitive DNA. In the first category are placed highly repeated, tandemly linked, simply sequences that usually are confined to the heterochromatin, whereas in the second are included shorter repetitive sequences that are inserted between genes that encode structural or enzymic proteins. These then represent intergenic spacers of a peculiar sort, which differ from most others in that they are transcribed. In fact, both strands of the dual DNA molecule in such regions may be represented in the transcripts, which are confined to the nuclei. Since each of these dispersed elements, consisting of eight tandemly arranged repeated subunits 77 to 79 base pairs in length, has been shown to be repeated 100,000 times in the *Xenopus* genome, it is difficult to propose a logical function for this class of elements.

Moreover, the repeated sequences themselves show the presence of extremely few mutational changes, whereas their flanking regions often have many. Interspersed repetitive DNA has been proposed to serve as a regulatory device for gene expression, but since the amount of particular families of this class of substances varies with the developmental stage and tissue, it is self-evident that some higher mechanism (the supramolecular genetic apparatus) is in turn needed to control their expression, and thus they, like others discussed earlier, become possible intermediaries, not the regulatory device proper. In different terms, these highly repeated elements may prove to serve for recognition, but only if it can be shown that the members of a given family of repeats are interspersed between members of those genes that are expressed during particular stages of development or within a given type of tissue. In view of the large numbers of a given set of repeated DNA sequences that have been reported, it is difficult to conceive that this possibility is other than highly remote. It is also pertinent to note that in the region flanking one such element that has been sequenced (Spohr *et al.*, 1981) are numerous combinations of A's and T's that correspond to the promoter signal, often along with -CA caplike dinucleotides located at a suitable distance. Yet these signals here are not known to induce transcription or capping—again emphasizing the nonmechanistic behavior of living molecular systems.

It is relevant to note that, while the genes for three small nuclear RNAs (U1, U2, and U3) are of universal occurrence among eukaryotic cells, pseudogenes complementary to all three are widely dispersed and abundantly repeated in the human genome (Van Arsdell *et al.*, 1981). In turn, these sequences are flanked wherever they occur by similar direct repetitive DNA sectors; consequently, it has been proposed that the three pseudogenes had undergone multiple translocations into new chromosomal loci, despite the lack of function on their part.

Reprogramming in Cancer Cells. During the induction of a cancerous condition in a given tissue, whether by a virus or a chemical or physical carcinogen, the affected cells undergo a number of changes in structure and physiology, a process known as transformation. In these procedures the alterations in gene expressions that occur are often retrogressive, so that embryonic or fetal proteins become synthesized. For example, hepatomas typically produce α-fetoprotein rather than albumin as normal adult livers do. Consequently, a portion of the transforming steps involves reverse differentiation in stepwise fashion, as in dedifferentiating tissues in various eukaryotes. Not all the changes are of this nature, however; in some cases, especially in those of viral origin, the genome of the infective organism in addition induces new types of programming, foreign to the native cells, but arising in the same manner. That is to say, the cell's supramolecular genetic apparatus is induced to undergo retrogressive reprogramming under the influence of the carcinogenic agents, including the proteins of the virus, and in the latter case, plus the inductive effects of the foreign genome. Thus, embryonic, fetal, and viral DNAs and proteins interact together to produce transformed cells. Such cells often have regained the developmental capacity for undergoing rapid division, a characteristic sometimes not expressed except under favorable conditions. The individual end products of the transformation are thus capable of developing new cancerous growth if they break free of the parental mass and are transported to other favorable organs of the body.

8.3. THE INCONSTANT GENE

In the foregoing discussion, it became evident that the genome is often under direct control of the supramolecular genetic apparatus, especially in quantitative changes of both a positive and negative nature. Because the changes in quantity did not always include the entire DNA complement, however, but characteristically involved only particular portions, they were also qualitative to a large degree. The present section provides data from several different sources to demonstrate that that same mechanism can effect alterations in the genic constitution of organisms in a very direct way.

8.3.1. Inconstant Immunoglobulin Genes

Portions of Chapter 7 reported the behavior of immunoglobulin genes in B lymphocytes after contact with antigen and other factors that induced those cells first to proliferate as they became altered to "memory cells." Then if these slightly modified lymphocytes were exposed to a second contact with the same antigen, they underwent further proliferation and increased in size to develop into plasma cells that secreted antibodies (immunoglobulins) specific against that foreign substance.

The More Obvious Qualitative Changes. As will be recalled, the discussion of the immunoglobulin gene structure (Chapter 7, Section 7.1.5) showed that some of the variability of the antibodies was often attained by several somatic recombinational events. In the λ light chain, it is true, no recombination of genes was involved, for only one genelet each for V_λ, J_λ, and C_λ domains existed. Construction of an Igλ polypeptide chain then merely involved transcription of these three sequences and the intervening segments into a precursorial mRNA, followed by enzymatic removal of the introns and, finally, translation. To the contrary, in Igκ an undetermined number of V_κ genelets existed, separated from a genelet for the C_κ region by four J_κ sequences and a J_κ pseudogene. Hence two rearrangements of a genelet sequence were required in preparing the pregene, the first choosing between one of many V_κ coding segments, while the remainder were not transcribed; the second involved the choice of one of the four active J_κ segments before transcription occurred. It has sometimes been claimed that the sectors that are not selected are deleted, but this view is proving to be simplistic (Cory *et al.*, 1980; Maki *et al.*, 1980).

In heavy-chain production, pretranscriptional events involve preliminary combination of a V_H to a D_H genelet and then one of the four J_H genelets to form the pregene for the V_H domain (Gough and Bernard, 1981); the resulting segment of DNA is then joined to a genelet for one of eight varieties of C_H region, either μ, γ, or so on. As will be recalled, during the earliest stages of B-cell formation, typically the μ genelet is selected. Then when an antigen becomes present, the B cell differentiates further by changing the type of immunoglobulin secreted; such "class switching" occurs in most mammals, the V_H gene then losing its connection to C_μ and characteristically becoming joined to C_γ or C_α. Both in the formation of the heavy and light chains, usually only one allele for a given gene family is expressed in a particular cell and its descendants, but the paternal component may be active in one lymphocyte population and the maternal in the other (Early and Hood, 1981). But a few appear able to express both sets of alleles, at least those for light genes (Cory *et al.*, 1980; Steinmetz and Zachau, 1980).

The foregoing activities are usually referred to as "somatic" rearrangements and allelic exclusion, without further examination of the mechanism involved (Gershenfeld *et al.*, 1981). The chromosomal region itself certainly is incapable of such multiple selective actions, nor is it likely that the RNA polymerase which does the transcription is able to perform them. So again the only available location for a suitable mechanism is in the cell soma. In other words, the supramolecular genetic apparatus conducts the selective expression of the respective alleles, choosing among the various J_L and V_H regions and joining the resulting pregene to the genelet for a constant domain. Once this pattern has been established within a given cell it does not change, except that class switching occurs under the influence of an external or internal stimulus, an antigen perhaps or a developmental state. Then it chooses another C_H gene-let, in some cases by excision of that for the μ chain, because reversal to IgM secretion sometimes does not occur. However, subsequent switches to other classes are often feasible, so that elimination of the remaining C_H genelets is not involved. These observations emphasize both the nonmechanistic nature of the gene and the unlikelihood that mere selective reading by the polymerase lies behind the recombinational events.

A More Profound Type of Change. An even more direct control by the supramolecular genetic apparatus over the genome is evidenced during the preparation of antibody to a given antigen. As shown by a number of investigations into this problem, the formulation of a specific idiotype includes what is called "somatic mutation" (Weigert *et al.*, 1970, 1978; Weigert and Riblet, 1976; Bernard *et al.*, 1978; Brack *et al.*, 1978; Valbuena *et al.*, 1978; Gearhart *et al.*, 1981), a principle that has become well established in immunological researches (Baltimore, 1981). The actual occurrence of this type of genetic mutation has been especially clearly documented by a study of the immune response to phosphorylcholine in BALB/c mice (Crews *et al.*, 1981). Nineteen immunoglobulins were found that bound this chemical, and the complete amino acid sequences of their V_H segments were established. Ten of these proved to have identical sequences in this region, while the remainder were variations that differed by one to eight residues from the common one (referred to as T15). Use of a cloned DNA segment complementary to the T15 sequence permitted the isolation of four V_H genelets from mouse sperm which proved to be homologous, one being identical to T15. Later comparisons of the four V_H genelets with the 19 V_H amino acid sequences demonstrated that all the latter must have arisen from the germline T15 V_H genelet, showing that virtually all the immune response to phosphorylcholine is derived from this single V_H coding sequence. Since nine had modifications of this prototype, it was stated that they were engendered by somatic mutation, for their differences could not be accounted for by recombinational events. Finally, it was shown that IgM chains expressed only the T15 V_H genelet, while all the mutants were found in IgA or IgG, so that the latter classes appear to display greater diversity than the former (Gearhart *et al.*, 1981). Similar experiments have been conducted in other strains of mice with precisely corresponding results (Bothwell *et al.*, 1981).

A Proposed Mechanism for Somatic Mutation. In order to understand fully the nature of such somatic mutations, it is well first to appreciate their relations to other types. As pointed out in Chapter 7, Section 7.2.1, vertebrate B lymphocytes do not gain the capacity for generating a diversity of antibodies until some time after hatching or birth, and therefore the genetic changes have a different origin than gametic mutations, which occur only in the gonads. Moreover, the production of antibody diversity is in response to an antigen, not such chemical or physical mutagens as nitrous acid or ionizing radiation, for only B lymphocytes undergo changes in this fashion. Furthermore, actual antibody formation occurs only on second contact with the antigen and under the influence of helper T cells (Chapter 7, Section 7.4.3). Therefore, it is clear that somatic mutagenesis involves an entirely different mechanism from gametic.

This observation is still further borne out by the nature of the variability that is induced, as set forth in Chapter 7, Section 7.1.3. The changes that occur in the V_H region during antibody formation are not random but are highly controlled. It will be recalled that in some sites of the four hypervariable regions, only four different amino acids occurred, in others five or six, and in a few as many as eight in the sequences provided in Table 7.8. At the same time as these regions were undergoing mutation, the several constant domains of the same immunoglobulins remained relatively free of change, in spite of all domains' having similar structures. Because of the inertness of DNA, the control mechanism again must be ascribed to the soma of the cell, that is, to the supramolecular genetic apparatus. In other words, this somatic mechanism has the ability both to induce mutations in the genome and to control the resulting changes in the DNA on a site-to-site basis, at least in the production of immunoglobulins. One can visualize that alterations in the programming of this apparatus are involved, under ordinary genetic control plus a feedback arrangement as elsewhere (Figure 8.3), but the actual nature of the reprogramming, as well as that of this somatic mechanism, should provide exciting and highly productive areas of research for many future investigators.

The Activities of the Supramolecular Genetic Mechanism. In summary, those cellular processes that seem to require the presence of an organized and programmed genetical mechanism outside the genome proper include the following that have been noted in the second and third volumes of this trilogy.

1. Governing transcription by selecting those genes to be transcribed at a given stage of development or period in circadian or other biorhythmic functions; this activity may include suppression of one member of a homologous chromosome pair, as the X chromosome of vertebrates.
2. In many cases preparing the genome for transcription by selecting among multiple like genelets and combining them to others to make pregenes and those into genes.
3. Regulating the processing of the precursorial transcripts.
4. Guiding translation of the mature transcriptive products.
5. Governing the posttranslational products. In eukaryotes transporting those products to such organelles as the dictyosomes, endoreticulum, peroxisomes, and so on for addition of carbohydrate side chains or other processing steps. Selective degradation of proteins, demonstrated recently to occur principally in the cytosol rather than in lysosomes, would be a negative aspect of this function (Bigelow *et al.*, 1981).
6. Conduction of those finished products to the site in the cell where

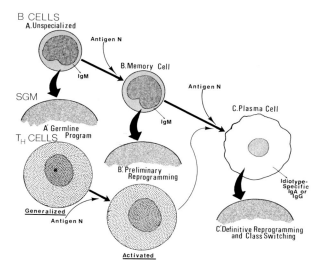

Figure 8.3. Role of the supramolecular genetic apparatus in immune reactions. The upper row of figures represents the B lymphocyte and its products, whereas the central set indicates some of the effects of specific antigens on the supramolecular genetic apparatus (SGM) during immunogenesis. Other parameters and/or cells, such as macrophages, also may exercise influences but are not shown in this diagram of major events.

needed. This would include guiding specific aminoacylated tRNAs to the site of formation of peptidoglycans and the like (Dillon, 1978, pp. 143, 235, and 236), placement of surface features of ciliates and other cells (Aufderheide *et al.*, 1980), as well as isozymes and structural proteins internally (Masters and Winzor, 1981).

7. Regulation of the polymerization and assembly of the macromolecules into their respective organelles, vesicles, and the like. Construction or replication of organelles, such as the centrioles.

8. Destroying organelles, microtubules, microfilaments, and other structures no longer needed; sometimes only depolymerization may be involved, with the monomeric units being transported to new sites as in 6 and 7.

9. Regulating the genome size by amplification (often of particular segments) or multiplication of ploidy and selective elimination of unwanted portions of or entire chromosomes.

10. Recombining selected regions of the chromatin during cell activities, as necessary.

11. Regulating and inducing somatic mutations on a site-by-site basis during development and immunological events, and perhaps in other activities or processes.

12. The opposite influence, maintenance of homology within a given

species among the genomic components of a multigene family as recently described in the mouth (Lalanne *et al.*, 1982), appear to be an additional function.

That these functions are conducted by an organized body within the soma of the cell, not merely by isolated independent enzyme systems, is evidenced particularly lucidly by the experiments on centrifuged fertilized ova reported in Chapter 3, Section 3.4.2. In spite of the strong centrifugation that displaced all internal organelles out of the typical animal–vegetal polar alignment, the treated cells regained the normal ovostratification as the embryo developed, oriented in normal relations to the typical axis.

8.3.2. Other Inconstancies

That somatic mutation may be a more widespread phenomenon in the development and daily functions of cells is beginning to be suggested by the results of several sets of researches. Because the investigators could not be expected to be aware of the well-documented but highly specialized knowledge just summarized from immunological sources, the data they obtained from developing embryos were interpreted in indefinite terms, such as resulting from translocations. However, the nature of the changes that were described later do not permit such an explanation.

Gene Changes during Embryogenesis. The presence of single-stranded regions (gaps) has long been known to occur throughout the genomes of a variety of organisms, which have proven to be of two types (Wortzman and Baker, 1981). The first class includes shorter gaps (under 1400 residues in length) that are associated with active sites of DNA replication. In the second class are found longer sequences containing up to 3000 nucleotides, many of which include genes for histones. In all cases, it was the antisense (minus) strand that was lacking in these gaps, which were found to be nonrandomly distributed in the genomes of sea urchin embryos (Wortzman and Baker, 1980). Similar single-stranded regions not associated with replication forks have also been described in mammalian DNA (Henson, 1978).

In a study on such structures in three early stages of development of the sea urchin (*S. purpuratus*), the single-stranded regions were shown to be in the form of hairpins, a number of which contained methylated nucleotides (Dickinson and Baker, 1978).* Comparisons of these hairpins derived from the morula, blastula, and gastrula stages revealed that sequence changes occurred *in vivo* within the majority of the adjacent single-stranded regions (Figure 8.4).

*The problem of how such loops are replicated during the synthesis of new DNA cannot be addressed here, because no evidence has been forthcoming that sheds light on a possible mechanism. The disclosure of how such consistent single-stranded regions are created, however, cannot fail both to extend immeasurably present appreciation of cell organization and provide a deeper insight into the nature of genetic processes.

A. ZYGOTE   B. BLASTULA C. GASTRULA D. FETAL   E. MATURE

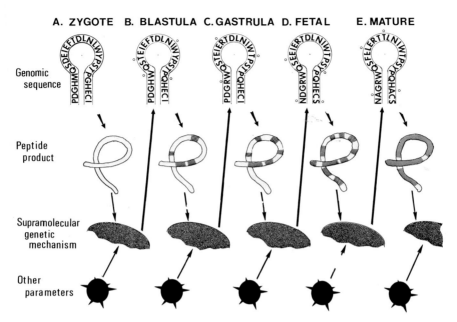

Figure 8.4. Suggested mode of somatic mutagenesis during development and differentiation. The genomic regions here are shown as hairpin loops, for thus far actual gene changes during embryogeny have been demonstrated only in such structures; however, they may eventually be shown to occur elsewhere also. For the sake of clarity, the genome is lettered as to the coded product, not in terms of codons. In the peptide products of those changing coding regions, the mutated sectors (in dark stipple) are only approximations. In the zygote (A) and early cleavage stages, the germline genomic sequences produce relatively primitive peptides, which together with positional effects and other parameters lead the supramolecular genetic mechanism to induce a few somatic mutations (indicated by small circles) in the genome. The resulting new polypeptides, plus other internal and external factors, lead the supramolecular genetic mechanism to induce additional somatic mutations in the genome of the blastula, and so on throughout development into the fetus, juvenile, adult, and senescent individuals.

Although such sequence changes were more frequent in loop-bearing methylated residues, they were present in the others also. These results were suggested to be produced by translocations rather than by hypermutation, but that interpretation is not in keeping with the data presented. Consequently, despite the present paucity of observations, one method of controlling the formation of alterations in the synthesis of proteins during embryogenesis is by way of somatic mutations comparable to those so clearly demonstrated to occur in immune reactions. Thus, the production of genome changes under the control of a programmed supramolecular genetic mechanism may be a more widespread phenomenon in biological processes than is currently indicated (Figure 8.4). Indeed comparable changes in genome structure have been reported in a protistan, in which several antigen genes of Trypanosoma are shown to fluctuate from day to day (Young *et al.*, 1982).

Programmed Mutagenesis in Other Processes. The author is not unaware that one of the most universal properties of living things, the capacity for undergoing evolutionary changes, might also in part involve programmed control of genomic primary structure by the supramolecular genetic apparatus. Although concrete evidence now is wanting, this absence very likely results more from a lack of awareness of the existence of such a device than from its nonoccurrence in the biological world. Indeed, the widespread and frequent presence of so-called mutator genes in organisms as diverse as bacteria, *Drosophila* and corn, among numerous others (Dillon, 1978b, p. 84), may be a reflection of this mutual feedback arrangement during development, both ontogenetic and evolutionary. Likewise the greatly differing abilities of organisms in exhibiting morphological diversity in response to geographical distribution (Dillon, 1966, 1970) may be attributed in part to a somatic control apparatus. It is similarly possible that the conservation of a given region in the nucleotidal sequence in one family of genes and numerous mutations in the same or comparable segment in a closely related cluster may be another manifestation of this control arrangement. For example, the 5'-terminal sector in exon 2 of the β family of hemoglobin genes is nearly invariant through the first 10 residues (Table 8.1). Yet in the α-family members there is almost no universal site homology in the same segment, in spite of its seeming to play the same functional role in support of the heme unit.

Moreover, a distinct possibility exists that this aspect of the supramolecular genetic apparatus also is as deeply involved in memory on the part of brain cells as it is in the production of memory cells during immune reactions and in others like those cells that remember omitted mitoses, for instance (Chapter 3, Section 3.4.2). Thus, the particular cerebral cortical cells may, when activated by stimulus-carrying neurons, undergo controlled mutagenesis, leading to the formation of a specific variety of protein that represents the information being stored. In addition, one can visualize comparable sets of processes to be associated with numerous other cellular and organismic activities for which no adequate explanation is currently available. Any such proposals would today be entirely speculative, but the concept of a second genetic mechanism guiding alterations in the primary structure of the genome by a complex feedback arrangement should open innumerable doors to suitable new lines of investigations and eventually permit the garnering of greater insight into that most complex biological unit, the cell, and its equally complicated genetical processes.

References

CHAPTER 1

Abe, T., Tanabe, Y., Kaneko, T., Mogi, K., and Hosoda, T. 1958. Immunochemical studies with radioactive isotope, similarly between vitellin and lipovitellin. *Proc. Soc. Exp. Biol. Med.* **98**:703–707.

Afzelius, B. A. 1955. The fine structure of the sea urchin spermatozoa as revealed by the electron microscope. *Z. Zellforsch. Mikrosk. Anat.* **42**:134–138.

Afzelius, B. A. 1972. Sperm morphology and fertilization biology. *In*: Beatty, R. A., and Gluecksohn-Waelsch, S., eds., *The Genetics of the Spermatozoon*, Edinburgh, University of Edinburgh, pp. 131–143.

Afzelius, B. A., ed. 1975. *The Functional Anatomy of the Spermatozoon*, Elmsford, N.Y., Pergamon Press.

Afzelius, B. A. 1977. Spermatozoa and spermatids of the crinoid *Antedon petasus*, with a note on primitive spermatozoa from deuterostome animals. *J. Ultrastruct. Res.* **59**:272–281.

Afzelius, B. A., and Mohri, H. 1966. Mitochondria respiring without exogenous substrate: A study of aged sea urchin spermatozoa. *Exp. Cell Res.* **42**:10–17.

Allen, B. M. 1911. The origin of the sex cells of *Amia* and *Lepidosteus*. *J. Morphol.* **22**:1–35.

Allen, M. J. 1961. A cytochemical study of the developing oocytes and attached nurse cells of the polychaetous annelid *Diopatra cuprea*. *Acta Embryol. Morphol. Exp.* **4**:219–238.

Alves, P., and Jonasson, J. 1978. New staining method for the detection of sister-chromatid exchanges in BrdU-labelled chromosomes. *J. Cell Sci.* **32**:185–195.

Amin, H., Richart, R. M., and Brinson, A. O. 1976. Preovulatory granulosa cells and steroidogenesis: An ultrastructural study in the rhesus monkey. *Obstet. Gynecol.* **47**:562–568.

Anderson, E. 1969. Oogenesis in the cockroach *Periplaneta americana*, with special reference to the specialization of the oolemma and the fate of coated vesicles. *J. Microsc. (Oxford)* **8**:721–738.

Anderson, E., and Huebner, E. 1968. Development of the oocyte and its accessory cells of the polychaete, *Diopatra cuprea* (Bosc). *J. Morphol.* **129**:89–125.

Anderson, L. M., and Telfer, W. H. 1969. A follicle cell contribution to the yolk spheres of moth oocytes. *Tissue Cell* **1**:633–644.

Anderson, W. A. 1968. Cytochemistry of sea urchin gametes. *J. Ultrastruct. Res.* **24**:398–411.

Anderson, W. A., and Personne, P. 1976. The molluscan spermatozoon, dynamic aspects of its structure and function. *Am. Zool.* **16**:293–313.

Ando, T., and Watanabe, S. 1969. A new method for fractionation of proteins and the amino acid sequences of salmine and three components of iridine. *Int. J. Protein Res.* **1**:221–224.

Angelier, N., and Lacroix, J. C. 1975. Complexes de transcription d'origines nucléolaire et chromosomique d'ovocytes de *Pleurodeles waltlii* et *P. poireti* (Urodèles). *Chromosoma* **51**:323–335.

Angelier, N., Hemon, D., and Bouteille, M. 1979. Mechanisms of transcription in nucleoli of amphibian oocytes as visualized by high-resolution autoradiography. *J. Cell Biol.* **80**:277–290.

Applebaum, S. W., James, T. C., Wreschner, D. H., and Tata, J. R. 1981. The preparation and characterization of locust vitellogenin messenger RNA and the synthesis of its complementary DNA. *Biochem. J.* **193**:209–216.

Arthur, C. G., Weide, C. M., Vincent, W. S., and Goldstein, E. S. 1979. mRNA sequence diversity during early embryogenesis in *Drosophila melanogaster*. *Exp. Cell Res.* **121**:87–94.

Avramova, Z., Dessev, G., and Tsanev, R. 1980. DNA-associated proteins of ram sperm nuclei. *FEBS Lett.* **118**:58–62.

Baca, M., and Zamboni, L. 1967. The fine structure of human follicular oocytes. *J. Ultrastruct. Res.* **19**:354–381.

Baccetti, B., and Afzelius, B. A. 1976. *The Biology of the Sperm Cell*, Basel, Karger.

Baccetti, B., and Dallai, R. 1977. The spermatozoon of onychophorans. 2. *Peripatoides leuckarti*. *Tissue Cell* **9**:563–566.

Baccetti, B., Dallai, R., Burrini, A., and Selmi, G. 1976. Fine structure of the spermatozoon of the onychophoran, *Peripatopsis*. *Tissue Cell* **8**:659–672.

Bachvarova, R. 1974. Incorporation of tritiated adenosine into mouse ovum RNA. *Dev. Biol.* **40**:52–58.

Baker, B. S., Carpenter, A. T. C., and Ripoll, P. 1978. The utilization during mitotic cell division of loci controlling meiotic recombination and disjunction in *D. melanogaster*. *Genetics* **90**:531–578.

Baker, T. G. 1970. Electron microscopy of the primary and secondary oocyte. *Adv. Biosci.* **6**:7–22.

Baker, T. G., and Neal, P. 1973. Initiation and control of meiosis and follicular growth in ovaries of the mouse. *Ann. Biol. Anim. Biochim. Biophys.* **13**:137–144.

Baker, T. G., and Neal, P. 1974. Oogenesis in human fetal ovaries maintained in organ culture. *J. Anat.* **117**:591–604.

Baker, T. G., and O, W. S. 1976. Development of the ovary and oogenesis. *Clin. Obstet. Gynecol.* **3**:3–26.

Barker, K. R., and Baker, C. L. 1970. Urodele spermateleosis: A comparative electron microscope study. *In*: Baccetti, B., ed., *Comparative Spermatology*, Rome, Accademia Nazionale dei Lincei, pp. 81–84.

Bast, R. E., and Telfer, W. H. 1976. Follicle cell protein synthesis and its contribution to the yolk of the cecropia moth oocyte. *Dev. Biol.* **52**:83–97.

Bawa, S. R. 1975. Comparative studies on the origin of the chromatoid body. *In*: Duckett, J. G., and Racey, P. A., eds., *The Biology of the Male Gamete*, New York, Academic Press, pp. 275–278.

Bedford, J. M. 1979. Evolution of the sperm maturation and sperm storage functions of the epididymis. *In*: Fawcett, D. W., and Bedford, J. M., eds., *The Spermatozoon*, Munich, Urban & Schwarzenberg, pp. 7–21.

Bedford, J. M., and Rifkin, J. M. 1979. An evolutionary view of the male reproductive tract and sperm maturation in a monotreme mammal—the echidna, *Tachyglossus aculeatus*. *Am. J. Anat.* **156**:207–230.

Bell, P. R. 1978. A microtubule–nuclear envelope complex in the spermatozoid of *Pteridium*. *J. Cell Sci.* **29**:189–195.

Bell, W. J. 1969. Dual role of juvenile hormone in the control of yolk formation in *Periplaneta americana*. *J. Insect Physiol.* **15**:1279–1290.

Bell, W. J., and Barth, R. H. 1971. Initiation of yolk deposition by juvenile hormone. *Nature New Biol.* **230**:220–221.

Benavente, R., and Wettstein, R. 1980. Ultrastructural characterization of the sex chromosomes during spermatogenesis of spiders having holocentric chromosomes and a long diffuse stage. *Chromosoma* **77**:69–81.

Benoit, J. 1930. Contribution à l'étude de la lignée germinale chez le poulet: Destruction précoce des gonocytes primaires par les rayons ultra-violets. *C. R. Soc. Biol.* **104**:1329–1331.

Benttinen, L. C., and Comb, D. G. 1971. Early and late histones during sea urchin development. *J. Mol. Biol.* **57**:355–358.

Bergink, E. W., and Wallace, R. A. 1974. Precursor–product relationship between amphibian vitellogenin and the yolk proteins, lipovitellin and phosvitin. *J. Biol. Chem.* **249**:2897–2903.

Bergink, E. W., Wallace, R. A., Van de Berg, J. A., Bos, E. S., Gruber, M., and Ab, G. 1974. Estrogen-induced synthesis of yolk proteins in roosters. *Am. Zool.* **14**:1177–1193.

Berrill, N.J., and Karp, G. 1976. *Development*, New York, McGraw-Hill.

Bird, M. M. 1980. The morphology of synaptic profiles in explants of foetal and neonatal mouse cerebral cortex maintained in a magnesium-enriched environment. *Cell Tissue Res.* **206**:115–122.

Bishop, D. W. 1961. Biology of spermatozoa. *In*: Young, W. G., ed., *Sex and Internal Secretions*, 3rd ed., Baltimore, Williams & Wilkins, Vol. 2, pp. 707–796.

Blackler, A. W. 1970. The integrity of the reproductive cell line in the Amphibia. *Curr. Top. Dev. Biol.* **5**:71–87.

Bleil, J. D., and Wassarman, P. M. 1980. Structure and function of the zona pellucida: Identification and characterization of the proteins of the mouse oocyte's zona pellucida. *Dev. Biol.* **76**:185–202.

Boitani, C., Geremia, R., Rossi, R., and Monesi, V. 1980. Electrophoretic pattern of polypeptide synthesis in spermatocytes and spermatids of the mouse. *Cell Differ.* **9**:41–49.

Bonnot, E. J. 1967. Le plan de l'organisation fondamentale de la spermatide de *Bryum capillare*. *C. R. Acad. Sci. Ser. D* **265**:958–961.

Borkhardt, B., and Olson, L. W. 1979. Meiotic prophase in diploid and tetraploid strains of *Allomyces macrogynus*. *Protoplasma* **100**:323–343.

Boss, J. M. N. 1954. Mitosis in cultures of newt tissue. II. Chromosome pairing in anaphase. *Exp. Cell Res.* **7**:225–231.

Boss, J. M. N. 1955. The pairing of somatic chromosomes: A survey. *Texas Rep. Biol. Med.* **13**:212–221.

Bournoure, L. 1939. *L'Origine des Cellules Réproductrices et le Problème de la Lignée Germinale*, Paris, Gauthier–Villars.

Brien, P., and Reniers-Decoen, M. 1951. La gamétogènese et l'intersexualité chez *Hydra attenuata*. *Ann. Soc. R. Zool. Belg.* **82**:285–327.

Brock, W. A., Trostle, P. K., and Meistrich, M. L. 1980. Meiotic synthesis of testis histones in the rat. *Proc. Natl. Acad. Sci. USA* **77**:371–375.

Brookes, V. J. 1969. The induction of yolk protein synthesis in the fat body of an insect, *Leucophaea maderae*, by an analog of the juvenile hormone. *Dev. Biol.* **20**:459–471.

Brooks, D. E. 1979. Biochemical environment of sperm maturation. *In*: Fawcett, D. W., and Bedford, J. M., eds., *The Spermatozoon*, Munich, Urban & Schwarzenberg, pp. 23–34.

Brown, D. D., and Dawid, I. B. 1968. Specific gene amplification in oocytes. *Science* **160**:272–280.

Brown, D. D., and Sugimoto, K. 1973. 5 S DNAs of *Xenopus laevis* and *Xenopus mulleri*: Evolution of a gene family. *J. Mol. Biol.* **78**:397–415.

Brown, D. D., and Weber, C. S. 1968. Unique DNA sequences homologous to 4S, 5S, and rRNA. *J. Mol. Biol.* **34**:681–697.

Brown, D. D., Wensink, P. C., and Jordan, E. 1971. Purification and some characteristics of 5 S DNA from *Xenopus laevis*. *Proc. Natl. Acad. Sci. USA* **68**:3175–3179.

Brown, W. V., and Bertke, E. M. 1974. *Textbook of Cytology*, 2nd ed., St. Louis, Mosby.

Brown, W. V., and Stack, S. M. 1968. Somatic pairing as a regular preliminary to meiosis. *Bull. Torrey Bot. Club* **95**:369–378.

Bruel, M. T. 1973. Localisation des gonocytes primaires chez le jeune embryon de poulet hybride Rhode-Whyandotte: Études histologiques et expérimentales. *Arch. Anat. Histol. Embryol. Norm. Exp.* **56**:51–54.

Brummett, A. R., and Dumont, J. N. 1977. Intracellular transport of vitellogenin in *Xenopus* oocytes. *Dev. Biol.* **60**:482–486.

Bulnheim, H. P. 1962. Untersuchungen zum Spermatozoendimorphismus von *Opalia crenimarginata* (Prosobranchia). *Z. Zellforsch. Mikrosk. Anat.* **56**:300–343.

Byers, B., and Goetsch, L. 1975. Electron microscopic observations on the meiotic karyotype of diploid and tetraploid *S. cerevisiae*. *Proc. Natl. Acad. Sci. USA* **72**:5056–5060.

Callan, H. G. 1963. The nature of lampbrush chromosomes. *Int. Rev. Cytol.* **15**:1–34.

Callan, H. G. 1967. The organization of genetic units in chromosomes. *J. Cell Sci.* **2**:1–7.

Callan, H. G., and Old, R. W. 1980. *In situ* hybridization to lampbrush chromosomes: A potential source of error exposed. *J. Cell Sci.* **41**:115–123.

Callen, J. C., Dennebouy, N., and Mounolou, J. C. 1980. Development of the mitochondrial mass and accumulation of mtDNA in previtellogenic stages of *Xenopus laevis* oocytes. *J. Cell Sci.* **41**:307–320.

Camatini, M., Saita, A., and Cotelli, F. 1974. Spermiogenesis of *Lithobius forficatus* at ultrastructural level. *Symp. Zool. Soc. London* **32**:231–235.

Camatini, M., Franchi, E., and Saita, A. 1977. Spermiogenesis in *Scutigera coleoptrata* (Chilopoda). *J. Submicrosc. Cytol.* **9**:373–387.

Camatini, M., Franchi, E., and Saita, A. 1979. Ultrastructural investigation of spermiogenesis in *Peripatopsis capensis* (Onychophora). *J. Morphol.* **159**:29–48.

Capco, D. G., and Jeffery, W. R. 1979. Origin and spatial distribution of maternal mRNA during oogenesis of an insect, *Oncopeltus fasciatus*. *J. Cell Sci.* **39**:63–76.

Carothers, Z. B. 1975. Comparative studies on spermatogenesis in bryophytes. *In*: Duckett, J. G., and Racey, P. A., eds., *The Biology of the Male Gamete*, New York, Academic Press, pp. 71–84.

Carothers, Z. B., and Kreitner, G. L. 1967. Studies of spermatogenesis in the Hepaticae. I. Ultrastructure of the Vierergruppe in *Marchantia*. *J. Cell Biol.* **33**:43–51.

Carpenter, A. T. C. 1975a. Electron microscopy of meiosis in *D. melanogaster* females. I. Structure, arrangement, and temporal change of the synaptonemal complex in wild-type. *Chromosoma* **51**:157–182.

Carpenter, A. T. C. 1975b. Electron microscopy of meiosis in *D. melanogaster* females. II. The recombination nodule—a recombination-associated structure at pachytene? *Proc. Natl. Acad. Sci. USA* **72**:3186–3189.

Carpenter, A. T. C. 1979a. Synaptonemal complex and recombination nodules in wild-type *D. melanogaster* females. *Genetics* **92**:511–541.

Carpenter, A. T. C. 1979b. Recombination nodules and synaptonemal complex in recombination-defective females of *Drosophila melanogaster*. *Chromosoma* **75**:259–292.

Challoner, S. 1975. Studies of oogenesis and follicular development in the golden hamster. 2. Initiation and control of meiosis *in vitro*. *J. Anat.* **119**:149–156.

Channing, C. P. 1979. Follicular non-steroidal regulators. *In*: Channing, C. P., Marsh, J. M., and Sadler, W. A., eds., *Ovarian Follicular and Corpus Luteum Function*, New York, Plenum Press, pp. 327–343.

REFERENCES FOR CHAPTER 1

Chapron, C., and Relexans, J. C. 1971. Connexions intercellulaires et évolution nucléaire au cours de la préméiose ovocytaire. *C. R. Acad. Sci.* **272**:3307–3310.

Chen, T. T. 1980. Vitellogenin in locusts (*Locusta migratoria*): Translation of vitellogenin in RNA in *Xenopus* oocytes and analysis of the polypeptide products. *Arch. Biochem. Biophys.* **201**:266–276.

Chen, T. T., Couble, P., DeLucca, F. L., and Wyatt, G. R. 1976. Juvenile hormone control of vitellogenin synthesis in *Locusta migratoria*. *In*: Gilbert, L. I., ed., *The Juvenile Hormones*, New York, Plenum Press, pp. 505–529.

Chen, T. T., Strahlendorf, P. W., and Wyatt, G. R. 1978. Vitellin and vitellogenin from locusts (*Locusta migratoria*). *J. Biol. Chem.* **253**:5325–5331.

Chen, T. T., Couble, P., Abu-Hakima, R., and Wyatt, G. R. 1979. Juvenile hormone-controlled vitellogenin synthesis in *Locusta migratoria* fat body. *Dev. Biol.* **69**:59–72.

Chouinard, L. 1973. An electron-microscope study of the extranucleolar bodies during growth of the oocyte in the prepubertal mouse. *J. Cell Sci.* **12**:55–69.

Christmann, J. L., Grayson, M. J., and Huang, R. C. C. 1977. Comparative study of hen yolk phosvitin and plasma vitellogenin. *Biochemistry* **16**:3250–3256.

Clarkson, S. G., Birnstiel, M. L., and Purdom, I. F. 1973. Clustering of tRNA genes of *Xenopus laevis*. *J. Mol. Biol.* **79**:411–429.

Clermont, Y. 1966a. Renewal of spermatogonia in man. *Am. J. Anat.* **118**:509–524.

Clermont, Y. 1966b. Spermatogenesis in man: A study of the spermatogonial population. *Fertil. Steril.* **17**:705–721.

Clermont, Y. 1970. Dynamics of human spermatogenesis. *In*: Rosenberg, E., and Paulsen, C. A., eds., *The Human Testes*, New York, Plenum Press, pp. 47–59.

Clermont, Y., and Rambourg, A. 1978. Evolution of the endoplasmic reticulum during rat spermiogenesis. *Am. J. Anat.* **151**:191–212.

Cognetti, G., Spinelli, G., and Vivoli, A. 1974. Synthesis of histones during sea urchin oogenesis. *Biochim. Biophys. Acta* **349**:447–455.

Cole, K., and Sheath, R. G. 1980. Ultrastructural changes in major organelles during spermatial differentiation in *Bangia* (Rhodophyta). *Protoplasma* **102**:253–279.

Colman, A. 1975. Transcription of DNAs of known sequence after injection into the eggs and oocytes of *Xenopus laevis*. *Eur. J. Biochem.* **57**:85–96.

Colman, A., Lane, C. D., Craig, R., Boulton, A., Mohun, T., and Morser, J. 1981. The influence of topology and glycosylation on the fate of heterologous secretory proteins made in *Xenopus* oocytes. *Eur. J. Biochem.* **113**:339–348.

Comings, D. E., and Okada, T. A. 1975. Mechanisms of chromosome banding. VI. Whole mount electron microscopy of banded metaphase chromosomes and a comparison with pachytene chromosomes. *Exp. Cell Res.* **93**:267–274.

Connell, C. J. 1978. A freeze-fracture and lanthanum tracer study of the complex junction between Sertoli cells of the canine testes. *J. Cell Biol.* **76**:57–75.

Connell, C. J. 1980. Blood-testis barrier formation and the initiation of meiosis in the dog. *In*: Steinberger, A., and Steinberger, E., eds., *Testicular Development, Structure, and Function*, New York, Raven Press, pp. 71–78.

Conner, M. K., Alarie, Y., and Dombroske, R. L. 1979. Sister chromatid exchange in murine alveolar macrophages, regenerating liver and bone marrow cells—a simultaneous multicellular *in vivo* assay. *Chromosoma* **74**:51–55.

Cook, W. H. 1961. Proteins of hen's egg yolk. *Nature (London)* **190**:1173–1175.

Cook, W. H. 1968. Macromolecular components of egg yolk. *In*: Carter, T. C., ed., *Egg Quality: A Study of the Hen's Egg*, Edinburgh, Oliver & Boyd, pp. 109–132.

Couble, P., Chen, T. T., and Wyatt, G. R. 1979. Juvenile hormone-controlled vitellogenin synthesis in *Locusta migratoria* fat body: Cytological development. *J. Insect Physiol.* **25**:327–337.

Czolowska, R. 1972. The fine structure of the "germinal cytoplasm" in the egg of *Xenopus laevis*. *Wilhelm Roux Arch. Dev. Biol.* **169**:335–344.

Darnbrough, C. H., and Ford, P. J. 1979. Turnover and processing of poly(A) in full-grown oocytes and during progesterone-induced oocyte maturation in *Xenopus laevis*. *Dev. Biol.* **71**:323–340.

Darnbrough, C. H., and Ford, P. J. 1981. Identification in *Xenopus laevis* of a class of oocyte-specific proteins bound to messenger RNA. *Eur. J. Biochem.* **113**:415–424.

Davidson, E. H. 1976. *Gene Activity in Early Development*, 2nd ed., New York, Academic Press.

Davies, P. L., Dixon, G. H., Ferrier, L. N., Gedamu, L., and Iatrou, K. 1976. The structure and function of protamine mRNA from developing trout testes. *Prog. Nucleic Acid Res. Mol. Biol.* **19**:135–155.

Denis, H., and Wegnez, M. 1977. Biochemical research on oogenesis: Oocytes and liver cells of the teleost fish *Tinca tinca* contain different kinds of 5 S RNA. *Dev. Biol.* **59**:228–236.

Denis, H., Picard, B., le Maire, M., and Clerot, J.-C. 1980. Biochemical research on oogenesis: The storage particles of the teleost fish *Tinca tinca*. *Dev. Biol.* **77**:218–223.

Diberardino, M. A. 1980. Genetic stability and modulation of metazoan nuclei transplanted into eggs and oocytes. *Differentiation* **17**:17–30.

Dickinson, H. G., and Heslop-Harrison, J. 1970. The ribosome cycle, nucleoli, and cytoplasmic nucleoids in the meiocytes of *Lilium*. *Protoplasma* **69**:187–200.

Dillon, L. S. 1978. *The Genetic Mechanism and the Origin of Life*, New York, Plenum Press.

Dillon, L. S. 1981. *Ultrastructure, Macromolecules, and Evolution*, New York, Plenum Press.

Dixon, G. H., Davies, P. L., Ferrier, L. N., Gedamu, L., and Iatrou, K. 1977. The expression of protamine genes in developing trout sperm cells. *In*: Ts'o, P., ed., *The Molecular Biology of the Mammalian Genetic Apparatus*, Amsterdam, Elsevier/North-Holland, pp. 356–379.

Doyle, W. L. 1933. Observations on spermiogenesis in *Sciara coprophila*. *J. Morphol.* **54**:477–485.

Dresser, M. E., and Moses, M. J. 1980. Synaptonemal complex karyotyping in spermatocytes of the Chinese hamster. IV. Light and electron microscopy of synapsis and nucleolar development by silver staining. *Chromosoma* **76**:1–22.

Dring, D. M. 1975. The male gamete in ascomycetes. *In*: Duckett, J. G., and Racey, P. A., eds., *The Biology of the Male Gamete*, New York, Academic Press, pp. 45–55.

Drury, K. C., and Schorderet-Slatkine, S. 1975. Effects of cycloheximide on the "autocatalytic" nature of the maturation promoting factor (MPF) in oocytes of *Xenopus laevis*. *C. R. Acad. Sci.* **280**:1273–1275.

Duckett, J. G. 1973. An ultrastructural study of the differentiation of the spermatozoid of *Equisetum*. *J. Cell Sci.* **12**:95–129.

Duckett, J. G. 1975. Spermatogenesis in pteridophytes. *In*: Duckett, J. G., and Racey, P. A., eds., *The Biology of the Male Gamete*, New York, Academic Press, pp. 97–127.

Duckett, J. G., and Bell, P. R. 1977. An ultrastructural study of the mature spermatozoid of *Equisetum*. *Philos. Trans. R. Soc. London Ser. B.* **277**:131–158.

Dumont, J. N. 1969. Oogenesis in the annelid *Enchytraeus albidus*, with special reference to the origin and cytochemistry of yolk. *J. Morphol.* **129**:317–344.

Dumont, J. N. 1972. Oogenesis in *Xenopus laevis* (Daudin): Stages of oocyte development in laboratory maintained animals. *J. Morphol.* **136**:153–180.

Dziadek, M., and Dixon, K. E. 1975. Mitosis in presumptive primordial germ cells in post-blastula embryos of *Xenopus laevis*. *J. Exp. Zool.* **192**:285–291.

Ecker, R. E. 1972. The regulation of protein synthesis in anucleate frog oocytes. *In*: Bonotto, S., Kirchmann, R., Goutier, R., and Maisin, J. R., eds., *Biology and Radiobiology of Anucleate Systems*, New York, Academic Press, pp. 165–179.

Etkin, L. D. 1978. Approaches to problems of gene regulation and cell type determination in amphibians. *Am. Zool.* **18**:215–224.

Etkin, L. D., and Maxson, R. E. 1980. The synthesis of authentic sea urchin transcriptional and translational products by sea urchin histone genes injected into *Xenopus laevis* oocytes. *Dev. Biol.* **75**:13–25.

Fargeix, N. 1966. Localisation des cellules germinales de l'embryon de canard au stage des premières paires de somites. *C. R. Acad. Sci.* **262**:2259–2262.

Fawcett, D. W., and Bedford, J. M., eds. 1979. *The Spermatozoon*, Munich, Urban & Schwarzenberg.

Felber, B. K., Maurhofer, S., Jaggi, R. B., Wyler, T., Wahli, W., Ryffel, G. U., and Weber, R. 1980. Isolation and translation *in vitro* of four related vitellogenin mRNAs of estrogen-stimulated *Xenopus laevis. Eur. J. Biochem.* **105**:17–24.

Finch, J. T., and Klug, A. 1976. Solenoidal model for superstructure in chromatin. *Proc. Natl. Acad. Sci. USA* **73**:1897–1901.

Follett, B. K., and Redshaw, M. R. 1968. The effects of oestrogens and gonadotropins on lipid and protein metabolism in *Xenopus laevis. J. Endocrinol.* **40**:439–456.

Follett, B. K., and Redshaw, M. R. 1974. The physiology of vitellogenesis. *In*: Lofts, B., ed., *The Physiology of Amphibia*, New York, Academic Press, Vol. II, pp. 219–308.

Folliot, R. 1979. Ultrastructural study of spermiogenesis of the anuran amphibian *Bombina variegata. In*: Fawcett, D. W., and Bedford, J. M., eds., *The Spermatozoon*, Munich, Urban & Schwarzenberg, pp. 333–339.

Ford, C. C., and Woodland, H. R. 1975. DNA synthesis in oocytes and eggs of *Xenopus laevis* injected with DNA. *Dev. Biol.* **43**:189–199.

Ford, P. J. 1972. RNA synthesis during oogenesis in *Xenopus laevis. In*: Biggers, J. D., and Schuetz, A. W., eds., *Oogenesis*, Baltimore, University Park Press, pp. 167–191.

Franzen, A. 1956. On spermiogenesis, morphology of the spermatozoon and biology of fertilization among invertebrates. *Zool. Bidr. Uppsala* **31**:355–482.

Franzen, A. 1970. Phylogenetic aspects of the morphology of the spermatozoa and spermiogenesis. *In*: Baccetti, B., ed., *Comparative Spermatology*, New York, Academic Press, pp. 29–46.

Fretter, V. 1953. Some aspects of egg laying in intertidal prosobranchs. *Br. J. Anim. Behav.* **1**:83–84.

Fritsch, F. E. 1952. *The Structure and Reproduction of the Algae*, London, Cambridge University Press, Vol. II.

Fuge, H. 1979. Synapsis, desynapsis, and formation of polycomplex-like aggregates in male meiosis of *Pales ferruginea. Chromosoma* **70**:353–373.

Furieri, P. 1975. The peculiar morphology of spermatozoon of *Bombina variegata* L. *Monit. Zool. Ital.* **9**:185–201.

Gall, J. G. 1955. On the sub-microscopic structure of chromosomes. *Brookhaven Symp. Biol.* **8**:17.

Gall, J. G., and Callan, H. G. 1962. ^{3}H-Uridine incorporation in lampbrush chromosomes. *Proc. Natl. Acad. Sci. USA* **48**:562–570.

Garber, R. C., and Aist, J. R. 1979. The ultrastructure of meiosis in *Plasmodiophora brassicae. Can. J. Bot.* **57**:2509–2518.

Genevès, L. 1968. Modalités de l'édification de l'appareil flagellaire des spermatozoides de *Polytrichum formosum. C. R. Acad. Sci. Ser. D.* **267**:849–852.

Geremia, R., Boitani, C., Conti, M., and Monesi, V. 1977. RNA synthesis in spermatocytes and spermatids and preservation of meiotic RNA during spermiogenesis in the mouse. *Cell Differ.* **5**:343–355.

Gifford, E. M., and Larson, S. 1980. Developmental features of the spermatogenous cell in *Ginkgo biloba. Am. J. Bot.* **67**:119–124.

Gilbert, A. B. 1971. The ovary. *In*: Bell, D. J., and Freeman, B. M., eds., *Physiology and Biochemistry of the Domestic Fowl*, New York, Academic Press, Vol. 3, pp. 1163–1208.

Gillies, C. B. 1979. The relationship between synaptonemal complexes, recombination nodules and crossing over in *Neurospora crassa* bivalents and translocation quadrivalents. *Genetics* **91**:1–17.

Goldberg, E. 1977. Isozymes in testes and spermatozoa. *In*: Ratazzi, M., Scandalios, J., and

Whitt, G., eds., *Isozymes: Current Topics in Biological and Medical Research*, New York, Liss, Vol. 1, pp. 79–124.

Goldstein, E. S. 1978. Translated and sequestered untranslated message sequences in *Drosophila* oocytes and embryos. *Dev. Biol.* **63**:59–96.

Goldstein, E. S., and Arthur, C. G. 1979. Isolation and characterization of cDNA complementary to transient maternal poly(A)⁺ RNA from the *Drosophila* oocyte. *Biochim. Biophys. Acta* **565**:265–274.

Gondos, B. 1970. Germ cell relationships in the developing rabbit ovary. *J. Embryol. Exp. Morphol.* **23**:419–426.

Gondos, B. 1978. Oogonia and oocytes in mammals. *In*: Jones, R. E., ed., *The Vertebrate Ovary*, New York, Plenum Press, pp. 83–120.

Gondos, B., and Zamboni, L. 1969. Ovarian development: The functional importance of germ cell interconnections. *Fertil. Steril.* **20**:176–189.

Gould, K. G. 1980. Scanning electron microscopy of the primate sperm. *Int. Rev. Cytol.* **63**:323–355.

Graham, C. F. 1966. The regulation of DNA synthesis and mitosis in multinucleate frog egg. *J. Cell Sci.* **1**:363–374.

Graham, C. F., Arms, K., and Gurdon, J. B. 1966. The induction of DNA synthesis by frog egg cytoplasm. *Dev. Biol.* **14**:349–381.

Grell, R. F., Oakberg, E. F., and Generoso, E. E. 1980. Synaptonemal complexes at premeiotic interphase in the mouse spermatocyte. *Proc. Natl. Acad. Sci. USA* **77**:6720–6723.

Grün, G. 1972. Über den Eidimorphismus und die Oogenese von *Dionophilus gyrociliatus* (Archiannelida). *Z. Zellforsch. Mikrosk. Anat.* **130**:70–92.

Gulyas, B. J. 1971. The rabbit zygote: Formation of annulate lamellae. *J. Ultrastruct. Res.* **35**: 112–126.

Gulyas, B. J. 1980. Cortical granules of mammalian eggs. *Int. Rev. Cytol.* **63**:357–392.

Gurdon, J. B. 1967. On the origin and persistence of a cytoplasmic state inducing nuclear DNA synthesis in frog's eggs. *Proc. Natl. Acad. Sci. USA* **58**:545–552.

Gurdon, J. B. 1968. Changes in somatic cell nuclei inserted into growing and maturing amphibian oocytes. *J. Embryol. Exp. Morphol.* **20**:401–414.

Gurdon, J. B. 1974. *The Control of Gene Expression in Animal Development*, London, Oxford University Press.

Gusse, M., and Chevaillier, P. 1980. Molecular structure of chromatin during sperm differentiation of the dogfish *Scyliorhinus caniculus* (L.). *Chromosoma* **77**:57–68.

Hadek, R. 1966. Cytoplasmic whorls in the golden hamster oocyte. *J. Cell Sci.* **1**:281–282.

Hagedorn, H. H., and Judson, C. L. 1972. Purification and site of synthesis of *Aedes aegypti* yolk protein. *J. Exp. Zool.* **182**:367–377.

Hanisch, J. 1970. Die Blastostyle- und Spermienentwicklung von *Eudendrium racemosum* Cavolini. *Zool. Jahrb. Anat. Ontog. Tiere* **87**:1–62.

Hanson, J., Randall, J. T., and Bayley, S. 1952. The microstructure of the spermatozoa of the snail, *Viviparus. Exp. Cell Res.* **3**:65–78.

Hardisty, M. W. 1978. Primordial germ cells and the vertebrate germ line. *In*: Jones, R. E., ed., *The Vertebrate Ovary*, New York, Plenum Press, pp. 1–45.

Harrison, R. A. P. 1975. Aspects of the enzymology of mammalian spermatozoa. *In*: Duckett, J. G., and Racey, P. A., eds., *The Biology of the Male Gamete*, New York, Academic Press, pp. 301–316.

Heald, P. J., and McLachlan, P. M. 1963. Isolation of phosvitin from the plasma of the laying hen. *Biochem. J.* **87**:571–576.

Heald, P. J., and McLachlan, P. M. 1965. The synthesis of phosvitin *in vitro* by slices of liver from the laying hen. *Biochem. J.* **94**:32–39.

Heilbrunn, L. V., Daugherty, K., and Wilber, K. M. 1939. Initiation of maturation in the frog egg. *Physiol. Zool.* **12**:97–100.

Heslop-Harrison, J. 1968. Wall development within the microspore tetrad of *Lilium longiflorum*. *Can. J. Bot.* **46**:1185–1192.

Hill, R. S. 1979. A quantitative electron-microscope analysis of chromatin from *Xenopus laevis* lampbrush chromosomes. *J. Cell Sci.* **40**:145–169.

Hill, R. S., and Macgregor, H. C. 1980. The development of lampbrush chromosome-type transcription in the early diplotene oocytes of *X. laevis*. *J. Cell Sci.* **44**:87–101.

Hinrichsen, M. J., and Blaquier, J. A. 1980. Evidence supporting the existence of sperm maturation in the human epididymis. *J. Reprod. Fertil.* **60**:291–294.

Hofstein, R., Hershkowitz, M., Gozes, I., and Samuel, D. 1980. The characterization and phosphorylation of an actin-like protein in synaptonemal membranes. *Biochim. Biophys. Acta* **624**:153–162.

Honda, B. M., Baillie, D. L., and Candido, E. P. M. 1975. Properties of chromatin subunits from developing trout testes. *J. Biol. Chem.* **250**:4643–4647.

Horesh, O., Simchen, G., and Friedmann, A. 1979. Morphogenesis of the synapton during yeast meiosis. *Chromosoma* **75**:101–115.

Hoskins, D. D., Stephens, D. T., and Hall, M. L. 1974. Cyclic adenosine 3′, 5′-monophosphate and protein kinase levels in developing bovine spermatozoa. *J. Reprod. Fertil.* **37**:131–133.

Hough-Evans, B. R., Wold, B. J., Ernst, S. G., Britten, R. J., and Davidson, E. H. 1977. Appearance and persistence of maternal RNA sequences in sea urchin development. *Dev. Biol.* **60**:258–277.

Hough-Evans, B. R., Ernst, S. G., Britten, R. J., and Davidson, E. H. 1979. RNA complexity in developing sea urchin oocytes. *Dev. Biol.* **69**:258–269.

Howards, S., Lechene, C., and Vigersky, R. 1979. The fluid environment of the maturing spermatozoon. *In*: Fawcett, D. W., and Bedford, J. M., eds., *The Spermatozoon*, Munich, Urban & Schwarzenberg, pp. 35–41.

Huebner, E., and Anderson, E. 1976. Comparative spiralian oogenesis—structural aspects: An overview. *Am. Zool.* **16**:315–343.

Huffman, D. M. 1968. Meiotic behavior in the mushroom *Collybia maculata* var. *scorzonerea*. *Mycologia* **60**:451–456.

Iatrou, K., and Dixon, G. H. 1977. The distribution of poly (A)$^+$ and poly (A)$^-$ protamine mRNA sequences in the developing trout testes. *Cell* **10**:433–441.

Iatrou, K., and Dixon, G. H. 1978. Protamine mRNA: Its life history during spermatogenesis in rainbow trout. *Fed. Proc.* **37**:2526–2533.

Iatrou, K., Spira, A. W., and Dixon, G. H. 1978. Protamine mRNA: Evidence for early synthesis in rainbow trout. *Dev. Biol.* **64**:82–98.

Iatrou, K., Gedamu, L., and Dixon, G. H. 1979. Protamine mRNA: Partial purification and characterization of a heterogeneous family of polyadenylated messenger components. *Can. J. Biochem.* **57**:945–956.

Ijiri, K., and Egami, N. 1975. Mitotic activity of germ cells during normal development of *Xenopus laevis* tadpoles. *J. Embryol. Exp. Morphol.* **34**:687–694.

Ikenishi, K., Kotani, M., and Tanabe, K. 1974. Ultrastructural changes associated with UV irradiation in the "germinal plasm" of *Xenopus laevis*. *Dev. Biol.* **36**:155–168.

Jacob, E. 1980. Characterization of cloned cDNA sequences derived from *Xenopus laevis* polyA(+) oocyte RNA. *Nucleic Acids Res.* **8**:1319–1337.

Jaggi, R. B., Felber, B. K., Maurhofer, S., Weber, R., and Ryffel, G. U. 1980. Four different vitellogenin proteins of *Xenopus* identified by translation *in vitro*. *Eur. J. Biochem.* **109**:343–347.

Jamieson, B. G. M. 1978. A comparison of spermiogenesis and spermatozoal ultrastructure in megascolecid and lumbricid earthworms. *Aust. J. Zool.* **26**:225–240.

Jamieson, B. G. M., and Daddow, L. 1979. An ultrasturctural study of microtubules and the acrosome in spermiogenesis of Tubificidae (Oligochaeta). *J. Ultrastruct. Res.* **67**:209–224.

Johnson, A. W., and Hnilica, L. S. 1971. Cytoplasmic and nuclear basic protein synthesis during early sea urchin development. *Biochim. Biophys. Acta* **246**:141–154.

Jonasson, J., Santesson, B., and Ström, A. 1980. Analysis of sister-chromatid exchanges and tumorigenicity in cell hybrids. *J. Cell Sci.* **42**:117–126.

Jones, R., and Glover, T. D. 1975. Interrelationships between spermatozoa, the epididymis and epididymal plasma. *In*: Duckett, J. G., and Racey, P. A., eds., *The Biology of the Male Gamete*, New York, Academic Press, pp. 367–384.

Jones, R. C. 1971. Studies of the structure of the head of boar spermatozoa from the epididymis. *J. Reprod. Fertil.* **13**(Suppl.):51–64.

Jones, R. C. 1975. Fertility and infertility in mammals in relation to sperm structure. *In*: Duckett, J. G., and Racey, P. A., eds., *The Biology of the Male Gamete*, New York, Academic Press, pp. 343–365.

Jordon, H. E. 1917. Embryonic history of the germ cells of the loggerhead turtle (*Caretta caretta*). *Publ. Carnegie Inst.* **251**:313–344.

Jukes, T. H., and Kay, H. D. 1932. The immunological behavior of the second protein (livetin) of hen's egg yolk. *J. Exp. Med.* **56**:469–482.

Kalt, M. R. 1973. Ultrastructural observations on the germ line of *Xenopus laevis*. *Z. Zellforsch. Mikrosk. Anat.* **138**:41–62.

Kalt, M. R. 1976. Morphology and kinetics of spermatogenesis in *Xenopus laevis*. *J. Exp. Zool.* **195**:393–408.

Kalt, M. R. 1977. Cytoplasmic inclusions in *Xenopus* spermatogenic cells: Ultrastructural and cytochemical analysis of the action of antimitotic agents on subcellular elements. *J. Cell Sci.* **28**:15–28.

Kalt, M. R., and Gall, J. G. 1974. Observations on early germ cell development and premeiotic rDNA amplification in *X. laevis*. *J. Cell Biol.* **62**:460–472.

Kalt, M. R., Pinney, H. E., and Graves, K. 1975. Inhibitor induced alterations of chromatid bodies in male germ line cells of *Xenopus laevis*. *Cell Tissue Res.* **161**:193–210.

Kanda, N., and Kato, H. 1979. *In vivo* sister chromatid exchange in cells of various organs of the mouse. *Chromosoma* **74**:299–305.

Kang, Y. H. 1974. Development of the zona pellucida in the rat oocyte. *Am. J. Anat.* **139**:535–566.

Kato, H. 1979. Preferential occurrence of sister chromatid exchanges at heterochromatin–euchromatin junctions in the wallaby and hamster chromosomes. *Chromosoma* **74**:307–316.

Kaye, J. S., and McMaster-Kaye, R. 1975. The fine structure and protein composition of developing spermatid nuclei. *In*: Duckett, J. G., and Racey, P. A., eds., *The Biology of the Male Gamete*, New York, Academic Press, pp. 227–237.

Keichline, L. D., and Wassarman, P. M. 1977. Developmental study of the structure of sea urchin embryo and sperm chromatin using micrococcal nuclease. *Biochim. Biophys. Acta* **475**:139–151.

Keichline, L. D., and Wassarman, P. M. 1979. Structure of chromatin in sea urchin embryos, sperm, and adult somatic cells. *Biochemistry* **18**:214–219.

Kemp, R. F. O. 1975. Oidia, plasmogamy and speciation in Basidiomycetes. *In*: Duckett, J. G., and Racey, P. A., eds., *The Biology of the Male Gamete*, New York, Academic Press, pp. 57–69.

Kerr, J. B., and Dixon, D. E. 1974. An ultrastructural study of germ plasm in spermatogenesis of *Xenopus laevis*. *J. Embryol. Exp. Morphol.* **32**:573–592.

Kessel, R. G., and Ganion, L. R. 1980a. Cytodifferentiation in the *Rana pipiens* oocyte. VI. The origin and morphogenesis of primary yolk precursor complexes. *J. Submicrosc. Cytol.* **12**:647–654.

Kessel, R. G., and Ganion, L. R. 1980b. Electron microscopic and autoradiographic studies on vitellogenesis in *Necturus maculosus*. *J. Morphol.* **164**:215–233.

Kierszenbaum, A. L., and Tres, L. L. 1974. Nucleolar and perichromosomal RNA synthesis during meiotic prophase in the mouse testis. *J. Cell Biol.* **60**:39–53.

King, R. C. 1970. The meiotic behavior of the *Drosophila* oocyte. *Int. Rev. Cytol.* **28**:125–168.

Klemperer, F. 1893. Über natürliche Immunität und ihre Verwertung für die Immunisierungstheräpie. *Arch. Exp. Pathol. Pharmakol.* **31**:356–382.

Kleve, M. G., and Clark, W. H. 1980. Association of actin with sperm centrioles: Isolation of centriolar complexes and immunofluorescent localization of actin. *J. Cell Biol.* **86**:87–95.

Kloetzel, P.-M., and Sommerville, J. 1981. Analysis and reconstruction of an RNP particle which stores 5 S RNA and tRNA in amphibian oocytes. *Nucleic Acids Res.* **9**:605–621.

Knox, R. B. 1976. Cell recognition and pattern formation in plants. *In*: Graham, C. F., and Wareing, P. F., eds., *The Developmental Biology of Plants and Animals*, Oxford, Blackwell, pp. 141–168.

Koeppe, J., and Ofengand, J. 1976. Juvenile hormone-induced biosynthesis of vitellogenin in *Leucophaea maderae*. *Arch. Biochem. Biophys.* **173**:100–113.

Korn, L. J., and Brown, D. D. 1978. Nucleotide sequences of *Xenopus borealis* oocyte 5S DNA: Comparisons of sequences that flank several related eucaryotic genes. *Cell* **15**:1145–1156.

Kostellow, A. B., and Morrill, G. A. 1977. Role of calcium and cyclic nucleotides in progesterone-induced meiotic maturation in *R. pipiens*. *Fed. Proc.* **36**:634.

Kowalski, D. T. 1965. Development and cytology of *Preussia typharum*. *Bot. Gaz.* **126**:123–130.

Kowalski, D. T. 1966. The morphology and cytology of *Preussia funiculata*. *Am. J. Bot.* **53**:1036–1041.

Krause, W. J., and Cutts, J. H. 1979. Pairing of spermatozoa in the epididymis of the opossum *Didelphis virginiana*: A scanning electron microscope study. *Arch. Histol. Jpn.* **42**:181–190.

Kressmann, A., Clarkson, S. G., Telford, J. L., and Birnstiel, M. L. 1978. Transcription of *Xenopus* tDNA^{Met} and sea urchin histone DNA injected into the *Xenopus* oocyte nucleus. *Cold Spring Harbor Symp. Quant. Biol.* **42**:1077–1082.

Kugrens, P. 1980. EM observations on the differentiation and release of spermatia in the marine red alga *Polysiphonia hendryi*. *Am. J. Bot.* **67**:519–528.

LaClaire, J. W., and West, J. A. 1978. Light- and electron-microscopic studies of growth and reproduction in *Cutleria*. *Protoplasma* **97**:93–110.

LaClaire, J. W., and West, J. A. 1979. Light- and electron-microscopic studies of growth and reproduction in *Cutleria* (Phaeophyta). II. Gametogenesis in the male plant of *C. hancocki*. *Protoplasma* **101**:247–267.

Lal, M., and Bell, P. R. 1975. Spermatogenesis in mosses. *In*: Duckett, J. G., and Racey, P. A., eds., *The Biology of the Male Gamete*, New York, Academic Press, pp. 85–95.

LaMarca, M. J., and Wassarman, P. M. 1979. Program of early development in the mammal: Changes in absolute rates of synthesis of ribosomal proteins during oogenesis and early embryogenesis in the mouse. *Dev. Biol.* **73**:103–119.

Lane, C. D. 1981. The fate of foreign proteins introduced into *Xenopus* oocytes. *Cell* **24**:281–282.

Lane, C. D., Champion, J., Haiml, L., and Kreil, G. 1981. The sequestration, processing and retention of honey-bee promellitin made in amphibian oocytes. *Eur. J. Biochem.* **113**:273–281.

Lange, L., and Olson, L. W. 1977. The zoospore of *Phlyctochytrium aestuarii*. *Protoplasma* **93**:27–43.

Lange, L., and Olson, L. W. 1978. The zoospore of *Synchytrium endobioticum*. *Can. J. Bot.* **56**:1229–1239.

Laskey, R. A., and Gurdon, J. B. 1973. Induction of polyoma DNA synthesis by injection into frog-egg cytoplasm. *Eur. J. Biochem.* **37**:467–471.

Laskowski, M., and Sealock, R. W. 1971. Protein proteinase inhibitors—Molecular aspects. *In*: Boyer, P. D., ed., *The Enzymes*, 3rd ed., New York, Academic Press, Vol. 3, pp. 376–473.

Lavallard, R. 1976. Données ultrastructurales sur la spermatogenèse chez *Peripatus accacioi*. *C. R. Acad. Sci. Ser. D.* **282**:461–464.

Lessie, P. E., and Lovett, J. S. 1968. Ultrastructural changes during sporangium formation and zoospore differentiation in *Blastocladiella emersonii*. *Am. J. Bot.* **55**:220–236.

Levine, N., and Marsh, D. J. 1971. Micropuncture studies of the electrochemical aspects of fluid and electrolyte transport in individual seminiferous tubules, the epididymis and the vas deferens in rats. *J. Physiol. (London)* **213**:557–570.

Lin, M. S. 1980. Sister chromatid exchanges in human cells and Chinese hamster cells. *Exp. Cell Res.* **127**:179–183.

Ling, V., and Dixon, G. H. 1970. The biosynthesis of protamine in trout testis. II. Polysome patterns and protein synthetic activities during testis maturation. *J. Biol. Chem.* **245**:3035–3042.

Ling, V., Trevithick, J. R., and Dixon, G. H. 1969. The biosynthesis of protamine in trout testis. I. Intercellular site of synthesis. *Can. J. Biochem.* **47**:51–60.

Linskens, H. F., and Kroh, M. 1967. In Kompatibiletät der Phanerogamen. *Encycl. Plant Physiol.* **18**:506–530.

Loones, M. T. 1979. *In vivo* effects of γ-irradiation on the functional architecture of the lampbrush chromosomes in *Pleurodeles* (Amphibia, Urodela). *Chromosoma* **73**:357–368.

Lovett, J. A., and Goldstein, E. S. 1977. The cytoplasmic distribution and characterization of poly(A)+ RNA in oocytes and embryos of *Drosophila*. *Dev. Biol.* **61**:70–78.

Lovett, J. S., Barstow, W. E., and Lassie, P. E. 1975. Growth and differentiation of the water mold *Blastocladiella emersonii*. *Bacteriol. Rev.* **39**:345–404.

Lu, B. C. 1967. Meiosis in *Coprinus lagopus*: A comparative study with light and electron microscopy. *J. Cell Sci.* **2**:529–536.

Lu, B. C., and Raju, N. B. 1970. Meiosis in *Coprinus*. II. Chromosome pairing and the lampbrush diplotene stage of meiotic prophase. *Chromosoma* **29**:305–316.

Luciani, J. M., and Stahl, A. 1971. Rapports des nucléoles avec les chromosomes méiotiques de l'ovocyte foetal humain. *C. R. Acad. Sci. Ser. D.* **273**:521–524.

McCully, K. A., Maw, W. A., and Common, R. H. 1959. Zone electrophoresis of the proteins of the fowl's serum and egg yolk. *Can. J. Biochem. Physiol.* **37**:1457–1468.

Macgregor, H. C., and Andrews, C. 1977. The arrangement and transcription of "middle repetitive" DNA sequences on lampbrush chromosomes of *Triturus*. *Chromosoma* **63**:109–126.

Macgregor, H. C., Mizuno, S., and Vlad, M. 1976. Chromosomes and DNA sequences in salamanders. *Chromosomes Today* **5**:331–339.

McMaster-Kaye, R., and Kaye, J. S. 1980a. Organization of chromatin during spermiogenesis: Beaded fibers, partly beaded fibers, and loss of nucleosome structure. *Chromosoma* **77**:41–46.

McMaster-Kaye, R., and Kaye, J. S. 1980b. Acrosomal bands: Specialized structures on the nuclear surface for holding the acrosomal granule. *J. Ultrastruct. Res.* **71**:233–248.

Magnusson, C. 1980. Role of cumulus cells for rat oocyte maturation and metabolism. *Gamete Res.* **3**:133–140.

Maguire, M. P. 1979. An indirect test for a role of the synaptonemal complex in the establishment of sister chromatid cohesiveness. *Chromosoma* **70**:313–321.

Malcolm, D. B., and Sommerville, J. 1974. The structure of chromosome-derived RNP in oocytes of *Triturus cristatus carnifex*. *Chromosoma* **48**:137–158.

Maller, J. L., Wu, M., and Gerhart, J. C. 1977. Changes in protein phosphorylation accompanying maturation of *X. laevis* oocytes. *Dev. Biol.* **58**:295–312.

Marcaillou, C., and Szöllösi, A. 1980. The "blood–testis" barrier in a nematode and a fish: A generalizable concept. *J. Ultrastruct. Res.* **70**:128–136.

Marushige, K., and Dixon, G. H. 1969. Developmental changes in chromosomal composition and template activity during spermatogenesis in trout testis. *Dev. Biol.* **19**:397–414.

Masui, Y. 1967. Relative roles of the pituitary, follicle cells, and progesterone in the induction of oocyte maturation in *Rana pipiens*. *J. Exp. Zool.* **166**:365–376.

Mauléon, P. 1975. Importance des différentes périodes ovogénétiques dans la gonade femelle d'embryon de brebis: Contrôle du changement de comportement mitotique en méiotique. *Ann. Biol. Anim. Biochim. Biophys.* **15**:725–737.

Mauléon, P., Devictor-Vuillet, M., and Luciani, J. M. 1976. The preloeptotene chromosome condensation and decondensation in the ovary of the sheep embryo. *Ann. Biol. Anim. Biochim. Biophys.* **16**:293–296.

May, F. E. B., and Knowland, J. 1980. The role of thyroxin in the transition of vitellogenin synthesis from noninducibility to inducibility during metamorphosis in *Xenopus laevis*. *Dev. Biol.* **77**:419–430.

Mermod, J. J., Schatz, G., and Crippa, M. 1980. Specific control of messenger translation in *Drosophila* oocyte and embryos. *Dev. Biol.* **75**:177–186.

Mertz, J., and Gurdon, J. B. 1977. Purified DNAs are transcribed after microinjection into *Xenopus* oocytes. *Nature (London)* **260**:116–120.

Metz, C. W. 1927. Chromosome behavior and genetic behavior in *Sciara*. II. Genetic evidence of selective segregation in *S. coprophila*. *Z. Indukt. Abstamm. Vererbungsl.* **45**:184–201.

Metz, C. W. 1938. Chromosome behavior, inheritance, and sex determination in *Sciara*. *An. Nat.* **72**:485–520.

Metz, C. W., and Schmuck, M. L. 1931. Studies on sex determination and the sex chromosome mechanism in *Sciara*. *Genetics* **16**:225–253.

Metz, C. W., Moses, M. S., and Hoppe, E. N. 1926. Chromosome behavior and genetic behavior in *Sciara*. I. Chromosome behavior in the spermatocyte divisions. *Z. Indukt. Abstamm. Vererbungsl.* **42**:237–267.

Meves, F. 1903. Über oligopyrene und apyrene Spermien und über ihre Entstehung nach Beobachtungen an *Paludina* und *Pygaera*. *Arch. Mikrosk. Anat. Entwicklungsmech.* **61**:1–84.

Millette, C. F. 1979. Appearance and partitioning of plasma membrane antigens during mouse spermatogenesis. *In*: Fawcett, D. W., and Bedford, J. M., eds., *The Spermatozoon*, Munich, Urban & Schwarzenberg, pp. 177–186.

Mizukami, I., and Gall, J. G. 1966. Centriole replication. II. Sperm formation in the fern, *Marsilea*, and the Cycad, *Zamia*. *J. Cell Biol.* **29**:97–111.

Moens, P. B. 1968. The structure and function of the synaptonemal complex in *Lilium longiflorum* sporocytes. *Chromosoma* **23**:418–451.

Moens, P. B., and Church, K. 1979. The distribution of synaptonemal complex material in metaphase I bivalents of *Locusta* and *Choealtis* (Orthoptera: Acrididae). *Chromosoma* **73**:247–254.

Moens, P. B., and Go, V. L. W. 1972. Intercellular bridges and division patterns of rat spermatogonia. *Z. Zellforsch. Mikrosk. Anat.* **127**:201–208.

Moestrup, O. 1975. Some aspects of sexual reproduction in eucaryotic algae. *In*: Duckett, J. G., and Racey, P. A., eds., *The Biology of the Male Gamete*, New York, Academic Press, pp. 23–35.

Mohun, T. J., Lane, C. D., Colman, A., and Wylie, C. C. 1981. The secretion of proteins *in vitro* from *Xenopus* oocytes and their accessory cells: A biochemical and morphological study. *J. Embryol. Exp. Morphol.* **61**:367–383.

Mok, C. C., Martin, W. G., and Common, R. H. 1961. A comparison of phosvitins prepared from hen's serum and hen's egg yolk. *Can. J. Biochem. Physiol.* **39**:109–117.

Monesi, V. 1964. Ribonucleic acid synthesis during mitosis and meiosis in the mouse testis. *J. Cell Biol.* **22**:521–532.

Monesi, V. 1965. Synthetic activities during spermatogenesis in the mouse: RNA and protein. *Exp. Cell Res.* **39**:197–224.

Monesi, V., Geremia, R., D'Agostino, A., and Boitani, C. 1978. Biochemistry of male germ cell differentiation in mammals: RNA synthesis in meiotic and post meiotic cells. *Curr. Top. Dev. Biol.* **12**:11–36.

Moor, R. M., Smith, M. W., and Dawson, R. M. C. 1980a. Measurement of intercellular coupling between oocytes and cumulus cells using intracellular markers. *Exp. Cell Res.* **126**:15–29.

Moor, R. M., Polge, C., and Willadsen, S. M. 1980b. Effect of follicular steroids on the maturation and fertilization of mammalian oocytes. *J. Embryol. Exp. Morphol.* **56**:319–335.

Moore, G. P. M., and Lintern-Moore, S. 1974. A correlation between growth and RNA synthesis in the mouse oocyte. *J. Cell Biol.* **60**:416–422.

Morgan, G. T. 1979. The time course of male meiosis in the red-backed salamander, *Plethodon cinereus*. *J. Cell Sci.* **38**:345–356.

Morrill, G. A., and Murphy, J. B. 1972. Role for protein phosphorylation in meiosis and in the early cleavage phase of amphibian embryonic development. *Nature (London)* **238**:282–284.

Moses, M. J., Karatsis, P. A., and Hamilton, A. E. 1979. Synaptonemal complex analysis of heteromorphic trivalents in *Lemur* hybrids. *Chromosoma* **70**:141–160.

Muckenthaler, F. A. 1964. Autoradiographic study of nucleic acid synthesis during spermatogenesis in the grasshopper, *Melanoplus differentialis*. *Exp. Cell Res.* **35**:531–547.

Muramatsu, M., Utakoji, T., and Sugano, H. 1968. Rapidly-labeled nuclear RNA in Chinese hamster testis. *Exp. Cell Res.* **53**:278–283.

Myles, D. G., and Bell, P. R. 1975. An ultrastructural study of the spermatozoid of the fern, *Marsilea vestiti*. *J. Cell Sci.* **17**:633–645.

Myles, D. G., and Hepler, P. K. 1977. Spermiogenesis in the fern *Marsilea*: Microtubules, nuclear shaping, and cytomorphogenesis. *J. Cell Sci.* **23**:57–83.

Nicolson, G. L., and Yanagimachi, R. 1979. Cell surface changes associated with the epididymal maturation of mammalian spermatozoa. *In*: Fawcett, D. W., and Bedford, J. M., eds., *The Spermatozoon*, Munich, Urban & Schwarzenberg, pp. 187–194.

Nicolson, G. L., Usui, N., Yanagimachi, R., Yanagimachi, H., and Smith, J. R. 1977. Lectin binding sites on the plasma membranes of rabbit spermatozoa. *J. Cell Biol.* **74**:950–962.

Norstog, K. 1975. The motility of cycad spermatozoids in relation to structure and function. *In*: Duckett, J. G., and Racey, P. A., eds., *The Biology of the Male Gamete*, New York, Academic Press, pp. 135–142.

Oakberg, E. F. 1968. Relationship between stage of follicular development and RNA synthesis in the mouse oocyte. *Mutat. Res.* **6**:155–165.

O'Brien, D. A., and Bellvé, A. R. 1980a. Protein constituents of the mouse spermatozoon. I. An electrophoretic characterization. *Dev. Biol.* **75**:386–404.

O'Brien, D. A., and Bellvé, A. R. 1980b. Protein constituents of the mouse spermatozoon. II. Temporal synthesis during spermatogenesis. *Dev. Biol.* **75**:405–418.

O'Connor, C. M., and Smith, L. D. 1976. Inhibition of oocyte maturation by theophylline: Possible mechanism of action. *Dev. Biol.* **52**:318–322.

Olins, A. L. 1977. ν bodies are close-packed in chromatin fibres. *Cold Spring Harbor Symp. Quant. Biol.* **42**:325–329.

Olson, L. W., Lange, L., and Reichle, R. 1978. The zoospore and meiospore of the aquatic phycomycete *Catenaria anquillulae*. *Protoplasma* **94**:53–71.

Opresko, L., Wiley, H. S., and Wallace, R. A. 1980. Differential postendocytotic compartmentation in *Xenopus* oocytes is mediated by a specifically bound ligand. *Cell* **22**:47–57.

O'Rand, M. G. 1979. Changes in sperm surface properties correlated with capacitation. *In*: Fawcett, D. W., and Bedford, J. M., eds., *The Spermatozoon*, Munich, Urban & Schwarzenberg, pp. 195–204.

O'Rand, M. G., and Romrell, L. J. 1980. Appearance of regional surface autoantigens during spermatogenesis: Comparison of anti-testis and anti-sperm autoantisera. *Dev. Biol.* **75**:431–441.

Ozaki, H. 1971. Developmental studies of sea urchin chromatin: Chromatin isolated from spermatozoa of *Strongylocentrotus purpuratus*. *Dev. Biol.* **26**:209–219.

Ozdzenski, W. 1967. Observations on the origin of primordial germ cells in the mouse. *Zool. Pol.* **17**:367–379.

Paddock, S. W., and Woolley, D. M. 1980. Helical conformation of dense fibers from mammalian spermatozoa. *Exp. Cell. Res.* **126**:199–206.

Pala, M. 1970. The embryonic history of the primordial germ cells in *Gambusia holbrookii* (Grd). *Boll. Zool.* **37**:49–62.

Pan, M. L. 1971. The synthesis of vitellogenin in the cecropia silkworm. *J. Insect Physiol.* **17**:677–689.

Pan, M. L., Bell, W. J., and Telfer, W. H. 1969. Vitellogenic blood protein synthesis by insect fat body. *Science* **165**:393–394.

Paolillo, D. J., Kreitner, G. L., and Reighard, J. A. 1968a. Spermatogenesis in *Polytrichum juniperinum*. I. The origin of the apical body and the elongation of the nucleus. *Planta* **78**:226–247.

Paolillo, D. J., Kreitner, G. L., and Reighard, J. A. 1968b. Spermatogenesis in *Polytrichum juniperinum*. II. The mature sperm. *Planta* **78**:248–261.

Parchman, L. G., and Lin, K. C. 1972. Nucleolar RNA synthesis during meiosis of lily microsporocytes. *Nature New Biol.* **239**:235–237.

Pathak, S., Lau, Y.-F., and Drwinga, H. L. 1979. Observations on the synaptonemal complex in Armenian hamster spermatocytes by light microscopy. *Chromosoma* **73**:53–60.

Peel, M. C., and Duckett, J. G. 1975. Studies of spermatogenesis in the Rhodophyta. *In*: Duckett, J. G., and Racey, P. A., eds., *The Biology of the Male Gamete*, New York, Academic Press, pp. 1–13.

Perlman, S. M., and Rosbash, M. M. 1978. Analysis of *Xenopus laevis* ovary and somatic cell polyadenylated RNA by molecular hybridization. *Dev. Biol.* **63**:197–212.

Perlman, S. M., Ford, P. J., and Rosbash, M. M. 1977. Presence of tadpole and adult globin RNA sequences in oocytes of *Xenopus laevis*. *Proc. Natl. Acad. Sci. USA* **74**:3835–3839.

Perry, M. M., and Gilbert, A. B. 1979. Yolk transport in the ovarian follicle of the hen (*Gallus domesticus*): Lipoprotein-like particles at the periphery of the oocyte in the rapid growth phase. *J. Cell Sci.* **39**:257–272.

Perry, R. P., and Kelley, D. E. 1973. Messenger RNA turnover in mouse L cells. *J. Mol. Biol.* **79**:681–696.

Peters, H., Levy, E., and Crone, M. 1962. DNA synthesis in oocytes of mouse embryos. *Nature (London)* **195**:915–916.

Peters, H., Levy, E., and Crone, M. 1965. Oogenesis in rabbits. *J. Exp. Zool.* **158**:169–180.

Phillips, D. M. 1966. Observations on spermiogenesis in the fungus gnat *Sciara coprophila*. *J. Cell Biol.* **30**:477–497.

Phillips, D. M. 1977. Mitochondrial disposition in mammalian spermatozoa. *J. Ultrastruct. Res.* **58**:144–154.

Phillips, D. M. 1980. Observations on mammalian spermiogenesis using surface replicas. *J. Ultrastruct. Res.* **72**:103–111.

Picard, B., and Wegnez, M. 1979. Isolation of a 7 S particle from *Xenopus laevis* oocytes: A 5 S RNA–protein complex. *Proc. Natl. Acad. Sci. USA* **76**:241–245.

Picard, B., le Maire, M., Wegnez, M., and Denis, H. 1980. Biochemical research on oogenesis: Composition of the 42-S storage particles of *X. laevis* oocytes. *Eur. J. Biochem.* **109**:359–368.

Pickett-Heaps, J. D. 1968. Ultrastructure and differentiation in *Chara*. IV. Spermatogenesis. *Aust. J. Biol. Sci.* **21**:655–690.

Pollister, A. W., and Pollister, P. F. 1943. The relation between centriole and centromere in atypical spermatogenesis of viviparid snails. *Ann. N.Y. Acad. Sci.* **45**:1–48.

Potter, H., and Dressler, D. 1980. DNA synaptase: An enzyme that fuses DNA molecules at a region of homology. *Proc. Natl. Acad. Sci. USA* **77**:2390–2394.

Preston, S. F., Deanin, G. G., Hanson, R. K., and Gordon, M. W. 1981. Tubulin: Tyrosine ligase in oocytes and embryos of *Xenopus laevis*. *Dev. Biol.* **81**:36–42.

Pukkila, P. J. 1975. Identification of the lampbrush chromosome loops which transcribe 5S rRNA in *Notophthalmus (Triturus) viridescens*. *Chromosoma* **53**:71–89.

Racey, P. A. 1972. Viability of bat spermatozoa after prolonged storage in the epididymis. *J. Reprod. Fertil.* **28**:303–307.

Racey, P. A. 1975. The prolonged survival of spermatozoa in bats. *In*: Duckett, J. G., and Racey, P. A., eds., *The Biology of the Male Gamete*, New York, Academic Press, p. 385–416.

Raghavan, V. 1976. Role of the generative cell in androgenesis in henbane. *Science* **191**:388–389.

Raghavan, V. 1978. Origin and development of pollen embryoids and pollen calluses in cultured anther segments of *Hyoscyamus niger* (henbane). *Am. J. Bot.* **65**:984–1002.

Raghavan, V. 1979. Embryogenic determination and RNA synthesis in pollen grains of *Hyoscyamus niger* (henbane). *Am. J. Bot.* **66**:36–39.

Ramirez, S. A., and Guajardo, M. 1980. A cytological and histochemical analysis of the ovarian follicle cells of the South Texas squid (*Loligo pealei*). *Tex. J. Sci.* **32**:43–54.

Redshaw, M. R., Follett, B. K., and Nicholls, T. J. 1969. Comparative effects of the oestrogens and other steroid hormones on serum lipids and proteins in *Xenopus laevis*. *J. Endocrinol.* **43**:47–53.

Reeves, R. 1978. Nucleosome structure of *Xenopus* oocyte amplified ribosomal genes. *Biochemistry* **17**:4908–4916.

Richards, A., and Thompson, J. T. 1921. The migration of the primary sex-cells of *Fundulus heteroclitus*. *Biol. Bull.* **40**:325–428.

Robbins, R. R., and Carothers, Z. B. 1978. Spermatogenesis in *Lycopodium*: The mature spermatozoid. *Am. J. Bot.* **65**:433–440.

Rodman, T. C., and Bachvarova, R. 1976. RNA synthesis in preovulatory mouse oocytes. *J. Cell Biol.* **70**:251–257.

Rodman, T. C., and Barth, A. H. 1979. Chromosomes of mouse oocytes in maturation: Differential trypsin sensitivity and amino acid incorporation. *Dev. Biol.* **68**:82–95.

Romrell, L. J., and O'Rand, M. G. 1978. Capping and ultrastructural localization of sperm surface isoantigens during spermatogenesis. *Dev. Biol.* **63**:76–93.

Roosen-Runge, E. C. 1977. *The Process of Spermatogenesis in Animals*, London, Cambridge University Press.

Rosbach, M., Ford, P. J., and Bishop, J. O. 1974. Analysis of the C-value paradox by molecular hybridization. *Proc. Natl. Acad. Sci. USA* **71**:3746–3750.

Rossen, J. M., and Westergaard, M. 1966. Meiosis and the time of meiotic chromosome replication in the ascomycete *Neottiella rutilans*. *C. R. Trav. Lab. Carlsberg* **35**:233–260.

Rubenstein, E. C. 1979. The role of an epithelial occlusion zone in the termination of vitellogenesis in *Hyalophora cecropia* ovarian follicles. *Dev. Biol.* **71**:115–127.

Ruhberg, H., and Storch, V. 1976. Zur Ultrastruktur von mannlichen Genital-trakt: Spermiocytogenesis und Spermien von *Peripatopsis moseleyi*. *Zoomorphologie* **85**:1–15.

Russell, L. D. 1980. Sertoli–germ cell interrelations: A review. *Gamete Res.* **3**:179–202.

Ryffel, G. U., Wyler, T., Muellener, D. B., and Weber, R. 1980. Identification, organization and processing intermediates of the putative precursors of *Xenopus* vitellogenin mRNA. *Cell* **19**:53–61.

Sagata, N., Shiokawa, K., and Yamana, K. 1980. A study on the steady-state population of poly(A)$^+$ RNA during early development of *Xenopus laevis*. *Dev. Biol.* **77**:431–448.

Sams, G. R., Bell, W. J., and Weaver, R. F. 1980. Vitellogenin: Its structure, synthesis and processing in the cockroach *Periplaneta americana*. *Biochim. Biophys. Acta* **609**:121–135.

Santos, A., Abreu, I., and Salema, R. 1979. Elaborate system of RER and degenerescence of tapetum during pollen development in some dicotyledons. *J. Submicrosc. Cytol.* **11**:99–107.

Schatz, F., and Ziegler, D. 1979. The role of follicle cells in *Rana pipiens* oocyte maturation induced by Δ^5-pregnenolone. *Dev. Biol.* **73**:59–67.

Scheer, U. 1981. Identification of a novel class of tandemly repeated genes transcribed on lampbrush chromosomes of *Pleurodeles waltlii*. *J. Cell Biol.* **88**:599–603.

Scheer, U., Franke, W. W., Trendelenburg, M. F., and Spring, H. 1976. Classification of loops of lampbrush chromosomes according to the arrangement of transcriptional complexes. *J. Cell Sci.* **22**:503–519.

Scheer, U., Sommerville, J., and Bustin, M. 1979a. Injected histone antibodies interfere with transcription of lampbrush chromosome loops in oocytes of *Pleurodeles*. *J. Cell Sci.* **40**:1–20.

Scheer, U., Spring, H., and Trendelenburg, M. F. 1979b. Organization of transcriptionally active chromatin in lampbrush chromosome loops. *In:* Busch, H., ed., *The Cell Nucleus*, New York, Academic Press, Vol. 7, pp. 3–47.

Schin, K. S. 1965. Core-strukturen in den meiotischen und post-meiotischen Kernen der Spermatogenese von *Gryllus domesticus*. *Chromosoma* **16**:436–452.

Schultz, R. M., Letourneau, G. E., and Wassarman, P. M. 1978a. Meiotic maturation of mouse oocytes *in vitro*: Protein synthesis in nucleate and anucleate oocyte fragments. *J. Cell Sci.* **30**:251–264.

Schultz, R. M., LaMarca, M. J., and Wassarman, P. M. 1978b. Absolute rates of protein synthesis during meiotic maturation of mammalian oocytes *in vitro*. *Proc. Natl. Acad. Sci. USA* **75**:4160–4164.

Schultz, R. M., Letourneau, G. E., and Wassarman, P. M. 1979a. Program of early development in the mammal: Changes in patterns and absolute rates of tubulin and total protein synthesis during oogenesis and early embryogenesis in the mouse. *Dev. Biol.* **68**:341–359.

Schultz, R. M., Letourneau, G. E., and Wassarman, P. M. 1979b. Program of early development in the mammal: Changes in patterns and absolute rates of tubulin and total protein synthesis during oocyte growth in the mouse. *Dev. Biol.* **73**:120–133.

Sconzo, G., Bono, D., Albanese, I., and Giudice, G. 1972. Studies on sea urchin oocytes. II. Synthesis of RNA during oogenesis. *Exp. Cell Res.* **72**:95–100.

Scott, S. E. M., and Sommerville, J. 1974. Location of nuclear proteins on the chromosomes of newt oocytes. *Nature (London)* **250**:680–682.

Selman, K., and Anderson, E. 1975. The formation and cytochemical characterization of cortical granules in ovarian oocytes of the golden hamster (*Mesocricetus auratus*). *J. Morphol.* **147**:251–274.

Selman, K., and Arnold, J. M. 1978. An ultrastructural and cytochemical analysis of oogenesis in the squid, *Loligo pealei*. *J. Morphol.* **152**:381–400.

Shih, R. 1975. Analyses of the amino acid pools, rates of protein synthesis and nuclear proteins of *Rana pipiens* oocytes and embryos. Ph.D. thesis, Purdue University.

Simon, D. 1960. Contribution à l'étude de la circulation et du transfert des gonocytes primaires dans les blastodermes d'oiseau cultivé *in vitro*. *Arch. Anat. Microsc. Morphol. Exp.* **49**:93–176.

Simpson, R. T., and Bergman, L. W. 1980. Structure of sea urchin sperm chromatin core particle. *J. Biol. Chem.* **255**:10702–10709.

Singleton, J. R. 1953. Chromosome morphology and the chromosome cycle in the ascus of *Neurospora crassa*. *Am. J. Bot.* **40**:124–144.

Slater, I., and Slater, D. W. 1979. Cell-free cytoplasmic polyadenylation of oogenic RNA. *Differentiation* **13**:109–115.

Smith, L. D., and Ecker, R. E. 1969. Cytoplasmic regulation in early events of amphibian development. *Proc. Can. Cancer Res. Conf.* **8**:103–129.

Smith, S. G. 1942. Polarization and progression and pairing. *Can. J. Res. Sect. D* **20**:221–229.

Söderström, K. O. 1981. The relationship between the nuage and the chromatoid body during spermatogenesis in the rat. *Cell Tissue Res.* **215**:425–430.

Söderström, K. O., and Parvinen, M. 1976. RNA synthesis in different stages of rat seminiferous epithelial cycle. *Mol. Cell. Endocrinol.* **5**:181–199.

Sommerville, J. 1979. Gene expression in lampbrush chromosomes. *FEBS Proc. Meet.* **51**:265–276.

Sommerville, J., and Malcolm, D. B. 1976. Transcription of genetic information in amphibian oocytes. *Chromosoma* **55**:183–208.

Sotelo, J. R., and Wettstein, R. 1966. Fine structure of meiotic chromosomes: Comparative study of nine species of insects. *Chromosoma* **20**:234–250.

Spiegelman, M., and Bennett, D. 1973. A light- and electron-microscopic study of primordial germ cells in the early mouse embryo. *J. Embryol. Exp. Morphol.* **30**:97–118.

Stack, S. M. 1973. The synaptonemal complex and the achiasmatic condition. *J. Cell Sci.* **13**:83–95.

Stack, S. M., and Brown, W. V. 1969. Somatic and premeiotic pairing of homologues in *Plantago ovalis*. *Bull. Torrey Bot. Club* **96**:143–149.

Stagni, A., and Lucchi, M. L. 1970. Ultrastructural observations on the spermatogenesis in *Hydra attenuata*. *In*: Baccetti, B., ed., *Comparative Spermatology*, New York, Academic Press, pp. 357–362.

Stahl, A., Luciani, J. M., Devictor, M., Capodano, A. M., and Gagné, R. 1975. Constitutive heterochromatin and micronucleoli in the human oocyte at the diplotene state. *Humangenetik* **26**:315–327.

Stay, B. 1965. Protein uptake in the oocytes of the cecropia moth. *J. Cell Biol.* **26**:49–62.

Stefanini, M., DeMartino, C., D'Agostino, A., Agrestini, A., and Monesi, V. 1974. Nucleolar activity of rat primary spermatocytes. *Exp. Cell Res.* **86**:166–170.

Storms, R., and Hastings, P. J. 1977. A fine structure analysis of meiotic pairing in *Chlamydomonas reinhardi*. *Exp. Cell Res.* **104**:39–46.

Strauch, A. R., Luna, E. J., and La Fountain, J. R. 1980. Biochemical analysis of actin in crane-fly gonial cells: Evidence for actin in spermatocytes and spermatids—but not sperm. *J. Cell Biol.* **86**:315–325.

Suominen, J., and Setchell, B. P. 1972. Enzymes and trypsin inhibitor in the rete testis fluid of rams and boars. *J. Reprod. Fertil.* **30**:235–245.

Swan, M. A., Linck, R. W., Ito, S., and Fawcett, D. W. 1980. Structure and function of the undulating membrane in spermatozoan propulsion in the toad *Bufo marinus*. *J. Cell Biol.* **85**:866–880.

Sykes, E. E., and Porter, D. 1981. Meiosis in the aquatic fungus *Catenaria allomycis*. *Protoplasma* **105**:307–320.

Szabo, P. L. 1967. Ultrastructure of the developing dog oocyte. *Anat. Rec.* **157**:330.

Szöllösi, D. 1967. Development of cortical granules and the cortical reactions in rat and hamster eggs. *Anat. Rec.* **159**:431–446.

Szöllösi, D. 1970. Changes of some cell organelles during oogenesis in mammals. *In*: Biggers,J. D., and Schuetz, A. W., eds., *Oogenesis*, Baltimore, University Park Press, pp. 47–64.

Tarlow, D. M., Watkins, P. A., Reed, R. E., Miller, R. S., Zwergel, E. E., and Lane, M. D. 1977. Lipogenesis and the synthesis and secretion of very low density lipoprotein by avian liver cells in nonproliferating monolayer culture: Hormonal effects. *J. Cell Biol.* **73**:332–353.

Tata, J. R. 1976. The expression of the vitellogenin gene. *Cell* **9**:1–14.

Tata, J. R., Baker, B. S., and Deeley, J. V. 1980. Vitellogenin as a multigene family. *J. Biol. Chem.* **255**:6721–6726.

Telfer, W. H. 1954. Immunological studies of insect metamorphosis. *J. Gen. Physiol.* **37**:539–558.

Telfer, W. H. 1960. The selective accumulation of blood proteins by the oocytes of saturnid moths. *Biol. Bull.* **118**:338–351.

Telfer, W. H. 1961. The route of entry and localization of blood proteins in the oocytes of saturnid moths. *J. Biophys. Biochem. Cytol.* **9**:743–759.

Telfer, W. H. 1965. The mechanism and control of yolk formation. *Annu. Rev. Entomol.* **10**:161–184.

Tenner, A. J., and Wallace, R. A. 1972. A cyclic AMP-stimulated protein kinase from amphibian ovary and oocytes. *Biochim. Biophys. Acta* **276**:416–424.

Threadgold, L. T. 1976. *The Ultrastructure of the Animal Cell*, Elmsford, N.Y., Pergamon Press.

Tongkao, D., and Chulavatnatol, M. 1979. Phosphorylation of microtubules of rat spermatozoa during epididymal maturation. *In*: Fawcett, D. W., and Bedford, J. M., eds., *The Spermatozoon*, Munich, Urban & Schwarzenberg, pp. 129–134.

Toth, R. 1974. Sporangial structure and zoosporogenesis in *Chorda tomentosa*. *J. Phycol.* **10**:170–185.

Toth, R., and Markey, D. 1973. Synaptonemal complexes in brown algae. *Nature (London)* **243**:236–237.

Tres, L. L. 1975. Nucleolar RNA synthesis of meiotic prophase spermatocytes in the human testes. *Chromosoma* **53**:141–151.

Tsafriri, A. 1978. Oocyte maturation in mammals. *In*: Jones, R. E., ed., *The Vertebrate Ovary*, New York, Plenum Press, pp. 409–442.

Tsafriri, A., and Channing, C. P. 1975a. An inhibitory influence of granulosa cells and follicular fluid upon porcine oocyte meiosis *in vitro*. *Endocrinology* **96**:922–927.

Tsafriri, A., and Channing, C. P. 1975b. Influence of follicular maturation and culture conditions on the meiosis of pig oocytes *in vitro*. *J. Reprod. Fertil.* **43**:149–152.

Turner, F. R. 1968. An ultrastructural study of plant spermatogenesis: Spermatogenesis in *Nitella*. *J. Cell Biol.* **37**:370–393.

Utakoji, T. 1966. Chronology of nucleic acid synthesis in meiosis of the male Chinese hamster. *Exp. Cell Res.* **42**:585–587.

Vanneman, A. S. 1917. The early history of the germ cells in the armadillo, *Tatusia novemcincta*. *Am. J. Anat.* **2**:341–363.

Varley, J. M., Macgregor, H. C., and Erba, H. P. 1980. Satellite DNA is transcribed on lampbrush chromosomes. *Nature (London)* **283**:686–688.

Vaudois, B., and Tourte, Y. 1979. Spermatogenesis in a pteridophyte. 1. First stages of the motile apparatus. *Cytobios* **24**:143–156.

Waddington, C. H. 1962. *New Patterns in Genetics and Development*, New York, Columbia University Press.

Wahli, W., Dawid, I. B., Wyler, T., Weber, R., and Ryffel, G. U. 1980. Comparative analysis of the structural organization of two closely related vitellogenin genes in *X. laevis*. *Cell* **20**:107–117.

Wallace, R. A. 1978. Oocyte growth in nonmammalian vertebrates. *In*: Jones, R. E., ed., *The Vertebrate Ovary*, New York, Plenum Press, pp. 469–502.

Wallace, R. A., and Jared, D. W. 1968. Estrogen induces lipophosphoprotein in serum of male *Xenopus laevis*. *Science* **160**:91–92.

Wallace, R. A., and Jared, D. W. 1969. Studies on amphibian yolk. *Dev. Biol.* **19**:498–526.

Wang, S. Y., and Williams, D. L. 1980. Identification, purification, and characterization of two distinct avian vitellogenins. *Biochemistry* **19**:1557–1563.

Ward, R. T. 1978. The origin of protein and fatty yolk in *Rana pipiens*. III. Intermitochondrial and primary vesicular yolk formation in frog oocytes. *Tissue Cell* **10**:515–524.

Wareing, P. F., and Graham, C. F. 1976. Nucleus and cytoplasm. *In*: Graham, C. F., and Wareing, P. F., eds., *The Developmental Biology of Plants and Animals*, Oxford, Blackwell, pp. 5–13.

Warren, T. G., and Mahowald, A. P. 1979. Isolation and partial chemical characterization of the three major yolk polypeptides from *D. melanogaster*. *Dev. Biol.* **68**:130–139.

Wartenberg, H. 1962. Elektronmikroskopische und Histochemische Studien über die Organogenese der Amphibieneizelle. *Z. Zellforsch. Mikrosk. Anat.* **58**:427–486.

Wassarman, P. M., and Letourneau, G. E. 1976. RNA synthesis in fully-grown mouse oocytes. *Nature (London)* **261**:73–74.

Wassarman, P. M., Schultz, R. M., and Letourneau, G. E. 1979. Protein synthesis during meiotic maturation of mouse oocytes *in vitro*. *Dev. Biol.* **69**:94–107.

Wasserman, W. J., and Masui, Y. 1975. Effects of cycloheximide on a cytoplasmic factor initiating meiotic maturation in *Xenopus* oocytes. *Exp. Cell Res.* **91**:381–388.

Wasserman, W. J., and Smith, L. D. 1978. Oocyte maturation in nonmammalian vertebrates. *In*: Jones, R. E., ed., *The Vertebrate Ovary*, New York, Plenum Press, pp. 443–468.

Webb, A. C., LaMarca, M. J., and Smith, L. D. 1975. Synthesis of mtRNA by full-grown and maturing oocytes of *Rana pipiens* and *Xenopus laevis*. *Dev. Biol.* **45**:44–55.

Wegnez, M., Denis, H., Mazabraud, A., and Clerot, J. C. 1978. Biochemical research on oogenesis: RNA accumulation during oogenesis of the dogfish *Scyliorhinus caniculus*. *Dev. Biol.* **52**:99–111.

White, M. J. D. 1946. The cytology of the Cecidomyidae (Diptera). II. The chromosome cycle and anomalous spermatogenesis of *Miastor*. *J. Morphol.* **79**:323–370.

Whitington, F. M., and Dixon, K. E. 1975. Quantitative studies of germ plasm and germ cells during early embryogenesis of *Xenopus laevis*. *J. Embryol. Exp. Morphol.* **33**:57–74.

Wiblet, M., Baltus, E., and Brachet, J. B. 1975. Méiose: Rôle d'une histone kinase dans la condensation des chromosomes d'oöcytes ovariens de *Xenopus laevis* et d'*Ambystoma mexicanum*. *C. R. Acad. Sci.* **281**:1891–1893.

Wieben, E. D., 1981. Regulation of the synthesis of lactate dehydrogenase-X during spermatogenesis in the mouse. *J. Cell Biol.* **88**:492–498.

Williams, J. 1962. Serum proteins and livetins of hen's egg yolk. *Biochem. J.* **83**:346–355.

Wilson, D., and Wilson, M. 1956. Biology of *Janthina*. *J. Mar. Biol. Assoc. U.K.* **35**:291–305.

Wischnitzer, S. 1966. The ultrastructure of the cytoplasm of the developing amphibian egg. *Adv. Morphol.* **5**:131–179.

Wolfe, S. L., and John, B. 1965. The organization and ultrastructure of male meiotic chromosomes in *Oncopeltus fasciatus*. *Chromosoma* **17**:85–103.

Wolgemuth, D. J., Jagiello, G. M., and Henderson, A. S. 1979. Quantitation of rRNA genes in fetal human oocyte nuclei using rRNA: DNA hybridization *in situ*. *Exp. Cell Res.* **118**:181–190.

Wong, P. Y. D., Au, C. L., and Ngai, H. K. 1979. Some characteristics of the salt and water transport in the rat epididymis. *In*: Fawcett, D. W., and Bedford, J. M., eds., *The Spermatozoon*, Munich, Urban & Schwarzenberg, pp. 57–63.

Wong, Y. C., Wong, P. Y. D., and Yeung, C. H. 1978. Ultrastructural correlation of water reabsorption in isolated rat cauda epididymis. *Experientia* **34**:485–487.

Woodland, H. R. 1974. Changes in the polysome content of developing *Xenopus laevis* embryos. *Dev. Biol.* **40**:90–101.

Woodland, H. R. 1979. The modifications of stored histones H3 and H4 during the oogenesis and early development of *Xenopus laevis*. *Dev. Biol.* **68**:360–370.

Woodland, H. R., and Wilt, F. H. 1980a. The functional stability of sea urchin histone mRNA injected into oocytes of *Xenopus laevis*. *Dev. Biol.* **75**:199–213.

Woodland, H. R., and Wilt, F. H. 1980b. The stability and translation of sea urchin histone mRNA molecules injected into *X. laevis* eggs and developing embryos. *Dev. Biol.* **75**:214–221.

Woods, F. A. 1902. Origin and migration of the germ cells in *Acanthias*. *Am. J. Anat.* **1**:307–320.

Wyatt, G. R., and Pan, M. C. 1978. Insect plasma proteins. *Annu. Rev. Biochem.* **47**:779–817.

Zamboni, L. 1970. Ultrastructure of mammalian oocytes and ova. *Biol. Reprod.* **2**(Suppl.):44–63.

Zamboni, L. 1974. Fine morphology of the follicle wall and the follicle cell–oocyte association. *Biol. Reprod.* **10**:125–149.

Zamboni, L., and Mastroianni, L. 1966. Electron microscopic studies on rabbit ova. I. The follicular oocyte. *J. Ultrastruct. Res.* **14**:95–117.

Zihler, J. 1972. Zur Spermatogeneses und Befruchtungsbiologie von *Hydra*. *Wilhelm Roux Arch. Dev. Biol.* **169**:239–267.

CHAPTER 2

Adesnik, M., Salditt, M., Thomas, W., and Darnell, J. E. 1972. Evidence that all mRNA molecules (except histone mRNA) contain poly(A) sequences and that the poly(A) has a nuclear function. *J. Mol. Biol.* **71**:21–30.

Afzelius, B. A. 1956. The ultrastructure of the cortical granules and their products in the sea urchin egg as studied with the electron microscope. *Exp. Cell Res.* **30**:93–97.

Afzelius, B. A. 1972a. Reactions of the sea urchin oocyte to foreign spermatozoa. *Exp. Cell Res.* **72**:25–33.

Afzelius, B. A. 1972b. Ultrastructure of species-foreign spermatozoa after penetrating the sea urchin oocyte. *Acta Embryol. Exp.* **1972**:123–133.

Aketa, K., Bianchetti, R., Marri, É., and Monroy, A. 1964. Hexose monophosphate level as a limiting factor for respiration in unfertilized sea urchin eggs. *Biochim. Biophys. Acta* **86**:211–215.

Allen, R. D. 1954. Fertilization and activation of sea urchin eggs in glass capillaries. *Exp. Cell Res.* **9**:157–167.

Anderson, E. 1968. Oocyte differentiation in the sea urchin, *Arbacia punctulata*, with particular reference to the origin of the cortical granules and their participation in the cortical reaction. *J. Cell Biol.* **37**:514–539.

Anderson, W. A. 1969. Nuclear and cytoplasmic DNA synthesis during early embryogenesis of *Paracentrotus lividus*. *J. Ultrastruct. Res.* **26**:95–110.

Austin, C. R. 1961. *The Mammalian Egg*, Oxford, Blackwell.

Austin, C. R. 1965. *Fertilization*, Englewood Cliffs, N.J., Prentice–Hall.

Austin, C. R., and Walton, A. 1960. Fertilisation. *In*: Parkes, A. S., ed., *Marshall's Physiology of Reproduction*, New York, Longmans, Green, Vol. 1, pp. 310–416.

Baca, M., and Zamboni, L. 1967. The fine structure of human follicular oocytes. *J. Ultrastruct. Res.* **19**:354–381.

Bagshaw, J. C., Acey, R., Helder, J. C., and Talley-Brown, S. J. 1980. RNA polymerases and transcriptional switches in developing *Artemia*. *In*: Persoone, G., Sorgeloos, P., Roels, O., and Jaspers, E., eds., *The Brine Shrimp Artemia*, Wetteren, Belgium, Universa Press, Vol. 2.

Ballinger, D. G., and Hunt, T. 1981. Fertilization of sea urchin eggs is accompanied by 40 S ribosomal subunit phosphorylation. *Dev. Biol.* **87**:277–285.

Bataillon, E., and Su, T. 1930. Études analytiques et experimentales sur les rhythmes cinétiques dans l'oeuf. *Arch. Biol.* **40**:441–540.

Bedford, J. M. 1968. Ultrastructural changes in the sperm head during fertilization in the rabbit. *Am. J. Anat.* **123**:329–358.

Bedford, J. M. 1972. An EM study of sperm penetration into the rabbit egg after natural mating. *Am. J. Anat.* **133**:213–254.

Bedford, J. M., and Cooper, G. W. 1978. Membrane fusion events in the fertilization of vertebrate eggs. *In*: Poste, G., and Nicolson, G. L., eds., *Membrane Fusion,* Amsterdam, Elsevier/North-Holland, pp. 65–125.

Bedford, J. M., and Cross, N. L. 1978. Normal penetration of rabbit spermatozoa through a trypsin- and acrosin-resistant zona pellucida. *J. Reprod. Fertil.* **54**:385–392.

Bendich, A., Borenfreund, E., and Sternberg, S. S. 1974. Penetration of somatic mammalian cells by sperm. *Science* **183**:857–859.

Black, R. E., Baptist, E., and Piland, J. 1967. Puromycin and cycloheximide inhibition of thymidine incorporation into the DNA of sea urchin eggs. *Exp. Cell Res.* **48**:431–439.

Blakeslee, A. F. 1904. Sexual reproduction in the Mucorineae. *Proc. Am. Acad. Arts Sci.* **40**:206–319.

Blankstein, L. A., and Kiefer, B. I. 1977. The relation of DNA and protein synthesis to the meiotic–mitotic transition in the zygote of *Urechis caupo*. *Dev. Biol.* **61**:1–10.

Bleil, J. D., and Wassarman, P. M. 1981. Mammalian sperm–egg interaction: Identification of a glycoprotein in mouse egg zonae pellucidae possessing receptor activity for sperm. *Cell* **20**:873–882.

Boveri, T. 1888. Über partielle Befruchtung. *Ber. Naturforsch. Ges. Freiburg im Breisgau* **4**:64–72.

Boveri, T. 1903. Über den Einfluss der Samenzellen auf die Larvencharactere der Echiniden. *Wilhelm Roux Arch. Entwicklungsmech. Org.* **16**:340–362.

Britckov, E. A. 1952. Über einige Besonderheiten der Pollenkeimung und das Wachstum der Pollenschläuche in den Fruchtblattgeweben. *Dokl. Akad. Nauk SSSR Ser. Biol.* **1**:121–134.

Brummett, A. R., and Dumont, J. N. 1981. Cortical vesicle breakdown in the fertilized eggs of *Fundulus heteroclitus*. *J. Exp. Zool.* **216**:63–79.

Burgess, D. R., and Schroeder, T. E. 1977. Polarized bundles of actin filaments within microvilli of fertilized sea urchin eggs. *J. Cell Biol.* **74**:1032–1037.

Chambers, E. L. 1939. The movement of the egg nucleus in relation to the sperm aster in the echinoderm egg. *J. Exp. Biol.* **16**:409–424.

Chambers, R. 1933. The manner of sperm entry in various marine ova. *J. Exp. Biol.* **10**:130–141.

Clark, W. H., Lynn, J. W., Yudin, A. I., and Persyn, H. O. 1980. Morphology of the cortical reaction in the eggs of *Penaeus aztecus*. *Biol. Bull.* **158**:175–186.

Colwin, A. L., and Colwin, L. H. 1955. Sperm entry and the acrosome filament (*Holothuria atra* and *Asterias amurensis*). *J. Morphol.* **97**:543–568.

Colwin, A. L., and Colwin, L. H. 1961. Changes in the spermatozoan during fertilization in *Hydroides hexagonus* (Annelida). 2. Incorporation with the egg. *J. Biophys. Biochem. Cytol.* **10**:255–274.

Colwin, A. L., and Colwin, L. H. 1963. Role of the gamete membranes in fertilization in *Saccoglossus kowalevskii* (Enteropneusta). 1. The acrosomal region and its changes in early stages of fertilization. *J. Cell Biol.* **19**:477–500.

Colwin, A. L., and Colwin, L. H. 1964. Role of the gamete membranes in fertilization. *In*: Lake, M., ed., *Symposium on Cellular Membranes in Development*, New York, Academic Press, pp. 233–279.

Colwin, L. H., and Colwin, A. L. 1956. The acrosome filament and sperm entry in *Thyone briareus* (Holothuria) and *Asterias*. *Biol. Bull.* **110**:243–255.

Colwin, L. H., and Colwin, A. L. 1961. Changes in the spermatozoan during fertilization in *Hydroides hexagonus* (Annelida). 1. Passage of the acrosomal region through the vitelline membrane. *J. Biophys. Biochem. Cytol.* **10**:231–254.

Colwin, L. H., and Colwin, A. L. 1963. Role of the gamete membranes in fertilization of *Saccoglossus kowalevskii* (Enteropneusta). II. Zygote formation by gamete membrane fusion. *J. Cell Biol.* **19**:501–518.

Colwin, L. H., and Colwin, A. L. 1967. Membrane fusion in relation to sperm–egg association. *In*: Metz, C. B., and Monroy, A., eds., *Fertilization*, New York, Academic Press, Vol. 1, pp. 295–367.

Cooper, D. C. 1940. Macrosporogenesis and embryology of the seed of *Phryma leptostachya*. *Am. J. Bot.* **28**:755–761.

Cooperstein, S. J. 1963. Reversible inactivation of cytochrome oxidase by disulphide bond reagents. *Anat. Anz.* **19**:280–287.

Dan, J. C., Ohori, Y., and Kushida, H. 1964. Studies on the acrosome. VII. Formation of the acrosomal process in sea urchin spermatozoa. *J. Ultrastruct. Res.* **11**:508–524.

Darnell, J. E., Jelinek, W. R., and Molloy, G. R. 1973. Biogenesis of mRNA: Genetic regulation in mammalian cells. *Science* **181**:1215–1221.

Das, N. K., and Barker, C. 1976. Mitotic chromosome condensation in the sperm nucleus during postfertilization maturation division in *Urechis* eggs. *J. Cell Biol.* **68**:155–159.

Dewel, W. C., and Clark, W. H. 1974. A fine structural investigation of surface specializations and the cortical reaction of the cnidarian *Bunodosoma cavernata*. *J. Cell Biol.* **60**:78–91.

Dillon, L. S. 1981. *Ultrastructure, Macromolecules, and Evolution*, New York, Plenum Press.

Dworkin, M. B., and Infante, A. A. 1978. RNA synthesis in unfertilized sea urchin eggs. *Dev. Biol.* **62**:247–257.

Eddy, E. M., and Shapiro, B. M. 1976. Changes in the topography of the sea urchin egg after fertilization. *J. Cell. Biol.* **71**:35–48.

Egrie, J. C., and Wilt, F. H. 1979. Changes in poly(A) polymerase activity during sea urchin embryogenesis. *Biochemistry* **18**:269–274.

Ellinger, M. S. 1978. The cell cycle and transplantation of blastula nuclei in *Bombina orientalis*. *Dev. Biol.* **65**:81–89.

Ellinger, M. S., and Carlson, J. T. 1978. Nuclear transplantation in *Bombina orientalis* and utilization of the *pale* mutation as a nuclear marker. *J. Exp. Zool.* **205**:353–359.

Endo, Y. 1961. Changes in the cortical layer of sea urchin eggs at fertilization as studied with the electron microscope. I. *Clypeaster japonicus*. *Exp. Cell Res.* **25**:383–397.

Epel, D. 1967. Protein synthesis in sea urchin eggs: A "late" response to fertilization. *Proc. Natl. Acad. Sci. USA* **57**:889–906.

Epel, D., Steinhardt, R. A., Humphreys, T., and Mazia, D. 1974. An analysis of the parietal metabolic derepression of sea urchin eggs by ammonia: The existence of independent pathways. *Dev. Biol.* **40**:245–255.

Flemming, W. 1881. Beiträge zur Kenntnis der Zelle und ihrer Lebenserscheinung. 3. *Arch. Mikrosk. Anat. Entwicklungsmech.* **20**:1–86.

Fol, H. 1879. Recherches sur la fécondation et le commencement de l'hénogenie chez diveris animaux. *Mem. Soc. Phys. Hist. Nat. Genève* **26**:89–250.

Ford, C. C., and Woodland, H. R. 1975. DNA synthesis in oocytes and eggs of *Xenopus laevis* injected with DNA. *Dev. Biol.* **43**:189–199.

Gabara, B., Gledhill, B. L., Croce, C. M., Cesarini, J. P., and Koprowski, H. 1973. Ultrastructure of rabbit spermatozoa after treatment with lysolecithin and in the presence of hamster somatic cells (37482). *Proc. Soc. Exp. Biol. Med.* **143**:1120–1124.

Gerassimova-Navashina, H. 1960. A contribution to the cytology of fertilization in flowering plants. *Nucleus (Calcutta)* **3**:111–120.

Gerassimova-Navashina, H. 1961. Fertilization and events leading up to fertilization, and their bearing on the origin of angiosperms. *Phytomorphology* **11**:139–146.

Giard, A. 1900. A propos de la parthénogénèse artificielle des oeufs d'echinodérmes. *C. R. Soc. Biol.* **52**:761–764.

Giudice, G. 1973. *Developmental Biology of the Sea Urchin Embryo*, New York, Academic Press.

Giudice, G., Vitorelli, M. L., and Monroy, A. 1962. Investigations on the protein metabolism during the early development of the sea urchin. *Acta Embryol. Morphol. Exp.* **5**:113–122.

Gledhill, B. L., Sawicki, W., Croce, C. M., and Koprowski, H. 1972. DNA synthesis in rabbit spermatozoa after treatment with lysolecithin and fusion with somatic cells. *Exp. Cell Res.* **73**:33–40.

Graham, C. F. 1966. The regulation of DNA synthesis and mitosis in multinucleate frog eggs. *J. Cell Sci.* **1**:363–374.

Grainger, J. L., Winkler, M. M., Shen, S. S., and Steinhardt, R. A. 1979. Intracellular pH controls protein synthesis rate in the sea urchin egg and early embryo. *Dev. Biol.* **68**:396–406.

Grey, R. D., Wolf, D. P., and Hedrick, J. L. 1974. Formation and structure of the fertilization envelope in *Xenopus laevis*. *Dev. Biol.* **36**:44–61.

Griffin, B. 1975. "Enigma variations" of mammalian mRNA. *Nature (London)* **255**:9.

Gulyas, B. J. 1974. Cortical granules in artificially activated (parthenogenetic) rabbit eggs. *Am. J. Anat.* **140**:577–582.

Gulyas, B. J. 1976. Ultrastructural observations on rabbit, hamster and mouse eggs following electrical stimulation *in vitro*. *Am. J. Anat.* **147**:203–218.

Gulyas, B. J. 1980. Cortical granules of mammalian eggs. *Int. Rev. Cytol.* **63**:357–392.

Gurdon, J. B. 1961. The transplantation of nuclei between two subspecies of *Xenopus laevis*. *Heredity* **16**:305–315.

Gurdon, J. B. 1968. Changes in somatic cell nuclei inserted into growing and maturing amphibian oocytes. *J. Embryol. Exp. Morphol.* **20**:401–414.

Gurdon, J. B. 1974. *The Control of Gene Expression in Animal Development*, Cambridge, Mass., Harvard University Press.

Gurdon, J. B. 1975. Nuclear transplantation and the cyclic reprogramming of gene expression. *In*: Reinert, J., and Holtzer, H., eds., *Cell Cycle and Cell Differentiation*, Berlin, Springer-Verlag, pp. 123–131.

Gurdon, J. B. 1976. The pluripotentiality of cell nuclei. *In*: Graham, C. F., and Wareing, P. F., eds., *The Developmental Biology of Plants and Animals*, Oxford, Blackwell, pp. 55–63.

Hadék, R. 1963. Submicroscopic changes in the penetrating spermatozoan of the rabbit. *J. Ultrastruct. Res.* **8**:161–169.

Hara, K. 1971. Cinematographic observation of "surface contraction waves" during the early cleavage of axolotl eggs. *Wilhelm Roux Arch. Dev. Biol.* **167**:183–186.

Hara, K., and Tydeman, P. 1979. Cinematographic observation of an "activation wave" (AW) on the locally inseminated eggs of *Xenopus laevis*. *Wilhelm Roux Arch. Dev. Biol.* **186**:91–94.

Hara, K., Tydeman, P., and Hengst, R. T. M. 1977. Cinematographic observation of "postfertilization" waves (PFW) on the zygote of *Xenopus laevis*. *Wilhelm Roux Arch. Dev. Biol.* **181**:189–192.

Hara, K., Tydeman, P., and Kirschner, M. 1980. A cytoplasmic clock with the same period as the division cycle in *Xenopus* eggs. *Proc. Natl. Acad. Sci. USA* **77**:462–466.

Harris, H. 1974. *Nucleus and Cytoplasm*, 3rd ed., London, Oxford University Press (Clarendon).

Harris, P. 1979. A spiral cortical fiber system in fertilized sea urchin eggs. *Dev. Biol.* **68**:525–532.

Harris, P., Osborn, M., and Weber, K. 1980a. Distribution of tubulin containing structures in the egg of the sea urchin *Strongylocentrotus purpuratus* from fertilization through first cleavage. *J. Cell Biol.* **84**:668–679.

Harris, P., Osborn, M., and Weber, K. 1980b. A spiral array of microtubules in the fertilized sea urchin egg cortex examined by indirect immunofluorescence and electron microscopy. *Exp. Cell Res.* **126**:227–236.

Hartmann, J. F., and Hutchison, C. F. 1981. Modulation of fertilization *in vitro* by peptides released during hamster sperm–zona pellucida interaction. *Proc. Natl. Acad. Sci. USA* **78**:1690–1694.

Hartmann, M. 1934. Untersuchungen über die Sexualität von *Ectocarpus siliculosus*. *Arch. Protistenkd.* **83**:110–153.

Hathaway, R. R. 1959. The effect of sperm on ^{35}S-labelled *Arbacia* fertilizin. *Biol. Bull.* **117**:395.

Hathaway, R. R. 1963. Activation of respiration in sea urchin spermatozoa by egg water. *Biol. Bull.* **125**:486–498.

Hathaway, R. R., and Metz, C. B. 1961. Interaction between *Arbacia* sperm and S^{35}-labelled fertilizin. *Biol. Bull.* **120**:360–369.

Hertwig, P. 1936. Artbastarde bei Tieren. *In*: Baur, E., and Hartmann, M., eds., *Handbuch der Vererbungswissenschaft*, Berlin, Verlag Gebr. Borntraeger, Vol. IIB.

Hickey, E. D., Weber, L. A., and Baglioni, C. 1976. Translation of RNA from unfertilized sea urchin eggs does not require methylation and is inhibited by 7-methyl-guanosine-5'-monophosphate. *Nature (London)* **261**:71–73.

Hiromoto, Y. 1962. Microinjection of the live spermatozoa into sea urchin eggs. *Exp. Cell Res.* **27**:416–426.

Hoffner, N. J., and DiBerardino, M. A. 1980. Developmental potential of somatic nuclei transplanted into meiotic oocytes of *Rana pipiens*. *Science* **209**:517–519.

Hudinaga, M. 1942. Reproduction, development, and rearing of *Pennaeus japonicus* Bate. *Jpn. J. Zool.* **10**:305–393.

Hultin, T. 1952. Incorporation of ^{15}N-labelled glycine and alanine into the proteins of developing sea urchin eggs. *Exp. Cell Res.* 3:494–496.

Hultin, T. 1953a. The amino acid metabolism of sea urchin embryos studied by means of N^{15}-labelled ammonium chloride and alanine. *Ark. Kemi* 5:543–552.

Hultin, T. 1953b. Incorporation of N^{15}-di-alanine into protein fractions of sea urchin embryos. *Ark. Kemi* 5:559–564.

Humphreys, T. 1971. Measurement of mRNA entering polysomes upon fertilization of sea urchin eggs. *Dev. Biol.* 26:201–208.

Hunter, R. H. F. 1967. Polyspermic fertilization in pigs during the luteal phase of the estrous cycle. *J. Exp. Zool.* 165:451–460.

Hutner, S. H., and Provasoli, L. 1951. The phytoflagellates. *In:* Lwoff, A., ed., *Biochemistry and Physiology of Protozoa,* New York, Academic Press, pp. 27–128.

Illmensee, K. 1972. Developmental potencies of nuclei from cleavage, preblastoderm and syncytial blastoderm transplanted into unfertilized eggs of *Drosophila melanogaster. Wilhelm Roux Arch. Dev. Biol.* 170:267–298.

Immers, J. 1961. The occurrence of sulphated mucopolysaccharide in the perivitelline liquid of *Echinus esculentus. Ark. Zool.* 13:299–306.

Ito, S. 1962. Resting potential and activation potential of the *Oryzias* egg. *Embryologia* 7:47–55.

Iwamatsu, T., and Ohta, T. 1978. EM observation on sperm penetration and pronuclear formation in the fish egg. *J. Exp. Zool.* 205:157–180.

Jaffe, L. A., and Robinson, K. R. 1978. Membrane potential of the unfertilized sea urchin egg. *Dev. Biol.* 62:215–228.

Jensen, W. A. 1965. The ultrastructure and histochemistry of the synergids of cotton. *Am. J. Bot.* 52:238–256.

Johnson, J. D., Epel, D., and Paul, M. 1976. Intracellular pH and activation of sea urchin eggs after fertilization. *Nature (London)* 262:661–664.

Kane, R. E. 1970. Direct isolation of the hyaline layer protein released from cortical granules of the sea urchin egg at fertilization. *J. Cell Biol.* 45:615–622.

Kane, R. E., and Hersh, R. T. 1959. The isolation and preliminary characterization of a major soluble protein of the sea urchin egg. *Exp. Cell Res.* 16:59–69.

Kao, C. Y. 1955. Changing electrical constants of the *Fundulus* egg surface. *Biol. Bull.* 109: 361.

Kapil, R. N., and Vasil, I. K. 1963. Ovule. *In:* Maheshwari, P., ed., *Recent Advances in Embryology of Angiosperms,* Delhi, International Society of Plant Morphologists, pp. 41–67.

Katagiri, C. 1974. A high frequency of fertilization in premature and mature coelomic toad eggs after enzymic removal of vitelline membrane. *J. Embryol. Exp. Morphol.* 31:573–587.

Katagiri, C., and Moriya, M. 1976. Spermatozoan response to the toad egg matured after removal of the germinal vesicle. *Dev. Biol.* 50:235–241.

Kaumeyer, J. F., Jenkins, N. A., and Raff, R. A. 1978. Messenger RNP particles in unfertilized sea urchin eggs. *Dev. Biol.* 63:266–278.

Köhler, E. 1930. Beobachtungen und Zoosporenaufschwemmungen von *Synchytrium endobioticum* (Schilb.) Perc. *Zentralbl. Bakteriol. Parasitenkd. Infekfionskr. Hyg.* (2) 82:1–10.

Kopečný, V., and Fléchon, J. E. 1981. Fate of acrosomal glycoproteins during the acrosomal reaction and fertilization: A light and electron microscope autoradiographic study. *Biol. Reprod.* 24:201–216.

Koyanagi, F., and Nishiyama, H. 1980. Phagocytosis of spermatozoa by the ovum of the domestic fowl, *Gallus gallus,* at the time of fertilization. *Cell Tissue Res.* 206:55–63.

Krane, S. M., and Crane, R. K. 1960. Changes in levels of triphosphopyridine nucleotide in marine eggs subsequent to fertilization. *Biochim. Biophys. Acta* 43:369–373.

Krishna, M., and Generoso, W. M. 1977. Timing of sperm penetration, pronuclear formation, pronuclear DNA synthesis, and first cleavage in naturally ovulated mouse eggs. *J. Exp. Zool.* 202:245–252.

Krystal, G. W., and Poccia, D. 1979. Control of chromosome condensation in the sea urchin egg. *Exp. Cell Res.* **123**:207–219.

Kunkle, M., Longo, F. J., and Magun, B. E. 1978a. Nuclear protein changes in the maternally and paternally derived chromatin at fertilization. *J. Exp. Zool.* **203**:371–380.

Kunkle, M., Magun, B. E., and Longo, F. J. 1978b. Analysis of isolated sea urchin nuclei incubated in egg cytosol. *J. Exp. Zool.* **203**:381–390.

Kusano, S. 1931. The life-history and physiology of *Synchytrium fulgens* Schroet., with special reference to its sexuality. *Jpn. J. Bot.* **5**:35–132.

Laser, H., and Rothschild, L. 1939. The metabolism of the eggs of *Psammechinus miliaris* during the fertilization reaction. *Proc. R. Soc. London Ser. B* **126**:539–557.

Lewin, R. 1950. Gamete behaviour in *Chlamydomonas. Nature (London)* **166**:76.

Lillie, F. R. 1913. Studies of fertilization. 5. The behavior of the spermatozoa of *Nereis* and *Arbacia* with special reference to egg-extractives. *J. Exp. Zool.* **14**:515–574.

Lillie, F. R. 1914. Studies on fertilization. 6. The mechanism of fertilization in *Arbacia. J. Exp. Zool.* **16**:523–590.

Linskens, H. F. 1969. Fertilization mechanisms in higher plants. *In:* Metz, C. B., and Monroy, A., eds., *Fertilization,* New York, Academic Press, Vol. 2, pp. 189–253.

Litchfield, J. B., and Whiteley, A. H. 1959. Studies on the mechanism of phosphate accumulation by sea urchin embryos. *Biol. Bull.* **117**:133–149.

Longo, F. J. 1973a. Fertilization: A comparative ultrastructural review. *Biol. Reprod.* **9**:149–215.

Longo, F. J. 1973b. An ultrastructural analysis of polyspermy in the surf clam, *Spisula solidissima. J. Exp. Zool.* **183**:153–180.

Longo, F. J. 1976a. Derivation of the membrane comprising the male pronuclear envelope in inseminated sea urchin eggs. *Dev. Biol.* **49**:347–368.

Longo, F. J. 1976b. An ultrastructural study of cross-fertilization [*Arbacia* ♂ × *Mytilus* ♀]. *J. Cell Biol.* **73**:14–26.

Longo, F. J. 1978. Insemination of immature sea urchin (*Arbacia punctulata*) eggs. *Dev. Biol.* **62**:271–291.

Longo, F. J. 1980. Organization of microfilaments in sea urchin (*Arbacia punctulata*) eggs at fertilization: Effects of cytochalasin B. *Dev. Biol.* **74**:422–433.

Longo, F. J., and Kunkle, M. 1977. Synthesis of RNA by male pronuclei of fertilized sea urchin eggs. *J. Exp. Zool.* **201**:431.

Longo, F. J., and Kunkle, M. 1978. Transformations of sperm nuclei upon insemination. *Curr. Top. Dev. Biol.* **12**:149–184.

Longo, F. J., and Plunkett, W. 1973. The onset of DNA synthesis and its relation to morphogenetic events of the pronuclei in activated eggs of the sea urchin, *Arbacia punctulata. Dev. Biol.* **30**:56–67.

Lovett, J. A., and Goldstein, E. S. 1977. The cytoplasmic districution and characterization of poly (A)⁺ RNA in oocytes and embryos of *Drosophila. Dev. Biol.* **61**:70–78.

McBlaine, P. J., and Carroll, E. J. 1980. Sea urchin egg hyaline layer: Evidence for the localization of hyaline on the unfertilized egg surface. *Dev. Biol.* **75**:137–147.

Machlis, L. 1958a. Evidence for a sexual hormone in *Allomyces. Physiol. Plant.* **11**:181–192.

Machlis, L. 1958b. A procedure for the purification of sirenin. *Nature (London)* **181**:1790–1791.

Machlis, L. 1963. *In:* Hisaw, F. L., ed., *Physiology of Reproduction,* Corvallis, Oregon State University Press, p. 79.

Machlis, L., and Rawitscher-Kunkel, E. 1967. Mechanisms of gametic approach in plants. *In:* Metz, C. B., and Monroy, A., eds., *Fertilization,* New York, Academic Press, Vol. 1, pp. 117–161.

Machlis, L., Nutting, W. H., Williams, M. W., and Rapoport, H. 1966. Production, isolation, and characterization of sirenin. *Biochemistry* **5**:2147–2152.

Maeno, T., Morita, H., and Kuwabara, M. 1956. Potential measurements on the eggs of Japanese killifish, *Oryzias latipes*. *Mem. Fac. Sci. Kyushu Univ.* **E2**:87–94.

Maggio, R., and Monroy, A. 1959. An inhibitor of cytochrome oxidase activity in the sea urchin egg. *Nature (London)* **184**:68–69.

Maheshwari, P. 1950. *Introduction to the Embryology of the Angiosperms,* New York, McGraw–Hill.

Mainx, F. 1931. Gametencopulation und Zygoten keimung bei *Hydrodictyon reticulatum*. *Arch. Protistenkd.* **75**:502–516.

Mar, H. 1980. Radial cortical fibers and pronuclear migration in fertilized and artificially activated eggs of *Lytechinus pictus*. *Dev. Biol.* **78**:1–13.

Marchand, B., and Mattei, X. 1976. Présence de flagelles spermatiques dans les sphères ovariennes des Eoacanthocéphales. *J. Ultrastruct. Res.* **56**:331–338.

Marchand, B., and Mattei, X. 1979. La fécondation chez les Acanthocéphales. I. Modifications ultrastructurales des sphères ovariennes et des spermatozoides après insémination des femelles de l'Acanthocéphale *Neoechinorhynchus agilis*. *J. Ultrastruct. Res.* **66**:32–39.

Marchand, B., and Mattei, X. 1980. Fertilization in Acanthocephala. II. Spermatozoon penetration of oocyte, transformation of gametes and elaboration of the fertilization membrane. *J. Submicrosc. Cytol.* **12**:95–105.

Mascarenhas, J. P., and Machlis, L. 1962. Chemotropic response of *Antirrhinum majus* pollen to calcium. *Nature (London)* **196**:292–293.

Mazia, D. 1937. The release of calcium in *Arbacia* eggs on fertilization. *J. Cell. Comp. Physiol.* **10**:291–304.

Mazia, D., Schatten, G., and Steinhardt, R. 1975. Turning on of activities in unfertilized eggs: Correlation with changes of the surface. *Proc. Natl. Acad. Sci. USA* **72**:4469–4473.

Metz, C. B. 1978. Sperm and egg receptors involved in fertilization. *Curr. Top. Dev. Biol.* **12**:107–147.

Meyerhof, P. G., and Masui, Y. 1979. Chromosome condensation activity in *Rana pipiens* eggs matured *in vivo* and in blastomeres arrested by cytostatic factors (CSF). *Exp. Cell Res.* **123**:345–353.

Miceli, D. C., del Pino, E. J., Barbieri, F. D., Mariano, M. I., and Raisman, J. S. 1977. The vitelline envelope-to-fertilization envelope transformation in the toad *Bufo arenarum*. *Dev. Biol.* **59**:101–110.

Miller, R. L. 1966. Chemotaxis during fertilization in the hydroid *Campanularia*. *J. Exp. Zool.* **162**:23–44.

Miller, R. L. 1974. Sperm behavior close to *Hydractinia* and *Ciona* eggs. *Am. Zool.* **14**:1250.

Miller, R. L. 1977. *In*: Adiyodi, K. G., and Adiyodi, P. G., eds., *Advances in Invertebrate Reproduction*, Karivellur, India, Peralana-Kenoth, Vol. 1, pp. 99–119.

Miller, R. L., and Nelson, L. 1962. Evidence of a chemotactic substance in the female gonangium of *Campanularia*. *Biol. Bull.* **123**:422.

Miller, R. L., and Tseng, C. Y. 1974. Properties and partial purification of the sperm attractant of *Tubularia*. *Am. Zool.* **14**:467–486.

Monroy, A. 1965. *Chemistry and Physiology of Fertilization*, New York, Holt, Rinehart & Winston.

Monroy, A., and Tyler, A. 1963. Formation of active ribosomal aggregates (polysomes) upon fertilization and development of sea urchin eggs. *Arch. Biochem. Biophys.* **103**:431–435.

Monroy, A., and Vittorelli, M. L. 1962. Utilization of ^{14}C-glucose for amino acids and protein synthesis by the sea urchin embryo. *J. Cell. Comp. Physiol.* **60**:285–288.

Monroy Oddo, A. 1946. Variations in Ca and Mg contents in *Arbacia* eggs as a result of fertilization. *Experientia* **2**:371–372.

Muthukrishnan, S., Both, G. W., Furuichi, Y., and Shatkin, A. J. 1975. 5′-Terminal 7-methylguanosine in eukaryotic mRNA is required for translation. *Nature (London)* **255**:33–37.

Nicosia, S. V., Wolf, D. P., and Inoue, M. 1977. Cortical granule distribution and cell surface characteristics in mouse eggs. *Dev. Biol.* **57**:56–74.

Noack, R. 1960. Die chemotropische Reaktionsfähigkeit der Pollenschläuche auf die Narbenitoffe der Blüten. *Z. Bot.* **48**:463–487.

Noda, Y. D., and Yanagimachi, R. 1976. Electron microscopic observations of guinea pig spermatozoa penetrating eggs in vitro. *Dev. Growth Differ.* **18**:15–23.

Nuccitelli, R. 1980a. The electrical changes accompanying fertilization and cortical vesicle secretion in the medaka egg. *Dev. Biol.* **76**:483–498.

Nuccitelli, R. 1980b. The fertilization potential is not necessary for the block to polyspermy or the activation of development in the medaka egg. *Dev. Biol.* **76**:499–504.

Ohnishi, T., and Sugiyama, M. 1963. Polarographic studies of oxygen uptake of sea urchin eggs. *Embryologia* **8**:79–88.

Okamura, F., and Nishiyama, H. 1978a. The passage of spermatozoa through the vitelline membrane in the domestic fowl, *Gallus gallus*. *Cell Tissue Res.* **188**:497–508.

Okamura, F., and Nishiyama, H. 1978b. Penetration of spermatozoon into the ovum and transformation of the sperm nucleus into the male pronucleus in the domestic fowl, *Gallus gallus*. *Cell Tissue Res.* **190**:89–98.

Okazaki, K. 1956a. Skeletal formation of sea urchin larvae. I. Effect of calcium concentration on the medium. *Biol. Bull.* **110**:320–333.

Okazaki, R. 1956b. On the possible role of high energy phosphate in the cortical change of sea urchin eggs. *Exp. Cell Res.* **10**:476–504.

Örström, Å., and Örström, M. 1942. Über die Bindung von Kalzium in Ei und Larve von *Paracentrotus lividus*. *Protoplasma* **36**:475–490.

Paolillo, D. J. 1981. The swimming sperms of land plants. *BioScience* **31**:367–373.

Pascher, A. 1931. Über Gruppenbildung und ''Geschlechtswechsel'' bei den Gameten einer Chlamydomonadine. *Jahrb. Wiss. Bot.* **75**:551–580.

Pasteels, J. J. 1965. Aspects structuraux de la fécondation reus au microscope électronique. *Arch. Biol.* **76**:463–509.

Pasteels, J. J., and de Harven, E. 1962. Étude au microscope électronique du cortex de l'oeuf de *Barnea candida* (Mollusque bivalve) et son évolution au moment de la fécondation, de la maturation et de la segmentation. *Arch. Biol. (Liège)* **73**:465–490.

Pfeffer, W. 1884. *Untersuch. Bot. Inst. Tubingen* **1**:363–481.

Phillips, S. G., Phillips, D. M., Dev, V. G., Miller, D. A., Van Diggelen, O. P., and Miller, O. J. 1976. Spontaneous cell hybridization of somatic cells present in sperm suspensions. *Exp. Cell. Res.* **98**:429–443.

Pikó, L. 1969. Gamete structure and sperm entry in mammals. *In*: Metz, C. B., and Monroy, A., eds., *Fertilization*, New York, Academic Press, pp. 325–403.

Plempel, M. 1960. Die zygotropische Reaktion bei Mucorineen. *Planta* **55**:254–258.

Poccia, D., Salik, J., and Krystal, G. 1981. Transitions in histone variants of the male pronucleus following fertilization and evidence for a maternal store of cleavage-stage histones in the sea urchin egg. *Dev. Biol.* **82**:287–296.

Racevskis, J., and Webb, T. E. 1974. Processing and release of rRNA from isolated nuclei: Analysis of the ATP-dependence and cytosol-dependence. *Eur. J. Biochem.* **49**:93–100.

Raff, E. C., and Raff, R. A. 1978. Tubulin and microtubules in the early development of the axolotl and other amphibia. *Am. Zool.* **18**:237–251.

Reiger, J. C., and Kafatos, F. C. 1977. Absolute rate of protein synthesis in sea urchins with specific activity measurements of radioactive leucine leucyl tRNA. *Dev. Biol.* **57**:270–283.

Richter-Landmann, W. 1959. Der Befruchtungsvorgang bei *Impatiens glanduligera* unter Berückeichtigung der plasmatischen Organelle von Spermazelle, Eizelle, und Zygote. *Planta* **53**:162–177.

Rosen, W. G. 1961. Studies on pollen tube chemotropism. *Am. J. Bot.* **48**:889–895.

Rosen, W. G. 1964. Chemotropism and fine structure of pollen tubes. *In*: Linskens, H. F., ed., *Pollen Physiology and Fertilization*, Amsterdam, North-Holland, pp. 159–169.

Sawicki, W., and Koprowski, H. 1971. Fusion of rabbit spermatozoa with somatic cells cultivated *in vitro*. *Exp. Cell Res.* **66**:145–151.

Schatten, G. 1981. The movements and fusion of the pronuclei at fertilization of the sea urchin *Lytechinus variegatus*: Time-lapse video microscopy. *J. Morphol.* **167**:231–247.

Schreiber, E. 1931. Über die geschlechtliche Fortpflanzung der Sphacelariales. *Ber. Dtsch. Bot. Ges.* **49**:235–240.

Schroeder, T. E. 1978. Microvilli on sea urchin eggs: A second burst of elongation. *Dev. Biol.* **64**:342–346.

Schroeder, T. E. 1979. Surface area change at fertilization: Resorption of the mosaic membrane. *Dev. Biol.* **70**:306–326.

Schultz, G. A., Clough, J. R., and Johnson, M. H. 1980. Presence of cap structures in the mRNA of mouse eggs. *J. Embryol. Exp. Morphol.* **56**:139–156.

Schultz, R. M., Letourneau, G. E., and Wassarman, P. M. 1979. Program of early development in the mammal: Changes in patterns and absolute rates of tubulin and total protein synthesis during oogenesis and early embryogenesis in the mouse. *Dev. Biol.* **68**:341–359.

Scopelliti, R., Senatori, O., Delpino, A., and Manelli, H. 1979. Ribosomi traslanti e non traslanti in alcuni stadi di sviluppo di *Bufo bufo*. *Atti Accad. Naz. Lincei* Ser. VIII, **6**:362–366.

Shellenbarger, D. L., and Shapiro, B. M. 1980. Effect of the inhibitors of ion movements, verapamil and tetraethylammonium, on fertilization of mouse eggs *in vitro*. *Gamete Res.* **3**:1–7.

Shen, S. S., and Steinhardt, R. A. 1980. Intracellular pH controls the development of new potassium conductance after fertilization of the sea urchin egg. *Exp. Cell Res.* **125**:55–61.

Shimizu, T. 1981. Cyclic changes in shape of a non-nucleate egg fragment of *Tubifex* (Annelida, Oligochaeta). *Dev. Growth Differ.* **23**:101–109.

Skoblina, M. N. 1974. Behavior of sperm nuclei injected into intact maturing and mature oocytes and into oocytes which matured after germinal vesicle removal. *Ontogenez* **5**:334–340.

Skoblina, M. N. 1976. Role of karyoplasm in the emergence of capacity of egg cytoplasm to induce DNA synthesis in transplanted sperm nuclei. *J. Embryol. Exp. Morphol.* **36**:67–72.

Slater, D. W., Slater, I., and Bollum, F. J. 1978. Cytoplasmic poly(A) polymerase from sea urchin eggs, merogons and embryos. *Dev. Biol.* **63**:94–110.

Slater, I., and Slater, D. W. 1974. Polyadenylation and transcription following fertilization. *Proc. Natl. Acad. Sci. USA* **71**:1103–1107.

Slater, I., Gillespie, D., and Slater, D. W. 1973. Cytoplasmic adenylation and processing of maternal RNA. *Proc. Natl. Acad. Sci. USA* **70**:406–411.

Smith, C., Brill, D., Bownes, M., and Ford, C. 1980. *Drosophila* nuclei replicate in *Xenopus* eggs. *J. Embryol. Exp. Morphol.* **55**:183–194.

Stambaugh, R., Brackett, B. G., and Mastroianni, L. 1969. Inhibition of *in vitro* fertilization of rabbit ova by trypsin inhibitors. *Biol. Reprod.* **1**:223–227.

Steffen, K. 1951. Zur Kenntnis der Befruchtungs vorganges bei *Impatiens glanduligera* Lundl. *Planta* **39**:175–244.

Steffen, K. 1953. Zytologische Untersuchungen an Pollenkorn und -schlauch. *Flora (Jena)* **140**:140–174.

Steinhardt, R. A., and Mazia, D. 1973. Development of K^+ conductance and membrane potential in unfertilized sea urchin eggs after exposure to NH_4OH. *Nature (London)* **241**:400–401.

Steinhardt, R. A., Shen, S., and Mazia, D. 1972. Membrane potential, membrane resistance and an energy requirement for the development of potassium conductance in the fertilization reaction of echinoderm eggs. *Exp. Cell Res.* **72**:195–203.

Steinhardt, R. A., Zucker, R., and Schatten, G. 1977. Intracellular calcium release at fertilization in the sea urchin egg. *Dev. Biol.* **58**:185–196.

Sugiyama, M. 1951. Re-fertilization of the fertilized eggs of the sea urchin. *Biol. Bull.* **101**:335–344.

Suzuki, N., Nomura, K., Ohtake, H., and Isaka, S. 1981. Purification and the primary structure of sperm-activating peptides from the jelly coat of sea urchin eggs. *Biochem. Biophys. Res. Commun.* **99**:1238–1244.

Szöllösi, D. G. 1962. Cortical granules: A general feature of mammalian eggs? *J. Reprod. Fertil.* **4**:223–224.

Szöllösi, D. G. 1967. Development of cortical granules and the cortical reaction in rat and hamster eggs. *Anat. Rec.* **159**:431–446.

Szöllösi, D. G., and Ris, H. 1961. Observation on sperm penetration in the rat. *J. Biophys. Biochem. Cytol.* **10**:275–283.

Thibault, C., and Gerard, M. 1970. Facteur cytoplasmique nécessaire à la formation de pronucleus mâle dans l'ovocyte de lapine. *C. R. Acad. Sci.* **270**:2025–2026.

Treigyte, G., and Gineitis, A. 1979. Specific changes in the biosynthesis and acetylation of nucleosomal histones in the early stages of embryogenesis of sea urchin. *Exp. Cell Res.* **121**:127–134.

Tsubo, Y. 1961. Chemotaxis and sexual behavior in *Chlamydomonas*. *J. Protozool.* **8**:114–121.

Tyler, A. 1948. On the chemistry of the fertilizin of the sea urchin *Strongylocentrotus purpuratus*. *Anat. Rec.* **101**(Suppl.):8–9.

Tyler, A. 1956. Physico-chemical properties of the fertilizin of the sea urchin *Arbacia punctulata* and the sand dollar *Echinarachinus parna*. *Exp. Cell Res.* **10**:377–386.

Tyler, A. 1960. Introductory remarks on the theory of fertilization. *In*: Ranzi, S., ed., *Symposium on Germ Cells and Development*, Pallanza, pp. 155–174.

Tyler, A. 1964. Studies on fertilization and early development. *Eng. Sci. Mag* **27**:17–20.

Tyler, A., and Hathaway, R. R. 1958. Production of ^{35}S-labelled fertilizin in eggs of *Arbacia punctulata*. *Biol. Bull.* **115**:369.

Tyler, A., Monroy, A., Kao, C. Y., and Grundfest, H. 1956. Membrane potential and resistance of the starfish egg before and after fertilization. *Biol. Bull* **111**:153–177.

Usui, N., and Yanagimachi, R. 1976. Behavior of hamster sperm nuclei incorporated into eggs at various stages of maturation, fertilization and early development. *J. Ultrastruct. Res.* **57**:276–288.

van Went, J., and Linskens, H. F. 1967. Die Entwicklung des sogenannten "Fadenapparates" in Embryosack von *Petunia hybrida*. *Genet. Breed. Res.* **37**:51–55.

Vasseur, E. 1947. The sulfuric acid content of the egg coat of the sea urchin *Strongylocentrotus droebachiensis* Müll. *Ark. Kemi Mineral. Geol.* **25B**:Nr 6.

Vasseur, E. 1949. The effect of sea urchin jelly coat solution and calcium ions on the oxygen uptake of sea urchin sperm. *Ark. Kemi* **1**:393–399.

Vazart, B. 1958. Differenciation des cellules sexuelles et fécondation chez les Phanérogames. *Protoplasmatologia* **7**:1–158.

Venezky, D. L., Angerer, L. M., and Angerer, R. C. 1981. Accumulation of histone repeat transcripts in the sea urchin egg pronucleus. *Cell* **24**:385–391.

von Beroldingen, C. H. 1981. The developmental potential of synchronized amphibian cell nuclei. *Dev. Biol.* **81**:115–126.

Warburg, O. 1910. Über die Oxydationen in lebenden Zellen nach Versuchen am Seeigelei. *Z. Physiol. Chem.* **66**:305–340.

Warburg, O. 1911. *Über die Oxydationen in lebenden Zellen nach Versuchen am Seeigelei*, Heidelberg, Rösaler & Herbert.

Weinberg, R. A. 1973. Nuclear RNA metabolism. *Annu. Rev. Biochem.* **42**:329–354.

Wilson, E. B. 1925. *The Cell in Development and Heredity*, 3rd ed., New York, Macmillan Co.

Wilt, F. H. 1973. Polyadenylation of maternal RNA of sea urchin eggs after fertilization. *Proc. Natl. Acad. Sci. USA* **70**:2345–2349.

Winkler, M. M., and Grainger, J. L. 1978. Mechanism of action of NH$_4$Cl and other weak bases in the activation of sea urchin eggs. *Nature (London)* **273**:236–238.

Wolf, D. E., Kinsey, W., Lennarz, W., and Edidin, M. 1981. Changes in the organization of the sea urchin plasma membrane upon fertilization: Indications from the lateral diffusion rates of lipid-soluble fluorescent dyes. *Dev. Biol.* **81**:133–138.

Wolf, D. P. 1974a. The cortical granule reaction in living eggs of the toad, *Xenopus laevis. Dev. Biol.* **36**:62–71.

Wolf, D. P. 1974b. On the contents of the cortical granules from *Xenopus laevis* eggs. *Dev. Biol.* **38**:14–29.

Wolf, D. P., Nishihara, T., West, D. M., Wyrick, R. E., and Hendrick, J. L. 1976. Isolation, physicochemical properties, and macromolecular composition of the vitelline and fertilization envelopes from *Xenopus laevis* eggs. *Biochemistry* **15**:3671–3678.

Yanagimachi, R. 1979. Sperm–egg association in mammals. *Curr. Top. Dev. Biol.* **12**:83–105.

Yanagimachi, R., and Noda, Y. D. 1970a. Electron microscope studies of sperm incorporation into the golden hamster egg. *Am. J. Anat.* **128**:429–462.

Yanagimachi, R., and Noda, Y. D. 1970b. Ultrastructural changes in the hamster sperm head during fertilization. *J. Ultrastruct. Res.* **31**:465–485.

Yanagimachi, R., and Usui, N. 1972. The appearance and disappearance of factors involved in sperm chromatin decondensation in the hamster egg. *J. Cell Biol.* **55**:293a.

Yanagimachi, R. Nicolson, G. L., Noda, Y. D., and Fujimoto, M. 1973. EM observations of the distribution of acidic anionic residues on hamster spermatozoa and eggs before and during fertilization. *J. Ultrastruct. Res.* **43**:344–353.

Yasbin, R., Sawicki, J., and MacIntyre, R. J. 1978. A developmental study of acid phosphatase-1 in *Drosophila melanogaster. Dev. Biol.* **63**:35–46.

Yasumasu, I., and Nakano, E. 1963. Respiratory level of sea urchin eggs before and after fertilization. *Biol. Bull.* **125**:182–187.

Yazaki, I. 1968. Immunological analysis of the calcium precipitable protein of sea urchin eggs. *Embryologia* **10**:131–141.

Young, C. W., Hendler, F. J., and Karnofsky, D. A. 1969. Synthesis of proteins for DNA replication and cleavage events in the sand dollar embryo. *Exp. Cell. Res.* **58**:15–26.

Yu, S.-F., and Wolf, D. P. 1981. Polyspermic mouse eggs can dispose of supernumerary sperm. *Dev. Biol.* **82**:203–210.

Zamboni, L. 1971. *Fine Morphology of Mammalian Fertilization*, New York, Harper & Row.

Zamboni, L. 1974. Fine morphology of the follicle wall and follicle cell–oocyte association. *Biol. Reprod.* **10**:125–149.

Zamboni, L., and Mastroianni, L. 1966. EM studies on rabbit ova. II. The penetrated tubal ovum. *J. Ultrastruct. Res.* **14**:118–132.

Zamboni, L., Stefanini, M., Ōura, C., and Smith, D. 1970. The pattern of sperm penetration into the mouse egg. *Proc. 7th Int. Congr. Electron Microsc.* **3**:663–664.

Zaneveld, L. J. D., Robertson, R. T., Kessler, M., and Williams, W. L. 1971. Inhibition of fertilization *in vivo* by pancreatic and seminal plasma trypsin inhibitors. *J. Reprod. Fertil.* **25**:387–392.

CHAPTER 3

Abelson, H. T., Johnson, L. F., Penman, S., and Green, H. 1974. Changes in RNA in relation to growth of the fibroblast. II. The lifetime of mRNA, rRNA, and tRNA in resting and growing cells. *Cell* **1**:161–165.

Abrams, R. 1951. Synthesis of nucleic acid purines in the sea urchin embryo. *Exp. Cell Res.* **2**:235–242.

Adamson, E. D., and Woodland, H. R. 1974. Histone synthesis in early amphibian development. *J. Mol. Biol.* **88**:263–285.

Adamson, E. D., and Woodland, H. R. 1977. Changes in the rate of histone synthesis during oocyte maturation and very early development in *Xenopus laevis. Dev. Biol.* **57**:136–149.

Agrell, I. 1958. A cytoplasmic production of RNA during the cell cycle of the micromeres in the sea urchin embryo. *Ark. Zool.* (2) **11**:435–440.

Amaldi, P. P., Felicetti, L., and Campioni, N. 1977. Flow of informational RNA from cytoplasmic poly(A)-containing particles to polyribosomes in *Artemia salina* cysts at early stages of development. *Dev. Biol.* **59**:49–61.

Anderson, K. V., and Lengyel, J. A. 1981. Changing rates of DNA and RNA synthesis in *Drosophila* embryos. *Dev. Biol.* **82**:127–138.

Arceci, R. J., and Gross, P. R. 1980. Histone gene expression: Progeny of isolated early blastomeres make the same change as in the embryo. *Science* **209**:607–609.

Arceci, R. J., Senger, D. R., and Gross, P. R. 1976. The programmed switch in lysine-rich histone synthesis at gastrulation. *Cell* **9**:171–178.

Arthur, C. G., Weide, C. M., Vincent, W. S., and Goldstein, E. S. 1979. mRNA sequence diversity during early embryogenesis in *Drosophila melanogaster*. *Exp. Cell Res.* **121**:87–94.

Azar, Y., and Eyal-Giladi, H. 1979. Marginal zone cells—The primitive streak-inducing component of the primary hypoblast in the chick. *J. Embryol. Exp. Morphol.* **52**:79–88.

Azar, Y., and Eyal-Giladi, H. 1981. Interaction of epiblast and hypoblast in the formation of the primitive streak and the embryonic axis in chick, as revealed by hypoblast-rotation experiments. *J. Embryol. Exp. Morphol.* **61**:133–144.

Bachvarova, R., and DeLeon, V. 1980. Polyadenylated RNA of mouse ova and loss of maternal RNA in early development. *Dev. Biol.* **74**:1–8.

Bagshaw, J. C., Acey, R., and Helder, J. C. 1980. RNA polymerases and transcriptional switches in developing *Artemia*. *In*: Persoone, G., Sorgeloos, P., Roels, O., and Jaspers, E., eds., *The Brine Shrimp Artemia*, Wetteren, Belgium, Universa Press.

Ballantine, J. E. M., Woodland, H. R., and Sturgess, E. A. 1979. Changes in protein synthesis during development of *Xenopus laevis*. *J. Embryol. Exp. Morphol.* **51**:137–153.

Barlow, P. W., and Sherman, M. I. 1972. The biochemistry of differentiation of mouse trophoblast: Studies on polyploidy. *J. Embryol. Exp. Morphol.* **27**:447–465.

Barth, L. G., and Barth, L. J. 1968. The role of sodium chloride in the process of induction by lithium chloride in cells of the *Rana pipiens* gastrula. *J. Embryol. Exp. Morphol.* **19**:387–396.

Batten, B. E., and Haar, J. L. 1979. Fine structural differentiation of germ layers in the mouse at the time of mesoderm formation. *Anat. Rec.* **194**:125–142.

Bellairs, R. 1979. The mechanism of somite segmentation in the chick embryo. *J. Embryol. Exp. Morphol.* **51**:227–243.

Bellairs, R., and Veini, M. 1980. An experimental analysis of somite segmentation in the chick embryo. *J. Embryol. Exp. Morphol.* **55**:93–108.

Bergami, M., Mansour, T. E., and Scarano, E. 1968. Properties of glycogen phosphorylase before and after fertilization in the sea urchin eggs. *Exp. Cell Res.* **49**:650–655.

Berrill, N. J., and Karp, G. 1976. *Development*, New York, McGraw–Hill.

Bevelander, G., and Nakahara, H. 1960. Development of the skeleton of the sand dollar. *Publ. Am. Assoc. Adv. Sci.* **64**:41–56.

Biggers, J. D., Whitten, W. K., and Whittingham, D. G. 1971. The culture of mouse embryos *in vitro*. *In*: Daniell, J. C., ed., *Methods in Mammalian Embryology*, San Francisco, Freeman, pp. 86–116.

Black, J. W., Duncan, W. A. M., Durant, C. J., Ganellin, C. R., and Parsons, E. M. 1972. Definition and antagonism of histamine H_2-receptors. *Nature (London)* **236**:385–390.

Borthwick, H. A. 1931. Carrot seed germination. *Proc. Am. Soc. Hortic. Sci.* **28**:310–314.

Bownes, M. 1975. A photographic study of development in the living embryo of *Drosophila melanogaster*. *J. Embryol. Exp. Morphol.* **33**:789–801.

Bownes, M., and Kalthoff, K. 1974. Embryonic defects in *Drosophila* eggs after partial irradiation at different wavelengths. *J. Embryol. Exp. Morphol.* **31**:329–345.

Brachet, J. 1977. An old enigma: The gray crescent of amphibian eggs. *Curr. Top. Dev. Biol.* **11**:133–186.

Brachet, J., Hanocq, F., and VanGansen, P. 1970. A cytochemical and ultrastructural analysis of *in vitro* maturation in amphibian oocytes. *Dev. Biol.* **21**:157–195.

Brady, T. 1973. Feulgen cytophotometric determination of the DNA content of the embryo proper and suspensor cells of *Phaseolus coccineus*. *Cell Differ.* **2**:65–75.

Brakel, C. L., and Blumenthal, A. B. 1977. Multiple forms of *Drosophila* embryo DNA polymerase: Evidence for proteolytic conversion. *Biochemistry* **16**:3137–3143.

Brandhorst, B. P. 1976. HnRNA of animal cells and its relationship to mRNA. *In*: McConkey, E. H., ed., *Protein Synthesis: A Series of Advances II*, New York, Dekker, pp. 1–67.

Brandhorst, B. P., and Bannet, M. 1978. Terminal completion of poly(A) synthesis in sea urchin embryos. *Dev. Biol.* **63**:421–431.

Brandhorst, B. P., Verma, D. P. S., and Fromson, D. 1979. Polyandenylated and non-polyandenylated mRNA fractions from sea urchin embryos code for the same abundant proteins. *Dev. Biol.* **71**:128–141.

Brandt, W. F., Strickland, W. N., Strickland, M., Carlisle, L., Woods, D., and von Holt, C. 1979. A histone programme during the life cycle of the sea urchin. *Eur. J. Biochem.* **94**:1–10.

Bravo, R., and Knowland, J. 1979. Classes of proteins synthesized in oocytes, eggs, embryos and differentiated tissues of *Xenopus laevis*. *Differentiation* **13**:101–108.

Brinster, R. L. 1973. Parental glucose phosphate isomerase activity in three-day mouse embryos. *Biochem. Genet.* **9**:187–191.

Bryant, P. J. 1979. Pattern formation, growth control and cell interactions in *Drosophila* imaginal discs. *Symp. Soc. Dev. Biol.* **37**:295–316.

Burnside, B., Kozak, C., and Kafatos, F. C. 1973. Tubulin determination by an isotope dilution vinblastine precipitation method. *J. Cell Biol.* **59**:755–767.

Busby, S., and Bakken, A. H. 1979. A quantitative electron microscopic analysis of transcription in sea urchin embryos. *Chromosoma* **71**:249–262.

Busby, S., and Bakken, A. H. 1980. Transcription in developing sea urchins: Electron microscopic analysis of cleavage, gastrula and prism stages. *Chromosoma* **79**:85–104.

Byrd, E. W., and Kasinsky, H. E. 1973. Histone synthesis during early embryogenesis in *Xenopus laevis*. *Biochemistry* **12**:246–253.

Byrd, E. W., and Kasinsky, H. E. 1974. Nuclear accumulation of newly synthesized histones in early *Xenopus* development. *Biochim. Biophys. Acta* **331**:430–441.

Calcarco, P. G., and Brown, E. H. 1969. An ultrastructural and cytological study of preimplantation development of the mouse. *J. Exp. Zool.* **171**:253–284.

Carroll, A. G., and Ozaki, H. 1979. Changes in the histones of the sea urchin *Strongylocentrotus purpuratus* at fertilization. *Exp. Cell Res.* **119**:307–315.

Cather, J. N., and Verdonk, N. H. 1974. The development of *Bithynia tentaculata* after removal of the polar lobe. *J. Embryol. Exp. Morphol.* **31**:415–422.

Cather, J. N., Verdonk, N.H., and Dohmen, M. R. 1976. Role of the vegetal body in the regulation of development in *Bithynia tentaculata* (Prosobranchia, Gastropoda). *Am. Zool.* **16**:455–468.

Chan, L. N., and Gehring, W. 1971. Determination of blastoderm cells in *Drosophila melanogaster*. *Proc. Natl. Acad. Sci. USA* **68**:2217–2221.

Chapman, V. M., Whitten, W. K., and Ruddle, F. H. 1971. Activation of glucose phosphate isomerase-1 (Gpi-1) in preimplantation stages of mouse embryo. *Dev. Biol.* **26**:153–158.

Childs, G., Maxson, R., and Kedes, L. H. 1979. Histone gene expression during sea urchin embryogenesis. *Dev. Biol.* **73**:153–173.

Church, R. B. 1970. Differential gene activity. *In*: Fraser, F. S., and McKusick, V. A., eds., *Congenital Malformations*, Amsterdam, Excerpta Medica, pp. 19–28.

Church, R. B., and Brown, I. R. 1972. Tissue specificity of genetic transcription. *In*: Ursprung,

H., ed., *Results and Problems in Cell Differentiation*, Berlin, Springer-Verlag, Vol. 3, pp. 11–24.

Clandinin, M. T., and Schultz, G. A. 1975. Levels and modifications of methionyl-tRNA in preimplantation rabbit embryos. *J. Mol. Biol.* **93**:517–528.

Clement, A. C. 1952. Experimental studies on germinal localization in *Ilyanassa*. I. The role of the polar lobe in determination of the cleavage pattern and its influence in later development. *J. Exp. Zool.* **121**:593–626.

Clement, A. C. 1971. *Ilyanassa. In*: Reverberi, G., ed., *Experimental Embryology of Marine and Fresh-water Invertebrates,* Amsterdam, North-Holland, pp. 188–214.

Clement, A. C. 1976. Cell determination and organogenesis in molluscan development: A reappraisal based on deletion experiments in *Ilyanassa. Am. Zool.* **16**:447–453.

Cognetti, G., Kedes, L. H., and Gross, P. R. 1969. Unpublished results. (*Fide* Cognetti *et al.*, 1974.)

Cognetti, G., Spinelli, G., and Vivoli, A. 1974. Synthesis of histones during sea urchin oogenesis. *Biochim. Biophys. Acta* **349**:447–455.

Cohen, L. H., Newrock, K. M., and Zweidler, A. 1975. Stage specific switches in histone synthesis during embryogenesis of the sea urchin. *Science* **190**:994–997.

Cohn, R. H., Lowry, J. C., and Kedes, L. H. 1976. Histone genes of the sea urchin *S. purpuratus* cloned in *E. coli. Cell* **9**:147–161.

Conklin, E. G. 1897. The embryology of *Crepidula. J. Morphol.* **13**:1–226.

Conklin, E. G. 1932. The embryology of Amphioxus. *J. Morphol.* **54**:69–151.

Costello, D. P. 1961. On the orientation of centrioles in dividing cells and its significance. *Biol. Bull.* **120**:285–312.

Costello, D. P., and Henley, C. 1976. Spiralian development: A perspective. *Am. Zool.* **16**:277–291.

Cowden, R. R., and Lehman, H. E. 1963. A cytochemical study of differentiation in early echinoid development. *Growth* **27**:185–197.

Crampton, H. E. 1896. Experimental studies on gastropod development. *Wilhelm Roux Arch.Entwicklungsmech. Org.* **3**:1–19.

Cremonini, R., and Cionini, P. G. 1977. Extra DNA synthesis in embryo suspensor cells of *Phaseolus coccineus. Protoplasma* **91**:303–313.

Crerar, M., and Pearlman, R. E. 1976. DNA polymerase from *Tetrahymena pyriformis. J. Biol. Chem.* **249**:3123–3131.

Croce, C. M., Talaveri, A., Basilico, C., and Miller, O. J. 1977. Suppression of production of mouse 28S rRNA in mouse–human hybrids segregating mouse chromosomes. *Proc. Natl. Acad. Sci. USA* **74**:694–697.

Dalcq, A., and Jones-Seaton, A. 1949. La répartition des éléments basophiles dans l'oeuf du rat et du lapin et son intérêt pour la morphologie. *Bull. Clin. Sci. Acad. R. Belg.* **35**:500–511.

Dan, K. 1960. Cytoembryology of echinoderms and amphibia. *Int. Rev. Cytol.* **9**:321–365.

Dan, K. 1978. Unequal division: Its cause and significance. *In*: Dirksen, E. R., Prescott, D. M., and Fox, C. F., eds., *Cell Reproduction: In Honor of Daniel Mazia*, New York, Academic Press, pp. 557–561.

Dan, K., and Nakajima, T. 1956. On the morphology of the mitotic apparatus isolated from echinoderm eggs. *Embryologia* **3**:187–194.

Dan, K., and Okazaki, K. 1956. Cytoembryological studies of sea urchins. III. Role of the secondary mesenchyme cells in the formation of the primitive gut in sea urchin larvae. *Biol. Bull.* **110**:29–42.

Dan, K., Ito, S., and Mazia, D. 1952. Study of the course of formation of the mitotic apparatus in *Arbacia* and *Mactra* by isolation techniques. *Biol. Bull.* **103**:292.

Dan, K., Noguchi, M., and Uemura, I. 1979. Studies on unequal division in sea urchin embryos: Inequality of ribosomal content. *In*: Ebert, J. D., and Okada, T. S., eds., *Mechanisms of Cell Change*, New York, Wiley, pp. 33–48.

Daniel, J. C., and Olson, J. D. 1966. Cell movement, proliferation and death in the formation of the embryonic axis of the rabbit. *Anat. Rec.* **156**:123–128.

Danilchik, M. V., and Hille, M. B. 1981. Sea urchin egg and embryo ribosomes: Differences in translational activity in a cell-free system. *Dev. Biol.* **84**:291–298.

Dan-Sohkawa, M., and Fujisawa, H. 1980. Cell dynamics of the blastulation process in the starfish, *Asterina pectinifera*. *Dev. Biol.* **77**:328–339.

Darnell, J. E. 1968. Ribonucleic acids from animal cells. *Bacteriol. Rev.* **32**:262–290.

Davidson, E. H., and Britten, R. J. 1979. Regulation of gene expression: Possible role of repetitive sequences. *Science* **204**:1052–1059.

Davidson, R. G., Nitowsky, H. M., and Childs, B. 1963. Demonstration of two populations of cells in the human female heterozygous for glucose-6-phosphate dehydrogenase variants. *Proc. Natl. Acad. Sci. USA* **50**:481–485.

Davies, J., and Wimsatt, W. A. 1966. Observation on the fine structure of the sheep placenta. *Acta Anat.* **65**:182–223.

De Feo, V. J. 1967. Decidualization. *In*: Wynn, R. M., ed., *Cellular Biology of the Uterus*, New York, Appleton–Century–Crofts, pp. 191–290.

Denny, P. C., and Tyler, A. 1964. Activation of protein biosynthesis in non-nucleate fragments of sea urchin eggs. *Biochem. Biophys. Res. Commun.* **11**:447–451.

Derrick, G. E. 1937. An analysis of the early development of the chick by means of the mitotic index. *J. Morphol.* **61**:257–284.

Dey, S. K., Villanueva, C., and Abdou, N. I. 1979a. Histamine receptors on rabbit blastocyst and endometrial cell membranes. *Nature (London)* **278**:648–649.

Dey, S. K., Johnson, D. C., and Santos, J. G. 1979b. Is histamine production by the blastocyst required for implantation in the rabbit? *Biol. Reprod.* **21**:1169–1173.

Dillon, L. S. 1978. *The Genetic Mechanism and the Origin of Life*, New York, Plenum Press.

Dillon, L. S. 1981. *Ultrastructure, Macromolecules, and Evolution*, New York, Plenum Press.

Dohmen, M. R., and Verdonk, N. H. 1979. The ultrastructure and role of the polar lobe in development of molluscs. *Symp. Soc. Dev. Biol.* **37**:3–27.

Dolecki, G. J., Duncan, R. F., and Humphreys, T. 1977. Complete turnover of poly(A) on maternal mRNA of sea urchin embryos. *Cell* **11**:339–344.

Dubroff, L. M. 1977. Oligouridylate stretches in heterogeneous nuclear RNA. *Proc. Natl. Acad. Sci. USA* **74**:2217–2221.

Dubroff, L. M. 1980. Oligomeric sequences in the cytoplasmic RNA of sea urchin embryos. *Biochim. Biophys. Acta* **607**:115–121.

Dubroff, L. M., and Nemer, M. 1975. Molecular classes of hnRNA in sea urchin embryos. *J. Mol. Biol.* **95**:455–476.

Dubroff, L. M., and Nemer, M. 1976. Developmental shifts in the synthesis of hnRNA classes in the sea urchin embryo. *Nature (London)* **260**:120–124.

Duncan, R., Dower, W., and Humphreys, T. 1975. Normal synthesis, transport and decay of mRNA in the absence of its translation. *Nature (London)* **253**:751–753.

Dworkin, M. B., and Infante, A. A. 1976. Relationship between the mRNA of polysomes and free ribonucleoprotein particles in the early sea urchin embryo. *Dev. Biol.* **53**:73–90.

Dworkin, M. B., Rudensey, L. M., and Infante, A. A. 1977. Cytoplasmic nonpolysomal RNP particles in sea urchin embryos and their relationship to protein synthesis. *Proc. Natl. Acad. Sci. USA* **74**:2231–2235.

Easton, D., and Chalkley, R. 1972. High-resolution electrophoretic analysis of the histones form embryos and sperm of *Arbacia punctulata*. *Exp. Cell Res.* **72**:502–508.

Ecker, R. E., and Smith, L. D. 1971. The nature and fate of *Rana pipiens* proteins synthesized during maturation and early cleavage. *Dev. Biol.* **24**:559–576.

Edström, J. E., and Lönn, V. 1976. Cytoplasmic zone analysis: RNA flow studied by micromanipulation. *J. Cell Biol.* **70**:562–572.

Ehrismann, R., Chiquet, M., and Turner, D. C. 1981. Mode of action of fibronectin in promoting chicken myoblast attachment. *J. Biol. Chem.* **256**:4056–4062.

Ellem, K. A. O., and Gwatkin, R. B. L. 1968. Patterns of nucleic acid synthesis in the early mouse embryo. *Dev. Biol.* **18**:311–330.

Ellinger, M. S. 1978. The cell cycle and transplantation of blastula nuclei in *Bombina orientalis*. *Dev. Biol.* **65**:81–89.

Emerson, C. P., and Humphreys, T. 1970. Regulation of DNA-like RNA and the apparent activation of rRNA synthesis in sea urchin embryos. *Dev. Biol.* **23**:86–112.

Eyal-Giladi, H., and Kochav, S. 1976. From cleavage to primitive streak formation: A complementary normal table and a new look at the first stages of the development of the chick. *Dev. Biol.* **49**:321–337.

Eyal-Giladi, H., Farbiasz, I., Ostrovsky, D., and Hochman, J. 1975. Protein synthesis in epiblast versus hypoblast during the critical stages of induction and growth of the primitive streak in the chick embryo. *Dev. Biol.* **45**:358–365.

Eyal-Giladi, H., Raveh, D., Feinstein, N., and Friedländer, M. 1979. Glycogen metabolism in the prelaid chick embryo. *J. Morphol.* **161**:23–38.

Felicetti, L., Amaldi, P. P., Moretti, S., Campioni, N., and Urbani, C. 1975. Intracellular distribution, sedimentation values and template activity of polyadenylic acid-containing RNA stored in *Artemia salina* cysts. *Cell Differ.* **4**:339–354.

Flickinger, R. A. 1980. The effect of heparin upon differentiation of ventral halves of frog gastrulae. *Wilhelm Roux Arch. Dev. Biol.* **188**:9–11.

Forino, L. M. C., Tagliasacchi, A. M., and Avanzi, S. 1979. Different structure of polytene chromosomes of *Phaseolus coccineus* suspensors during early embryogenesis. *Protoplasma* **101**:231–246.

Forman, D., and Slack, J. M. W. 1980. Determination and cellular commitment in the embryonic amphibian mesoderm. *Nature (London)* **286**:492–493.

Freeman, G. 1979. The multiple roles which cell division can play in the localization of developmental potential. *Symp. Soc. Dev. Biol.* **37**:53–76.

Frels, W. I., and Chapman, V. M. 1980. Expression of the maternally derived X chromosome in the mural trophoblast of the mouse. *J. Embryol. Exp. Morphol.* **56**:179–190.

Friedman, P. A., Platzer, E. G., and Carroll, E. J. 1980. Tubulin characterization during embryogenesis of *Ascaris suum*. *Dev. Biol.* **76**:47–57.

Fromson, D., and Verma, D. P. S. 1976. Translation of nonpolyadenylated mRNA of sea urchin embryos. *Proc. Natl. Acad. Sci. USA* **73**:148–151.

Galau, G. A., Britten, R. J., and Davidson, E. H. 1974. A measurement of the sequence complexity of polysomal mRNA in sea urchin embryos. *Cell* **2**:9–21.

Galau, G. A., Lipson, E. D., Britten, R. J., and Davidson, E. H. 1977. Synthesis and turnover of polysomal mRNAs in sea urchin embryos. *Cell* **10**:415–432.

Gardner, R. L., and Lyon, M. F. 1971. X chromosome inactivation studied by injection of a single cell into the mouse blastocyst. *Nature (London)* **231**:385–386.

Gardner, R. L., and Papaioannou, V. E. 1975. Differentiation in the trophectoderm and inner cell mass. *Symp. Br. Soc. Dev. Biol.* **2**:107–132.

Gebhardt, D. O. F., and Nieuwkoop, P. D. 1964. The influence of lithium on the competence of the ectoderm in *Ambystoma mexicanum*. *J. Embryol. Exp. Morphol.* **12**:317–331.

Gibbins, J. R., Tilney, L. G., and Porter, K. H. 1969. Microtubules in the formation and development of the primary mesenchyme in *Arbacia*. *J. Cell Biol.* **41**:201–226.

Gipson, I. 1974. Electron microscopy of early cleavage furrows in the chick blastodisc. *J. Ultrastruct. Res.* **49**:331–347.

Giudice, G. 1973. *Developmental Biology of the Sea Urchin Embryo*, New York, Academic Press.

Glišin, V. R., and Glišin, M. V. 1964. RNA metabolism following fertilization in sea urchin eggs. *Proc. Natl. Acad. Sci. USA* **52**:1548–1553.

Golbus, M. S., Calarco, P. G., and Epstein, C. F. 1973. The effects of inhibitors of RNA synthesis (α-amanitin and actinomycin D) on preimplantation mouse embryogenesis. *J. Exp. Zool.* **186**:207–216.

Goldstein, E. S., and Arthur, C. G. 1979. Isolation and characterization of cDNA complementary to transient maternal poly(A)$^+$ RNA from *Drosophila* oocyte. *Biochim. Biophys. Acta* **565**:265–274.

Green, L. H., Brandis, J. W., Turner, F. R., and Raff, R. A. 1975. Cytoplasmic microtubule proteins of the embryo of *Drosophila melanogaster*. *Biochemistry* **14**:4487–4491.

Gross, K. W., Jacobs-Lorena, M., Baglioni, C., and Gross, P. R. 1973: Cell-free translation of maternal mRNA from sea urchin eggs. *Proc. Natl. Acad. Sci. USA* **70**:2614–2618.

Gross, P. R., and Cousineau, G. H. 1963. Effect of actinomycin D on macromolecule synthesis and early development in sea urchin eggs. *Biochem. Biophys. Res. Commun.* **10**:321–326.

Gross, P. R., Malkin, L. I., and Moyer, W. A. 1964. Templates for the first proteins of embryonic development. *Proc. Natl. Acad. Sci. USA* **51**:407–414.

Gross, P. R., Kraemer, K., and Malkin, L. I. 1965. Base composition of RNA synthesized during cleavage of the sea urchin embryo. *Biochem. Biophys. Res. Commun.* **18**:569–575.

Grunstein, M. 1978. Hatching in the sea urchin *Lytechinus pictus* is accompanied by a shift in histone H4 gene activity. *Proc. Natl. Acad. Sci. USA* **75**:4135–4139.

Grunstein, M., and Grunstein, J. E. 1977. The histone H4 gene of *S. purpuratus* DNA and mRNA sequences at the 5′ end. *Cold Spring Harbor Symp. Quant. Biol.* **42**:1083–1092.

Grunstein, M., Diamond, K. E., Knoppel, E., and Grunstein, J. E. 1981. Comparison of the early histone H4 gene sequence of *Strongylocentrotus purpuratus* with maternal, early, and late histone H4 mRNA sequences. *Biochemistry* **20**:1216–1223.

Guerrier, P., and van den Biggelaar, J. A. M. 1979. Intracellular activation and cell interactions in so-called mosaic embryos. *INSERM Symp.* **10**:29–36.

Guerrier, P., van den Biggelaar, J. A. M., van Dongen, C. A. M., and Verdonk, N. H. 1978. Significance of the polar lobe for the determination of dorsoventral polarity in *Dentalium vulgare*. *Dev. Biol.* **63**:233–242.

Gussek, D. J., and Hedrick, J. L. 1972. The enzymatic characteristics and control of glycogen phosphorylase during early amphibian development. *J. Biol. Chem.* **247**:6603–6609.

Gustafson, T., and Kinnander, H. 1956a. Gastrulation in the sea urchin larva studied by aid of time-lapse cinematography. *Exp. Cell Res.* **10**:733–734.

Gustafson, T., and Kinnander, H. 1956b. Microaquaria for time-lapse cinematographic studies of morphogenesis in swimming larvae and observations on sea urchin gastrulation. *Exp. Cell Res.* **11**:36–51.

Gustafson, T., and Wolpert, L. 1961a. Studies on the cellular basis of morphogenesis in the sea urchin embryo. *Exp. Cell Res.* **24**:64–79.

Gustafson, T., and Wolpert, L. 1961b. Cellular mechanisms in the morphogenesis of the sea urchin larva. *Exp. Cell Res.* **22**:509–520.

Gustafson, T., and Wolpert, L. 1962. Cellular mechanisms in the morphogenesis of the sea urchin larva. *Exp. Cell Res.* **27**:260–279.

Gustafson, T., and Wolpert, L. 1963. The cellular basis of morphogenesis and sea urchin development. *Int. Rev. Cytol.* **15**:139–214.

Gustafson, T., and Wolpert, L. 1967. Cellular movement and contact in sea urchin morphogenesis. *Biol. Rev.* **42**:442–498.

Gwatkin, R. B. L. 1966. Defined media and development of mammalian eggs *in vitro*. *Ann. N.Y. Acad. Sci.* **139**:79–90.

Halperin, W., and Jensen, W. A. 1967. Ultrastructural changes during growth and embryogenesis in carrot cell cultures. *J. Ultrastruct. Res.* **18**:428–443.

Hamburger, V., and Hamilton, H. L. 1951. A series of normal stages in the development of the chick embryo. *J. Morphol.* **88**:49–92.

Hansmann, I., Gebauer, J., Bihl, L., and Grimm, T. 1978. Onset of nucleolus organizer activity in early mouse embryogenesis and evidence for its regulation. *Exp. Cell Res.* **114**:263–268.

Hara, K. 1977. The cleavage pattern of the axolotl egg studied by cinematography and cell count-ing. *Wilhelm Roux Arch. Dev. Biol.* **181**:73–87.

Hara, K., and Boterenbrood, E. C. 1977. Refinement of Harrison's normal table for the morula and blastula of the axolotl. *Wilhelm Roux Arch. Dev. Biol.* **181**:89–93.

Hille, M. B., Hall, D. C., Yablonka-Reuveni, Z., Danilchik, M. V., and Moon, R. T. 1981. Translational control in sea urchin eggs and embryos: Initiation is rate limiting in blastula stage embryos. *Dev. Biol.* **86**:241–249.

Hirsh, D. 1979. Temperature sensitive maternal effect mutants of early development in *Caenorhabditis elegans*. *Symp. Soc. Dev. Biol.* **37**:149–165.

Hoffman, L. H., and Olson, G. E. 1980. Crystalline inclusions in the rabbit blastocyst. Evidence for microtubular aggregates. *Exp. Cell Res.* **127**:1–14.

Hogan, B., and Gross, P. R. 1971. The effect of protein synthesis inhibition on the entry of mRNA into the cytoplasm of sea urchin embryos. *J. Cell Biol.* **49**:692–701.

Holmes, D. S., Cohn, R. H., Kedes, L. H., and Davidson, N. 1977. Positions of sea urchin (*Strongylocentrotus purpuratus*) histone genes relative to restriction endonuclease sites on the chimeric plasmids pSp2 and pSp17. *Biochemistry* **16**:1504–1512.

Horiuchi, R., Yaoi, Y., and Amano, N. 1972. RNA synthesis in cultured chick embryo cells in growing and confluent phases. *Dev. Growth Differ.* **14**:185–195.

Hörstadius, S. 1939. The mechanism of sea urchin development, studied by operative methods. *Biol. Rev.* **14**:132–179.

Hsu, Y. C. 1973. Differentiation *in vitro* of mouse embryos to the stage of early somite. *Dev. Biol.* **33**:403–411.

Hsu, Y. C. 1980. Embryo growth and differentiation factors in embryonic sera of mammals. *Dev. Biol.* **76**:465–474.

Huber, G. C. 1915. The development of the albino rat, *Mus norvegicus albinus*. *J. Morphol.* **26**:247–358.

Huebner, E., Tobe, S. S., and Davey, K. G. 1975. Structural and functional dynamics of oogenesis in *Glossina austeni*: Vitellogenesis with special reference to the follicular epithelium. *Tissue Cell* **7**:535–558.

Hunt, C. V., and Avery, G. B. 1971. Increased levels of DNA during trophoblast giant-cell formation in mice. *J. Reprod. Fertil.* **25**:85–91.

Iwai, K., Hayashi, H., and Ishikawa, K. 1972. Calf thymus lysine- and serine-rich histone. III. Complete amino acid sequence and its implication for interactions of histones with DNA. *J. Biochem.* **72**:357–367.

Jäckle, H. 1979. Degradation of maternal poly(A)-containing RNA during early embryogenesis of an insect (*Smittia* sp., Chironomidae, Diptera). *Wilhelm Roux Arch. Dev. Biol.* **187**:179–193.

Jäckle, H., and Kalthoff, K. 1979. RNA and protein synthesis in developing embryos of *Smittia* spec. (Chironomidae, Diptera). *Wilhelm Roux Arch. Dev. Biol.* **187**:283–305.

Jackson, V., Shires, A., Granner, D., and Chalkley, R. 1975. Studies on highly metabolically active acetylation and phosphorylation of histones. *J. Biol. Chem.* **250**:4856–4863.

Jackson, V., Shires, A., Tanphaichitr, N., and Chalkley, R. 1976. Modifications to histones immediately after synthesis. *J. Mol. Biol.* **104**:471–483.

Jaffe, L. F. 1966. Electrical currents through the developing *Fucus* egg. *Proc. Natl. Acad. Sci. USA* **56**:1102–1109.

Jaffe, L. F. 1968. Localization in the developing *Fucus* egg and the general role of localizing currents. *Adv. Morphog.* **7**:295–328.

Jelinek, W., Adesnik, M., Salditt, M., Sheiness, D., Wall, R., Molloy, G., Phillipson, L., and Darnell, J. E. 1973. Further evidence on the nuclear origin and transfer to the cytoplasm of poly(A) sequences in mammalian cell RNA. *J. Mol. Biol.* **75**:515–532.

Jensen, W. A. 1963. Cell development during plant embryogenesis. *Brookhaven Symp. Biol.* **16**:179–202.

Johnson, A. W., and Hnilica, L. S. 1971. Cytoplasmic and nuclear basic protein synthesis during early sea urchin development. *Biochim. Biophys. Acta* **246**:141–154.

Johnson, L. F., Levis, R., Abelson, H. T., Green, H., and Penman, S. 1976. Changes in RNA in relation to growth of the fibroblast. *J. Cell Biol.* **71**:933–938.

Jolly, J., and Férester-Tadié, M. 1936. Recherches sur l'oeuf du rat et de la souris. *Arch. Anat. Microsc. Morphol. Exp.* **32**:323–390.

Kalf, G. F., Maguire, R. F., Metrione, R. M., and Koszalka, T. R. 1980. DNA replication by isolated rat trophoblast nuclei. *Dev. Biol.* **77**:253–270.

Kalthoff, K. 1979. Analysis of a morphogenetic determinant in an insect embryo (*Smittia* sp.). *Symp. Soc. Dev. Biol.* **37**:97–126.

Karkas, J. D., Margulies, L., and Chargaff, E. 1975. A DNA polymerase from embryos of *Drosophila melanogaster. J. Biol. Chem.* **250**:8657–8663.

Karp, G. C., and Solursh, M. 1974. Acid mucopolysaccharide metabolism, the cell surface, and primary mesenchyme cell activity in the sea urchin embryo. *Dev. Biol.* **41**:110–123.

Kauffman, S. A. 1977. Chemical patterns, compartments and a binary epigenetic code in *Drosophila. Am. Zool.* **17**:631–648.

Kedes, L. H., and Birnstiel, M. L. 1971. Reiteration and clustering of DNA sequences complementary to histone mRNA. *Nature New Biol.* **230**:165–169.

Kedes, L. H., Cohn, R. H., Lowry, J. C., Chang, A. C. Y., and Cohen, S. N. 1975. The organization of sea urchin histone genes. *Cell* **6**:359–369.

Keller, R. E. 1980. The cellular basis of epiboly: An SEM study of deep-cell rearrangement during gastrulation in *Xenopus laevis. J. Embryol. Exp. Morphol.* **60**:201–234.

Kinoshita, S., and Saiga, H. 1979. The role of proteoglycan in the development of sea urchins. *Exp. Cell Res.* **123**:229–236.

Kirschner, M. W., and Gerhart, J. C. 1981. Spatial and temporal changes in the amphibian egg. *BioScience* **31**:381–388.

Klag, J. J., and Ubbels, G. A. 1975. Regional morphological and cytochemical differentiation in the fertilized egg of *Discoglossus pictus. Differentiation* **3**:15–20.

Kochar, S., Ginsburg, M., and Eyal-Giladi, H. 1980. From cleavage to primitive streak formation: A complementary normal table and a new look at the first stages of the development of the chick. II. Microscopic anatomy and cell population dynamics. *Dev. Biol.* **79**:296–308.

Kojima, S., and Wilt, F. H. 1969. Rate of nuclear RNA turnover in sea urchin embryos. *J. Mol. Biol.* **40**:235–246.

Kozak, L. P., and Quinn, P. J. 1975. Evidence for dosage compensation of an X-linked gene in the 6-day embryo of the mouse. *Dev. Biol.* **45**:65–73.

Kunkel, N. S., and Weinberg, E. S. 1978. Histone gene transcripts in the cleavage and mesenchyme blastula embryo of the sea urchin *S. purpuratus. Cell* **14**:313–326.

Kunkel, N. S., Hemminki, K., and Weinberg, E. S. 1978. Size of histone gene transcripts in different embryonic stages of the sea urchin, *Strongylocentrotus purpuratus. Biochemistry* **17**:2591–2598.

LaMarca, M. J., and Wassarman, P. M. 1979. Program of early development in the mammal: Changes in absolute rates of synthesis of ribosomal proteins during oogenesis and early embryogenesis in the mouse. *Dev. Biol.* **73**:103–119.

Landström, U., and Løvtrup, S. 1979. Fate maps and cell differentiation in the amphibian embryo—An experimental study. *J. Embryol. Exp. Morphol.* **54**:113–130.

Laufer, J. S., Bazzicalupo, P., and Wood, W. B. 1980. Segregation of developmental potential in early embryos of *Caenorhabditis elegans. Cell* **19**:569–577.

Lawrence, P. A., and Morata, G. 1979. Pattern formation and compartments in the tarsus of *Drosophila. Symp. Soc. Dev. Biol.* **37**:317–323.

LeBlanc, J., and Brick, I. 1981. Morphological aspects of adhesion and spreading behavior of amphibian blastula and gastrula cells. *J. Embryol. Exp. Morphol.* **61**:145–163.

Lev, Z., Thomas, T. L., Lee, A. S., Angerer, R. C., Britten, R. J., and Davidson, E. H. 1980.

Developmental expression of two cloned sequences coding for rare sea urchin embryo messages. *Dev. Biol.* **76**:322–340.

Levey, I. L., Troike, D. E., and Brinster, R. L. 1977. Effects of α-amanitin on development of mouse ova in culture. *J. Reprod. Fertil.* **50**:147–150.

Levey, I. L., Stull, G. B., and Brinster, R. L. 1978. Poly(A) and synthesis of polyadenylated RNA in the preimplantation mouse embryo. *Dev. Biol.* **64**:140–148.

Lewin, B. 1975a. Units of transcription and translation: The relationship between hnRNA and mRNA. *Cell* **4**:11–20.

Lewin, B. 1975b. Units of transcription and translation: Sequence components of hnRNA and mRNA. *Cell* **4**:77–93.

Lifton, R. P., and Kedes, L. H. 1976. Size and sequence homology of masked maternal and embryonic histone mRNAs. *Dev. Biol.* **48**:47–55.

Loeb, L. A. 1974. Eucaryotic DNA polymerases. *Enzymes* **10**:173–209.

Loomis, L. W., Rossomando, E. F., and Chang, L. M. S. 1976. DNA polymerase of *Dictyostelium discoideum*. *Biochim. Biophys. Acta* **425**:469–477.

Louie, A. J., and Dixon, G. H. 1972. Synthesis, acetylation and phosphorylation of histone IV on its binding to DNA during spermatogenesis in trout. *Proc. Natl. Acad. Sci. USA* **69**:1975–1979.

Løvtrup, S., Landström, U., and Løvtrup-Rein, H. 1978. Polarities, cell differentiation and primary induction in the amphibian embryo. *Biol. Rev.* **53**:1–42.

Lyon, M. F. 1972. X-chromosome inactivation and developmental patterns in mammals. *Biol. Rev.* **47**:1–35.

McClintock, B. 1978. Development of the maize endosperm as revealed by clones. *Symp. Soc. Dev. Biol.* **36**:217–237.

McColl, R. S., and Aronson, A. I. 1978. Changes in transcription patterns during early development of the sea urchin. *Dev. Biol.* **65**:126–138.

McMahon, D. 1974. Chemical messengers in development: A hypothesis. *Science* **185**:1012–1021.

Mahowald, A. P., Allis, C. D., Karrer, K. M., Underwood, E. M., and Waring, G. L. 1979. Germ plasm and pole cells of *Drosophila*. *Symp. Soc. Dev. Biol.* **37**:127–146.

Malacinski, G. M., Chung, H. M., and Asashima, M. 1980. The association of primary embryonic organizer activity with the future dorsal side of amphibian eggs and early embryos. *Dev. Biol.* **77**:449–462.

Manes, C. 1971. Nucleic acid synthesis in preimplantation rabbit embryos. II. Delayed synthesis of rRNA. *J. Exp. Zool.* **176**:87–96.

Manner, H. W. 1964. *Elements of Comparative Vertebrate Embryology,* New York, Macmillan Co.

Mar, H. 1980. Radial cortical fibers and pronuclear migration in fertilized and artificially activated eggs of *Lytechinus pictus*. *Dev. Biol.* **78**:1–13.

Margulies, L., and Chargaff, E. 1973. Survey of DNA polymerase activity during the early development of *Drosophila melanogaster*. *Proc. Natl. Acad. Sci. USA* **70**:2946–2950.

Marsland, D. 1956. Protoplasmic contractility in relation to gel structure: Temperature–pressure experiments on cytokinesis and amoeboid movement. *Adv. Morphog.* **7**:295–328.

Marsland, D., and Landau, J. V. 1954. The mechanics of cytokinesis: Temperature–pressure studies on the cortical gel system in various marine eggs. *J. Exp. Zool.* **125**:507–539.

Meier, S. 1979. Development of the chick embryo mesoblast: Formation of the embryonic axis and establishment of the metameric pattern. *Dev. Biol.* **73**:25–45.

Meier, S. 1981. Development of the chick embryo mesoblast: Morphogenesis of the prechordal plate and cranial segments. *Dev. Biol.* **83**:49–61.

Merlino, G. T., Water, R. D., Moore, G. P., and Kleinsmith, L. J. 1981. Change in expression of the actin gene family during early sea urchin development. *Dev. Biol.* **85**:505–508.

Migeon, B. R. 1972. Stability of X chromosomal inactivation in human somatic cells. *Nature (London)* **239**:87–89.

Migeon, B. R. 1978. Clonal analysis of development: X-inactivation and cell communication as determinants of female phenotype. *Symp. Soc. Dev. Biol.* **36**:205–215.

Migeon, B. R., Norum, R. A., and Corsaro, C. M. 1974. Isolation and analysis of somatic hybrids derived from two human diploid cells. *Proc. Natl. Acad. Sci. USA* **71**:937–941.

Milcarek, C., Price, R. P., and Penman, S. 1974. The metabolism of a poly(A)⁻ mRNA fraction in HeLa cells. *Cell* **3**:1–10.

Miller, D. A., Dev, V. G., Tantravahi, R., and Miller, O. J. 1976. Suppression of human nucleolus organizer activity in mouse–human somatic hybrid cells. *Exp. Cell Res.* **101**:235–243.

Miller, L. 1978. Relative amounts of newly synthesized poly(A)⁺ and poly(A)⁻ mRNA during development of *Xenopus laevis*. *Dev. Biol.* **64**:118–129.

Miller, O. J., Miller, D. A., Dev, V. G., Tantravahi, R., and Croce, C. M. 1976. Expression of human and suppression of mouse nucleolus organizer activity in mouse–human somatic cell hybrids. *Proc. Natl. Acad. Sci. USA* **73**:4531–4535.

Mintz, B. 1964. Synthetic processes and early development in the mammalian egg. *J. Exp. Zool.* **157**:85–100.

Molloy, G. R., Thomas, W. L., and Darnell, J. E. 1972. Occurrence of uridylate-rich oligonucleotide regions in hnRNA of HeLa cells. *Proc. Natl. Acad. Sci. USA* **69**:3684–3688.

Monné, L., and Hårde, S. 1951. On the formation of the blastocoel and similar embryonic cavities. *Ark. Zool.* (2) **1**:463–469.

Moon, R. T., and Morrill, J. B. 1979. Further studies on the electrophoretically mobile acid phosphatases of the developing embryo of *Lymnaea palustris*. *Acta Embryol. Exp.* **1979**:3–15.

Moore, A. R., and Burt, A. S. 1939. On the locus and nature of forces causing gastrulation in embryos of *Dendraster excentricus*. *J. Exp. Zool.* **82**:159–171.

Morgan, T. H. 1927. *Experimental Embryology,* New York, Columbia University Press.

Morrill, J. B., Blair, C. A., and Larsen, W. J. 1973. Regulative development in the pulmonate gastropod, *Lymnaea palustris*, as determined by blastomere deletion experiments. *J. Exp. Zool.* **183**:47–56.

Mulnard, J. 1955. Contribution à la connaissance des enzymes dans l'ontogenèse. *Arch. Biol.* **66**:527–685.

Nagl, W. 1970. Temperature-dependent functional structures in the polytene chromosomes of *Phaseolus*, with special reference to the nucleolus organizers. *J. Cell Sci.* **6**:87–107.

Nagl, W. 1972. Giant sex chromatin in endopolyploid trophoblast nuclei of the rat. *Experientia* **28**:217–218.

Nagl, W., Peschke, C., and van Gyseghem, R. 1976. Heterochromatin underreplication in *Tropaeolum* embryogenesis. *Naturwissenschaften* **4**:198.

Nakazato, H., Kopp, D., and Edmonds, M. 1973. Localization of the poly(A) sequences in mRNA and in hnRNA of HeLa cells. *J. Biol. Chem.* **248**:1472–1476.

Nalbandov, A. V. 1971. Endocrine control of implantation. *In*: Blandau, R. J., ed., *The Biology of the Blastocyst*, Chicago, University of Chicago Press, pp. 383–392.

Nemer, M. 1962. Characteristics of the utilization of nucleosides by embryos of *Paracentrotus lividus*. *J. Biol. Chem.* **237**:143–149.

Nemer, M., Graham, M., and Dubroff, L. M. 1974. Co-existence of nonhistone mRNA species lacking and containing polyadenylic acid in sea urchin embryos. *J. Mol. Biol.* **89**:435–454.

Newrock, K. M., and Raff, R. A. 1975. Polar lobe specific regulation of translation in embryos of *Ilyanassa obsoleta*. *Dev. Biol.* **42**:242–261.

Newrock, K. M., Alfageme, C. R., Nardi, R. V., and Cohen, L. H. 1977. Histone changes during chromatin remodeling in embryogenesis. *Cold Spring Harbor Symp. Quant. Biol.* **42**:421–431.

Newrock, K. M., Cohen, L. H., Hendricks, M. B., Donnelly, R. J., and Weinberg, E. S. 1978. Stage specific mRNAs coding for subtypes of H2A and H2B histones in the sea urchin embryo. *Cell* **14**:327–336.

Nieuwkoop, P. D. 1969. The formation of the mesoderm in urodelean amphibians. *Wilhelm Roux Arch. Entwicklungsmech. Org.* **163**:298–315.

Nieuwkoop, P. D. 1977. Origin and establishment of embryonic polar axes in amphibian development. *Curr. Top. Dev. Biol.* **11**:115–132.

Nüsslein-Volhard, C. 1979. Maternal effect mutations that alter the spatial coordinates of the embryo of *Drosophila melanogaster*. *Symp. Soc. Dev. Biol.* **37**:185–211.

Okazaki, K. 1956. Skeletal formation of sea urchin larvae. I. Effect of calcium concentration on the medium. *Biol. Bull.* **110**:320–333.

Okazaki, K. 1962. Skeleton formation of sea urchin larvae. IV. Correlation in shape of spiculae and matrix. *Embryologia* **7**:21–38.

Okazaki, K. 1965. Skeleton formation of sea urchin larvae. V. Continuous observation of the process of matrix formation. *Exp. Cell Res.* **11**:548–559.

O'Melia, A. F. 1979a. Quantitative measurements of rates of 5S RNA and tRNA synthesis in sea urchin embryos. *Differentiation* **15**:97–105.

O'Melia, A. F. 1979b. The synthesis of 5S RNA and its regulation during early sea urchin development. *Dev. Growth Differ.* **21**:99–103.

O'Melia, A. F., and Villee, C. A. 1972. De novo synthesis of tRNA and 5S RNA in cleaving sea urchin embryos. *Nature (London)* **289**:51–52.

Paradiso, P., and Schofield, P. 1976. Changes in tRNA nucleotidyltransferase activity during embryonic development in *X. laevis*. *Exp. Cell Res.* **100**:9–14.

Parks, H. B. 1936. Cleavage patterns in *Drosophila* and mosaic formation. *Ann. Entomol. Soc. Am.* **29**:350–392.

Pearson, M. 1974. Polyteny and the functional significance of the polytene cell cycle. *J. Cell Sci.* **15**:457–479.

Peltz, R., and Giudice, G. 1967. The control of skeletal differentiation in sea urchin embryos: A molecular approach. *Biol. Bull.* **133**:479.

Pikó, L. 1970. Synthesis of macromolecules in early mouse embryos cultured *in vitro*: RNA, DNA, and a polysaccharide component. *Dev. Biol.* **21**:257–279.

Raff, E. C. 1977. Microtubule proteins in axolotl eggs and developing embryos. *Dev. Biol.* **58**:56–75.

Raff, E. C., and Raff, R. A., 1978. Tubulin and microtubules in the early development of the axolotl and other amphibia. *Am. Zool.* **18**:237–251.

Raff, R. A. 1975. Regulation of microtubule synthesis and utilization during early embryonic development of the sea urchin. *Am. Zool.* **15**:661–678.

Raff, R. A., and Kaumeyer, J. F. 1973. Soluble microtubule proteins of the sea urchin embryo: Partial characterization of the proteins and behavior of the pool in early development. *Dev. Biol.* **32**:309–320.

Randolph, L. F. 1936. Developmental morphology of the caryopsis in maize. *J. Agric. Res.* **53**:881–916.

Raveli, D., Friedländer, M., and Eyal-Giladi, H. 1976. Nucleolar ontogenesis in the uterine chick germ correlated with morphogenetic events. *Exp. Cell Res.* **100**:195–203.

Regier, J. C., and Kafatos, F. C. 1977. Absolute rates of protein synthesis in sea urchins with specific activity measurements of radioactive leucine and leucyl-tRNA. *Dev. Biol.* **57**:270–283.

Rickoll, W. L. 1976. Cytoplasmic continuity between embryonic cells and the primitive yolk sac during early gastrulation in *D. melanogaster*. *Dev. Biol.* **49**:304–310.

Rizzino, A., and Sherman, M. I. 1979. Development and differentiation of mouse blastocyst in serum-free medium. *Exp. Cell Res.* **121**:221–233.

Roeder, R. G. 1974. Multiple forms of DNA-dependent RNA polymerase in *Xenopus laevis*. *J. Biol. Chem.* **249**:249–256.

Romeo, G., and Migeon, B. R. 1975. Stability of X chromosomal inactivation in human somatic cells transformed by SV-40. *Humangenetik* **29**:165–170.

Rosenquist, G. C. 1966. A radioautographic study of labelled grafts in the chick blastoderm: Development from primitive streak stages to stage 12. *Contrib. Embryol. Carnegie Inst. Washington* **38**:71–110.

Rossant, J., and Papaioannou, V. E. 1977. The biology of embryogenesis. *In*: Sherman, M. I., ed., *Concepts in Mammalian Embryogenesis,* Cambridge, Mass., MIT Press, pp. 1–36.

Roth, J. S. 1964. Biological information in a single strand of DNA. *Nature (London)* **202**:182–183.

Ruderman, J. V., and Gross, P. R. 1974. Histones and histone synthesis in sea urchin development. *Dev. Biol.* **36**:286–298.

Ruderman, J. V., Baglioni, C., and Gross, P. R. 1974. Histone mRNA and histone synthesis during embryogenesis. *Nature (London)* **247**:36–38.

Sagata, N., Shiokawa, K., and Yamana, K. 1980. A study of the steady-state population of poly(A)$^+$ RNA during early development of *Xenopus laevis*. *Dev. Biol.* **77**:431–448.

Sawicki, J. A., and MacIntyre, R. J. 1978. Localization at the ultrastructural level of maternally derived enzyme and determination of the time of paternal gene expression for acid phosphatase-1 in *D. melanogaster*. *Dev. Biol.* **63**:47–58.

Saxén, C., and Toivonen, S. 1962. *Primary Embryonic Induction*, Englewood Cliffs, N.J., Prentice–Hall.

Schmidt, B. A., Kelly, P. T., May, M. C., Davis, S. E., and Conrad, G. W. 1980. Characterization of actin from fertilized eggs of *Ilyanassa obsoleta* during polar lobe formation and cytokinesis. *Dev. Biol.* **76**:126–140.

Schubiger, G., and Wood, W. J. 1977. Determination during early embryogenesis in *Drosophila melanogaster*. *Am. Zool.* **17**:565–576.

Schultz, G. A., Manes, C., and Hahn, W. E. 1973. Synthesis of RNA containing polyadenylic acid sequences in preimplantation rabbit embryos. *Dev. Biol.* **30**:418–426.

Schultz, R. M., Letourneau, G. E., and Wassarman, P. M. 1979. Program of early development in the mammal: Changes in patterns and absolute rates of tubulin and total protein synthesis during oocyte growth in the mouse. *Dev. Biol.* **73**:120–133.

Seale, R. L., and Aronson, A. I. 1973. Chromatin-associated proteins of the developing sea urchin embryo. I. Kinetics of synthesis and characterization of nonhistone proteins. *J. Mol. Biol.* **75**:633–645.

Selenka, E. 1884. *Die Blätter umkehrung im Ei der Nagathiere*, Weisbaden.

Sellens, M. H., and Sherman, M. I. 1980. Effects of culture conditions on the developmental programme of mouse blastocyst. *J. Embryol. Exp. Morphol.* **56**:1–22.

Senatori, O., Delpino, A., Scopelliti, R., and Manelli, H. 1979. Protein content of ribosome subunits during *Bufo bufo* development. *Acta Embryol. Exp.* **1979**:29–38.

Shalgi, R., and Sherman, M. I. 1979. Scanning electron microscopy of the surface of normal and implantation-delayed mouse blastocysts during development *in vitro*. *J. Exp. Zool.* **210**:69–80.

Shepherd, G. W., and Flickinger, R. 1979. Post-transcriptional control of mRNA diversity in frog embryos. *Biochim. Biophys. Acta* **563**:413–421.

Sherman, M. I. 1975. The culture of cells derived from mouse blastocysts. *Cell* **5**:343–349.

Sherman, M. I., and Wudl, L. R. 1976. The implanting mouse blastocyst. *In*: Poste, G., and Nicolson, G. L., eds., *The Cell Surface in Animal Embryogenesis and Development*, Amsterdam, North-Holland, pp. 81–125.

Sherman, M. I., Shalgi, R., Rizzino, A., Sellens, M. H., Gay, S., and Gay, R. 1979. Changes in the surface of the mouse blastocyst at implantation. *Ciba Found. Ser.* **64**:33–52.

Shih, R. J., Smith, L. D., and Keem, K. 1980. Rates of histone synthesis during early development of *Rana pipiens*. *Dev. Biol.* **75**:329–342.

Shiokawa, K., and Pogo, A. O. 1974. The role of cytoplasmic membranes in controlling the transport of nuclear mRNA and initiation of protein synthesis. *Proc. Natl. Acad. Sci. USA* **71**:2658–2662.

Shiokawa, K., Yasuda, Y., and Yamana, K. 1977. Transport of different RNA species from the nucleus to the cytoplasm in *Xenopus laevis* neurula cells. *Dev. Biol.* **59**:259–262.

Shiokawa, K., Misumi, Y., Yasuda, Y., Nishio, Y., Kurata, S., Sameshima, M., and Yamana, K. 1979. Synthesis and transport of various RNA species in developing embryos of *Xenopus laevis*. *Dev. Biol.* **68**:503–514.

Sierra, J. M., Meier, D., and Ochoa, J. 1974. Effect of development on the translation of messenger RNA in *Artemia salina* embryos. *Proc. Natl. Acad. Sci. USA* **71**:2693–2697.

Singh, U. N. 1968. Rate of flow of rapidly labelled RNA from nucleus to cytoplasm during embryonic development of sea urchin. *Exp. Cell Res.* **53**:537–543.

Skoultchi, A., and Gross, P. R. 1973. Maternal histone mRNA: Detection by molecular hybridization. *Proc. Natl. Acad. Sci. USA* **70**:2840–2844.

Skreb, N., Svajger, A., and Levak-Svajger, B. 1976. Developmental potentialities of the germ layers in mammals. *In*: O'Connor, M., ed., *Embryogenesis in Mammals, Ciba Found. Symp.* **40**:27–45.

Slater, D. W., Slater, I., and Gillespie, D. 1972. Postfertilization synthesis of polyadenylic acid in sea urchin embryos. *Nature (London)* **240**:333–337.

Slater, D. W., Gillespie, D., and Slater, I. 1973. Cytoplasmic adenylation and processing of maternal RNA. *Proc. Natl. Acad. Sci. USA* **70**:406–411.

Smith, L. D., and Ecker, R. E. 1970. Foundations for the expression of developmental potential. *In*: Hanley, E. W., ed., *RNA in Development*, Salt Lake City, University of Utah Press, pp. 355–379.

Snow, M. H. L. 1977. Gastrulation in the mouse: Establishment of cell populations in the epiblast of t^{w18}/t^{w18} embryos. *J. Embryol. Exp. Morphol.* **42**:293–303.

Snow, M. H. L. 1978. Proliferation centres in embryonic development. *In*: Johnson, M. H., ed., *Development in Mammals*, Amsterdam, North-Holland, Vol. 3, pp. 337–362.

Sonnenblick, B. P. 1950. The early embryology of *Drosophila melanogaster*. *In*: Demerec, M., ed., *Biology of Drosophila*, New York, Wiley, pp. 62–167.

Spemann, H., and Mangold, H. 1924. Über Induktion von Embryonalanlagen durch Implantation artfremder Organisatoren. *Wilhelm Roux Arch. Entwicklungsmech. Org.* **100**:599–638.

Spirin, A. S., and Nemer, M. 1965. Messenger RNA in early sea urchin embryos: Cytoplasmic particles. *Science* **150**:214–217.

Spratt, N. T., and Haas, H. 1962. Integrative mechanisms in development of the early chick blastoderm. *J. Exp. Zool.* **149**:75–102.

Stearns, L. W. 1974. *Sea Urchin Development: Cellular and Molecular Aspects,* Stroudsburg, Pa., Dowden, Hutchinson & Ross.

Steffenson, D. M. 1968. A reconstruction of cell development in the shoot apex of maize. *Am. J. Bot.* **55**:354–369.

Street, H. E. 1976. Experimental embryogenesis—The totipotency of cultured plant cells. *In*: Graham, C. F., and Wareing, P. F., eds., *The Developmental Biology of Plants and Animals*, Oxford, Blackwell, pp. 73–90.

Sturgess, E. A., Ballantine, J. E. M., Woodland, H. R., Mohum, P. R., Lane, C. D., and Dimitriadis, G. J. 1980. Actin synthesis during the early development of *Xenopus laevis*. *J. Embryol. Exp. Morphol.* **58**:303–320.

Sures, I. S., Maxam, A., Cohn, R. H., and Kedes, L. H. 1976. Identification and location of the histone H2A and H3 genes by sequence analysis of sea urchin *S. purpuratus* DNA cloned in *E. coli*. *Cell* **9**:495–502.

Sures, I. S., Lowry, J. C., and Kedes, L. H. 1978. The DNA sequence of sea urchin *S. purpuratus* H2A, H2B, and H3 histone coding and spacer regions. *Cell* **15**:1033–1044.

Surrey, S., and Nemer, M. 1976. Methylated blocked 5′ terminal sequences of sea urchin embryo mRNA classes containing and lacking poly(A). *Cell* **9**:589–595.

Surrey, S., Ginzburg, I., and Nemer, M. 1979. Ribosomal RNA synthesis in pre- and post-gastrula-stage sea urchin embryos. *Dev. Biol.* **71**:83–99.

Sussman, P., and Betz, T. W. 1978. Embryonic stages: Morphology, timing, and variance in the toad *Bombina orientalis*. *Can. J. Zool.* **56**:1540–1545.

Suzuki, N., and Mano, Y. 1974. Phosphorylation of deoxyribonucleosides and DNA synthesis in early cleaving embryos of the sea urchin. *J. Biochem.* **75**:1349–1362.

Takagi, N. 1974. Differentiation of X chromosomes in the early female mouse embryos. *Exp. Cell Res.* **86**:127–135.

Takagi, N., and Sasaki, M. 1975. Preferential inactivation of the paternally derived X chromosome in the extraembryonic membrane of the mouse. *Nature (London)* **256**:640–642.

Takagi, N., Wake, N., and Sasaki, M. 1978. Cytologic evidence for preferential inactivation of the paternally derived X chromosome in XX mouse blastocysts. *Cytogenet. Cell Genet.* **20**:240–248.

Tanaka, Y. 1976. Effects of the surfactants on the cleavage and further development of the sea urchin embryos. *Dev. Growth Differ.* **18**:113–122.

Thoma, F., Koller, T., and Klug, A. 1979. Involvement of histone H1 in the organization of the nucleosome and of the salt-dependent superstructures of chromatin. *J. Cell Biol.* **83**:403–427.

Thomas, C., Heilporn-Pohl, V., Hanocq, F., Pays, E., and Boloukhère, M. 1980. Changes in "template-bound" and "free" RNA polymerase activities in isolated nuclei from *Xenopus laevis* embryos. *Exp. Cell Res.* **127**:63–73.

Trinkhaus, J. P. 1965. Mechanisms of morphogenetic movements. *In: International Conference on Organogenesis,* Baltimore, Holt, Reinhart & Winston, pp. 55–104.

Turner, R. F., and Mahowald, A. P. 1976. Scanning EM of *Drosophila* embryogenesis. *Dev. Biol.* **50**:95–108.

Ubbels, G. A., and Hengst, R. T. M. 1978. A cytochemical study of the distribution of glycogen and mucosubstances in the early embryo of *Ambystoma mexicanum*. *Differentiation* **10**:109–122.

Underwood, E. M., Caulton, J. H., Allis, C. D., and Mahowald, A. P. 1980. Developmental fate of pole cells in *D. melanogaster*. *Dev. Biol.* **77**:303–314.

Van Blerkom, J., and Manes, C. 1977. The molecular biology of the preimplantation embryo. *In:* Sherman, M. I., ed., *Concepts in Mammalian Embryogenesis*, Cambridge, Mass., MIT Press, pp. 37–94.

van den Biggelaar, J. A. M., and Guerrier, P. 1979. Dorsoventral polarity and mesentoblast determination as concomitant results of cellular interactions in the mollusk *Patella vulgata*. *Dev. Biol.* **68**:462–471.

van Helden, P. D., Strickland, W. N., Brandt, W. F., and von Holt, C. 1979. The complete amino acid sequence of histone H2B from the mollusk *Patella granatina*. *Eur. J. Biochem.* **93**:71–78.

Verdonk, N. H. 1968. The relation of the two blastomeres to the polar lobe in *Dentalium*. *J. Embryol. Exp. Morphol.* **20**:101–105.

Villee, C. A., Lowens, M., Gordon, M., Leonard, E., and Rich, A. 1949. The incorporation of P[32] into the nucleoproteins and phosphoproteins of the developing sea urchin embryo. *J. Cell. Comp. Physiol.* **33**:93–112.

Vogt, W. 1929. Gestaltungsanlayse am Amphibienkeim mit örthlicker Vitalfärbung. *Wilhelm Roux Arch. Entwicklungsmech. Org.* **120**:384–706.

Waddington, C. H. 1966. Mendel and the study of development [of an embryonic cell]. *Proc. R. Soc. London Ser. B* **164**:219–229.

Wake, N., Takagi, M., and Sasaki, M. 1976. Non-random inactivation of X chromosome in the rat yolk sac. *Nature (London)* **262**:580–581.

Wallace, H. 1960. The development of anucleate embryos of *Xenopus laevis*. *J. Embryol. Exp. Morphol.* **8**:405–413.

Weinberg, E. S., Overton, G. C., Shutt, R. H., and Reeder, R. H. 1975. Histone gene arrangement in the sea urchin, *Stronglyocentrotus purpuratus*. *Proc. Natl. Acad. Sci. USA* **72**:4815–4819.

West, M. H. P., and Bonner, W. M. 1980. Histone 2A, a heteromorphous family of eight protein species. *Biochemistry* **19**:3238–3245.

Wiley, L. M., and Eglitis, M. A. 1980. Effects of colcemid on cavitation during mouse blastocoele formation. *Exp. Cell Res.* **127**:89–101.

Wilson, E. B. 1892. The cell-lineage of *Nereis*. *J. Morphol.* **6**:361–480.

Wilson, E. B. 1904a. Experimental studies on germinal localization. I. The germ-regions in the egg of *Dentalium*. *J. Exp. Zool.* **1**:1–72.

Wilson, E. B. 1904b. Experimental studies on germinal localization. II. Experiments on the cleavage-mosaic in *Patella* and *Dentalium*. *J. Exp. Zool.* **1**:197–268.

Wilson, E. B. 1929. The development of egg-fragments in annelids. *Wilhelm Roux Arch. Entwicklungsmech. Org.* **117**:179–210.

Wilt, F. H. 1973. Polyadenylation of maternal RNA of sea urchin eggs after fertilization. *Proc. Natl. Acad. Sci. USA* **70**:2345–2349.

Wintersberger, U. 1974. Absence of a low-molecular-weight DNA polymerase from nuclei of the yeast, *S. cerevisiae*. *Eur. J. Biochem.* **50**:197–202.

Wolpert, L. 1969. Positional information and the spatial pattern of cellular differentiation. *J. Theor. Biol.* **25**:1–47.

Wolpert, L., and Gustafson, T. 1961. Studies on the cellular basis of morphogenesis of the sea urchin embryo: The formation of the blastula. *Exp. Cell Res.* **25**:374–382.

Wolpert, L., and Mercer, E. H. 1963. An electron microscope study of the development of the sea urchin embryo and its radial polarity. *Exp. Cell Res.* **30**:280–300.

Woodland, H. R. 1979. The modification of stored histones H3 and H4 during the oogenesis and early development of *Xenopus laevis*. *Dev. Biol.* **68**:360–370.

Woodland, H. R., and Ballantine, J. E. M. 1981. Paternal gene expression in developing hybrid embryos of *Xenopus laevis* and *Xenopus borealis*. Personal communication.

Woodland, H. R., and Graham, C. F. 1969. RNA synthesis during early development of the mouse. *Nature (London)* **221**: 327–332.

Wu, M., Holmes, D. S., Davidson, N., Cohn, R., and Kedes, L. H. 1976. The relative positions of sea urchin histone genes on the chimeric plasmids pSp2 and pSp17 as studied by electron microscopy. *Cell* **9**:163–169.

Wudl, L., and Chapman, V. 1976. The expression of β-glucuronidase during preimplantation development of mouse embryos. *Dev. Biol.* **48**:104–109.

Yasbin, R., Sawicki, J., and MacIntyre, R. J. 1978. A developmental study of acid phosphatase-1 in *Drosophila melanogaster*. *Dev. Biol.* **63**:35–46.

Yasumasu, I. 1960. Quantitative determination of hatching enzyme activity of the sea urchin blastulae. *J. Fac. Sci. Univ. Tokyo Ser. 4* **9**:39–47.

Yasumasu, I. 1963. Inhibition of the hatching enzyme formation during embryogenesis of the sea urchin by chloramphenicol, 8-aza-guanine, and 5-bromo-uracil. *Sci. Pap. Coll. Gen. Educ. Univ. Tokyo* **13**:211–246.

Youn, B. W., and Malacinski, G. M. 1981. Axial structure development in ultraviolet-irradiated (notochord-defective) amphibian embryos. *Dev. Biol.* **83**:339–352.

Young, E. M., and Raff, R. A. 1979. Messenger RNP particles in developing sea urchin embryos. *Dev. Biol.* **72**:24–40.

Yurowitzky, Y. G., and Milman, L. S. 1972. Changes in enzyme metabolism during oocyte maturation in a teleost *Misgurnus fossilis*. *Wilhelm Roux Arch. Dev. Biol.* **171**:48–54.

Zalokar, M., and Erk, I. 1976. Division and migration of nuclei during early embryogenesis of *Drosophila melanogaster*. *J. Microsc. Biol. Cell* **25**:97–106.

Zeikus, J. G., Taylor, M. W., and Buck, C. A. 1969. Transfer RNA changes associated with early development and differentiation of the sea urchin, *Strongylocentrotus purpuratus*. *Exp. Cell Res.* **57**:74–78.

Zybina, E. V. 1961. Endomitosis and polyteny of trophoblast giant cells. *Dokl. Akad. Nauk SSSR* **140**:1177–1180 (in Russian).

Zybina, E. V. 1963. Cytophotometric determination of DNA content in nuclei of trophoblast giant cells. *Dokl. Acad. Nauk SSSR* **153**:1428–1431 (in Russian).

Zybina, E. V. 1970. Anomalies of polyploidization of the cells of the trophoblast. *Tsitologiya* **12**:1081–1091 (in Russian).

CHAPTER 4

Abelev, G. I. 1971. Alpha-fetoprotein in ontogenesis and its association with malignant tumours. *Adv. Cancer Res.* **14**:295–357.

Abraham, E. C., Cope, N. D., Braziel, N. N., and Huisman, T. H. J. 1979. On the chromatographic heterogeneity of human fetal hemoglobin. *Biochim. Biophys. Acta* **577**:159–169.

Abramovich, D. R., Baker, T. G., and Neal, P. 1974. Effect of human chorionic gonadotropin on testosterone secretion by the fetal human testes in organ culture. *J. Endocrinol.* **60**:179–185.

Ackerman, G. A. 1962. Electron microscopy of the bursa of Fabricius of the embryonic chick with particular reference to the lympho-epithelial nodules. *J. Cell Biol.* **13**:127–146.

Ackerman, G. A. 1965. The epithelial origin of the lymphocytes in the thymus of the embryonic hamster. *Anat. Rec.* **152**:35–54.

Ackerman, G. A. 1970. Structural studies of the lymphocyte and lymphocyte development. *In*: Gordon, A. S., ed., *Regulation of Hematopoiesis*, New York, Appleton–Century–Crofts, Vol. 2, pp. 1297–1337.

Ackerman, G. A., Grasso, J. A., and Knouff, R. A. 1961. Erythropoiesis in the early mammalian embryonic liver as revealed by electron microscopy. *Lab Invest.* **10**:787–796.

Adler, C. P., and Costabel, V. 1975. Cell number in human heart atrophy, hypertrophy, and under the influence of cytostatics. *Recent Adv. Stud. Card. Struct. Metab.* **6**:343–355.

Affara, N. A., Robert, B., Jacquet, M., Buckingham, M. E., and Gros, F. 1980a. Changes in gene expression during myogenic differentiation. I. Regulation of mRNA sequences expressed during myotube formation. *J. Mol. Biol.* **140**:441–458.

Affara, N. A., Daubas, P., Weydert, A., and Gros, F. 1980b. Changes in gene expression during myogenic differentiation. II. Identification of the proteins encoded by myotube-specific complementary DNA sequences. *J. Mol. Biol.* **140**:459–470.

Ahrens, P. B., Solursh, M., Reiter, R. S., and Singley, C. T. 1979. Position-related capacity for differentiation of limb mesenchyme in cell culture. *Dev. Biol.* **69**:436–450.

Aizawa, S., Mitsui, Y., Kurimoto, F., and Nomura, K. 1980. Cell surface changes accompanying aging in human diploid fibroblasts. *Exp. Cell Res.* **127**:143–157.

Allen, E. R. 1978. Development of vertebrate skeletal muscle. *Am. Zool.* **18**:101–111.

Amphlett, G. W., Syska, H., and Perry, S. V. 1976. The polymorphic forms of tropomyosin and troponin in developing rabbit skeletal muscle. *FEBS Lett.* **63**:22–25.

Amprino, R. 1965. Aspects of limb morphogenesis in the chicken. *In*: DeHaan, R. L., and Ursprung, H., eds., *Organogenesis*, New York, Holt, Rinehart & Winston, pp. 255–281.

Amsellem, J., and Nicaise, G. 1980. Ultrastructural study of muscle cells and their connections in the digestive tract. *J. Submicrosc. Cytol.* **12**:219–231.

Anderson, H., Chacko, S., Abbott, J., and Holtzer, H. 1970. The loss of phenotypic traits by differentiated cells *in vitro*. *Am. J. Pathol.* **60**:289–312.

Archer, R. K. 1970. Regulatory mechanisms in eosinophil leukocyte production, release, and distribution. *In*: Gordon, A. S., ed., *Regulation of Hematopoiesis*, New York, Appleton–Century–Crofts, Vol. 2, pp. 917–941.

Arnold, H. H., and Siddiqui, M. A. Q. 1979. Control of embryonic development: Isolation and purification of chick heart myosin light chain mRNA and quantitation with a cDNA probe. *Biochemistry* **18**:647–654.

Awai, M., Okada, S., Takebayashi, J., Kubo, T., Inoue, M., and Seno, S. 1968. Studies on the mechanism of denucleation of the erythroblast. *Acta Haematol.* **39**:193–209.

Bank, A., Rifkind, R. A., and Marks, P. A. 1970. Regulation of globin synthesis. *In*: Gordon, A. S., ed., *Regulation of Hematopoiesis*, New York, Appleton–Century–Crofts, Vol. 1, pp. 701–729.

Bantle, J. A., and Tassava, R. A. 1974. The neurotrophic influence on RNA precursor incorporation into polyribosomes of regenerating adult newt forelimbs. *J. Exp. Zool.* **189**:101–113.

Barker, J. E. 1980. Hemoglobin switching in sheep: Characteristics of BFU-E derived colonies from fetal liver. *Blood* **56**:495–500.

Barker, J. E., Pierce, J. E., and Nienhuis, A. W. 1980. Hemoglobin switching in sheep: A comparison of the erythropoietin-induced switch to HbC and the fetal to adult hemogloin switch. *Blood* **56**:488–494.

Bartelmez, S. H., Dodge, W. H., Mahmoud, A. A. F., and Bass, D. A. 1980. Stimulation of eosinophil production *in vitro* by eosinophilopoietin and spleen-cell-derived eosinophil growth-stimulating factor. *Blood* **56**:706–711.

Bast, R. E., Singer, M., and Ilan, J. 1979. Nerve-dependent changes in content of ribosomes, polysomes, and nascent peptides in newt limb regenerates. *Dev. Biol.* **70**:13–26.

Beams, H. W., and Kessel, R. G. 1966. Electron microscope and ultracentrifugation studies on the rat reticulocyte. *Am. J. Anat.* **118**:471–508.

Benoff, S., and Nadal-Ginard, B. 1980. Transient induction of poly(A)-short myosin heavy chain mRNA during terminal differentiation of L_6E_9 myoblasts. *J. Mol. Biol.* **140**:283–298.

Bernhard, W., and Granboulan, N. 1968. Electron microscopy of the nucleolus in vertebrate cells. *In*: Dalton, A. J., and Haguenau, J., eds., *Ultrastructure in Biological Systems*, New York, Academic Press, Vol. 3, pp. 81–149.

Berrill, N. J., and Karp, G. 1976. *Development*, New York, McGraw–Hill.

Bertles, J. F. 1970. The occurrence and significance of fetal hemoglobins. *In*: Gordon, A. S., ed., *Regulation of Hematopoiesis*, New York, Appleton–Century–Crofts, Vol. 1, pp. 731–765.

Bertles, J. F. 1974. Human fetal hemoglobin: Significance in disease. *Ann. N.Y. Acad. Sci.* **241**:638–652.

Bester, A. J., Kennedy, D. S., and Heywood, S. M. 1975. Two classes of translational control RNA: Their role in the regulation of protein synthesis. *Proc. Natl. Acad. Sci. USA* **72**:1523–1527.

Beug, H., and Graf, T. 1977. Isolation of clonal strains of chicken embryo fibroblasts. *Exp. Cell Res.* **107**:417–428.

Bischoff, R. 1979. Tissue culture studies on the origin of myogenic cells during muscle regeneration in the rat. *In*: Mauro, A., ed., *Muscle Regeneration*, New York, Raven Press, pp. 13–29.

Bishop, S. P., and Hine, P. 1974. Cardiac muscle cytoplasmic and nuclear changes during canine neonatal growth. *Recent Adv. Stud. Card. Struct. Metab.* **8**:77–98.

Block, E. 1967. The conversion of 7-^{3}H-pregnenolone and 4-^{14}C-progesterone to testosterone and androstenedione by mammalian fetal testes *in vitro*. *Steroids* **9**:415–430.

Bornstein, P., Ehrlich, H. P., and Wyke, A. W. 1972. Procollagen: Conversion of the precursor to collagen by a neutral protease. *Science* **175**:544–546.

Boström, S. L., and Johansson, G. 1972. Enzyme activity patterns in white and red muscle of the eel (*Anguilla anguilla*) at different developmental stages. *Comp. Biochem. Physiol.* **42B**:533–542.

Bragg, P. W., Dym, H. P., and Heywood, S. M. 1980. Embryonic chick myosin heavy chain mRNA is poly(A)$^+$. *FEBS Lett.* **113**:177–182.

Brinkmann, A. O. 1977. Testosterone synthesis *in vitro* by the fetal testis of the guinea pig. *Steroids* **29**:861–873.

Brodsky, W. Y., Arefyeva, A. M., and Uryvaeva, I. V. 1980. Mitotic polyploidization of mouse heart myocytes during the first postnatal week. *Cell Tissue Res.* **210**:133–144.

Broyles, R. H., Johnson, G. M., Maples, P. B., and Kindell, G. R. 1981. Two erythropoietic microenvironments and two larval red cell lines in bullfrog tadpoles. *Dev. Biol.* **81**:299–314.

Brunst, V. V. 1950. Influence of X-rays on limb regeneration in urodele amphibians. *Q. Rev. Biol.* **25**:1–29.

Bryant, S. V., French, V., and Bryant, P. J. 1981. Distal regeneration and symmetry. *Science* **212**:993–1002.

Bucher, N. L. R. 1963. Regeneration of mammalian liver. *Int. Rev. Cytol.* **15**:245–300.

Buckingham, M. E., Caput, D., Cohen, A., Whalen, R. G., and Gros, F. 1974. The synthesis and stability of cytoplasmic mRNA during myoblast differentiation in culture. *Proc. Natl. Acad. Sci. USA* **71**:1466–1470.

Buhl, A. E., Pasztor, L. M., and Resko, J. A. 1979. Sex steroids in guinea pig fetuses after sexual differentiation of the gonads. *Biol. Reprod.* **21**:905–908.

Bühler, R. H. O., and Kägi, J. H. R. 1974. Human hepatic metallothioneins. *FEBS Lett.* **39**:229–234.

Bunn, H. F., Gabbay, K. H., and Gallop, P. M. 1978. The glycosylation of hemoglobin: Relevance to diabetes mellitus. *Science* **200**:21–27.

Burnstock, G. 1970. Structure of smooth muscle and its innervation. *In*: Bülbring, E., Brading, A. F., Jones, A. W., and Tomita, T., eds., *Smooth Muscle*, Baltimore, Williams & Wilkins, pp. 1–69.

Butler, E. G. 1933. The effects of X-irradiation on limb regeneration of the fore limb of *Amblystoma* larvae. *J. Exp. Zool.* **65**:271–316.

Cagnioni, M., Fantini, F., Morace, G., and Ghetti, A. 1965. Failure of testosterone propionate to induce the early-androgen syndrome in rats previously injected with progesterone. *J. Endocrinol.* **33**:527–528.

Caplan, A. I., Niedergang, C., Okazaki, H., and Mandel, P. 1979. Poly(ADP ribose) levels as a function of chick limb mesenchymal cell development as studied *in vitro* and *in vivo*. *Dev. Biol.* **72**:102–109.

Capone, R. J., Weinreb, E. L., and Chapman, G. B. 1964. Electron microscope studies on normal human myeloid elements. *Blood* **23**:300–320.

Cardenas, J. M., Bandman, E., and Strohman, R. C. 1978. Hybrid isozymes of pyruvate kinase appear during avian cardiac development. *Biochem. Biophys. Res. Commun.* **80**:593–599.

Carlson, B. M. 1968. Regeneration of the completely excised gastrocnemius muscle in the frog and rat from minced muscle fragments. *J. Morphol.* **125**:447–472.

Carlson, B. M. 1978. Types of morphogenetic phenomena in vertebrate regenerating systems. *Am. Zool.* **18**:869–882.

Carlsson, R. N. K., and Ingvarsson, B. I. 1979. Localization of α-fetoprotein and albumin in pig liver during fetal and neonatal development. *Dev. Biol.* **73**:1–10.

Carpenter, K. L., and Turpen, J. B. 1979. Experimental studies on hematopoiesis in the pronephros of *Rana pipiens*. *Differentiation* **14**:167–174.

Castro-Malaspina, H., Gay, R. E., Resnick, G., Kapoor, N., Meyers, P., Chiarieri, D., McKenzie, S., Broxmeyer, H. E., and Moore, M. A. S. 1980. Characterization of human bone marrow fibroblast colony-forming cells (CFU-F) and their progeny. *Blood* **56**:289–301.

Ceico, A. 1964. Electron microscopic observations of young rat liver. *Z. Zellforsch. Mikrosk. Anat.* **62**:717–742.

Chacko, S. 1979. Cardiac muscle differentiation and growth in developing chick embryos. *In*: Mauro, A., ed., *Muscle Regeneration*, New York, Raven Press, pp. 363–381.

Chedid, A., and Nair, V. 1974. Ontogenesis of cytoplasmic organelles in rat hepatocytes and the effects of prenatal phenobarbital on endoplasmic reticulum development. *Dev. Biol.* **39**:49–62.

Chi, J. C., Fellini, S. A., and Holtzer, H. 1975. Differences among myosins synthesized in nonmyogenic cells, presumptive myoblasts, and myoblasts. *Proc. Natl. Acad. Sci. USA* **72**:4999–5003.

Clements, J. A., Reyes, F. I., Winters, J. S. D., and Faiman, C. 1976. Studies on human sexual development. III. Fetal pituitary and serum and amniotic fluid concentrations of LH, CG, and FSH. *J. Clin. Endocrinol. Metab.* **42**:9–19.

Colbert, D. A., Tedeschi, M. V., Atryzek, V., and Fausto, N. 1977. Diversity of poly(A) mRNA sequences in normal and 12-hr regenerating liver. *Dev. Biol.* **59**:111–123.

Cole, R. J., Regan, T., White, S. L., and Cheek, E. M. 1975. The relationship between erythropoietin-dependent cellular differentiation and colony-forming ability in prenatal haemopoietic tissue. *J. Embryol. Exp. Morphol.* **34**:575–588.

Colonno, R. J. 1981. Accumulation of newly synthesized mRNAs in response to human fibroblast (β) interferon. *Proc. Natl. Acad. Sci. USA* **78**:4763–4766.

Comings, D. E. 1966. The inactive X-chromosome. *Lancet* **1966**(2):1137–1138.

Conrad, G. W., Hart, G. W., and Chen, Y. 1977a. Differences *in vitro* between fibroblast-like cells from cornea, heart, and skin of embryonic chicks. *J. Cell Sci.* **26**:119–137.

Conrad, G. W., Hamilton, C., and Haynes, E. 1977b. Differences in glycosaminoglycans synthesized by fibroblast-like cells from chick cornea, heart, and skin. *J. Biol. Chem.* **252**:6861–6870.

Craig, M. L., and Russell, E. S. 1964. A development change in haemoglobins correlated with an embryonic red cell population in the mouse. *Dev. Biol.* **10**:191–201.

Cunha, G. R. 1975. Age-dependent loss of sensitivity of female urogenital sinus to androgenic conditions as a function of the epithelial–stromal interaction in mice. *Endocrinology* **97**:665–673.

Cutts, J. H., Krause, W. J., and Leeson, C. R. 1980. Changes in the erythrocytes of the developing opossum, *Didelphis virginiana*. *Blood Cells* **6**:55–62.

Dallner, G., Siekovitz, P., and Palade, G. E. 1965. Synthesis of microsomal membranes and their enzymic constituents in developing rat liver. *Biochem. Biophys. Res. Commun.* **20**:135–141.

Dallner, G., Siekovitz, P., and Palade, G. E. 1966a. Biogenesis of endoplasmic reticulum membranes. I. Structural and chemical differentiation in developing rat hepatocytes. *J. Cell Biol.* **30**:73–96.

Dallner, G., Siekovitz, P., and Palade, G. E. 1966b. Biogenesis of endoplasmic reticulum membranes. II. Synthesis of constitutive microsomal enzymes in developing rat hepatocytes. *J. Cell Biol.* **30**:97–117.

Dearlove, G. E., and Stocum, D. L. 1974. Denervation-induced changes in soluble protein content during forelimb regeneration in adult newt, *Notophthalmus viridescens*. *J. Exp. Zool.* **190**:317–327.

de la Chapelle, A., Fantoni, A., and Marks, P. A. 1969. Differentiation of mammalian somatic cells: DNA synthesis and haemoglobin synthesis in foetal mice. *Proc. Natl. Acad. Sci. USA* **63**:812–819.

DeLuca, S., Heinegård, D., Hascall, V. C., Kimura, J. H., and Caplan, A. I. 1977. Chemical and physical changes in proteoglycans during development of chick limb bud chondrocytes grown *in vitro*. *J. Biol. Chem.* **252**:6600–6608.

Dessau, W., von der Mark, H., von der Mark, K., and Fischer, S. 1980. Changes in the patterns of collagens and fibronectin during limb-bud chondrogenesis. *J. Embryol. Exp. Morphol.* **57**:51–60.

Detwiler, S. R., and van Dyke, R. H. 1934. The development and functions of dedifferentiated fore limbs in *Amblystoma*. *J. Exp. Zool.* **68**:321–346.

Devlin, R. B., and Emerson, C. P. 1978. Coordinate regulation of contractile protein synthesis during myoblast differentiation. *Cell* **13**:599–611.

Devlin, R. B., and Emerson, C. P. 1979. Coordinate accumulation of contractile protein mRNAs during myoblast differentiation. *Dev. Biol.* **69**:202–216.

Dhoot, G. K., and Perry, S. V. 1979. Distribution of polymorphic forms of troponin components and tropomyosin in skeletal muscle. *Nature (London)* **278**:714–716.

Dillon, L. S. 1981. *Ultrastructure, Macromolecules, and Evolution*, New York, Plenum Press.

Dinsmore, C. E. 1974. Morphogenetic interactions between minced limb muscle and transplanted blastemas in the axolotl. *J. Exp. Zool.* **187**:223–232.

DiPersio, J. F., Brennan, J. K., and Lichtman, M. A. 1978. Granulocyte growth modulators elaborated by human cell lines. *ICN–UCLA Symp. Mol. Cell. Biol.* **10**:433–444.

Doetschman, T. C., Dym, H. P., Siegel, E. J., and Heywood, S. M. 1980. Myoblast stored myosin heavy chain transcripts are precursors to the myotube polysomal myosin heavy chain mRNAs. *Differentiation* **16**:149–162.

Dover, G. J., and Boyer, S. H. 1981. Quantitation of hemoglobins within individual red cells: Asynchronous biosynthesis of fetal and adult hemoglobin during erythroid maturation in normal subjects. *Blood* **56**:1082–1091.

Dresden, M. H. 1969. Denervation effects on newt limb regeneration: DNA, RNA, and protein synthesis. *Dev. Biol.* **19**:311–320.

Dresler, S. L., Runkel, D., Stenzel, P., Brimhall, B., and Jones, R. T. 1974. Multiplicity of the hemoglobin α chains in dogs and variations among related species. *Ann. N.Y. Acad. Sci.* **241**:411–415.

Drews, U., Kocher-Becker, U., and Drews, U. 1972. The induction of visceral cartilage from cranial neural crest by pharyngeal endoderm in hanging drop cultures and the locomotory behavior of the neural crest cells during cartilage differentiation. *Wilhelm Roux Arch. Dev. Biol.* **171**:17–37.

Durante, M. 1956. Cholinesterase in the development of *Ciona intestinalis* (Ascidia). *Experientia* **12**:307–308.

Dyche, W. J. 1979. A comparative study of the differentiation and involution of the Mullerian duct and Wolffian duct in the male and female fetal mouse. *J. Morphol.* **162**:175–210.

Ebbe, S. 1970. Megakaryocytopoiesis. *In*: Gordon, A. S., ed., *Regulation of Hematopoiesis*, New York, Appleton–Century–Crofts, Vol. 2, pp. 1587–1610.

Edgerton, V. R. 1978. Mammalian muscle fiber types and their adaptability. *Am. Zool.* **18**:113–125.

Elgin, S. C. R., and Weintraub, H. 1975. Chromosomal proteins and chromatin structure. *Annu. Rev. Biochem.* **44**:725–774.

Elias, H. 1955. Origin and early development of the liver in various vertebrates. *Acta Hepatol.* **3**:1–56.

Emerson, C. P. 1977. Control of myosin synthesis during myoblast differentiation. *In: Pathogenesis of Human Muscular Dystrophies*, Proc. 5th Int. Conf. Musc. Dyst. Assoc., Durango, Colorado, 1976, pp. 799–809.

Emerson, C. P., and Beckner, S. K. 1975. Activation of myosin synthesis in fusing and mononucleated myoblasts. *J. Mol. Biol.* **93**:431–447.

Eppenberger, H. M., Eppenberger, M., Richterich, R., and Aebi, H. 1964. The ontogeny of creatine kinase isozymes. *Dev. Biol.* **10**:1–16.

Epperlein, H. H. 1974. The ectomesenchymal–endodermal interaction system (EEIS) of *Triturus alpestris* in tissue culture. I. Observations on attachment, migration, and differentiation of neural crest cells. *Differentiation* **2**:151–168.

Epperlein, H. H., and Lehmann, R. 1975. Ectomesenchymal–endodermal interaction system of *Triturus alpestris* in tissue culture. 2. Observations on differentiation of visceral cartilage. *Differentiation* **4**:159–174.

Erslev, A. J., Kansu, E., and Caro, J. 1978. The biogenesis and metabolism of erythropoietin. *ICN–UCLA Symp. Mol. Cell. Biol.* **10**:1–14.

Erslev, A. J., Caro, J., Kansu, E., and Silver, R. 1980. Renal and extrarenal erythropoietin production in anaemic rats. *Br. J. Haematol.* **45**:65–72.

Fantoni, A., de la Chapelle, A., Chui, D., Rifkind, R. A., and Marks, P. A. 1969. Control mechanism of the conversion from synthesis of embryonic to adult haemoglobin. *Ann. N.Y. Acad. Sci.* **165**:194–204.

Filburn, C. R. 1969. Changes in acid phosphatase isozymes during *Xenopus* tail resorption. *Am. Zool.* **9**:1128–1129.

Filburn, C. R. 1973. Acid phosphatase isozymes of *Xenopus laevis* tadpole tails. I. Separation and partial characterization. *Arch. Biochem. Biophys.* **159**:683–693.

Filburn, C. R., and Vanable, J. W. 1973. Acid phosphatase isozymes of *Xenopus laevis* tadpole tails. II. Changes in activity during tail regression. *Arch. Biochem. Biophys.* **159**:694–703.

Finch, R. A. 1969. The influence of the nerve on lower jaw regeneration in the adult newt (*Triturus viridescens*). *J. Morphol.* **129**:401–414.

Flavin, M., Duprat, A. M., and Rosa, J. 1979. Ontogenic changes in the haemoglobins of the salamander, *Pleurodeles waltlii*. *Cell Differ.* **8**:405–410.

Ford, C. E., Hamerton, J. L., Barnes, D. W. H., and Loutit, J. F. 1956. Cytological identification of radiation-chimaeras. *Nature (London)* **177**:452–454.

Forsberg, J. G. 1973. Cervicovaginal epithelium: Its origin and development. *Am. J. Obstet. Gynecol.* **115**:1025–1043.

Forsyth, J. 1946. The histology of anuran limb regeneration. *J. Morphol.* **79**:287–317.

Frank, G., and Weeds, A. G. 1974. The amino acid sequence of the alkali light chains of rabbit skeletal-muscle myosin. *Eur. J. Biochem.* **44**:317–334.

Friar, P. M., Strasberg, P. M., Freeman, K. B., and Peterson, A. C. 1979. Mitochondrial malic enzyme in mosaic skeletal muscle of mouse chimeras. *Biochem. Genet.* **17**:693–713.

Fritz, P. J., White, E. L., and Pruitt, K. M. 1975. Intracellular turnover of lactate dehydrogenase isozymes. *In*: Market, C. L., ed., *Isozymes*, New York, Academic Press, Vol. 3, pp. 347–358.

Gabbiani, G., Schmid, E., Winter, S., Chaponnier, C., de Chastonay, C., Vanderkerckhove, J., Weber, K., and Franke, W. W. 1981. Vascular smooth muscle cells differ from other smooth muscle cells: Predominance of vimentin filaments and a specific α-type actin. *Proc. Natl. Acad. Sci. USA* **78**:298–302.

Galli, F. E., and Wasserman, G. F. 1973. Steroid synthesis by gonads of 7- and 10-day-old chick embryos. *Gen. Comp. Endocrinol.* **21**:77–83.

García, A. M. 1964. Feulgen-DNA values in megakaryocytes. *J. Cell Biol.* **20**:342–345.

Garrett, D. M., and Conrad, G. W. 1979. Fibroblast-like cells from embryonic chick corena, heart, and skin are antigenically distinct. *Dev. Biol.* **70**:50–70.

Gartner, T. K., and Podleski, T. R. 1975. Evidence that a membrane bound lectin mediates fusion of L₆ myoblasts. *Biochem. Biophys. Res. Commun.* **67**:972–978.

Gartner, T. K., and Podleski, T. R. 1976. Evidence that the type and specific activity of lectins control fusion of L₆ myoblasts. *Biochem. Biophys. Res. Commun.* **70**:1142–1149.

Geiduschek, J. B., and Singer, S. J. 1979. Molecular changes in the membranes of mouse erythroid cells accompanying differentiation. *Cell* **16**:149–163.

Gelfand, E. W., Dosch, H. M., and Shore, A. 1978. The role of the thymus and thymus microenvironment in T-cell differentiation. *ICN–UCLA Symp. Mol. Cell. Biol.* **10**:277–293.

Gitlin, D. 1975. Normal biology of α-fetoprotein. *Ann. N.Y. Acad. Sci.* **259**:7–16.

Glücksmann, A. 1951. Cell death in normal vertebrate ontogeny. *Biol. Rev.* **26**:59–86.

Goldsmith, P. K. 1981. Postnatal development of some membrane-bound enzymes of rat liver and kidney. *Biochim. Biophys. Acta* **672**:45–56.

Goldstein, M. A., Claycomb, W. C., and Schwartz, A. 1973. DNA synthesis and mitosis in well-differentiated mammalian cardiocytes. *Science* **183**:212–213.

Goldstein, M. A., Schroeter, J. P., and Sass, R. L. 1979. The Z lattice in canine cardiac muscle. *J. Cell Biol.* **83**:187–204.

Goldstein, M. A., Stromer, M. H., Schroeter, J. P., and Sass, R. L. 1980. Optical reconstruction of nemaline rods. *Exp. Neurol.* **70**:83–97.

Goldwasser, E., and Inana, G. 1978. Molecular aspects of the initiation of erythropoiesis. *ICN–UCLA Symp. Mol. Cell. Biol.* **10**:15–35.

Goode, D. 1975. Mitosis of embryonic heart muscle cells *in vitro. Cytobiologie Z. Exp. Zellforsch.* **11**:203–229.

Gordon, A. S., and Zanjani, E. D. 1970. Some aspects of erythropoietin physiology. *In:* Gordon, A. S., ed., *Regulation of Hematopoiesis*, New York, Appleton–Century–Crofts, Vol. 1, pp. 413–457.

Gorin, M. B., Cooper, D. L., Eiferman, F., van de Rijn, P., and Tilghman, S. M. 1981. The evolution of α-fetoprotein and albumin. I. A comparison of the primary amino acid sequences of mammalian α-fetoprotein and albumin. *J. Biol. Chem.* **256**:1954–1959.

Goy, R. W., Bridson, W. E., and Young, W. C. 1964. Period of maximum susceptibility of the prenatal female guinea pig to masculinizing actions of testosterone propionate. *J. Comp. Physiol. Psychol.* **57**:166–174.

Gratzer, W. B., and Allison, A. C. 1960. Multiple haemoglobins. *Biol. Rev.* **35**:459–506.

Grim, M., and Carlson, B. M. 1979. The formation of muscles in regenerating limbs of the newt after denervation of the blastema. *J. Embryol. Exp. Morphol.* **54**:99–111.

Grobstein, C. 1955. Tissue disaggregation in relation to determination and stability of cell type. *Ann. N.Y. Acad. Sci.* **60**:1095–1106.

Groenendijk-Huijbers, M. M. 1962. The cranio-caudal regression of the right Müllerian duct in the chick embryo as studied by castration experiments and estrogen treatment. *Anat. Rec.* **142**:9–20.

Gross, J., and Kirk, D. 1958. The heat precipitation of collagen from neutral salt solutions. *J. Biol. Chem.* **233**:355–360.

Gross, S. R., and Bromwell, K. 1977. Postnatal development of phosphorylase kinase in mouse skeletal muscle. *Arch. Biochem. Biophys.* **184**:1–11.

Grüneberg, H. 1963. *The Pathology of Development: A Study of Inherited Skeletal Disorders in Animals*, New York, Wiley.

Gudernatsch, J. F. 1912. *Wilhelm Roux Arch. Entwicklungsmech. Org.* **35**:457–483.

Guichard, A., Cedard, L., and Haffen, K. 1973. Aspect comparatif de la synthèse de steroides sefuels par les gonades embryonnaires de poulet à differents stades du développement: L'étude en culture organotypique à partir de précurseurs radioactifs. *Gen. Comp. Endocrinol.* **20**:16–28.

Haffen, K. 1975. Sex differentiation of avian gonads *in vitro. Am. Zool.* **15**:257–272.

Hågå, P., and Kristiansen, S. 1981. Role of the kidney in foetal erythropoiesis: Erythropoiesis and erythropoietin levels in newborn mice with renal agenesis. *J. Embryol. Exp. Morphol.* **61**:165–173.

Hall, B. K., and Tremaine, R. 1979. Ability of neural crest cells from the embryonic chick to differentiate into cartilage before their migration away from the neural tube. *Anat. Rec.* **194**:469–476.

Hamburger, V. 1938. Morphogenetic and axial self-differentiation of transplanted limb primordia of 2-day chick embryos. *J. Exp. Zool.* **77**:379–399.

Hamburger, V. 1939. The development and innervation of transplanted limb primordia of chick embryos. *J. Exp. Zool.* **80**:347–390.

Hamburger, V., and Hamilton, H. L. 1951. A series of normal stages in the development of the chick embryo. *J. Morphol.* **88**:49–92.

Hamerman, D., Todaro, G. J., and Green, H. 1965. The production of hyaluronate by spontaneously established cell lines and viral transformed lines of fibroblastic origin. *Biochim. Biophys. Acta* **101**:343–351.

Hamilton, H. L. 1952. *Lillie's Development of the Chick*, New York, Holt.

Hamilton, T. H. 1961. Studies on the physiology of urogenital differentiation in the chick embryo. *J. Exp. Zool.* **146**:265–274.

Hampé, A. 1960. Sur l'induction et la compétance dans les relations entre l'épiblaste et le mésenchyme de la patte de poulet. *J. Embryol. Exp. Morphol.* **8**:246–250.

Hannah, R., Simkins, R., and Eisen, H. J. 1980. Synthesis of α-fetoprotein and albumin by fetal mouse liver cultured in chemically defined medium. *Dev. Biol.* **77**:244–252.

Hardingham, T. E., Fitton-Jackson, S., and Muir, H. 1972. Replacement of proteoglycans in embryonic chick cartilage in organ culture after treatment with testicular hyaluronidase. *Biochem. J.* **129**:101–112.

Harkins, R. N., Black J. A., and Rittenberg, M. B. 1977. M_2 isozyme of pyruvate kinase from human kidney as the product of a separate gene. *Biochemistry* **16**:3831–3837.

Harris, M., ed. 1974. *Poly(ADP-ribose): An International Symposium*, U.S. Department of Health, Education and Welfare, Publication 74-477.

Harrison, R. G. 1904. An experimental study of the relation of the nervous system to the developing musculature in the embryo of the frog. *Am. J. Anat.* **3**:197–220.

Harrison, R. G. 1907. Experiments in transplanting limbs and their bearing upon the problems of the development of nerves. *J. Exp. Zool.* **4**:239–281.

Harrison, R. G. 1921. On relations of symmetry in transplanted limbs. *J. Exp. Zool.* **32**:1–136.

Hascall, V. C., and Heinegård, D. 1974. Aggregation of cartilage proteoglycans. *J. Biol. Chem.* **249**:4232–4241.

Hay, D. A., and Low, F. N. 1972. The fine structure of progressive stages of myocardial mitosis in chick embryos. *Am. J. Anat.* **134**:175–202.

Hay, E. D. 1958. The fine structure of blastema cells and differentiating cartilage cells in regenerating limbs of *Amblystoma* larvae. *J. Biophys. Biochem. Cytol.* **4**:583–591.

Hay, E. D. 1959. Electron microscopic observations of muscle dedifferentiation in regenerating *Amblysoma* limbs. *Dev. Biol.* **1**:555–585.

Hay, E. D., and Fischman, D. A. 1961. Origin of the blastema in regenerating limbs of the newt *Triturus viridescens*. *Dev. Biol.* **3**:26–59.

Hayashi, J., Ishimoda, T., and Hirabayashi, T. 1977. On the heterogeneity and organ specificity of chicken tropomyosins. *J. Biochem.* **81**:1487–1495.

Hessler, A. C., and Landesman, R. 1981. An investigation of the prolactin–thyroxine synergism in newt limb regeneration. *J. Morphol.* **167**:103–108.

Heywood, S. M., and Kennedy, D. S. 1976. Purification of myosin translational control RNA and its interaction with myosin mRNA. *Biochemistry* **15**:3314–3319.

Hirai, K. I., Nagata, K., Maeda, M., and Ichikawa, Y. 1979. Changes in ultrastructure and enzyme activities during differentiation of myeloid leukemia cells to normal macrophages. *Exp. Cell Res.* **124**:269–283.

Hirakow, R., and Krause, W. J. 1980. Postnatal differentiation of ventricular myocardial cells of the opossum (*Didelphis virginiana* Kerr) and T-tubule formation. *Cell Tissue Res.* **210**:95–100.

Hirsch, F. W., Nall, K. N., Busch, F. N., Morris, H. P., and Busch, H. 1978a. Comparison of abundant cytosol proteins in rat liver, Novikoff hepatoma, and Morris hepatoma by two-dimensional gel electrophoresis. *Cancer Res.* **38**:1514–1522.

Hirsch, F. W., Nall, K. N., Spohn, W. H., and Busch, H. 1978b. Enrichment of special Novikoff hepatoma and regenerating liver mRNA by hybridization to cDNA cellulose. *Proc. Natl. Acad. Sci. USA* **75**:1736–1739.

Hodgson, G. S. 1967. Effect of vinblastine and 4-amino-N^{10}-methyl-pteroylglutamic acid on the erythropoietin responsive cell. *Proc. Soc. Exp. Biol. Med.* **125**:1206–1209.

Hodgson, G. S. 1970. Mechanism of action of erythropoietin. *In*: Gordon, A. S., ed., *Regulation of Hematopoiesis*, New York, Appleton–Century–Crofts, Vol. 1, pp. 459–469.

Hoh, J. F. Y. 1979. Developmental changes in chicken skeletal myosin isoenzymes. *FEBS Lett.* **98**:267–270.

Hoh, J. F. Y., and Yeoh, G. P. S. 1979. Rabbit skeletal myosin isoenzymes from fetal, fast-twitch and slow-twitch muscles. *Nature* (*London*) **280**:321–323.

Hoh, J. F. Y., McGrath, P. A., and White, R. I. 1976. Electrophoretic analysis of multiple forms of myosin in fast-twitch and slow-twitch muscles of the chick. *Biochem. J.* **157**:87–95.

Holder, N. 1978. The onset of osteogenesis in the developing chick limb. *J. Embryol. Exp. Morphol.* **44**:15–29.

Holder, N., Tank, P. W., and Bryant, S. V. 1980. Regeneration of symmetrical forelimbs in the axolotl, *Ambystoma mexicanum*. *Dev. Biol.* **74**:302–314.

Hollyday, M., and Hamburger, V. 1976. Reduction of naturally occurring motor neuron loss by enlargement of the periphery. *J. Comp. Neurol.* **170**:311–320.

Hollyday, M., and Mendell, L. 1976. Analysis of moving supernumerary limbs of *Xenopus laevis*. *Exp. Neurol.* **51**:316–329.

Holmes, L. B., and Trelstad, R. L. 1977. Patterns of cell polarity in the developing mouse limb. *Dev. Biol.* **59**:164–173.

Holmes, L. B., and Trelstad, R. L. 1980. Cell polarity in precartilage mouse limb mesenchyme cells. *Dev. Biol.* **78**:511–520.

Holtfreter, J. 1968. Mesenchyme and epithelia in inductive and morphogenetic processes. *In*: Fleischmajer, R., ed., *Epithelial–Mesenchymal Interactions*, Baltimore, Williams & Wilkins, pp. 1–30.

Holtzer, H., Abbott, J., Lash, H., and Holtzer, S. 1960. The loss of phenotypic traits by differentiated cells *in vitro*. I. Dedifferentiation of cartilage cells. *Proc. Natl. Acad. Sci. USA* **46**:1533–1542.

Holtzer, H., Croop, J., Dienstman, S., Ishikawa, H., and Somlyo, A. P. 1975. Effects of cytochalasin B and colcemide on myogenic cultures. *Proc. Natl. Acad. Sci. USA* **72**:513–517.

Horn, E. C. 1942. An analysis of neutron and X-ray effects on regeneration of the forelimb of larval *Amblystoma*. *J. Morphol.* **71**:185–219.

Hörstadius, S. 1950. *The Neural Crest: Its Properties and Derivatives in Light of Experimental Research*, London, Oxford University Press.

Hostetler, J. R., and Ackerman, G. A. 1966. The relationship between the histological localization of alkaline phosphatase activity and appearance of lymphocytes in lymphocytic tissue of the embryonic and neonatal rabbit. *Anat. Rec.* **156**:191–214.

Hsu, L., Trupin, G. L., and Roisen, F. J. 1979. The role of satellite cells and myonuclei during myogenesis *in vitro*. *In*: Mauro, A., ed., *Muscle Regeneration*, New York, Raven Press, pp. 115–120.

Hsu, T. C. 1962. Differential rate in RNA synthesis between euchromatin and heterochromatin. *Exp. Cell Res.* **27**:332–334.

Hudson, G. 1960. Eosinophil populations in blood and bone marrow of normal pigs. *Am. J. Physiol.* **198**:1171–1173.

Huehns, E. R., Flynn, F. V., Butler, E. A., and Beaven, G. H. 1961. Two new haemoglobin variants in a very young human embryo. *Nature (London)* **189**:496–497.

Huhtaniemi, I. T., Korenbrot, C. C., and Jaffe, R. B. 1977. HCG binding and stimulation of testosterone biosynthesis in the human fetal testes. *J. Clin. Endocrinol. Metab.* **44**:963–967.

Hurle, J. M., and Lafarga, M. 1978. Cytokinesis in developing cardiac muscle cells: An ultrastructural study in the chick embryo. *Rev. Biol. Cell.* **33**:195–198.

Hurle, J. M., and Ojeda, J. L. 1979. Cell death during the development of the truncus and conus of the chick embryo heart. *J. Anat.* **129**:427–439.

Hurle, J. M., Lafarga, M., and Ojeda, J. L. 1977. Cytological and cytochemical studies of the necrotic area of the bulbus of the chick embryo heart: Phagocytosis by developing myocardial cells. *J. Embryol. Exp. Morphol.* **41**:161–170.

Hurle, J. M., Lafarga, M., and Ojeda, J. L. 1978. *In vivo* phagocytosis by developing myocardial cells: An ultrastructural study. *J. Cell Sci.* **33**:363–369.

Hynes, R. O. 1976. Cell surface proteins and malignant transformation. *Biochim. Biophys. Acta* **458**:73–107.

Ibsen, K. H., Murray, L., and Marles, S. W. 1976. Electrofocusing and kinetic studies of adult and embryonic chicken pyruvate kinases. *Biochemistry* **15**:1064–1073.

Innis, M. A., and Miller, D. L. 1977. A quantitation of rat α-fetoprotein mRNA with a complementary DNA probe. *J. Biol. Chem.* **252**:8469–8475.

Innis, M. A., and Miller, D. L. 1980. α-Fetoprotein gene expression. *J. Biol. Chem.* **255**:8994–8996.

Iscove, N. N. 1978. Erythropoietin-independent stimulation of early erythropoiesis in adult marrow cultures by conditioned media from lectin-stimulated mouse spleen cells. *ICN–UCLA Symp. Mol. Cell. Biol.* **10**:37–52.

Javois, L. C., and Iten, L. E. 1981. Position of origin of donor posterior chick wing bud tissue transplanted to an anterior host site determines the extra structures formed. *Dev. Biol.* **82**:329–342.

Javois, L. C., Iten, L. E., and Murphy, D. J. 1981. Formation of supernumerary structures by the embryonic chick wing depends on the position and orientation of a graft in a host limb bud. *Dev. Biol.* **82**:343–349.

Johnson, M. A., Mastaglia, F. L., Montgomery, A. G., Pope, B., and Weeds, A. G. 1980. Changes in myosin light chains in the rat soleus after thyroidectomy. *FEBS Lett.* **110**:230–235.

Johnston, I. A., Ward, P. S., and Goldspink, G. 1975. Studies on the swimming musculature of the rainbow trout. I. Fibre types. *J. Fish Biol.* **7**:451–458.

Johnston, M. C. 1966. A radioautographic study of the migration and fate of cranial neural crest cells in the chick embryo. *Anat. Rec.* **156**:143–156.

Jones, C. L. 1979. The morphogenesis of the thigh of the mouse with special reference to tetrapod muscle homologies. *J. Morphol.* **162**:275–310.

Jost, A. 1947. Expériences de décapitation de l'embryon de lapin. *C. R. Acad. Sci.* **225**:322–324.

Jost, A. 1970. Hormonal factors in the sex differentiation of the mammalian foetus. *Philos. Trans. R. Soc. London Ser. B* **259**:119–131.

Jost, A., Vigier, B., Prépin, J., and Perchellet, J. P. 1973. Studies on sex differentiation in mammals. *Recent Prog. Horm. Res.* **29**:1–35.

Jurand, A. 1965. Ultrastructural aspects of early development of the forelimb buds in the chick and mouse. *Proc. R. Soc. London Ser. B* **162**:387–405.

Just, J. J., Schwager, J., Weber, R., Fey, H., and Pfister, H. 1980. Immunological analysis of hemoglobin transition during metamorphosis of normal and isogenic *Xenopus*. *Wilhelm Roux Arch. Dev. Biol.* **188**:75–80.

Kabat, D. 1974. The switch from fetal to adult hemoglobin in humans: Evidence suggesting a role for γ–β gene linkage. *Ann. N.Y. Acad. Sci.* **241**:119–131.

Karasawa, K., Kimata, K., Ito, K., Kato, Y., and Suzuki, S. 1979. Morphological and biochemical differentiation of limb bud cells cultured in chemically defined medium. *Dev. Biol.* **70**:287–305.

Karlsson, B. W. 1970. Fetoprotein and albumen levels in the blood serum of developing neonatal pigs. *Biol. Neonate* **34**:259–268.

Karrer, H. E., and Cox, J. 1960. EM observations on developing chick embryo liver: Golgi complex and its possible role in the formation of glycogen. *J. Ultrastruct. Res.* **4**:149–165.

Karrer, H. E., and Cox, J. 1961. EM observations on chick embryo liver: Glycogen, bile canaliculi, inclusion bodies and hematopoiesis. *J. Ultrastruct. Res.* **5**:116–141.

Kawai, N., Nishiyama, F., and Hirano, H. 1979. Changes of lectin-binding sites on the embryonic muscle cell surface in the developing ascidian, *Halocynthia aurantium*. *Exp. Cell Res.* **122**:293–304.

Keller, L. R., and Emerson, C. P. 1980. Synthesis of adult myosin light chains by embryonic muscle culture. *Proc. Natl. Acad. Sci. USA* **77**:1020–1024.

Keller, R. H., Calvanico, N. J., and Tomasi, T. B. 1976. Immunosuppressive properties of AFP: Role of estrogens. *In*: Fishman, W. H., and Sell, S., eds. *Onco Developmental Gene Expression*, New York, Academic Press, pp. 287–295.

Kelly, A. M., and Chacko, S. 1976. Myofibril organization and mitosis in cultured cardiac muscle cells. *Dev. Biol.* **48**:421–430.

Kennedy, D. S., Siegel, E., and Heywood, S. M. 1978. Purification of myosin mRNP translational control RNA and its inhibition of myosin and globin messenger translation. *FEBS Lett.* **90**:209–214.

Keppler, D., Lesch, R., Reutter, W., and Decker, K. 1968. Experimental hepatitis induced by D-galactosamine. *Exp. Mol. Pathol.* **9**:279–290.

Kioussis, D., Eiferman, F., van de Rijn, P., Gorin, M. B., Ingram, R. S., and Tilghman, S. M. 1981. The evolution of α-fetoprotein and albumin genes in the mouse. II. The structures of the α-fetoprotein and albumin genes in the mouse. *J. Biol. Chem.* **256**:1960–1967.

Klee, H. J., DiPetro, D., Fournier, M. J., and Fischer, M. S. 1978. Characterization of tRNA from liver of the developing amphibian *Rana catesbeiana*. *J. Biol Chem.* **253**:8074–8080.

Kleihauer, E., and Stöffler, G. 1968. Embryonic hemoglobins of different animal species. *Mol. Gen. Genet.* **101**:59–69.

Kleinebeckel, K. 1979. Movements of supernumerary hindlimbs after innervation by single lumbar spinal nerves of *Xenopus laevis*. *Experientia* **35**:506–507.

Klingman, D., and Nameroff, M. 1980a. Analysis of the myogenic lineage in chick embryos. I. Studies on the terminal cell division. *Exp. Cell Res.* **125**:201–210.

Klingman, D., and Nameroff, M. 1980b. Analysis of the myogenic lineage in chick embryos. II. Evidence for a deterministic lineage in the final stages. *Exp. Cell Res.* **127**:237–247.

Klotz, C., Swynghedauw, B., Mendes, H., Marotte, F., and Leger, J. J. 1981. Evidence for new forms of cardiac myosin heavy chains in mechanical heart overloading and in ageing. *Eur. J. Biochem.* **115**:415–421.

Ko, D. S., Page, R. C., and Narayanan, A. S. 1977. Fibroblast heterogeneity and prostaglandin regulation of subpopulations. *Proc. Natl. Acad. Sci. USA* **74**:3429–3432.

Konigsberg, I. R. 1971. Diffusion-mediated control of myoblast fusion. *Dev. Biol.* **26**:133–152.

Korneliussen, H., Dahl, H. A., and Paulsen, J. E. 1978. Histochemical definition of muscle fibre types in the trunk musculature of a teleost fish (cod, *Gadus morhua*). *Histochemistry* **55**:1–16.

Kosher, R. A., and Savage, M. P. 1980. Studies on the possible role of cAMP in limb morphogenesis and differentiation. *J. Embryol. Exp. Morphol.* **56**:91–105.

Kovach, J. S., Marks, P. A., Russell, E. S., and Epler, H. 1967. Erythroid cell development in fetal mice: Ultrastructural characteristics and hemoglobin synthesis. *J. Mol. Biol.* **25**:131–142.

Krasner, G. N., and Bryant, S. V. 1980. Distal transformation from double-half forearms in the axolotl *Ambystoma mexicanum*. *Dev. Biol.* **74**:315–325.

Kuroda, M., and Masaki, T. 1980. Extractability of actin and actinlike protein from myosin-removed myofibrils of skeletal muscle. *J. Biochem.* **88**:605–608.

Lajtha, L. G. 1970 Stem cell kinetics. *In*: Gordon, A. S., ed., *Regulation of Hematopoiesis*, New York, Appleton–Century–Crofts, Vol. 1, pp. 111–131.

Lajtha, L. G., Pozzi, L. V., Schofield, R., and Fox, M. 1969. Kinetic properties of haemopoietic stem cells. *Cell Tissue Kinet.* **2**:39–49.

Lamb, A. H. 1976. The projection patterns of the ventral horn to the hind limb during development. *Dev. Biol.* **54**:82–99.

Lamb, A. H. 1977. Neuronal death in the development of the somatotopic projections of the ventral horn in *Xenopus*. *Brain Res.* **134**:145–150.

Lamb, A. H. 1979a. Ventral horn cell counts in a *Xenopus* with naturally occurring supernumerary hind limbs. *J. Embryol. Exp. Morphol.* **49**:13–16.

Lamb, A. H. 1979b. Evidence that some developing limb motoneurons die for reasons other than peripheral competition. *Dev. Biol.* **71**:8–21.

Lee-Huang, S., Sierra, J. M., Naranjo, R., Filipowicz, W., and Ochoa, S. 1977. Eucaryotic oligonucleotides affecting mRNA translation. *Arch. Biochem. Biophys.* **180**:276–287.

Leibovitch, M. P., Leibovitch, S. A., Harel, J., and Kruh, J. 1979. Changes in the frequency and diversity of mRNA populations in the course of myogenic differentiation. *Eur. J. Biochem.* **98**:321–326.

Leknes, I. L. 1980. Ultrastructure of atrial endocardium and myocardium in three species of Gadidae (Teleostei). *Cell Tissue Res.* **210**:1–10.

Le Lièvre, C. 1974. Rôle des cellules mesectodermiques issues des crètes neurales céphaliques dans la formation des arcs branchiaux et du squelette viscéral. *J. Embryol. Exp. Morphol.* **31**:453–477.

Le Lièvre, C. 1978. Participation of neural crest derived cells in the genesis of the skull in birds. *J. Embryol. Exp. Morphol.* **47**:17–37.

Lemanski, L. F., Marx, B. S., and Hill, C. S. 1977. Evidence for abnormal heart induction in cardiac-mutant salamanders (*Ambystoma mexicanum*). *Science* **196**:894–896.

Lemanski, L. F., Paulson, D. J., and Hill, C. S. 1979. Normal anterior endoderm corrects the heart defect in cardiac mutant salamanders (*Ambystoma mexicanum*). *Science* **204**:860–862.

Lemanski, L. F., Fuldner, R. A., and Paulson, D. J. 1980. Immunofluorescence studies for myosin, α-actinin and tropomyosin in developing hearts of normal and cardiac lethal mutant Mexican axolotls, *Ambystoma mexicanum*. *J. Embryol. Exp. Morphol.* **55**:1–15.

Lentz, T. L. 1969. Cytological studies of muscle dedifferentiation and differentiation during limb regeneration of the newt *Triturus*. *Am. J. Anat.* **124**:447–480.

Levine, R. F. 1980. Isolation and characterization of normal human megakaryocytes. *Br. J. Haematol.* **45**:487–497.

Liao, W. S., Conn, A. R., and Taylor, J. M. 1980. Changes in rat α_1-fetoprotein and albumin mRNA levels during fetal and neonatal development. *J. Biol. Chem.* **255**:10036–10039.

Linsenmayer, T. F., Toole, B. P., and Trelstad, R. L. 1973. Temporal and spatial transitions in collagen types during embryonic chick limb development. *Dev. Biol.* **35**:232–239.

Littau, V. C., Allfrey, V. G., Frenster, J. H., and Mirsky, A. E. 1964. Active and inactive regions of nuclear chromatin as revealed by EM radiography. *Proc. Natl. Acad. Sci. USA* **52**:93–100.

Loomis, W. F., Wahrmann, J. P., and Luzzati, D. 1973. Temperature-sensitive variants of an established myoblast line. *Proc. Natl. Acad. Sci. USA* **70**:425–429.

Lough, J., and Ingram, V. M. 1978. Change in a nuclear phosphoprotein during *in vitro* myogenesis. *Exp. Cell Res.* **114**:349–356.

Lowey, S., and Risby, D. 1971. Light chains from fast and slow muscle myosins. *Nature (London)*:**234**:81–85.

Lowy, P. H. 1970. Preparation and chemistry of erythropoietin. *In*: Gordon, A. S., ed., *Regulation of Hematopoiesis*, New York, Appleton–Century–Crofts, Vol. 1, pp. 395–412.

Lufti, A. 1971. The fate of chondrocytes during cartilage erosion in the growing tibia in the domestic fowl (*Gallus domesticus*). *Acta Anat.* **79**:27–35.

Luzzatto, A. C. 1981. Hepatocyte differentiation during early fetal development in the rat. *Cell Tissue Res.* **215**:133–142.

Lyon, J. B. 1970. The X-chromosome and the enzymes controlling muscle glycogen: Phosphorylase kinase. *Biochem. Genet.* **4**:169–185.

McCulloch, E. A. 1970. Control of hematopoiesis at the cellular level. *In*: Gordon, A. S. ed., *Regulation of Hematopoiesis*, New York, Appleton–Century–Crofts, Vol. 1, pp. 133–159.

McEwen, B. S., Lieberburg, I., Macluskey, N., and Plapinger, L. 1976. Interactions of testosterone and estradiol with the neonatal rat brain protective mechanism and possible relationship to sexual differentiation. *Ann. Biol. Anim. Biochim. Biophys.* **16**:471–478.

Maden, M. 1976. Blastemal kinetics and pattern formation during amphibian limb regeneration. *J. Embryol. Exp. Morphol.* **36**:561–574.

Maden, M. 1979a. Neurotropic and X-ray blocks in the blastemal cell cycle. *J. Embryol. Exp. Morphol.* **50**:169–173.

Maden, M. 1979b. The role of irradiated tissue during pattern formation in the regeneration limb. *J. Embryol. Exp. Morphol.* **50**:235–242.

Maden, M. 1980. Intercalary regeneration in the amphibian limb and the rule of distal transformation. *J. Embryol. Exp. Morphol.* **56**:201–209.

Maden, M., and Goodwin, B. C. 1980. Experiments on developing limb buds of the axolotl, *Ambystoma mexicanum*. *J. Embryol. Exp. Morphol.* **57**:177–187.

Maden, M., and Wallace, H. 1976. How X-rays inhibit amphibian limb regeneration. *J. Exp. Zool.* **197**:105–113.

Mailman, M. L., and Dresden, M. H. 1979. Denervation effects on newt limb regeneration: Collagen and collagenase. *Dev. Biol.* **71**:60–70.

Malpoix, P. 1964. Influence of extraneous RNA on the differentiation of haematopoietic tissue in chick embryos. *Nature (London)* **203**:520–521.

Man, N. T., Morris, G. E., and Cole, R. J. 1980a. Two-dimensional gel analysis of nuclear proteins during muscle differentiation *in vitro*. I. Changes in nuclear protein content. *Exp. Cell Res.* **126**:375–382.

Man, N. T., Morris, G. E., and Cole, R. J. 1980b. Two-dimensional gel analysis of nuclear proteins during muscle differentiation *in vitro*. II. Changes in protein phosphorylation. *Exp. Cell Res.* **126**:383–390.

Manasek, F. J. 1968. Mitosis in developing cardiac muscle. *J. Cell Biol.* **37**:191–196.

Manasek, F. J. 1969. Myocardial cell death in the embryonic chick ventricle. *J. Embryol. Exp. Morphol.* **21**:271–284.

Markert, C. L., and Ursprung, H. 1962. The ontogeny of isozyme patterns of lactate dehydrogenase in the mouse. *Dev. Biol.* **5**:363–381.

Marks, P. A., and Rifkind, R. A. 1972. Protein synthesis: Its control in erythropoiesis. *Science* **175**:955–961.

Masseyeff, R., Gilli, J., Krebs, B., Calluaud, A., and Bonet C. 1975. Evolution of α-fetoprotein serum levels throughout life in humans and rats, and during pregnancy in the rat. *Ann. N.Y. Acad. Sci.* **259**:17–28.

Matsuda, G., Suzuyama, Y., Maita, T., and Umegane, T. 1977. The L-2 light chain of chicken skeletal muscle myosin. *FEBS Lett.* **84**:53–56.

Mauro, A. 1961. Satellite cells of skeletal muscle fibers. *J. Biophys. Biochem. Cytol.* **9**:493–495.

Metcalf, D., and Moore, M. A. S. 1971. *Haemopoietic Cells*, Amsterdam, North-Holland.

Midttun, B. 1980. Ultrastructure of atrial and ventricular myocardium in the pike *Esox lucius* and mackerel *Scomber scombrus* L. *Cell Tissue Res.* **211**:41–50.

Miller, M. M., Klotz, J. L., and Teplitz, R. L. 1979. Characterization of a chick embryonic erythrocyte antigen using immunochemical electron microscopy. *Exp. Cell Res.* **124**:159–169.

Milojević, B. D. 1924. Beiträge zum Frage über die Determination der Regenerate. *Wilhelm Roux Arch. Entwicklungsmech. Org.* **103**:80–94.

Milunsky, A., Spielvogel, C., and Kanfer, J. N. 1972. Lysosomal enzyme variations in cultured normal skin fibroblasts. *Life Sci.* **11**:1101–1107.

Mirand, E. A., and Murphy, G. P. 1980. Extrarenal erythropoietin activity in man and experimental animals. *In*: Gordon, A. S., ed., *Regulation of Hematopoiesis*, New York, Appleton–Century–Crofts, Vol. 1, pp. 495–518.

Miura, Y., and Wilt, F. H. 1970. The formation of blood islands in dissociated-reaggregated chick embryo yolk sac cells. *Exp. Cell Res.* **59**:217–226.

Moore, M. A. S., and Metcalf, D. 1970. Ontogeny of the hematopoietic system: Yolk sac origin of *in vivo* and *in vitro* colony forming cells in the developing mouse embryo. *Br. J. Haematol.* **18**:279–296.

Moore, M. A. S., and Owen, J. J. T. 1965. Chromosome marker studies on the development of the haematopoietic system in the chick embryo. *Nature (London)* **208**:965, 989–990.

Moore, M. A. S., and Owen, J. J. T. 1966. Experimental studies on the development of the bursa of Fabricius. *Dev. Biol.* **14**:40–51.

Moore, M. A. S., and Owen, J. J. T. 1967a. Stem cell migration in developing myeloid and lymphoid systems. *Lancet* **1967(2)**:958–959.

Moore, M. A. S., and Owen, J. J. T. 1967b. Experimental studies on the development of the thymus. *J. Exp. Med.* **126**:715–725.

Moore, M. A. S., McNeill, T. A., and Haskill, J. S. 1970. Density distribution analysis of *in vivo* and *in vitro* colony forming cells in developing fetal liver. *J. Cell. Physiol.* **75**:181–192.

Moore, M. A. S., Kurland, J., and Broxmeyer, H. E. 1976. The granulocytic and monocytic stem cell. *In*: Cairnie, A. B., Lala, P. K., and Osmund, D. G., eds., *Stem Cells of Renewing Cell Populations*, New York, Academic Press, pp. 181–188.

Morris, N. P., Fessler, L. I., Weinstock, A., and Fessler, J. H. 1975. Procollagen assembly and secretion in embryonic chick bone. *J. Biol. Chem.* **250**:5719–5726.

Morzlock, F. V., and Stocum, D. L. 1972. Neural control of RNA synthesis in regenerating limbs of the adult newt *Triturus viridescens*. *Wilhelm Roux Arch. Dev. Biol.* **171**:170–180.

Moss, F. P., and Leblond, C. P. 1971. Satellite cells as the source of nuclei in muscles of growing rats. *Anat. Rec.* **170**:421–436.

Moss, P. S., and Strohman, R. C. 1976. Myosin synthesis by fusion-arrested chick embryo myoblasts in cell culture. *Dev. Biol.* **48**:431–437.

Mourelle, M., and Rubalcava, B. 1981. Regeneration of the liver after carbon tetrachloride. *J. Biol. Chem.* **256**:1656–1660.

Muguruma, M., Muguruma, Y., and Fukazawa, T. 1980. Contribution of Z-line constituents to the formation of contraction bands of chicken myofibrils on addition of Mg^{2+}-ATP. *J. Biochem.* **88**:145–149.

Muller, C. J. 1961. *Molecular Evolution*, Assem, The Netherlands, Van Gorcum.

Murgita, R. A., Goidl, E. A., Kontiainen, S., and Wigzell, H. 1977. α-Fetoprotein induces suppressor T cells *in vitro*. *Nature (London)* **1267**:257–259.

Myklebust, R., Dalen, H., and Saetersdal, T. S. 1980. A correlative transmission and scanning electron microscope study of the pigeon myocardial cell. *Cell Tissue Res.* **207**:31–41.

Naftolin, F., Ryan, K. J., and Petro, Z. 1971. Aromatization of androstenedione by the diencephalon. *J. Clin. Endocrinol. Metab.* **33**:368–370.

Nag, A. C. 1972. Ultrastructure and ATPase activity of red and white muscle fibres of the caudal region of a fish, *Salmo gairdneri*. *J. Cell Biol.* **55**:42–57.

Nag, A. C., and Foster, J. D. 1981. Myogenesis in the adult mammalian skeletal muscle *in vitro*. *J. Anat.* **132**:1–18.

Nakeff, A., and Bryan, J. E. 1978. Megalokaryocyte proliferation and its regulation as revealed by CFU-M analysis. *ICN–UCLA Symp. Mol. Cell. Biol.* **10**:241–259.

Nameroff, M., and Holtzer, H. 1967. The loss of phenotypic traits by differentiated cells. IV. Changes in polysaccharides produced by dividing chondrocytes. *Dev. Biol.* **16**:250–281.

Nayak, N. C., and Mital, I. 1977. The dynamics of α-fetoprotein and albumin synthesis in human and rat liver during normal ontogeny. *Am. J. Pathol.* **86**:359–374.

Newman, S. A. 1977. Lineage and pattern in the developing wing bud. *In*: Ede, D. A., Hinchcliffe, J. R., and Balls, M., eds., *Vertebrate Limb and Somite Morphogenesis*, London, Cambridge University Press, pp. 181–197.

Newman, S. A. 1980. Fibroblast progenitor cells of the embryonic chick limb. *J. Embryol. Exp. Morphol.* **56**:191–200.

Newman, S. A., and Frisch, H. L. 1979. Dynamics of skeletal pattern formation in developing chick limb. *Science* **205**:662–668.

Nist, C., von der Mark, K., Hay, E. D., Olsen, B. R., Bornstein, P., Ross, R., and Dehm, P. 1975. Location of procollagen in chick corneal and tendon fibroblasts with ferritin-conjugated antibodies. *J. Cell Biol.* **65**:75–87.

Nogami, H., and Urist, M. R. 1970. A substratum of bone matrix for differentiation of mesenchymal cells in chondro-osseous tissues *in vitro*. *Exp. Cell Res.* **63**:404–410.

Novák, E., Drummond, G. I., Skála, J., and Hahn, P. 1972. Developmental changes in cAMP, protein kinase, phosphorylase kinase, and phosphorylase in liver, heart, and skeletal muscle of the rat. *Arch. Biochem. Biophys.* **150**:511–518.

Nunzi, M. G., Burighel, P., and Schiaffino, S. 1979. Muscle cell differentiation in the ascidean heart. *Dev. Biol.* **68**:371–380.

Nute, P. E. 1974. Multiple hemoglobin α-chain loci in monkeys, apes, and man. *Ann. N.Y. Acad. Sci.* **241**:39–60.

Oberpriller, J., and Oberpriller, J. C. 1971. Mitosis in adult newt ventricle. *J. Cell Biol.* **49**:560–563.

Obinata, T., Hasegawa, T., Masaki, T., and Hayashi, T. 1976. The subunit structure of myosin from skeletal muscle of the early chick embryo. *J. Biochem.* **79**:521–531.

Obinata, T., Shimada, Y., and Matsuda, R. 1979. Troponin in embryonic chick skeletal muscle cells *in vitro*. *J. Cell Biol.* **81**:59–66.

Odell, T. T., Jackson, C. W., and Gosslee, D. G. 1965. Maturation of rat megakaryocytes studied by microspectrophotometric measurement of DNA. *Proc. Soc. Exp. Biol. Med.* **119**:1194–1199.

Ojeda, J. L., and Hurle, J. M. 1975. Cell death during the formation of tubular heart of the chick embryo. *J. Embryol. Exp. Morphol.* **33**:523–534.

Olsen, B. R., Berg, R. A., Kishida, Y., and Prockop, D. J. 1975. Further characterization of embryonic tendon fibroblasts and use of immunoferritin techniques to study collagen biosynthesis. *J. Cell Biol.* **64**:340–355.

O'Neill, M. C., and Stockdale, F. E. 1972. Differentiation without cell division in cultured skeletal muscle. *J. Cell Biol.* **29**:410–417.

Ontell, M. 1974. Muscle satellite cells: A validated technique for light microscopic identification and a quantitative study of changes in their population following denervation. *Anat. Rec.* **178**:211–228.

Ordahl, C. P., and Caplan, A. I. 1978. High diversity in the poly(A) RNA populations of embryonic myoblasts. *J. Biol. Chem.* **253**:7683–7691.

Ordahl, C. P., Kioussis, D., Tilghman, S. M., Ovitt, C. E., and Fornwald, J. 1980. Molecular cloning of developmentally regulated, low-abundance mRNA sequences from embryonic muscle. *Proc. Natl. Acad. Sci. USA* **77**:4519–4523.

Orlic, D. 1970. Ultrastructural analysis of erythropoiesis. *In*: Gordon, A. S., ed., *Regulation of Hematopoiesis*, New York, Appleton–Century–Crofts, Vol. 1, pp. 271–296.

Osculati, F., Amati, S., Petrini, E., Franceschini, F., and Cinti, S. 1978. Ultrastructural investigation of the Purkinje fibers of rabbit's and cat's hearts. *J. Submicrosc. Cytol.* **10**:185–197.

Ovadia, M., Parker, C. H., and Lash, J. W. 1980. Changing patterns of proteoglycan synthesis during chondrogenic differentiation. *J. Embryol. Exp. Morphol.* **56**:59–70.

Owen, J. J. T., and Ritter, M. A. 1969. Tissue interaction in the development of thymus lymphocytes. *J. Exp. Med.* **129**:431–437.

Owen, J. J. T., Raff, M. C., and Cooper, M. D. 1976. Studies of the generation of B-lymphocytes in the mouse embryo. *Eur. J. Immunol.* **5**:468–473.

Paone, D. B., Cutts, J. H., and Krause, W. J. 1975. Megakaryocytopoiesis in the liver of the developing opossum, *Didelphis virginiana*. *J. Anat.* **120**:239–252.

Parker, R. C. 1932a. The fundamental characteristics of nine races of fibroblasts. *Science* **76**:219–220.

Parker, R. C. 1932b. The stability of functionally distinct races of fibroblasts. *Science* **76**:446–447.

Paterson, B., and Strohman, R. C. 1972. Myosin synthesis in cultures of differentiating chick embryo skeletal muscle. *Dev. Biol.* **29**:113–138.

Peachey, L. D. 1965. Sarcoplasmic reticulum and transverse tubules of the frog's sartorius. *J. Cell Biol.* **25**:209–233.

Pearson, H. A. 1974. Pathophysiology of thalassemias. *Ann. N.Y. Acad. Sci.* **241**:274–279.

Pelloni-Muller, G., Ermini, M., and Jenny, F. 1976. Changes in myosin light and heavy chain stoichiometry during development of rabbit fast, slow and cardiac muscle. *FEBS Lett.* **70**:113–117.

Peschle, C., Tallarida, G., Leone, G., and Condorelli, M. 1967. Richerche sul fattore eritropoietico renale. V. Estrazione di un fattore renale generante eritropoietino dopo incubazione con plasma omologo. *Prog. Med. (Rome)* **23**:911–919.

Peschle, C., Migliaccio, G., Covelli, A., Lettieri, F., Migliaccio, A. R., Condorelli, M., Comi, P., Pozzoli, M. L., Giglioni, B., Ottolenghi, S., Cappellini, M. D., Polli, E., and Gianni,A. M. 1980. Hemoglobin synthesis in individual bursts from normal adult blood: All bursts and subcolonies synthesize $^G\gamma$- and $^A\gamma$-globin chains. *Blood* **56**:218–226.

Pescitelli, M. J., and Stocum, D. L. 1981. Nonsegmental organization of positional information in regenerating *Ambystoma* limbs. *Dev. Biol.* **82**:69–85.

Peters, T. 1975. Serum albumin. *In*: Putnam, F. W., ed., *The Plasma Proteins*, New York, Academic Press, Vol. 1, pp. 133–181.

Pexieder, T. 1972. The tissue dynamics of heart morphogenesis. I. The phenomena of cell death. *Z. Anat. Entwicklungsgesch.* **138**:241–254.

Playfair, J. H. L., and Cole, L. J. 1965. Quantitative studies on colony-forming units in isogenic radiation chimaeras. *J. Cell. Comp. Physiol.* **65**:7–18.

Podleski, T. R., Greenberg, I., and Nichols, S. C. 1979a. Studies on lectin activity during myogenesis. *Exp. Cell Res.* **122**:305–316.

Podleski, T. R., Greenberg, I., Schlessinger, J., and Yamada, K. M. 1979b. Fibronectin delays the fusion of L_6 myoblasts. *Exp. Cell Res.* **122**:317–326.

Polezhaev, L. 1936. La valeur de la structure de l'organe et les capacités du blastème régénératif dans le processus de la détermination du régénérat. *Bull. Biol. Fr. Belg.* **70**:54–85.

Polezhaev, L. 1972. *Loss and Restoration of Regenerative Capacity*, Cambridge, Mass., Harvard University Press.

Price, D., Ortiz, E., and Zaaijer, J. J. P. 1967. Organ culture studies of hormone secretion in endocrine glands of fetal guinea pigs. III. The relation of testicular hormones to sex differentiation of the reproductive ducts. *Anat. Rec.* **157**:27–42.

Proudfoot, N. J., Shander, M. H. M., Manley, J. L., Gefter, M. L., and Maniatis, T. 1980. Structure and *in vitro* transcription of human globin genes. *Science* **209**:1329–1336.

Raeside, J. I., and Middleton, A. T. 1979. Development of testosterone secretion in the fetal pig testis. *Biol. Reprod.* **21**:985–989.

Reiners, J. J., and Busch, H. 1980. Transcriptional and posttranscriptional modulation of cytoplasmic RNAs in regenerating liver and Novikoff hepatoma. *Biochemistry* **19**:833–841.

Revel, J. P., and Hay, E. D. 1963. An autoradiographic and electron microscopic study of collagen synthesis in differentiating cartilage. *Z. Zellforsch. Mikrosk. Anat.* **61**:110–144.

Rich, I. N., and Kubanek, B. 1979. The ontogeny of erythropoiesis in the mouse detected by the erythroid colony-forming technique. *J. Embryol. Exp. Morphol.* **50**:57–74.

Richardson, B. J., and Russell, E. M. 1969. Changes with age in the proportion of nucleated red blood cell types and in the type of haemoglobin in kangaroo pouch young. *Aust. J. Exp. Biol. Med. Sci.* **47**:563–580.

Richmond, A., and Elmer, W. A. 1980. Purification of a mouse embryo extract component which enhances chondrogenesis *in vitro*. *Dev. Biol.* **76**:366–383.

Rifkind, R. A., Cantor, L. N., Cooper, M., Levy, J., Maniatis, G. M., Bank, A., and Marks, P. A. 1974. Ontogeny of erythropoiesis in the fetal mouse. *Ann. N.Y. Acad. Sci.* **241**:113–118.

Rigaudiere, N. 1977. Evolution des teneurs en testosterone et dihydrotestosterone dans le plasma, le testicule et l'ovaire chez le cobaye au cours de lavie foetale. *C. R. Acad. Sci.* **285**:989–992.

Riordan, J. R., and Richards, V. 1980. Human fetal liver contains both zinc- and copper-rich forms of metallothionein. *J. Biol. Chem.* **255**:5380–5383.

Rosenberg, S. A., Speiss, P. J., and Schwarz, S. 1980. *In vitro* growth of murine T-cells. IV. Use of T-cell growth factor to clone lymphoid cells. *Cell. Immunol.* **54**:293–306.

Rosse, W. F., and Waldmann, T. A. 1966. Factors controlling erythropoiesis in birds. *Blood* **27**:654–661.

Rosse, W. F., Waldmann, T. A., and Hull, E. 1963. Factors stimulating erythropoiesis in frogs. *Blood* **22**:66–72.

Roy, R. K., Sreter, F. A., and Sarkar, S. 1979a. Changes in tropomyosin subunits and myosin light chains during development of chicken and rabbit striated muscles. *Dev. Biol.* **69**:15–30.

Roy, R. K., Mabuchi, K., Sarkar, S., Mis, C., and Sreter, F. A. 1979b. Changes in tropomyosin subunit pattern in chronic electrically stimulated rabbit fast muscles. *Biochem. Biophys. Res. Commun.* **89**:181–187.

Rubenstein, N. A., and Holtzer, H. 1979. Fast and slow muscles in tissue culture synthesize only fast myosin. *Nature (London)* **280**:323–325.

Rubenstein, N. A., Pepe, F., and Holtzer, H. 1977. Myosin types during development of embryonic chicken fast and slow muscles. *Proc. Natl. Acad. Sci. USA* **74**:4524–4527.

Rucknagel, D. L., and Winter, W. P. 1974. Duplication of structural genes for hemoglobin α and β chains in man. *Ann. N.Y. Acad. Sci.* **247**:80–92.

Rudolph, R., and Woodard, M. 1978. Spatial orientation of microtubules in contractile fibroblasts *in vivo*. *Anat. Rec.* **191**:169–182.

Rugh, R. 1968. *The Mouse: Reproduction and Development*, Minneapolis, Minn., Burgess, pp. 253–259.

Rumyantsev, P. P. 1972. Electron microscope study of the myofibril partial disintegration and recovery in the mitotically dividing cardiac muscle cells. *Z. Zellforsch. Mikrosk. Anat.* **129**:471–499.

Ruoslahti, E., and Engvall, E. 1980. Complexing of fibronectin glycosaminoglycans and collagen. *Biochim. Biophys. Acta* **631**:350–358.

Rushbrook, J. I., and Stracher, A. 1979. Comparison of adult, embryonic, and dystrophic myosin heavy chains from chicken muscle by sodium dodecyl sulfate/polyacrylamide gel electrophoresis and peptide mapping. *Proc. Natl. Acad. Sci. USA* **76**:4331–4334.

Rytömaa, T. 1960. Organ distribution and histochemical properties of eosinophil granulocytes in rat. *Acta Pathol. Scand.* **50**(Suppl. 140):1–118.

Saetersdal, T., Ødegården, S., Rotevatn, S., and Engedal, H. 1980. Atrial specific granules of the human auricle in embryogenesis, tissue culture, and hypertrophy. *Cell Tissue Res.* **209**:345–351.

Sainte-Marie, G., and Sin, Y. M. 1970. Morphologic aspects and kinetics of the formation of neutrophils and eosinophils. *In*: Gordon, A. S., ed., *Regulation of Hematopoiesis*, New York, Appleton–Century–Crofts, Vol. 2, pp. 1109–1142.

Sala-Trepat, J. M., Dever, J., Sargent, T. D., Thomas, K., Sell, S., and Bonner, J. 1979. Changes in expression of albumin and α-fetoprotein genes during rat liver development and neoplasia. *Biochemistry* **18**:2167–2178.

Sarkar, S., Sreter, F. A., and Gergeley, J. 1971. Light chains of myosins from white, red and cardiac muscles. *Proc. Natl. Acad. Sci. USA* **68**:946–950.

Sartore, S., Gorza, L., Bormioli, S. P., Libera, L. D., and Schiaffino, S. 1981. Myosin types and fiber types in cardiac muscle. 1. Ventricular myocardium. *J. Cell Biol.* **88**:226–233.

Satoh, N. 1979. On the 'clock' mechanism determining the time of tissue-specific enzyme development during ascidean embryogenesis. *J. Embryol. Exp. Morphol.* **54**:131–139.

Saunders, J. W. 1948. The proximo-distal sequence of origin of the parts of the chick wing and the role of the ectoderm. *J. Exp. Zool.* **108**:363–403.

Saunders, J. W. 1966. Death in embryonic systems. *Science* **154**:604–612.

Saunders, J. W., and Fallon, J. F. 1966. Cell death in morphogenesis. *In*: Locke, M., ed., *Major Problems in Developmental Biology*, New York, Academic Press, pp. 289–314.

Scadding, S. R. 1977. Phylogenic distribution of limb regeneration capacity in adult Amphibia. *J. Exp. Zool.* **202**:57–69.

Schiltz, J. R., and Ward, S. 1980. Effects of chick embryo extract fractions on collagen and glycosaminoglycan metabolism by chick chondroblasts. *Biochim. Biophys. Acta* **628**:343–354.

Schiltz, J. R., Mayne, R., and Holtzer, H. 1973. Synthesis of collagen and glycosaminoglycans by dedifferentiated chondroblasts in culture. *Differentiation* **1**:97–108.

Schmidt, A. 1969. *Cellular Biology of Vertebrate Regeneration and Repair*, Chicago, University of Chicago Press.

Scholla, C. A., Tedeschi, M. V., and Fausto, N. 1980. Gene expression and the diversity of polysomal mRNA sequences in regenerating liver. *J. Biol. Chem.* **255**:2855–2860.

Schotté, O. E., and Hummel, K. P. 1939. Lens induction at the expense of regenerating tissues of amphibians. *J. Exp. Zool.* **80**:131–166.

Schreiber, G., Rotermund, H. M., Maeno, H., Weigand, K., and Lesch, R. 1969. The proportion of the incorporation of leucine into albumin to that into total protein in rat liver and hepatoma Morris 5123TC. *Eur. J. Biochem.* **10**:355–361.

Schreiber, G., Lesch, R., Weinssen, U., and Zähringer, J. 1970. The distribution of albumin synthesis throughout the liver lobule. *J. Cell Biol.* **47**:285–289.

Schroeder, W. A., and Huisman, T. H. J. 1974. Multiple cistrons for fetal hemoglobins in man. *Ann. N.Y. Acad. Sci.* **241**:70–79.

Schroeder, W. A., Huisman, T. H. J., Brown, A. K., Uy, R., Bouver, N. G., Lerch, P. O., Shelton, J. R., Shelton, J. B., and Apell, G. 1971. Postnatal changes in the chemical heterogeneity of human fetal hemoglobin. *Pediatr. Res.* **5**:493–499.

Scornik, O. A., and Botbol, V. 1976. Role of changes in protein degradation in the growth of regenerating livers. *J. Biol. Chem.* **251**:2891–2897.

Scott-Savage, P., and Hall, B. K. 1979. The timing of the onset of osteogenesis in the tibia of the embryonic chick. *J. Morphol.* **162**:453–464.

Scott-Savage, P., and Hall, B. K. 1980. Differentiation ability of the tibial periosteum from the embryonic chick. *Acta Anat.* **106**:129–140.

Searls, R. L. 1965. An autoradiographic study of the uptake of S^{35} sulfate during the differentiation of limb bud cartilage. *Dev. Biol.* **11**:155–168.

Searls, R. L. 1973, Chondrogenesis. *In*: Coward, S. J., ed., *Developmental Regulation*, New York, Academic Press, pp. 219–250.

Sell, S. 1974. The catabolism of α_1-fetoprotein and albumin in rats bearing Morris hepatoma 7777. *Cancer Res.* **34**:1608–1611.

Shainberg, A., Yagil, G., and Yaffe, D. 1971. Alterations of enzymatic activities during muscle differentiation *in vitro*. *Dev. Biol.* **25**:1–29.

Shambaugh, J., and Elmer, W. A. 1980. Analysis of glycosaminoglycans during chondrogenesis of normal and brachypod mouse limb mesenchyme. *J. Embryol. Exp. Morphol.* **56**:225–238.

Shimada, Y., and Obinata, T. 1977. Polarity of actin filaments at the initial stage of myofibril assembly in myogenic cells *in vitro*. *J. Cell Biol.* **72**:777–785.

Sholl, S. A., and Goy, R. W. 1978. Androgen and estrogen synthesis in the fetal guinea pig gonad. *Biol. Reprod.* **18**:160–169.

Shreiner, D. P., Weinberg, J., and Enoch, D. 1980. Plasma thrombopoietic activity in humans with normal and abnormal platelet counts. *Blood* **56**:183–188.

Shyamala, G., and Gorski, J. 1967. Interrelationship of estrogen receptors in the nucleus and cytosol. *J. Cell Biol.* **35**:125A–126A.

Shyamala, G., and Gorski, J. 1969. Estrogen receptors in the rat uterus. *J. Biol. Chem.* **244**:1097–1103.

Siegel, C. D. 1970. Possible hematopoietic mechanisms in nonmammalian vertebrates. *In*: Gordon, A. S., ed., *Regulation of Hematopoiesis*, New York, Appleton–Century–Crofts, Vol. 1, pp. 67–76.

Simpkins, H., Thompson, L. M., Waldeck, N., Gross, D. S., and Mooney, D. 1981. Conformational changes in rat liver chromatin after liver regeneration. *Biochem. J.* **193**: 671–678.

Simpson, C. F., and Kling, J. M. 1967. The mechanism of denucleation in circulating erythroblasts. *J. Cell Biol.* **35**:237–245.

Singer, M. 1952. The influence of the nerve in regeneration of the amphibian extremity. *Q. Rev. Biol.* **27**:169–199.

Singer, M. 1974. Neurotrophic control of limb regeneration in the newt. *Ann. N.Y. Acad. Sci.* **228**:308–321.

Singer, M., and Caston, J. D. 1972. Neurotrophic dependence of macromolecular synthesis in the early limb regenerate of the newt. *J. Embryol. Exp. Morphol.* **28**:1–11.

Singer, M., and Craven, L. 1948. The growth and morphogenesis of the regenerating forelimb of adult *Triturus* following denervation at various stages of development. *J. Exp. Zool.* **108**:272–308.

Singer, M., and Ilan, J. 1977. Nerve-dependent regulation of absolute rates of protein synthesis in newt limb regenerates. *Dev. Biol.* **57**:174–187.

Sippel, A. E., Kurtz, D. T., Morris, H. P., and Feigelson, P. 1976. Comparison of *in vivo* translation rates and mRNA levels of α_{2v}-globulin in rat liver and Morris hepatoma 5123D. *Cancer Res.* **36**:3588–3593.

Skutelsky, E., and Danon, D. 1967. An electron microscope study of nuclear elimination from the late erythroblast. *J. Cell Biol.* **33**:625–635.

Skutelsky, E., and Farquhar, M. G. 1976. Variations in distribution of Con A receptor sites and anionic groups during red cell differentiation in the rat. *J. Cell Biol.* **71**:218–231.

Slack, J. M. W. 1976. Determination of polarity in the amphibian limb. *Nature (London)* **261**:44–46.

Slack, J. M. W. 1980a. Regulation and potency in the forelimb rudiment of the axolotl embryo. *J. Embryol. Exp. Morphol.* **57**:203–217.

Slack, J. M. W. 1980b. Morphogenetic properties of the skin in axolotl limb regeneration. *J. Embryol. Exp. Morphol.* **58**::265–288.

Slater, C. R. 1976. Control of myogenesis *in vitro* by chick embryo extract. *Dev. Biol.* **50**:264–284.

Smith, P. B. 1980. Postnatal development of glycogen- and cyclic AMP-metabolizing enzymes in mammalian skeletal muscle. *Biochim. Biophys. Acta* **628**:19–25.

Snell, K. 1974. Pathways of gluconeogenesis from L-serine in the neonatal rat. *Biochem. J.* **142**:433–436.

Snell, K. 1980. Liver enzymes of serine metabolism during neonatal development of the rat. *Biochem. J.* **190**:451–455.

Snow, M. H. 1979. Origin of regenerating myoblasts in mammalian skeletal muscle. *In*: Mauro, A., ed., *Muscle Regeneration*, New York, Raven Press, pp. 91–100.

Sohal, G. S., and Holt, R. K. 1980. Role of innervation on the embryonic development of skeletal muscle. *Cell Tissue Res.* **210**:383–393.

Solursh, M., and Reiter, R. S. 1980. Evidence for histogenic interactions during *in vitro* limb chondrogenesis. *Dev. Biol.* **78**:141–150.

Solursh, M., Reiter, R. S., Ahrens, P. B., and Pratt, R. M. 1979. Increase in levels of cAMP during avian limb chondrogenesis *in vitro*. *Differentiation* **15**:183–186.

Sommer, J. R., and Johnson, E. A. 1968. Cardiac muscle: A comparative study of Purkinje fibers and ventricular fibers. *J. Cell Biol.* **36**:497–526.

Sommer, J. R., Wallace, N. R., and Junker, J. 1980. The intermediate cisternae of the sarcoplasmic reticulum of skeletal muscle. *J. Ultrastruct. Res.* **71**:126–142.

Stark, R., and Searls, R. 1973. A description of chick wing development and a model of morphogenesis. *Dev. Biol.* **33**:138–153.

Stocum, D. L. 1968a. The urodele limb regeneration blastema: A self-organizing system. I. Differentiation *in vitro*. *Dev. Biol.* **18**:441–456.

Stocum, D. L. 1968b. The urodele limb regeneration blastema: A self-organizing system. II. Morphogenesis and differentiation of autografted whole and fractional blastemas. *Dev. Biol.* **18**:457–480.

Stocum, D. L. 1975a. Outgrowth and pattern formation during limb ontogeny and regeneration. *Differentiation* **3**:167–182.

Stocum, D. L. 1975b. Regulation after proximal or distal transposition of limb regeneration blastemas and determination of the proximal boundary of the regenerate. *Dev. Biol.* **45**:112–136.

Stocum, D. L. 1978. Regeneration of symmetrical hindlimbs in larval salamanders. *Science* **200**:790–793.

Strandholm, J. J., Cardenas, J. M., and Dyson, R. D. 1975. Pyruvate kinase isozymes in adult and fetal tissue of chicken. *Biochemistry* **14**:2242–2246.

Strandholm, J. J., Dyson, R. D., and Cardenas, J. M. 1976. Bovine pyruvate isozymes and hybrid isozymes. *Arch. Biochem. Biophys.* **173**:125–131.

Studitsky, A. N. 1963. Dynamics of the development of myogenic tissue under conditions of explantation and transplantation. *In*: Rose, G. G., ed., *Cinemicrography in Cell Biology*, New York, Academic Press, pp. 171–200.

Sugavara, S., Tsuneoka, K., and Shikita, M. 1980. Colony-stimulating factor and the proliferation of X-irradiated myeloid stem cells. *Biochem. Biophys. Res. Commun.* **96**:1488–1493.

Suleiman, S. A., Jones, G. L., Singh, H., and Labrecque, D. R. 1980. Changes in lysosomal cathepsins during liver regeneration. *Biochim. Biophys. Acta* **627**:17–22.

Summerbell, D. 1974. A quantitative analysis of the effect of excision of the AER from the chick limb bud. *J. Embryol. Exp. Morphol.* **32**:651–660.

Summerbell, D., and Stirling, R. V. 1981. The innervation of dorsoventrally reversed chick wings: Evidence that motor axons do not actively seek out their appropriate targets. *J. Embryol. Exp. Morphol.* **61**:233–247.

Taban, C. H., Constantinidis, J., Cathieni, M., and Guntern, R. 1977. Présence de catécholamines dans le nerf et la blastème de triton observée à l'histofluorescence. *Acta Anat.* **99**:234.

Taban, C. H., Cathieni, M., Guntern, R., and Constantinidis, J. 1978. Histofluorescence of monoamines in newt forelimb regenerates. *Wilhelm Roux Arch. Dev. Biol.* **185**:79–94.

Takami, H., and Busch, H. 1979. Two-dimensional gel electrophoretic comparison of proteins of nuclear fractions of normal liver and Novikoff hepatoma. *Cancer Res.* **39**:507–518.

Takami, H., Busch, F. N., Morris, H. P., and Busch, H. 1979. Comparison of salt-extractable nuclear proteins of regenerating liver, fetal liver, and Morris hepatomas 9618A and 3924A. *Cancer Res.* **39**:2096–2105.

Tank, P. W. 1978. The occurrence of supernumerary limbs following blastemal transplantation in the regenerating forelimb of the axolotl *Ambystoma mexicanum. Dev. Biol.* **62**:143–161.

Tank, P. W. 1979. Positional information in the forelimb of the axolotl: Experiments with double-half tissues. *Dev. Biol.* **73**:11–24.

Tarbutt, R. G., and Cole, R. J. 1970. Cell population kinetics of erythroid tissue in the liver of foetal mice. *J. Embryol. Exp. Morphol.* **24**:429–446.

Tauber, R., and Reutter, W. 1978. Protein degradation in the plasma membrane of regenerating liver and Morris hepatomas. *Eur. J. Biochem.* **83**:37–45.

Tavassoli, M., and Crosby, W. H. 1973. Fate of the nucleus of the marrow erythroblast. *Science* **179**:912–913.

Teichberg, V. I., Silman, I., Beutsch, D. D., and Resheff, G. 1975. A β-D-galactoside binding protein from electric organ tissue of *Electrophorus electricus. Proc. Natl. Acad. Sci. USA* **72**:1383–1387.

Teng, C. S., and Teng, C. T. 1975a. Studies on sex organ development: Isolation and characterization of an oestrogen receptor from chick Müllerian duct. *Biochem. J.* **150**:183–190.

Teng, C. S., and Teng, C. T. 1975b. Studies on sex-organ development: Ontogeny of cytoplasmic oestrogen receptor in chick Müllerian duct. *Biochem. J.* **150**:191–194.

Teng, C. S., and Teng, C. T. 1976. Studies on sex-organ development: Oestrogen receptor translocation in the developing chick Müllerian duct. *Biochem. J.* **154**:1–9.

Teng, C. S., and Teng, C. T. 1978. Studies on sex-organ development. *Biochem. J.* **172**:361–370.

Teng, C. T., and Teng, C. S. 1977. Studies on sex-organ development: The hormonal regulation of steroidogenesis and adenosine 3′ : 5′-cyclic monophosphate in embryonic-chick ovary. *Biochem. J.* **162**:123–124.

Terasawa, T., Ogawa, M., Porter, P. N., and Karam, J. D. 1980. $^G\gamma$ and $^A\gamma$ globin-chain biosynthesis by adult and umbilical cord blood erythropoietic bursts and reticulocytes. *Blood* **56**:93–97.

Thornton, C. S. 1938. The histogenesis of muscle in the regenerating forelimb of larval *Amblystoma punctatum. J. Morphol.* **62**:17–47.

Thornton, C. S. 1970. Amphibian limb regeneration and its relation to nerves. *Am. Zool.* **10**:113–118.

Thorogood, P. V., and Hinchliffe, J. R. 1975. An analysis of the condensation process during chondrogenesis in the embryonic chick hind limb. *J. Embryol. Exp. Morphol.* **33**:581–606.

Till, J. E., McCulloch, E. A., and Siminovitch, L. 1964. Isolation of variant cell lines during serial transplantation of hematopoietic cells derived from fetal liver. *J. Natl. Cancer Inst.* **33**:707–720.

Tillack, T. W., Boland, R., and Martonosi, A. 1974. The ultrastructure of developing sarcoplasmic reticulum. *J. Biol. Chem.* **249**:624–633.

Trampusch, H. A. L. 1951. Regeneration inhibited by X-rays and its recovery. *K. Ned. Akad. Wet. Amsterdam* **C54**:373–385.

Trampusch, H. A. L. 1958. The action of X-rays on the morphogenetic field. *K. Ned. Akad. Wet. Amsterdam* **C61**:417–430.

Trampusch, H. A. L. 1966. Regeneration from interocular grafts. *Arch. Zool. Ital.* **51**:787–822.

Trelstad, R. L. 1971. Vacuoles in the embryonic chick corneal epithelium, an epithelium which produces collagen. *J. Cell Biol.* **48**:689–694.

Trelstad, R. L., and Hayashi, K. 1979. Tendon collagen fibrillogenesis: Intracellular subassemblies and cell surface changes associated with fibril growth. *Dev. Biol.* **71**:228–242.

Trelstad, R. L., Hayashi, K., and Toole, B. P. 1974. Epithelial collagens and glycosaminoglycans in the embryonic cornea. *J. Cell Biol.* **62**:815–830.

Trotter, J. A., and Nameroff, M. 1976. Myoblast differentiation *in vitro*: Morphological differentiation of mononucleated myoblasts. *Dev. Biol.* **49**:548–555.

Trupin, G. L. 1979. The identification of myogenic cells in regenerating skeletal muscle. I. Early anuran regenerates. *Dev. Biol.* **68**:59–71.

Trupin, G. L., and Hsu, L. 1979. The identification of myogenic cells in regenerating skeletal muscle. II. Early mammalian regenerates. *Dev. Biol.* **68**:72–81.

Trupin, G. L., Hsu, L., and Hsieh, Y. H. 1979. Satellite cell mimics in regenerating skeletal muscle. *In*: Mauro, A., ed., *Muscle Regeneration*, New York, Raven Press, pp. 101–114.

Tse, T. P. H., Morris, H. P., and Taylor, J. M. 1978. Molecular basis of reduced albumin synthesis in Morris hepatoma 7777. *Biochemistry* **17**:3121–3127.

Turner, D. C., Gmür, R., Lebherz, H. G., Siegrist, M., Wallimann, T., and Eppenberger, H. M. 1976. Differentiation in cultures derived from embryonic chicken muscle. *Dev. Biol.* **48**:284–291.

Turpen, J. B. 1980. Early embryogenesis of hematopoietic cells in *Rana pipiens. In*: Horton, J. D., ed., *Development and Differentiation of Vertebrate Lymphocytes*, Amsterdam, Elsevier/North-Holland, pp. 15–24.

Turpen, J. B., Volpe, E. P., and Cohen, N. C. 1973. Ontogeny and peripheralization of thymic lymphocytes. *Science* **182**:931–933.

Turpen, J. B., Turpen, C. J., and Flajnik, M. 1979. Experimental analysis of hematopoietic cell development in the liver of larval *Rana pipiens. Dev. Biol.* **69**:466–479.

Ullrick, W. C., Toselli, P. A., Saide, J. D., and Phear, W. P. C. 1977a. Fine structure of the vertebrate Z-disc. *J. Mol. Biol.* **115**:61–74.

Ullrick, W. C., Toselli, P. A., Chase, D., and Dasse, K. 1977b. Are there extensions of thick filaments to the Z line in vertebrate and invertebrate striated muscle? *J. Ultrastruct. Res.* **60**:263–271.

Umanski, E. 1937. Untersuchung des Regenerationsvorganges bei Amphibien mittels ausschaltung der Einzelnen gewebe durch Röntgenbestrahlung. *Biol. Zh.* **6**:757–758.

Umanski, E. 1938. The regeneration potencies of axolotl skin studied by means of exclusion of the regeneration capacity of tissues through exposure to X-rays. *Bull. Biol. Med. Exp.* **6**:141–145.

Upholt, W. B., Vertel, B. M., and Dorfman, A. 1979. Translation and characterization of mRNAs in differentiating chicken cartilage. *Proc. Natl. Acad. Sci. USA* **76**:4847–4851.

Urist, M. R., Dowell, T. A., Hay, P. H., and Strates, B. S. 1968. Inductive substrates for bone formation. *Clin. Orthop.* **59**:59–96.

Urist, M. R., Iwata, H., Ceccotti, P. L., Dorfman, R. L., Boyd, S. D., McDowell, R. M., and Chien, C. 1973. Bone morphogenesis in implants of insoluble bone gelatine. *Proc. Natl. Acad. Sci. USA* **70**:3511–3515.

Urist, M. R., Granstein, R., Nogami, H., Svenson, L., and Murphy, R. 1977. Transmembrane bone morphogenesis across multiple-walled diffusion chambers. *Arch. Surg. (Chicago)* **112**:612–619.

Urist, M. R., Terashima, Y., Nakagawa, M., and Stamos, C. 1978. Cartilage tissue differentiation from mesenchymal cells derived from nature muscle in tissue culture. *In Vitro* **14**:697–706.

Urist, M. R., Mikulski, A., and Lietze, A. 1979. Solubilized and insolubilized bone morphogenetic protein. *Proc. Natl. Acad. Sci. USA* **76**:1828–1832.

Vainchenker, W., Testa, U., Dubart, A., Beuzard, Y., Breton-Gorius, J., and Rosa, J. 1980. Acceleration of the hemoglobin switch in cultures of neonate erythroid precursors by adult cells. *Blood* **56**:541–548.

Valet, J. P., Marceau, N., and Deschênes, J. 1981. Restricted specialization of differentiating hepatocytes in terms of albumin and α-fetoprotein production. *Cell Biol. Int. Rep.* **5**:307–314.

van der Rhee, H. J., van der Burgh-de Winter, C. P. M., and Daems, W. T. 1979. The differentiation of monocytes into macrophages, epitheloid cells, and multinucleated giant cells in subcutaneous granulomas. I. Fine structure. *Cell Tissue Res.* **197**:355–379.

VanDenbos, G., and Frieden, E. 1976. DNA synthesis and turnover in the bullfrog tadpole during metamorphosis. *J. Biol. Chem.* **251**:4111–4114.

Vanderkerckhove, J., and Weber, K. 1979. The complete amino acid sequence of actins from bovine aorta, heart, fast skeletal muscle and rabbit slow skeletal muscle. *Differentiation* **14**:123–133.

Vasan, N. S., and Lash, J. W. 1977. Heterogeneity of proteoglycans in developing chick limb cartilage. *Biochem. J.* **164**:179–183.

Vasan, N. S., and Lash, J. W. 1979 Monomeric and aggregate proteoglycans in the chondrogenic differentiation of embryonic chick limb buds. *J. Embryol. Exp. Morphol.* **49**:47–59.

Vbrová, G. 1963. Changes in motor reflexes produced by tentomy. *J. Physiol. (London)* **169**:513–526.

Vedvick, T. S., Wheeler, S. A., and Koenig, H. M. 1980. Switching of the nonallelic forms of fetal hemoglobin during late gestation. *Blood* **56**:732–735.

Veis, A., Anesey, J., and Mussell, S. 1967. A limiting microfibril model for the three-dimensional arrangement within collagen fibers. *Nature (London* **215**:931–934.

Vertel, B. M., and Fischman, D. A. 1976. Myosin accumulation in mononucleated cells of chick muscle cultures. *Dev. Biol.* **48**:438–445.

von der Mark, H., and von der Mark, K. 1979. Isolation and characterization of collagen A and B chains from chick embryos. *FEBS Lett.* **99**:101–105.

von der Mark, H., von der Mark, K., and Gay, S. 1976. Study of differential collagen synthesis during development of the chick embryo by immunofluorescence. *Dev. Biol.* **48**:237–249.

von der Mark, K. 1979. Immunological and biochemical studies of collagen type transition during *in vitro* chondrogenesis of chick limb mesodermal cells. *J. Cell Biol.* **73**:736–747.

Wahli, W., Abraham, I., and Weber, R. 1978. Retention of the differentiated state by larval *Xenopus* liver cells in primary culture. *Wilhelm Roux Arch. Dev. Biol.* **185**:235–248.

Wallace, H., and Maden, M. 1976. Irradiation inhibits the regeneration of aneurogenic limbs. *J. Exp. Zool.* **195**:353–358.

Watabe, H. 1974. Purification and chemical characterization of α-fetoprotein from rat and mouse. *Int. J. Cancer* **13**:377–388.

Watanabe, A., Taketa, K., and Kosaka, K. 1975. Microheterogeneity of rat α-fetoprotein. *Ann. N.Y. Acad. Sci.* **259**:95–108.

Watanabe, K., Sasaki, F., Takahama, H., and Iseki, H. 1980. Histogenesis and distribution of red and white muscle fibres of urodelan larvae. *J. Anat.* **130**:83–96.

Weber, R. 1962. Induced metamorphosis in isolated tails of *Xenopus* larvae. *Experientia* **18**:84–85.

Weinstock, M. 1972. Collagen formation—Observations on its intracellular packaging and transport. *Z. Zellforsch. Mikrosk. Anat.* **129**:455–470.

Weinstock, M. 1977. Centrosymmetrical crossbanded structures in the matrix of rat incisor predentin and dentin. *J. Ultrastruct. Res.* **61**:218–229.

Weiss, E., Gross, V., and Heinrich, P. C. 1976. Changes in chromatin during the development of liver cell injury induced by galactosamine. *FEBS Lett.* **64**:193–196.

Weiss, L. 1970. The histology of the bone marrow. *In*: Gordon, A. S., ed., *Regulation of Hematopoiesis,* New York, Appleton–Century–Crofts, Vol. 1, pp. 79–92.

Weiss, P. 1925. Unabhängigkeit der Extremititätenregeneration vom Skelett (bei *Triton cristatus*). *Arch. Mikrosk. Anat. Entwicklungsmech.* **104**:359–394.

Weiss, P. 1927. Potenzprüfung am Regenerationsblastem. *Wilhelm Roux Arch. Entwicklungsmech. Org.* **122**:379–394.

Weiss, P. 1941. Nerve patterns: The mechanics of nerve growth. *Growth* **5**:163–203.

Weniger, J. P., and Zeis, A. 1971. Biosynthèsis d'oestrogènes par les ébauches gonadiques de poulet. *Gen. Comp. Endocrinol.* **16**:391–395.

Wertz, R. L., and Donaldson, D. J. 1979. Effects of X-rays on nerve-dependent (limb) and nerve-independent (jaw) regeneration in the adult newt, *Notophthalmus viridescens.* *J. Embryol. Exp. Morphol.* **53**:315–325.

Wetzel, B. K. 1970a. The fine structure and cytochemistry of developing granulocytes, with special reference to the rabbit. *In*: Gordon, A. S., ed., *Regulation of Hematopoiesis,* New York, Appleton–Century–Crofts, Vol. 2, pp. 769–817.

Wetzel, B. K. 1970b. The comparative fine structure of normal and diseased mammalian granulocytes. *In*: Gordon, A. S., ed., *Regulation of Hematopoiesis,* New York, Appleton–Century–Crofts, Vol. 2, pp. 819–872.

Whittaker, J. R. 1973. Segregation during ascidian embryogenesis of egg cytoplasmic information for tissue-specific enzyme development. *Proc. Natl. Acad. Sci. USA* **70**:2096–2100.

Whittaker, J. R., Ortolani, G., and Farinella-Ferruza, N. 1977. Autonomy of acetylcholinesterase differentiation in muscle cells of ascidian embryos. *Dev. Biol.* **55**:196–200.

Wilkinson, J. M. 1978. The components of troponin from chicken fast skeletal muscle: A comparison of troponin T and troponin I from breast and leg muscle. *Biochem. J.* **169**:229–238.

Wilkinson, J. M. 1980. Troponin C from rabbit slow skeletal and cardiac muscle is the product of a single gene. *Eur. J. Biochem.* **103**:179–188.

Wilkinson, J. M., and Grand, R. J. A. 1978. Comparison of amino acid sequence of troponin I from different striated muscles. *Nature (London)* **271**:31–35.

Williams, N., and Eger, R. R. 1978. Purification and characterization of clonable murine granulocyte-macrophage precursor cell populations. *In*: Golde, D. W., Cline, M. J., Metcalf, D., and Fox, C. F., eds., *Hematopoietic Cell Differentiation,* New York, Academic Press, pp. 385–398.

Wilt, F. H. 1967. The control of embryonic hemoglobin synthesis. *Adv. Morphog.* **6**:89–125.

Wilt, F. H. 1974. The beginnings of erythropoiesis in the yolk sac of the chick embryo. *Ann. N.Y. Acad. Sci.* **241**:99–112.

Wolff, Et., and Wolff, Em. 1947. Sur les stades de réceptivité aux hormones femelles des gonades et des voies genitales chez l'embryon de poulet mâle. *C. R. Séances Soc. Biol.* **141**:415–416.

Wolff, Et., and Wolff, Em. 1951. The effects of castration on bird embryos. *J. Exp. Zool.* **116**:59–97.

Woodroofe, M. N., and Lemanski, L. F. 1981. Two actin variants in developing axolotl heart. *Dev. Biol.* **82**:172–179.

Yamada, K. M., and Olden, K. 1978. Fibronectins—Adhesive glycoproteins of cell surface and blood. *Nature (London)* **275**:179–184.

Yntema, C. L. 1959. Regeneration in sparsely innervated and aneurogenic forelimbs of *Ambystoma* larvae. *J. Exp. Zool.* **140**:101–124.

Yoffey, J. M. 1980. Transitional cells of hemopoietic tissues: Origin, structure, and development potential. *Int. Rev. Cytol.* **62**:311–359.

Zeichner, M., and Breitkreutz, D. 1978. Isolation of low molecular weight RNAs from connective tissue. *Arch. Biochem. Biophys.* **188**:410–417.

Zevin-Sonkin, D., and Yaffe, D. 1980. Accumulation of muscle-specific RNA sequences during myogenesis. *Dev. Biol.* **74**:326–334.

Zucker-Franklin, D. 1980. Ultrastructural evidence for the common origin of human mast cells and basophils. *Blood* **56**:534–540.

Zuckerman, S. 1940. The histogenesis of tissues sensitive to oestrogens. *Biol. Rev.* **15**:231–271.

Zwilling, E. 1961. Limb morphogenesis. *Adv. Morphog.* **1**:301–329.

CHAPTER 5

Agabian, N., Evinger, M., and Parker, G. 1979. Generation of asymmetry during development: Segregation of type-specific proteins in *Caulobacter. J. Cell Biol.* **81**:123–136.

Ahmed, Z. U., and Kamara, O. P. 1975. DNA content of dormant barley leaf nuclei and the synthesis of RNA and DNA during germination, *FEBS Lett.* **51**:277–280.

Ajtkhozhin, M. A., Doshchanov, K. I., and Akhanov, A. U. 1976. Informosomes as a stored form of mRNA in wheat embryo. *FEBS Lett.* **66**:124–126.

Allis, C. D., Glover, C. V. C., and Gorovsky, M. A. 1979. Micronuclei of *Tetrahymena* contain two types of histone H₃. *Proc. Natl. Acad. Sci. USA* **76**:4857–4861.

Allis, C. D., Glover, C. V. C., Bowen, J. K., and Gorovsky, M. A. 1980a. Histone variants specific to the transcriptionally active, amitotically dividing macronucleus of the unicellular eucaryote, *Tetrahymena thermophila. Cell* **20**:609–617.

Allis, C. D., Bowen, J. K., Abraham, G. N., Glover, C. V. C., and Gorovsky, M. A. 1980b. Proteolytic processing of histone H3 in chromatin: A physiologically regulated event in *Tetrahymena* micronuclei. *Cell* **20**:55–64.

Alton, T. H., and Brenner, M. 1979. Comparisons of proteins synthesized by anterior and posterior regions of *Dictyostelium discoideum* pseudoplasmodia. *Dev. Biol.* **71**:1–7.

Alton, T. H., and Lodish, H. F. 1977. Developmental changes in mRNAs and protein synthesis in *Dictyostelium discoideum. Dev. Biol.* **60**:180–206.

Ammermann, D. 1971. Morphology and development of the macronuclei of the ciliates *Stylonychia mytilus* and *Euplotes aediculatus. Chromosoma* **33**:209–238.

Ammermann, D., Steinbrück, G., von Berger, L., and Hennig, W. 1974. The development of the macronucleus in the ciliated protozoan *Stylonychia mytilus. Chromosoma* **45**:401–429.

Arima, K., and Oka, T. 1965. Cyanide resistance in *Achromobacter. J. Bacteriol.* **90**:734–743.

Arnaud, M., Mahler, I., Halvorson, H. O., Boschwitz, H., and Keynan, A. 1980. *In vitro* translation of mRNA from sporulating and nonsporulating strains of *B. subtilis. J. Bacteriol.* **142**:1045–1048.

Aspart, L., Cooke, R., and Delseny, M. 1979. Stability of polyadenylic and polyadenylated ribonucleic acids in radish (*Raphanus sativus*) seedlings. *Biochim. Biophys. Acta* **564**:43–54.

Bagshaw, J. C., Bernstein, R. S., and Bond, B. H. 1978. DNA-dependent RNA polymerases from *Artemia salina*: Decreasing polymerase activities and number of polymerase II molecules in developing larvae. *Differentiation* **10**:13–21.

Bakalkin, G. Y., Kalnov, S. L., Galkin, A. B., Zubatov, A. S., and Luzikov, V. N. 1978. The lability of the products of mitochondrial protein synthesis in *Saccharomyces cerevisiae. Biochem. J.* **170**:569–576.

Basha, S. M. M., and Beevers, L. 1976. Glycoprotein metabolism in the cotyledons of *Pisum sativum. Plant Physiol.* **57**:93–97.

Batts-Young, B., Maizels, N., and Lodish, H. F. 1977. Precursors of rRNA in the cellular slime mold, *Dictyostelium discoideum. J. Biol. Chem.* **252**:3952–3960.

Batts-Young, B., Lodish, H. F., and Jacobson, A. 1980. Similarity of the primary sequences of rRNAs isolated from vegetative and developing cells of *Dictyostelium discoideum. Dev. Biol.* **78**:352–364.

Bayen, M., and Dalmon, J. 1976. 5-Methylcytosine in *Chlorella pyrenoidosa* DNAs. *Biochim. Biophys. Acta* **432**:273–280.

Berking, S. 1977. Bud formation in hydra: Inhibition by an endogenous morphogen. *Wilhelm Roux Arch. Dev. Biol.* **181**:215–225.

Berking, S. 1979. Analysis of head and foot formation in *Hydra* by means of an endogenous inhibitor. *Wilhelm Roux Arch. Dev. Biol.* **186**:189–210.

Beug, H., Katz, F. E., and Gerisch, G. 1973. Dynamics of antigenic membrane sites relating to cell aggregation in *Dictyostelium discoideum. J. Cell Biol.* **56**:647–658.

Biedermann, M., and Drews, G. 1968. Trennung der Thylakoidbausteine einiger Athiorhodaceae durch Gelelektrophorese. *Arch. Mikrobiol.* **61**:48–58.

Biedermann, M., Drews, G., Marx, R., and Schröder, J. 1967. Der Einfluss des Sauerstoff partialdruckes und der Antibiotica Actinomycin und Puromycin. *Arch. Mikrobiol.* **56**:133–147.

Birndorf, H. C., D'Alessio, J., and Bagshaw, J. C. 1975. DNA-dependent RNA-polymerases from *Artemia* embryos: Characterization of polymerases I and II from nauplius larvae. *Dev. Biol.* **45**:34–43.

Blumberg, D. D., and Lodish, H. F. 1980a. Complexity of nuclear and polysomal RNAs in growing *Dictyostelium discoideum* cells. *Dev. Biol.* **78**:268–284.

Blumberg, D. D., and Lodish, H. F. 1980b. Changes in the mRNA population during differentiation of *Dictyostelium discoideum. Dev. Biol.* **78**:285–300.

Blumberg, D. D., and Lodish, H. F. 1981. Changes in the complexity of nuclear RNA during development of *Dictyostelium discoideum. Dev. Biol.* **81**:74–80.

Bode, H. G., and David, C. N. 1978. Regulation of a multipotent stem cell, the interstitial cell of *Hydra. Prog. Biophys. Mol. Biol.* **33**:189–206.

Bode, H. G., Flick, K. M., and Smith, G. S. 1976. Regulation of interstitial cell differentiation in *Hydra attenuata*. I. Homeostatic control of interstitial cell population size. *J. Cell Sci.* **20**:29–46.

Bonner, J. T. 1947. Evidence for the formation of cell aggregates by chemotaxis in the development of the slime mold *Dictyostelium discoideum. J. Exp. Zool.* **106**:1–26.

Bonner, J. T. 1949. The demonstration of acrosin in the later stages of development of the slime mold *Dictyostelium discoideum. J. Exp. Zool.* **110**:259–271.

Bonner, J. T. 1957. A theory of the control of differentiation in the cellular slime molds. *Q. Rev. Biol.* **32**:232–246.

Bonner, J. T. 1967. *The Cellular Slime Molds,* Princeton, N.J., Princeton University Press.

Brambl, R. M. 1975. Characteristics of developing mitochondrial genetic and respiratory functions in germinating fungal spores. *Biochim. Biophys. Acta* **396**:175–186.

Brambl, R. M. 1977. Mitochondrial biogenesis during fungal spore germination: Development of cytochrome *c* oxidase activity. *Arch. Biochem. Biophys.* **182**:273–281.

Brambl, R. M. 1980. Mitochondrial biogenesis during the fungal spore germination. *J. Biol. Chem.* **255**:7673–7680.

Brambl, R. M., and Josephson, M. 1977. Mitochondrial biogenesis during fungal spore germination. *J. Bacteriol.* **129**:291–297.

Brambl, R. M., and Van Etten, J. L. 1970. Protein synthesis during fungal spore germination. V. Evidence that the ungerminated conidiospores of *B. theobromae* contain mRNA. *Arch. Biochem. Biophys.* **137**:442–452.

Brenner, M. 1978. Cyclic AMP levels and turnover during development of the cellular slime mold *Dictyostelium discoideum. Dev. Biol.* **64**:210–223.

Campbell, R. D. 1976. Elimination of *Hydra* interstitial and nerve cells by means of colchicine. *J. Cell Sci.* **21**:1–13.

Campbell, R. D. 1979. Development of *Hydra* lacking interstitial and nerve cells (''epithelial hydra''). *Symp. Soc. Dev. Biol.* **37**:267–293.

Castor, L. N., and Chance, B. 1959. Photochemical determinations of the oxidases of bacteria. *J. Biol. Chem.* **234**:1587–1592.

Chapman, A. G., and Atkinson, D. E. 1977. Adenine nucleotide concentrations and turnover rates: Their correlation with biological activity in bacteria and yeast. *Adv. Microbiol. Physiol.* **15**:253–306.

Chen, D., Schultz, G., and Katchalski, E. 1971. Early rRNA transcription and appearance of cytoplasmic ribosomes during germination of the wheat embryo. *Nature New Biol.* **231**:69–72.

Cheung, S. C., Kobayashi, G. S., Schlessinger, D., and Medoff, G. 1974. RNA metabolism during morphogenesis in *Histoplasma capsulatum. J. Gen. Microbiol.* **82**:301–307.

Church, B. D., and Halvorson, H. 1957. Intermediate metabolism of aerobic spores. *J. Bacteriol.* **73**:470–476.

Clark, R. L., and Steck, T. L. 1979. Morphogenesis in *Dictyostelium*: An orbital hypothesis. *Science* **204**:1163–1168.

Cleffmann, G. 1968. Regulierung der DNS-Menge in Makronucleus von *Tetrahymena. Exp. Cell Res.* **50**:193–207.

Cleffmann, G. 1975. Amount of DNA produced during extra S-phases in *Tetrahymena. J. Cell Biol.* **66**:204–209.

Cleffmann, G. 1980. Chromatin elimination and the genetic organization of the macronucleus in *Tetrahymena thermophila. Chromosoma* **78**:313–325.

Cocucci, S. M., and Sussman, M. 1970. RNA in cytoplasmic and nuclear fractions of cellular slime mold amebas. *J. Cell Biol.* **45**:399–407.

Cost, H. B., and Gray, E. D. 1967. Rapidly labelled RNA synthesis during morphogenesis. *Biochim. Biophys. Acta* **138**:601–604.

Cotter, D. A., and Raper, K. B. 1966. Spore germination in *Dictyostelium discoideum. Proc. Natl. Acad. Sci. USA* **56**:880–887.

Cotter, D. A., and Raper, K. B. 1968. Properties of germinating spores of *Dictyostelium discoideum. J. Bacteriol.* **96**:1680–1689.

Cotter, D. A., Morin, J. W., and O'Connell, R. W. 1976. Spore germination in *Dictyostelium discoideum. Arch. Microbiol.* **108**:93–98.

Cuming, A. C., and Lane, B. G. 1978. Wheat embryo ribonucleates. XI. Conserved mRNA in dry wheat embryos and its relation to protein synthesis during early imbibition. *Can. J. Biochem.* **56**:365–369.

Cuming, A. C., and Lane, B. G. 1979. Protein synthesis in imbibing wheat embryos. *Eur. J. Biochem.* **99**:217–224.

D'Alesandro, M. M., Jaskot, R. H., and Dunham, V. L. 1980. Soluble and chromatin-bound DNA polymerases in developing soybean. *Biochem. Biophys. Res. Commun.* **94**:233–239.

D'Alessio, J. M., and Bagshaw, J. C. 1977. DNA-dependent RNA polymerases from *Artemia salina*. IV. Appearance of nuclear RNA polymerase activity during pre-emergence development of encysted embryos. *Differentiation* **8**:53–56.

D'Alessio, J. M., and Bagshaw, J. C. 1979. DNA-dependent RNA polymerases from *Artemia salina*. *Dev. Biol.* **70**:71–81.

David, C. N., and Gierer, A. 1974. Cell cycle kinetics and development of *Hydra attentuata*. III. Nerve and nematocyte differentiation. *J. Cell Sci.* **16**:359–375.

David, C. N., and Plotnick, I. 1980. Distribution of interstitial stem cells in *Hydra*. *Dev. Biol.* **76**:175–184.

Davis-Mancini, K., Lopez, I. P., and Hageman, J. H. 1978. Benzeneboronic acid selectively inhibits the sporulation of *Bacillus subtilis*. *J. Bacteriol.* **136**:625–630.

DeJesus, T. G. S., and Gray, E. D. 1971. Isoaccepting tRNA species in differing morphogenetic states of *Rhodopseudomonas spheroides*. *Biochim. Biophys. Acta* **254**:419–428.

Delseny, M., Aspart, L., and Guitton, Y. 1977. Disapperance of stored polyadenylic acid and mRNA during early germination of radish (*Raphanus sativus*) embryo axes. *Planta* **135**:125–128.

Deltour, R. 1970. Synthèse et translocations de RNA dans les cellules radiculaires de *Zea mays* au début de la germination. *Planta* **92**:235–239.

Deltour, R., and Jacqmard, A. 1974. Relation between water stress and DNA synthesis during germination of *Zea mays* L. *Ann. Bot.* **38**:529–534.

Deltour, R., Gautier, A., and Fakan, J. 1979. Ultrastructural cytochemistry of the nucleus in *Zea mays* embryos during germination. *J. Cell Sci.* **40**:43–62.

Deltour, R., Fransolet, S., and Loppes, R. 1981. Inorganic phosphate accumulation and phophatan activity in the nucleus of maize embryo root cells. *J. Cell Sci.* **47**:77–90.

Dillon, L. S. 1978. *The Genetic Mechanism and the Origin of Life*, New York, Plenum Press.

Dillon, L. S. 1981. *Ultrastructure, Macromolecules, and Evolution*, New York, Plenum Press.

Dini, F., and Luporini, P. 1979. Preconjugant cell interaction and cell cycle in the ciliate *Euplotes crassus*. *Dev. Biol.* **69**:506–516.

Dobrzanska, M., and Buchowicz, J. 1976. High molecular weight UMP-rich RNA of germinating wheat embryo. *Biochim. Biophys. Acta* **432**:73–79.

Doerder, F. P., and DeBault, L. E. 1978. Life cycle variation and regulation of macronuclear DNA content in *Tetrahymena thermophila*. *Chromosoma* **69**:1–19.

Dowbenko, D. J., and Ennis, H. L. 1980. Regulation of protein synthesis during spore germination in *Dictyostelium discoideum*. *Proc. Natl. Acad. Sci. USA* **77**:1791–1795.

Dunkle, L. D., Van Etten, J. L., and Brambl, R. M. 1972. Mitochondrial DNA synthesis during fungal spore germination. *Arch. Mikrobiol.* **85**:225–232.

Dzięgielewski, T., Kedzierski, W., and Pawetkiewicz, J. 1979. Levels of aminoacyl-tRNA synthetases, tRNA nucleotidyl-transferase and ATP in germinating lupin seeds. *Biochim. Biophys. Acta* **564**:37–42.

Edwards, S. W., and Lloyd, D. 1978. Oscillations of respiration and adenine nucleotides in synchronous cultures of *Acanthamoeba castellani*: Mitochondrial respiratory control *in vivo*. *J. Gen. Microbiol.* **108**:197–204.

Edwards, S. W., and Lloyd, D. 1980. Oscillations in protein and RNA content during synchronous growth of *Acanthamoeba castellani*. *FEBS Lett.* **109**:21–26.

Elsevier, S. M., Lipps, H. J., and Steinbrück, G. 1978. Histone genes in macronuclear DNA of the ciliate *Stylonychia mytilus*. *Chromosoma* **69**:291–306.

Esau, K. 1978. The protein inclusions in sieve elements of cotton (*Gossypium hirsutum* L.). *J. Ultrastruct. Res.* **63**:224–235.

Evinger, M., and Agabian, N. 1979. *Caulobacter crescentus* nucleoid: Analysis of sedimentation behavior and protein composition during the cell cycle. *Proc. Natl. Acad. Sci. USA* **76**:175–178.

Fakan, S., and Deltour, R. 1981. Ultrastructural visualization of nucleolar organizer activity during early germination of *Zea mays* L. In press.

Farnsworth, P. 1973. Experimentally induced aberrations in the pattern of differentiation in the cellular slime mold *Dictyostelium discoideum*. *J. Embryol. Exp. Morphol.* **31**:435–451.

Filipowicz, W., Furuichi, Y., Sierra, J. M., Muthukrishnan, S., Shatkin, A. J., and Ochoa, S. 1976. A protein binding the methylated 5′-terminal sequence, m⁷GpppN, of eurkaryotic mRNA. *Proc. Natl. Acad. Sci. USA* **:**1559–1563.

Forsee, W. T., Valkovitch, G., and Elbein, A. D. 1976. Glycoprotein biosynthesis in plants. *Arch. Biochem. Biophys.* **174**:469–479.

Frankel, J. 1973. The positioning of ciliary organelles in hypotrich ciliates. *J. Protozool.* **20**:8–18.

Frazier, W. A., Rosen, S. D., Reitherman, R. W., and Barondes, S. H. 1975. Purification and comparison of two developmentally regulated lectins from *Dictyostelium discoideum*. *J. Biol. Chem.* **250**:7714–7721.

Freiburg, M. 1981. Functional states of RNA polymerase in the macronucleus of *Tetrahymena pyriformis* and their dependence on culture growth. *J. Cell Sci.* **47**:267–275.

Fujisawa, T., and David, C. N. 1981. Commitment during nematocyte differentiation in *Hydra*. *J. Cell Sci.* **48**:207–222.

Fujishima, M., and Watanabe, T. 1981. Transplantation of germ nuclei in *Paramecium caudatum*. III. Role of germinal micronucleus in vegetative growth. *Exp. Cell Res.* **132**:47–56.

Furusawa, I., Nishiguchi, M., Tani, M., and Ishida, N. 1977. Evidence of early protein synthesis essential to the spore germination of *Colletotrichum lagenarium*. *J. Gen. Microbiol.* **101**:307–310.

Gerisch, G. 1979. Control circuits in cell aggregation and differentiation of *Dictyostelium discoideum*. *In*: Ebert, J. D., and Okada, T. S., eds., *Mechanisms of Cell Change*, New York, Wiley, pp. 225–239.

Gilder, J., and Cronshaw, J. 1973. Adenosine triphosphatase in the phloem of *Cucurbita*. *Planta* **110**:189–204.

Gliddon, R. 1966. Ciliary organelles and associated fiber systems in *Euplotes eurystomus*. *J. Cell Sci.* **1**:439–448.

Gomes, S. L., Mennucci, L., and da Costa Maia, J. C. 1978. Adenylate cyclase activity and cyclic AMP metabolism during cytodifferentiation of *Blastocladiella emersonii*. *Biochim. Biophys. Acta* **541**:190–198.

Gorovsky, M. A., and Keevert, J. B. 1975. Absence of histone F1 in a mitotically dividing, genetically inactive nucleus. *Proc. Natl. Acad. Sci. USA* **72**:2672–2676.

Gorovsky, M. A., Glover, C., Johmann, C. A., Keevert, J. B., Mathis, D. J., and Samuelson, M. 1978. Histones and chromatin structure in *Tetrahymena* macro- and micronuclei. *Cold Spring Harbor Symp. Quant. Biol.* **42**:493–503.

Gray, E. D. 1967. Studies on the adaptive formation of photosynthetic structures in *Rhodopseudomonas sphaeroides*. *Biochim. Biophys. Acta* **138**:550–563.

Grim, J. N. 1967. Ultrastructure of pellicular and ciliary structures of *Euplotes eurystomus*. *J. Protozool.* **14**:625–633.

Grimes, G. W. 1972. Cortical structure in nondividing and cortical morphogenesis in dividing *Oxytricha fallax*. *J. Protozool.* **19**:428–445.

Grimes, G. W. 1973. Differentiation during encystment and excystment in *Oxytricha fallax*. *J. Protozool.* **20**:92–104.

Grimes, G. W., and Adler, J. A. 1976. The structure and development of the dorsal bristle complex of *Oxytricha fallax* and *Stylonychia pustulata*. *J. Protozool.* **23**:135–143.

Grimes, G. W., and L'Hernault, S. W. 1978. The structure and morphogenesis of the ventral ciliature in *Paurostyla hymenophora*. *J. Protozool.* **25**:65–74.

Grimes, G. W., and L'Hernault, S. W. 1981. Cytogeometrical determination of ciliary pattern formation in the hypotrich ciliate *Stylonychia mytilus*. *Dev. Biol.*

Grimmelikhuijzen, C. J. P. 1979. Properties of the foot activator from *Hydra*. *Cell Differ.* **8**:267–273.

Grimmelikhuijzen, C. J. P., and Schaller, H. C. 1977. Isolation of a substance activating foot formation in hydra. *Cell Differ.* **6**:297–305.

Guha, S., and Szulmajster, J. 1977. Specific alteration of the 30S ribosomal subunits of *B. subtilis* during sporulation. *J. Bacteriol.* **131**:866–871.

Guilfoyle, T. J., and Malcolm, S. 1980. The amounts, subunit structures, and template-engaged activities of RNA polymerases in germinating soybean axes. *Dev. Biol.* **78**:113–125.

Hanlin, R. T. 1976. Phialide and conidium development in *Aspergillus clavatus*. *Am. J. Bot.* **63**:144–155.

Hereford, L. M., and Rosbash, M. 1977. Number and distribution of polyadenylated RNA sequences in yeast. *Cell* **10**:453–462.

Hiatt, V. S., and Snyder, L. A. 1973. Phenylalanine transfer RNA species in early development of barley. *Biochim. Biophys. Acta* **324**:57–68.

Hoefert, L. L. 1979. Ultrastructure of developing sieve elements in *Thlaspi arvense* L. I. The immature state. *Am. J. Bot.* **66**:925–932.

Hoefert, L. L. 1980. Ultrastructure of developing sieve elements in *Thlaspi arvense*. II. Maturation. *Am. J. Bot.* **67**:194–201.

Holloman, D. W. 1969. Biochemistry of germination in *Peronospora tabacina* (Adam) condia: Evidence for the existence of stable mRNA. *J. Gen. Microbiol.* **55**:267–274.

Holmes, P. K., and Levinson, H. S. 1967. Metabolic requirements for microcycle sporogenesis of *Bacillus megaterium*. *J. Bacteriol.* **94**:434–440.

Hotta, Y., and Hecht, N. 1971. Methylation of Lilium DNA during the meiotic cycle. *Biochim. Biophys. Acta* **238**:50–59.

Hultin, T., and Morris, J. E. 1968. The ribosomes of encysted embryos of *Artemia salina* during cryptobiosis and resumption of development. *Dev. Biol.* **17**:143–164.

Hussey, C., Losick, R., and Sonenshein, A. L. 1971. Ribosomal RNA synthesis is turned off during sporulation of *Bacillus subtilis*. *J. Mol. Biol.* **57**:59–70.

Inouye, M., Inouye, S., and Zusman, D. R. 1979. Gene expression during development of *Myxococcus xanthus*: Pattern of protein synthesis. *Dev. Biol.* **68**:579–591.

Jacquet, M., Part, D., and Felenbok, B. 1981. Changes in the polyadenylated mRNA population during development of *Dictyostelium discoideum*. *Dev. Biol.* **81**:155–166.

Jakob, K. M. 1972. RNA synthesis during the DNA synthesis period of the first cell cycle in the root meristem of germinating *Vicia faba*. *Exp. Cell Res.* **72**:370–376.

Jansing, R. L., Stein, J. L., and Stein, G. S. 1977. Activation of histone gene transcription by nonhistone chromosomal proteins in WI-38 human diploid fibroblasts. *Proc. Natl. Acad. Sci. USA* **74**:173–177.

Johmann, C. A., and Gorovsky, M. A. 1976. Purification and characterization of the histones associated with the macronucleus of *Tetrahymena*. *Biochemistry* **15**:1249–1256.

Johnson, C. B., Holloway, B. R., Smith, H., and Grierson, D. 1973. Isozymes of acid phosphates in germinating peas. *Planta* **115**:1–10.

Josephson, M., and Brambl, R. 1980. Mitochondrial biogenesis during fungal spore germination. *Biochim. Biophys. Acta* **606**:125–137.

Juliani, M. H., and da Costa Maia, J. C. 1979. Cyclic AMP-dependent and -independent protein kinases of the water mold, *Blastocladiella emersonii*. *Biochim. Biophys. Acta* **567**:347–356.

Juliani, M. H., Brochetto, M. R., and da Costa Maia, J. C. 1980. Changes in cAMP binding and protein kinase activities during growth and differentiation of *Blastocladiella emersonii*. *Cell Differ.* **8**:421–430.

Kahl, G., Schäfer, W., and Wechselberger, M. 1979. Changes in nonhistone chromosomal proteins during the development of potato tubers: Their involvement in wound- and hormone-induced processes. *Plant Cell Physiol.* **20**:1217–1228.

Kaur, S., and Jayaraman, K. 1979. Appearance of polyadenylated RNA species during sporulation in *Bacillus polymyxa*. *Biochem. Biophys. Res. Commun.* **86**:331–339.

Kay, R. R. 1979. Gene expression in *Dictyostelium discoideum*: Mutually antagonistic roles of cyclic-AMP and ammonia. *J. Embryol. Exp. Morphol.* **52**:171–182.

Kay, R. R., Town, C. D., and Gross, J. D. 1979. Cell differentiation in *Dictyostelium discoideum*. *Differentiation* **13**:7–14.

Kedzierski, W., and Pawelkiewicz, J. 1977. Effect of seed germination on levels of tRNA aminoacylation. *Phytochemistry* **16**:503–504

Keiding, J., and Andersen, H. A. 1978. Regulation of ribosomal RNA synthesis in *Tetrahymena pyriformis*. *J. Cell Sci.* **31**:13–23.

Keith, G., Rogg, H., Dirheimer, G., Menichi, B., and Heyman, T. 1976. Post-transcriptional modification of tyrosine tRNA as a function of growth in *B. subtilis*. *FEBS Lett.* **61**:120–123.

Kessin, R. H. 1973. RNA metabolism during vegetative growth and morphogenesis of the cellular slime mold, *Dictyostelium discoideum*. *Dev Biol.* **31**:242–251.

Kessler, D. 1967. Nucleic acid synthesis during and after mitosis in the slime mold, *Physarum polycephalum*. *Exp. Cell Res.* **45**:676–680.

Kish, V. M., and Kleinsmith, L. J. 1974. Nuclear protein kinases: Evidence for their heterogeneity, tissue specificity, substrate specificities, and differential responses to cAMP. *J. Biol. Chem.* **249**:750–760.

Kleinsmith, L. J. 1975. Phosphorylation of non-histone proteins in the regulation of chromosomal structure and function. *J. Cell. Physiol.* **85**:459–475.

Konijn, T. M. 1972. Cyclic AMP as a first messenger. *Adv. Cyclic Nucleotide Res.* **1**:17–31.

Konijn, T. M. 1974. The chemotactic effect of cAMP and its analogues in the Acrasiae. *Antibiot. Chemother. Basel* **19**:96–110.

Kumar, B. V., McMillan, R. A., Medoff, G., Gutwein, M., and Kobayashi, G. 1980. Comparison of the RNA polymerases from both phases of *Histoplasma capsulatum*. *Biochemistry* **19**:1080–1087.

Lauth, M. R., Spear, B. B., Heumann, J., and Prescott, D. M. 1976. DNA of ciliated protozoa: DNA sequence diminution during macromolecular development of *Oxytricha*. *Cell* **7**:67–74.

Lawn, R. M., Heumann, J. M., Herrick, G., and Prescott, D. M. 1973. The gene-size DNA molecules in *Oxytricha*. *Cold Spring Harbor Symp. Quant. Biol.* **2**:483–492.

Lerner, M. R., and Steitz, J. A. 1979. Antibodies to small nuclear RNAs complexed with proteins are produced by patients with systemic lupus erythematosus. *Proc. Natl. Acad. Sci. USA* **76**:5495–5499.

Lerner, M. R., Boyle, J. A., Mount, S. M., Wolin, S. J., and Steitz, J. A. 1980. Are snRNPs involved in splicing? *Nature (London)* **283**:220–224.

Li, S. C., and Li, Y. T. 1970. Studies on the glycosidases of jack bean meal. *J. Biol. Chem.* **245**:5153–5160.

Lipps, H. J., and Steinbrück, G. 1978. Free genes for rRNAs in the macronuclear genome of the ciliate *Stylonychia mytilus*. *Chromosoma* **69**:21–26.

Loomis, W. F. 1975. *Dictyostelium discoideum: A Developmental System*, New York, Academic Press.

Loomis, W. F. 1979. Biochemistry of aggregation in *Dictyostelium*. *Dev. Biol.* **70**:1–12.

Lovett, J. S. 1975. Growth and differentiation of the water mold *Blastocladiella emersonii*: Cytodifferentiation and the role of RNA and protein synthesis. *Bacteriol. Rev.* **39**:345–404.

Luporini, P., and Dallai, R. 1980. Sexual interaction of *Euplotes crassus*: Differentiation of cellular surfaces in cell-to-cell union. *Dev. Biol.* **77**:167–177.

Luporini, P., and Dini, F. 1975. Reationships between cell cycle and conjugation in three hypotrichs. *J. Protozool.* **22**:541–544.

Luporini, P., and Giachetti, C. 1980. Multiconjugant complexes of *Euplotes crassus*: An instance of coordination of nuclear events. *J. Protozool.* **27**:108–112.

Luporini, P., Bracchi, P., and Esposito, F. 1979. Specific contact-dependent cell-to-cell communication during preconjugant interaction of the ciliate *Euplotes crassus*. *J. Cell Sci.* **39**:201–213.

McClean, D. K., and Warner, A. H. 1971. Aspects of nucleic acid metabolism during development of the brine shrimp *Artemia salina*. *Dev. Biol.* **24**:88–105.

MacKechnie, I., and Hanson, R. S. 1968. Microcycle sporogenesis of *Bacillus cereus* in a chemically defined medium. *J. Bacteriol.* **95**:355–359.

McMillan, R. A., and Arceneaux, J. L. 1975. Alteration of tyrosine isoaccepting tRNA species in wild-type and asporogenous strains of *Bacillus subtilis*. *J. Bacteriol.* **122**:526–531.

McTavish, C., and Sommerville, J. 1980. Macronuclear DNA organization and transcription in *Paramecium primaurelia*. *Chromosoma* **78**:147–164.

Margolskee, J. P., and Lodish, H. F. 1980. The regulation of the synthesis of actin and two other proteins induced early in *Dictyostelium discoideum* development. *Dev. Biol.* **74**:50–64.

Marin, F. T. 1977. Regulation of development in *Dictyostelium discoideum*. II. Regulation of early cell differentiation by amino acid starvation and intercellular interaction. *Dev. Biol.* **60**:389–395.

Marin, F. T., Goyette-Boulay, M., and Rothman, F. G. 1980. Regulation of development in *Dictyostelium discoideum*. III. Carbohydrate-specific intercellular interactions in early development. *Dev. Biol.* **80**:301–312.

Melera, P. W. 1971. Nucleic acid metabolism in germinating onion. I. Changes in root tip nucleic acid during germination. *Plant Physiol.* **48**:73–81.

Menichi, B., and Heyman, T. 1976. Study of tyrosine tRNA modification in relation to sporulation in *Bacillus subtilis*. *J. Bacteriol.* **127**:268–280.

Mercer, J. A., and Soll, D. R. 1980. The complexity and reversibility of the timer for the onset of aggregation in *Dictyostelium*. *Differentiation* **16**:117–124.

Merrick, W. C., and Dure, L. S. 1972. The developmental biochemistry of cotton seed embryogenesis and germination. *J. Biol. Chem.* **247**:7988–7999.

Meyer, H., Mayer, E., and Hamel, E. 1971. Acid phosphatase in germinating lettuce—Evidence for partial activation. *Physiol. Plant.* **24**:95–101.

Milhausen, M., and Agabian, N. 1981. Regulation of polypeptide synthesis during *Caulobacter crescentus* development: 2-dimensional gel analysis. *J. Bacteriol.* **148**:163–173.

Miyake, A. 1978. Cell communication, cell union, and initiation of meiosis in ciliate conjugation. *Curr. Top. Dev. Biol.* **12**:37–82.

Muller, K., and Gerisch, G. 1978. A specific glycoprotein as the target site of adhesion blocking Fab in aggregating *Dictyostelium discoideum* cells. *Nature (London)* **274**:445–449.

Murray, C. D., Pun, P., and Strauss, N. 1974. Template specificity changes of DNA-dependent RNA polymerase in *B. subtilis* during sporulation. *Biochem. Biophys. Res. Commun.* **60**:295–303.

Murti, K. G. 1973. Electron-microscopic observations on the macronuclear development in *Stylonychia mytilus* and *Tetrahymena pyriformis*. *J. Cell Sci.* **13**:479–509.

Newell, P. C., Ellington, J. S., and Sussman, M. 1969. Synchrony of enzyme accumulation in a population of differentiating slime mold cells. *Biochim. Biophys. Acta* **177**:610–614.

Ng, A. M. L., Smith, J. E., and McIntosh, A. F. 1973. Conidiation of *Aspergillus niger* in continuous culture. *Arch. Mikrobiol.* **88**:119–126.

Nilsson, M. O., and Hultin, T. 1974. Characteristics and intracellular distribution of messenger-like RNA in encysted embryos of *Artemia salina*. *Dev. Biol.* **38**:138–149.

Nuske, J., and Eschrich, W. 1976. Synthesis of P-protein in mature phloem of *Cucurbita maxima*. *Planta* **132**:109–118.

Oberhäuser, R., and Kollmann, R. 1977. Cytochemische Charakterizierung des sogenannten "Freien Nucleolus" als Proteinkörper in den Siebelementen von *Passiflora coerulea*. *Z. Pflanzenphysiol.* **84**:61–75.

Oliver, P. T. P. 1972. Conidiophore and spore development in *Aspergillus nidulans*. *J. Gen. Microbiol.* **73**:45–54.

Otto, J. J., and Campbell, R. D. 1977. Budding in *Hydra attenuata*: Bud stages and fate map. *J. Exp. Zool.* **200**:417–428.

Palatnik, C. M., Storti, R. V., and Jacobson, A. 1979. Fractionation and functional analysis of newly synthesized and decaying mRNAs from vegetative cells of *Dictyostelium discoideum*. *J. Mol. Biol.* **128**:371–395.

Palatnik, C. M., Storti, R. V., Capone, A. K., and Jacobson, A. 1980. Messenger RNA stability in *Dictyostelium discoideum*: Does poly(A) have a regulatory role? *J. Mol. Biol.* **141**:99–118.

Payne, P. I. 1976. The long-lived mRNA of flowering plant seeds. *Biol. Rev.* **51**:339–363.

Peumans, W. J., Carlier, A. R., and Caers, L. I. 1978. Sedimentation properties of preformed messenger particles in dry rye embryo extracts. *Planta* **140**:171–176.

Peumans, W. J., Caers, L. I., and Carlier, A. R. 1979. Some aspects of the synthesis of long-lived RNPs in developing rye embryos. *Planta* **144**:485–490.

Pittilo, R. M., Ball, S. J., and Hutchison, W. M. 1980. The ultrastructural development of the macrogamete of *Eimeria stiedai*. *Protoplasma* **104**:33–41.

Preer, J. R., and Preer, L. B. 1979. The size of macromolecular DNA and its relationship to models for maintaining genic balance. *J. Protozool.* **26**:14–18.

Prescott, D. M. 1955. Relations between cell growth and cell division. *Exp. Cell Res.* **9**:328–337.

Prescott, D. M., and Murti, K. G. 1973. Chromosome structure in ciliated protozoans. *Cold Spring Harbor Symp. Quant. Biol.* **38**:609–618.

Pudek, M. R., and Bragg, P. D. 1974. Inhibition by cyanide of the respiratory chain oxidases of *E. coli*. *Arch. Biochem. Biophys.* **164**:682–693.

Randolph, L. F. 1936. Developmental morphology of the caryopsis in maize. *J. Agric. Res.* **53**:881–916.

Reitherman, R. W., Rosen, S. D., Frazier, W. A., and Barondes, S. H. 1975. Cell surface species-specific high affinity receptors for discoidin: Developmental regulation in *Dictyostelium discoideum*. *Proc. Natl. Acad. Sci. USA* **72**:3541–3545.

Rejman, E., and Buchowicz, J. 1973. RNA synthesis during the germination of wheat seed. *Phytochemistry* **12**:271–276.

Rhaese, H. J., and Groscurth, R. 1976. Control of development: Role of regulatory nucleotides synthesized by membranes of *Bacillus subtilis* in initiation of sporulation. *Proc. Natl. Acad. Sci. USA* **73**:331–335.

Rickenberg, H. V., Rahmsdorf, H. J., Campbell, A., North, M. J., Kwasniak, J., and Ashworth, J. M. 1975. Inhibition of development in *Dictyostelium discoideum* by sugars. *J. Bacteriol.* **124**:212–219.

Ro-Choi, T. S., and Busch, H. 1974. Low-molecular-weight nuclear RNA's. *In*: Busch, H., ed., *The Cell Nucleus*, New York, Academic Press, Vol. 3, pp. 151–208.

Rosen, S. D., Kafka, J. A., Simpson, D. L., and Barondes, S. H. 1973. Developmentally regulated, carbohydrate-binding protein in *Dictyostelium discoideum*. *Proc. Natl. Acad. Sci. USA* **70**:2554–2557.

Sacks, P. G., and Davis, L. E. 1980. Developmental dominance in *Hydra*. I. The basal disk. *Dev. Biol.* **80**:454–465.

Sakakibara, Y., Saito, H., and Ikeda, Y. 1965. Incorporation of radioactive amino acids and bases into nucleic acid and protein fractions of germinating spores of *Bacillus subtilis*. *J. Gen. Appl. Microbiol.* **11**:243–254.

Salamone, M. F., and Nachtway, D. S. 1979. Formation and fate of extranuclear chromatin bodies in *Tetrahymena*. *J. Protozool.* **26**:227–231.

Sanyal, S. 1966. Bud determination in hydra. *Indian J. Exp. Biol.* **4**:88–92.

Schaap, P., van der Molen, L., and Konijn, T. M. 1981. Development of the simple cellular slime mold *Dictyostelium minutum*. *Dev. Biol.* **85**:171–179.

Schaeffer, P., Millet, J., and Aubert, J. P. 1965. Catabolic repression of bacterial sporulation. *Proc. Natl. Acad. Sci. USA* **54**:704–711.

Schäfer, W., and Kahl, G. 1982. Phosphorylation of chromosomal proteins in resting and wounded potato (*Solanum tuberosum*) tuber tissue. *Plant Cell. Physiol.* **23**:137–146.

Schaller, H. C., and Gierer, A. 1973. Distribution of the head-activating substance in *Hydra* and its localization in membranous particles in nerve cells. *J. Embryol. Exp. Morphol.* **29**:39–52.

Schaller, H. C., Grimmelikhuijzen, C. J. P., Schmidt, T., and Bode, H. 1979a. Morphogenetic substances in nerve-depleted *Hydra. Wilhelm Roux Arch. Dev. Biol.* **187**:323–328.

Schaller, H. C., Schmidt, T., and Grimmelikhuijzen, C. J. P. 1979b. Separation and specificity of action of four morphogens from hydra. *Wilhelm Roux Arch. Dev. Biol.* **186**:139–150.

Schaller, H. C., Rau, T., and Bode, H. 1980. Epithelial cells in nerve-free hydra produce morphogenetic substances. *Nature (London)* **283**:589–591.

Scherbaum, H., Louderback, A. L., and Jahn, T. L. 1958. The formation of subnuclear aggregates in normal and synchronized protozoan cells. *Biol. Bull.* **115**:269–275.

Schmidt, T., and Schaller, H. C. 1976. Evidence for a foot-inhibiting substance in *Hydra. Cell Differ.* **5**:151–159.

Sekar, V., Wilson, S. P., and Hageman, J. H. 1981. Induction of *Bacillus subtilis* sporulation by nucleosides: Inosine appears to be sporogen. *J. Bacteriol.* **145**:489–493.

Setlow, P. 1975. Protein metabolism during germination of *Bacillus megaterium* spores. *J. Biol. Chem.* **250**:631–637.

Setlow, P., and Kornberg, A. 1970a. Biochemical studies of bacterial sporulation and germination. XXII. Energy metabolism in early stages of germination of *Bacillus megaterium* spores. *J. Biol. Chem.* **245**:3637–3644.

Setlow, P., and Kornberg, A. 1970b. Biochemical studies of bacterial sporulation and germination. XXIII. Nucleotide metabolism during spore germination. *J. Biol. Chem.* **245**:3645–3652.

Setlow, P., and Primus, G. 1975. Protein metabolism during germination of *Bacillus megaterium* spores. I. Protein synthesis and amino acid metabolism. *J. Biol. Chem.* **250**:623–630.

Sexton, R., Cronshaw, J., and Hall, J. L. 1971. A study of the biochemistry and cytochemical localization of β-glycerophosphatase activity in root tips of maize and pea. *Protoplasma* **73**:417–441.

Shepard, D. C. 1965. Production and elimination of excess DNA in ultraviolet irradiated *Tetrahymena. Exp. Cell Res.* **38**:570–579.

Shostak, S., and Kankel, D. 1967. Morphogenetic movements during budding in *Hydra. Dev. Biol.* **15**:451–463.

Sierra, J. M., Filipowicz, W., and Ochoa, S. 1976. Messenger RNA in undeveloped and developing *Artemia salina* embryos. *Biochem. Biophys. Res. Commun.* **69**:181–189.

Singhal, R. P., and Vold, B. 1976. Changes in tRNAs of *B. subtilis* during different growth phases. *Nucleic Acids Res.* **3**:1249–1261.

Siu, C. H., Lerner, R., Ma, G., Firtel, R., and Loomis, W. F. 1976. Developmentally regulated proteins of the plasma membrane of *Dictyostelium discoideum. J. Mol. Biol.* **100**:157–178.

Slobin, L. I., and Möller, W. 1977. The heavy form of EFI in *Artemia salina* embryos is functionally analogous to a complex of bacterial factors EF-Tu and EF-Ts. *Biochem. Biophys. Res. Commun.* **74**:356–365.

Sloma, A., and Smith, I. 1979. RNA synthesis during spore germination in *Bacillus subtilis. Mol. Gen. Genet.* **175**:113–120.

Smith, J. E., Anderson, J. G., Deans, S. G., and Davis, B. 1977. Asexual development in *Aspergillus. In*: Smith, J. E., and Pateman, J. A., eds., *Genetics and Physiology of Aspergillus*, New York, Academic Press, pp. 23–58.

Smith, L., White, D. C., Sinclair, P., and Chance, B. 1970. Rapid reactions of cytochromes of *Hemophilus parainfluenzae* on additions of substrates or oxygen. *J. Biol. Chem.* **245**:5096–5100.

Srinivasan, V. R., and Halvorson, H. O. 1963. Endogenous factor in the sporogenesis in bacteria. *Nature (London)* **197**:100–101.

Stein, G. S., Park, W., Thrall, C., Mans, R., and Stein, J. L. 1975. Regulation of cell-cycle stage-specific transcription of histone genes from chromatin by nonhistone chromosomal proteins. *Nature (London)* **257**:764–767.

Stein, G. S., Stein, J. L., Kleinsmith, L. J., Park, W., Jansing, R. L., and Thompson, J. A.

1976. Nonhistone chromosomal proteins and histone gene transcription. *Prog. Nucleic Acid Res. Mol. Biol.* **19**:421–445.

Sturani, E., Costantini, M. G., Martegani, E., and Alberghina, L. 1979. Level and turnover of poly(A)-containing RNA in *Neurospora crassa* in different steady states of growth. *Eur. J. Biochem.* **99**:1–7.

Sudo, S., and Dworkin, M. 1973. Comparative biology of prokaryotic resting cells. *Adv. Microbiol. Physiol.* **9**:153–224.

Sugiyama, T., and Fujisawa, T. 1978. Genetic analysis of developmental mechanisms in *Hydra*. II. Isolation and characterization of an interstitial cell-deficient strain. *J. Cell Sci.* **29**:35–52.

Sussman, M., and Brackenbury, R. 1976. Biochemical and molecular genetic aspects of cellular slime mold development. *Annu. Rev. Plant Physiol.* **27**:229–265.

Sweet, W. J., and Peterson, J. A. 1978. Changes in cytochrome content and electron transport pattern in *Pseudomonas putida* as a function of growth phase. *J. Bacteriol.* **133**:217–224.

Tannreuther, G. 1919. The migration of reproductive organs from parents to buds in *Hydra*. *Biol. Bull.* **37**:418–422.

Testa, D., and Rudner, R. 1975. Synthesis of ribosomal RNA during sporulation in *Bacillus subtilis*. *Nature (London)* **254**:630–632.

Theiss, G., and Follmann, H. 1980. 5-Methylcytosine formation in wheat embryo DNA. *Biochem. Biophys. Res. Commun.* **94**:291–297.

Thompson, E. W., and Lane, B. G. 1980. Relation of protein synthesis in imbibing wheat embryos to the cell-free translational capacities of bulk mRNA from dry and imbibing embryos. *J. Biol. Chem.* **255**:5965–5970.

Thompson, J. A., Stein, J. L., Kleinsmith, L. J., and Stein, G. S. 1976. Activation of histone gene transcription by nonhistone chromosomal phosphoproteins. *Science* **194**:428–431.

Timberlake, W. E. 1980. Developmental gene regulation in *Aspergillus nidulans*. *Dev. Biol.* **78**:497–510.

Toda, K., Ono, K. I., and Ochiai, H. 1980. Surface labeling of membrane glycoproteins and their drastic changes during development of *Dictyostelium discoideum*. *Eur. J. Biochem.* **111**:377–388.

Tokunaga, M., Tokunaga, J., and Harada, K. 1973. Scanning and transmission electron microscopy of sterigma and conidiospore formation in *Aspergillus* group. *J. Electron Microsc.* **22**:27–38.

Trewavas, A. 1976. Post-translational modification of proteins by phosphorylation. *Annu. Rev. Plant Physiol.* **27**:349–374.

Vale, V. L., Gomes, S. L., Maia, J. C. C., and Mennucci, L. 1976. Transient cyclic AMP accumulation in germinating zoospores of *Blastocladiella emersonii*. *FEBS Lett.* **67**:189–192.

Van de Walle, C. 1971. MAK column chromatography of the first RNA synthesized during germination of *Zea mays* embryos. *FEBS Lett.* **16**:219–222.

Vanyushin, B. F., and Belozerskii, A. N. 1959. A comparative study of the composition of DNA in higher plants. *Dokl. Akad. Nauk SSSR* **127**:196–199.

Varner, J. E. 1965. Seed development and germination. *In*: Bonner, J., and Varner, J. E., eds., *Plant Biochemistry*, New York, Academic Press, pp. 763–792.

Varnum, B., and Soll, D. R. 1981. Chemoresponsiveness to cAMP and folic acid during growth, development, and dedifferentiation in *Dictyostelium discoideum*. *Differentiation* **18**:151–160.

Venugopal, G., and David, C. N. 1981a. Nerve commitment in *Hydra*. I. Role of morphogenetic signals. *Dev. Biol.* **83**:353–360.

Venugopal, G., and David, C. N. 1981b. Nerve commitment in *Hydra*. II. Localization of commitment in S phase. *Dev. Biol.* **83**:361–365.

Verni, F., Rosati, G., and Luporini, P. 1978. Preconjugant cell–cell interaction in the ciliate *Euplotes crassus*: A possible role of the ciliary ampules. *J. Exp. Zool.* **204**:171–179.

Vold, B. S. 1974. Degree of completion of 3′-terminus of transfer ribonucleic acids of *Bacillus subtilis* 168 at various developmental stages and asporogenous mutants. *J. Bacteriol.* **117**:1361–1362.

Vold, B. S. 1978. Post-transcriptional modifications of the anticodon loop region: Alterations in isoaccepting species of tRNAs during development in *B. subtilis*. *J. Bacteriol.* **135**:124–132.

Vold, B. S., and Sypherd, P. S. 1968. Modification in transfer RNA during the differentiation of wheat seedlings. *Proc. Natl. Acad. Sci. USA* **59**:453–458.

Walbot, V. 1972. Development and differentiation of haploid *Lycopersicon esculentum* (tomato). *Planta* **108**:161–171.

Wallace, L. J., and Frazier, W. A. 1979. Photoaffinity labeling of cyclic-AMP- and AMP-binding proteins of differentiating *Dictyostelium discoideum* cells. *Proc. Natl. Acad. Sci. USA* **76**:4250–4254.

Wanek, N., Marcum, B. A., and Campbell, R. D. 1980. Histological structure of epithelial hydra and evidence for the complete absence of interstitial and nerve cells. *J. Exp. Zool.* **212**:1–11.

Wang, T. Y., Kostraba, N. C., and Newman, R. S. 1976. Selective transcription of DNA mediated by nonhistone proteins. *Prog. Nucleic Acid Res. Mol. Biol.* **19**:447–462.

Webster, G. 1971. Morphogenesis and pattern formation in hydroids. *Biol. Rev.* **46**:1–46.

Weinberg, R. A., and Penman, S. 1968. Small molecular weight monodisperse nuclear RNA. *J. Mol. Biol.* **38**:289–304.

Wenzler, H., and Brambl, R. M. 1978. *In vitro* translation of poly(A)-containing RNAs from dormant and germinating spores of the fungus *Botryodiplodia theobromae*. *J. Bacteriol.* **135**:1–9.

Wielgat, B., and Kahl, G. 1979. Gibberellic acid activates chromatin-bound DNA-dependent RNA polymerase in wounded potato tuber tissue. *Plant Physiol.* **64**:867–871.

Wielgat, B., Wechselberger, M., and Kahl, G. 1979. Age-dependent variations in transcriptional response to wounding and gibberellic acid in a higher plant. *Planta* **147**:205–209.

Wise, J. A., and Weiner, A. M. 1980. Dictyostelium small nuclear RNA D2 is homologous to rat nucleolar RNA U3 and is encoded by a dispersed multigene family. *Cell* **22**:109–118.

Wise, J. A., and Weiner, A. M. 1981. The small nuclear RNAs of the cellular slime mold *Dictyostelium discoideum*. *J. Biol. Chem.* **256**:956–963.

Wolpert, L., Hicklin, J., and Hornbruch, A. 1971. Positional information and pattern regulation in regeneration of hydra. *Symp. Soc. Exp. Biol.* **25**:391–417.

Wolpert, L., Hornbruch, A., and Clarke, M. R. B. 1974. Positional information and positional signalling in hydra. *Am. Zool.* **14**:647–663.

Yao, M., and Gorovsky, M. A. 1974. Comparison of the sequences of macro- and micronuclear DNA of *Tetrahymena pyriformis*. *Chromosoma* **48**:1–48.

Yi, C. K. 1981. Increase in β-*N*-acetylglucosaminidase activity during germination of cotton seeds. *Plant Physiol.* **67**:68–73.

Zieve, G., and Penman, S. 1976. Small RNA species of the HeLa cell: Metabolism and subcellular localization. *Cell* **8**:19–31.

Zimmermann, C. R., Orr, W. C., Leclerc, R. F., Barnard, E. C., and Timberlake, W. E. 1980. Molecular cloning and selection of genes regulated in *Aspergillus* development. *Cell* **21**:709–715.

Zonneveld, B. J. M. 1977. Biochemistry and ultrastructure of sexual development in *Aspergillus*. *In*: Smith, J. E., and Pateman, J. A., eds., *Genetics and Physiology of Aspergillus*, New York, Academic Press, pp. 59–80.

CHAPTER 6

Adler, W. H., Takiguchi, T., and Smith, R. T. 1971. Effect of age upon primary alloantigen recognition by mouse spleen cells. *J. Immunol.* **107**:1357–1362.

Albertsson, P. Å., and Baird, G. D. 1962. Counter-current distribution of cells. *Exp. Cell Res.* **28**:296–322.

Albrecht, E. D. 1981. Effect of aging and adrenocorticotropin on adrenal Δ^5-3β-hydroxysteroid dehydrogenase activity in male rats. *Exp. Aging Res.* **7**:11–15.

Albrecht, E. D., Koos, R. D., and Wehrenberg, W. B. 1977. Aging and adrenal Δ^5-3β-hydroxy-steroid dehydrogenase in female mice. *J. Endocrinol.* **73**:193–194.

Arutyunyan, G. S., Mashkovskii, M. D., and Roshchina, L. F. 1964. Pharmacological properties of melatonin. *Fed. Proc.* **23**:T1330–T1332.

Aschoff, J. 1955. Jahresperiodik der Fortpflanzung bei Warmblütern. *Stud. Gen.* **8**:742–776.

Axelrod, J. A., and Weissbach, H. 1961. Purification and properties of hydroxyindole-*O*-methyl-transferase. *J. Biol. Chem.* **236**:211–213.

Axelrod, J. A., and Zatz, M. 1977. The β-adrenergic receptor and the regulation of circadian rhythms in the pineal gland. *In*: Litwack, G., ed., *Biochemical Actions of Hormones*, New York, Academic Press, Vol. 4, pp. 249–268.

Bakke, J. L., and Lawrence, N. 1965. Circadian periodicity in thyroid stimulating hormone titer in the rat hypophysis and serum. *Metabolism* **14**:841–843.

Balthazart, J., and Hendrick, J. 1976. Annual variation in reproductive behavior, testosterone, and plasma FSH levels in the Rouen duck *Anas platyrhynchos*. *Gen. Comp. Endocrinol.* **28**:171–183.

Barchas, J., DaCosta, F., and Spector, S. 1967. Acute pharmacology of melatonin. *Nature (London)* **214**:919–920.

Barkman, R. C. 1978. The use of otolith growth rings to age young Atlantic silversides, *Menidia menidia*. *Trans. Am. Fish. Soc.* **107**:790–792.

Barnett, A. 1969. Cell division: A second circadian clock system in *Paramecium multimicronu-cleatum*. *Science* **164**:1417–1419.

Bates, R. W., Riddle, O., and Lahr, E. L. 1937. Mechanism of the antigonadal action of prolactin in adult pigeons. *Am. J. Physiol.* **119**:610–614.

Bayliss, M. T., and Ali, S. Y. 1978. Age-related changes in the composition and structure of human articular-cartilage proteoglycans. *Biochem. J.* **176**:683–693.

Beaupain, R., Icard, C., and Macieira-Coelho, A. 1980. Changes in DNA alkali-sensitive sites during senescence and establishment of fibroblasts *in vitro*. *Biochim. Biophys. Acta* **606**:251–261.

Benoit, J. 1936. Facteurs externes et internes de l'activité sexuelle. *Bull. Biol. Fr. Belg.* **70**:487–533.

Berger, J. 1980. Circannual rhythms in the blood picture of laboratory rats. *Folia Haematol. Leipzig* **107**:54–60.

Berger, J. 1981. Seasonal variations in reticulocyte counts in blood of laboratory mice and rats. *Z. Versuchstierkd.* **23**:8–12.

Berthold, P., and Querner, U. 1981. Genetic basis of migratory behavior in European warblers. *Science* **212**:77–79.

Berumen, L., and Macieira-Coelho, A. 1977. Changes in albumin uptake during the lifespan of human fibroblasts *in vitro*. *Mech. Aging Dev.* **6**:165–172.

Bianchi, D. E. 1964. An endogenous circadian rhythm in *Neurospora crassa*. *J. Gen. Microbiol.* **35**:437–445.

Binkley, S. A. 1974. Pineal and melatonin: Circadian rhythms and body temperatures of sparrows. *In*: Scheving, L. E., Halberg, F., and Pauly, J. E., eds., *Chronobiology*, Tokyo, Igaku Shoin, pp. 582–585.

Birks, E. K., and Ewing, R. D. 1981a. Characterization of hydroxyindole-*O*-methyltransferase (HIOMT) from the pineal gland of chinook salmon (*Oncorhynchus tshawytscha*). *Gen. Comp. Endocrinol.* **43**:269–276.

Birks, E. K., and Ewing, R. D. 1981b. Photoperiod effects on hydroxyindole-*O*-methyltransferase activity in the pineal gland of chinook salmon (*Oncorhynchus tshawytscha*). *Gen. Comp. Endocrinol.* **43**:277–283.

Bolla, R., and Brot, N. 1975. Age dependent changes in enzymes involved in macromolecular synthesis in *Turbatrix aceti*. *Arch. Biochem. Biophys.* **169**:227–236.

Bortels, H. 1959. Synchronbeobachtungen über Beziehungen physikalischchemischer und mikrobiologischer Renktionen zu Luftdruckänderungen in und bei Braunschweig. *Arch. Meteorol. Geophys. Bioklimatol. Ser. B* **9**:464–486.

Boyd, E. 1932. The weight of the thymus gland in health and disease. *Am. J. Dis. Child.* **43**:1162–1214.

Bradbury, E. M., Inglis, R. J., and Matthews, H. R. 1974. Control of cell division by very lysine rich histone (F1) phosphorylation. *Nature (London)* **247**:257–261.

Brady, J. 1969. How are insect circadian rhythms controlled? *Nature (London)* **223**:781–784.

Breaux, C. B., and Meier, A. H. 1971. Diurnal periodicity in the effectiveness of prolactin to inhibit metamorphosis in *Rana pipiens* tadpoles. *Am. Midl. Nat.* **85**:267–271.

Brody, S., and Martins, S. A. 1976. Circadian rhythms in *Neurospora*: The role of unsaturated fatty acids. *In*: Hastings, J. W., and Schweiger, H. G., eds., *The Molecular Basis of Circadian Rhythms*, Berlin, Dahlem Konferenzen, pp. 245–246 (abstract).

Brown, A. J. P., and Hardman, N. 1980. Utilization of polyadenylated mRNA during growth and starvation in *Physarum polycephalum*. *Eur. J. Biochem.* **110**:413–420.

Brown, A. J. P., and Hardman, N. 1981. The effect of age on the properties of poly(A)-containing mRNA in *Physarum polycephalum*. *J. Gen. Microbiol.* **122**:143–150.

Brown, F. A. 1978. Interrelations between biological rhythms and clocks. *In:* Samis, H. V., and Capobianco, S., eds., *Aging and Biological Rhythms,* New York, Plenum Press, pp. 215–234.

Bruce, V. G., 1970. The biological clock in *Chlamydomonas reinhardi. J. Protozool.* **17**:328–334.

Bruce, V. G., 1972. Mutants of the biological clock in *Chlamydomonas reinhardi. Genetics* **70**:537–548.

Bruce, V. G., 1974. Recombinants between clock mutants of *Chlamydomonas reinhardi. Genetics* **77**:221–230.

Bruce, V. G., 1976. Clock mutants. *In:* Hastings, J. W., and Schweiger, H. G., eds., *The Molecular Basis of Circadian Rhythms,* Berlin, Dahlem Konferenzen, pp. 339–351.

Bruce, V. G., and Pittendrigh, C. S. 1957. Resetting the euglena clock with a single light stimulus. *Am. Nat.* **92**:295–306.

Bünning, E. 1936. Die endonome Tagesrhymik als Grundlage der photoperiodischen Reaktion. *Ber. Dtsch. Bot. Ges.* **54**:590–607.

Bünning, E. 1973. *The Physiological Clock,* revised 3rd ed., Berlin, Springer-Verlag.

Bunt, A. H. 1971. Enzymatic digestion of synaptic ribbons in amphibian retinal photoreceptors. *Brain Res.* **25**:571–577.

Burnet, F. M. 1970. *Immunological Surveillance,* Elmsford, N.Y., Pergamon Press.

Burns, E. R., Scheving, L. E., and Tsai, T. 1972. Circadian rhythm in uptake of tritiated thymidine by kidney, parotid, and duodenum of isoproterenol-treated mice. *Science* **175**:71–73.

Cahn, R. D., Kaplan, N. O., Levine, L., and Zwilling, E. 1962. Nature and development of lactic dehydrogenases. *Science* **136**:962–969.

Campbell, R. R., Etches, R. J., and Leatherland, J. F. 1981. Seasonal changes in plasma prolactin concentration and carcass lipid levels in the lesser snow goose (*Anser caerulescens caerulescens*). *Comp. Biochem. Physiol.* **68A**:653–657.

Chadwick, C. S. 1940. Identity of prolactin with water drive factor in *Triturus viridescens. Proc. Soc. Exp. Biol. Med.* **45**:335–337.

Chan, A. C., Ng, S. K. C., and Walter, I. G. 1976. Reduced DNA repair during differentiation of a myogenic cell line. *J. Cell Biol.* **70**:685–691.

Chetsanga, C. J., and Liskiwskyi, M. 1979. Decrease in specific activity of heart and muscle aldolase in old mice. *Int. J. Biochem.* **8**:753–756.

Chetsanga, C. J., Tuttle, M., Jacoboni, A., and Johnson, C. 1977. Age-associated structural alterations in senescent mouse brain DNA. *Biochim. Biophys. Acta* **474**:180–187.

Cleaver, J. E. 1977. Nucleosome structure controls rates of excision repair in DNA of human cells. *Nature (London)* **270**:451–453.

Comfort, A. 1979. *The Biology of Senescence,* 3rd ed., Amsterdam, Elsevier.

Cremer, T., Werdan, K., Stevenson, A. F. G., Lehner, K., and Messerschmidt, O. 1981. Aging *in vitro* and D-glucose uptake kinetics of diploid human fibroblasts *J. Cell. Physiol.* **106**:99–108.

Cuello, A. C., and Tramezzani, J. H. 1969. The epiphysis cerebri of the Weddell seal: Its remarkable size and glandular pattern. *Gen. Comp. Endocrinol.* **12**:154–164.

Cunningham, A. J. 1976. Self-tolerance maintained by active suppressor mechanisms. *Transplant. Rev.* **31**:23–43.

Cusick, F. J., and Cole, H. 1959. An improved method of breeding golden hamsters. *Tex. Rep. Biol. Med.* **17**:201–204.

Deitzner, G. F., Kempf, O., Fischer, S., and Wagner, E. 1974. Rhythmic control of enzymes involved in the tricarboxylic-acid cycle and the oxidative pentose-phosphate pathway in *Chenopodium rubrum* L. *Planta* **117**:29–41.

Dell'Orco, R. T., and Anderson, L. E. 1981. Unscheduled DNA synthesis in human diploid cells of different donor ages. *Cell Biol. Int. Rep.* **5**:359–364.

Díaz-Jouanen, E., Strickland, R. G., and Williams, R. C. 1975. Studies of human lymphocytes in the newborn and the aged. *Am. J. Med.* **58**:620–628.

Dieckmann, C., and Brody, S. 1980. Circadian rhythms in *Neurospora crassa:* Oligomycin-resistant mutations affect periodicity. *Science* **207**:896–898.

Dikstein, S. 1971. Stimulability, adenosine triphosphatases and their control by cellular redox processes. *Naturwissenschaften* **58**:439–443.

Dillon, L. S. 1978. *The Genetic Mechanism and the Origin of Life,* New York, Plenum Press.

Dillon, L. S. 1981. *Ultrastructure, Macromolecules, and Evolution,* New York, Plenum Press.

Donham, R. S. 1979. Annual cycle of plasma LH and sex hormones in male and female mallards. *Biol. Reprod.* **21**:1273–1285.

Donofrio, R. J., and Reiter, R. J. 1972. Depressed pituitary prolactin levels in blinded anosmic female rats: Role of the pineal gland. *J. Reprod. Fertil.* **31**:159–162.

Dons, R. F., Corash, L. M., and Gorden, P. 1981. The insulin receptor is an age-dependent integral component of the human erythrocyte membrane. *J. Biol. Chem.* **256**:2982–2987.

Dunkelberger, D. G., Dean, J. M., and Watabe, N. 1980. The ultrastructure of the otolithic membrane and otolith in the juvenile mummichog, *Fundulus heteroclitus. J. Morphol.* **163**:367–377.

Dunn, G. R., and Stevens, L. C. 1970. Determination of sex of teratomas derived from early mouse embryos. *J. Natl. Cancer Inst.* **44**:99–105.

Dusseau, J., and Meier, A. H. 1971. Diurnal and seasonal variation of plasma adrenal steroid hormone in the white-throated sparrow, *Zonotrichia albicollis. Gen. Comp. Endocrinol.* **16**:399–408.

Edmunds, L. N., and Adams, K. J. 1981. Clocked cell cycle clocks. *Science* **211**:1002–1013.

Edmunds, L. N., Sulzman, F. M., and Walther, W. G. 1974. Circadian oscillations in enzyme activity in *Euglena* and their relation to the circadian rhythm of cell division. *In:* Scheving, L. E., Halberg, F., and Pauly, J. E., eds., *Chronobiology,* Tokyo, Igaku Shoin, pp. 61–66.

Eguchi, E., Waterman, T. H., and Akiyama, J. 1973. Localization of the violet and yellow receptor cells in the crayfish retinula. *J. Gen. Physiol.* **62**:355–374.

Ellison, N., Weller, J. L., and Klein, D. C. 1972. Development of a circadian rhythm in the activity of pineal serotonin N-acetyltransferase. *J. Neurochem.* **19**:1335–1341.

Esser, K., and Kuenen, R. 1967. *Genetics of Fungi,* Berlin, Springer-Verlag.

Etkin, W., and Gona, A. G. 1967. Antagonism between prolactin and thyroid hormone in amphibian development. *J. Exp. Zool.* **165**:249–258.

Evans, L. T., and King, R. W. 1969. Role of phytochrome in photoperiodic induction of *Pharbitis nil. Z. Pflanzenphysiol.* **60**:277–288.

Farner, D. S. 1970. Predictive functions in the control of annual cycles. *Environ. Res.* **3**:119–131.

Feldman, J. F., and Hoyle, M. N. 1973. Isolation of circadian clock mutants of *Neurospora crassa*. *Genetics* **75**:605–613.

Feldman, J. F., and Hoyle, M. N. 1974. A direct comparison between circadian and non-circadian rhythms in *Neurospora*. *Plant Physiol.* **53**:928–930.

Feldman, J. F., Hoyle, M. N., and Shelgren, J. 1973. Carcadian clock mutants of *Neurospora crassa*: Genetic and physiological characteristics. *Genetics* **74**:S77–S78.

Fellini, S. A., Pacifici, M., and Holtzer, H. 1981. Changes in the sulfated proteoglycans synthesized by "aging" chondrocytes. II. Organ-cultured vertebral columns. *J. Biol. Chem.* **256**:1038–1043.

Fondeville, J. C., Borthwick, H. A., and Hendricks, S. D. 1966. Leaflet movement of *Mimosa pudica* L. indicative of phytochrome action. *Planta* **69**:357–364.

Frosch, S., and Wagner, E. 1973. Endogenous rhythmicity and energy transduction. II. Phytochrome action and the conditioning of rhythmicity of adenylate kinase, NAD- and NADP-linked glyceraldehyde-3-phosphate dehydrogenase in *Chenopodium rubrum* by temperature and light intensity cycles during germination. *Can. J. Bot* **51**:1521–1528.

Frosch, S., Wagner, E., and Cumming, E. G. 1973. Endogenous rhythmicity and energy transduction. I. Rhythmicity in adenylate kinase, NAD- and NADP-linked glyceraldehyde-3-phosphate dehydrogenase in *Chenopodium rubrum*. *Can. J. Bot.* **51**:1355–1362.

Fry, M., Loeb, L. A., and Martin, G. M. 1981. On the activity and fidelity of chromatin-associated hepatic DNA polymerase-β in aging murine species of different life spans. *J. Cell. Physiol.* **106**:435–444.

Fujimoto, M., Kanaya, A., Nakabou, Y., and Hagihira, H. 1978. Circadian rhythm in the ornithine decarboxylase activity of rat small intestine. *J. Biochem.* **83**:237–242.

Gaston, S., and Menaker, M. 1968. Pineal function: The biological clock in the sparrow? *Science* **160**:1125–1127.

Gaubatz, J., Ellis, M., and Chalkley, R. 1979. The structural organization of mouse chromatin as a function of age. *Fed. Proc.* **38**:1973–1978.

Gerisch, G. 1976. Cyclic-AMP oscillation and signal transmission in aggregating *Dictyostelium* cells. *In*: Hastings, J. W., and Schweiger, H. G., eds., *The Molecular Basis of Circadian Rhythms*, Berlin, Dahlem Konferenzen, pp. 433–440.

Glick, D., Ferguson, R. B., Greenberg, L. I., and Halberg, F. 1961. Circadian studies on succinic dehydrogenase, pantothenate and biotin of rodent adrenal. *Am. J. Physiol.* **200**:811–814.

Goldsmith, P. K., and Stetten, M. R. 1979. Different developmental changes in latency for two functions of a single membrane bound enzyme—Glucose-6-phosphate activities as a function of age. *Biochim. Biophys. Acta* **583**:133–147.

Gorski, R. A., Mennin, S. P., and Kubo, K. 1975. The neural and hormonal bases of the reproductive cycle of the rat. *In*: Hedlund, L. W., Franz, J. M., and Kenny, A. D., eds., *Biological Rhythms and Endocrine Function*, New York, Plenum Press, pp. 115–153.

Goss, R. J. 1980. Photoperiod control of antler cycles in deer. V. Reversed seasons. *J. Exp. Zool.* **211**:101–105.

Grant, W. C. 1961. Special aspects of the metamorphic process—Second metamorphosis. *Am. Zool.* **1**:163–171.

Grant, W. C., and Grant, J. A. 1958, Water drive studies on hypo-physectomized effects of *Diemyctylus viridescens*. Part 1. The role of lactogenic hormone. *Biol. Bull.* **114**:1–9.

Gupta, S. K., and Rothstein, M. 1976. Phosphoglycerate kinase from young and old *Turbatrix aceti*. *Biochim. Biophys. Acta* **445**:632–644.

Gwinner, E., Turek, F. W., and Smith, Z. D. 1971. Extraocular light perception in photoperiodic responses of the white-crowned sparrow (*Zonotrichia leucophrys*) and of the golden-crowned sparrow (*Z. atricapilla*). *Z. Vgl. Physiol.* **75**:323–331.

Haase, E., Sharp, P. J., and Paulke, E. 1975a. Annual cycle of plasma luteinizing hormone concentrations in wild mallard drakes. *J. Exp. Zool.* **194**:553–558.

Haase, E., Sharp. P. J., and Paulke, E. 1975b. Seasonal changes in plasma LH levels in domestic ducks. *J. Reprod. Fertil.* **44**:591–594.

Hafner, G. S., Hammond-Soltis, G., and Tokarski, T. 1980. Diurnal changes of lysosome-related bodies in the crayfish photoreceptor cells. *Cell Tissue Res.* **206**:319–332.

Halaban, R., and Hillman, W. S. 1974. Photoperiodic time measurement in a short-day-plant: Effects of the external medium. *In:* Scheving, L. E., Halberg, F., and Pauly, J. E., eds., *Chronobiology,* Tokyo, Igaku Shoin, pp. 666–670.

Halberg, F., Halberg, F., and Giese, A. 1974. Circannual biochemical and gonadal index rhythms of marine invertebrates *In:* Scheving, L. E., Halberg, F., and Pauly, J. E., eds., *Chronobiology,* Tokyo, Igaku Shoin, pp. 703–708.

Harley, C. B., Pollard, J. W., Chamberlain, J. W., Stanners, C. P., and Goldstein, S. 1980. Protein synthetic errors do not increase during aging of cultured human fibroblasts. *Proc. Natl. Acad. Sci. USA* **77**:1885–1889.

Harold, F. M. 1972. Conservation and transformation of energy by bacterial membranes. *Bacteriol. Rev.* **36**:172–230.

Hart, R. W., and Modak, S. P. 1980. Aging and changes in genetic information. *In*: Oota, K., Makinodan, T., Iriki, M., and Baker, L. S., eds., *Aging Phenomena: Relationships around Different Levels of Organization,* New York, Plenum Press, pp. 123–137.

Hart, R. W., and Setlow, R. B. 1974. Correlation between deoxyribonucleic acid excision-repair and life-span in a number of mammalian species. *Proc. Natl. Acad. Sci. USA* **71**:2169–2173.

Hastings, J. W. 1959. Unicellular clocks. *Annu. Rev. Microbiol.* **13**:297–312.

Hayflick, L. 1965. The limited *in vitro* lifetime of human diploid cell strains. *Exp. Cell Res.* **37**:614–636.

Hayflick, L., and Moorhead, P. S. 1961. The serial cultivation of human diploid cell strains. *Exp. Cell Res.* **25**:585–621.

Hendricks, S. B., and Borthwick, H. A. 1967. The function of phytochrome in regulation of plant growth. *Proc. Natl. Acad. Sci. USA* **58**:2125–2130.

Hirokawa, K., Hatakeyawa, S., and Sado, T. 1978. *XIth Int. Congr. Gerontol., Tokyo, Symp. Immune System* p. 2.

Hishikawa, Y., Cramer, H., and Kichlo, W. 1969. Natural and melatonin-induced sleep in young chickens—A behavioral and electrographic study. *Exp. Brain Res.* **7**:84–94.

Hochberg, M. L., and Sargent, M. L. 1974. Rhythms of enzyme activity associated with circadian conidiation in *Neurospora crassa. J. Bacteriol.* **121**:1164–1175.

Hogan, B. L. M. 1976. Changes in the behavior of teratocarcinoma cells cultivated in *in vitro. Nature (London)* **263**:136–137.

Hsueh, A. J. W., Erickson, G. F., and Lu, K. H. 1979. Changes in uterine estrogen receptor and morphology in aging female rats. *Biol. Reprod.* **21**:793–800.

Huang, H. H., Marshall, S., and Meites, J. 1976a. Capacity of old versus young female rats to secrete LH, FSH, and prolactin. *Biol. Reprod.* **14**:538–543.

Huang, H. H., Steger, R. W., Bruni, J. F., and Meites, J. 1976b. Patterns of sex steroid and gonadotropin secretion in aging female rats. *Endocrinology* **103**:1855–1859.

Hung, C. Y., Perkins, E. H., and Yang, W. K. 1975. Age-related refractoriness of PHA-induced lymphocyte transformation. *Mech. Aging Dev.* **4**:103–112.

Illnerová, H. 1971. Effect of environmental lighting on serotonin rhythm in rat pineal gland during postnatal development. *Life Sci.* **10**:583–590.

Ito, T., and Matsushima, S. 1968. Electron microscopic observations on the mouse pineal, with particular emphasis on its secretory nature. *Arch. Histol. Jpn.* **30**:1–15.

Jacklet, J. W. 1969. Circadian rhythm of optic nerve impulses recorded in darkness from isolated eye of *Aplysia. Science* **164**:562–563.

Jacklet, J. W. 1974. A circadian rhythm from a population of interacting neurons in the eye of *Aplysia. In*: Scheving, L. E., Halberg, F., and Pauly, J. E., eds., *Chronobiology,* Tokyo, Igaku Shoin, pp. 67–71.

Jacklet, J. W. 1981. Circadian timing by endogenous oscillators in the nervous system: Toward cellular mechanisms. *Biol. Bull.* **160**:199–227.

Jackson, B. 1959. Time-associated variations of mitotic activity in livers of young rats. *Anat. Rec.* **134**:365–377.

Jerebzoff, S. 1976. Metabolic steps involved in periodicity. *In*: Hastings, J. W., and Schweiger, H. G., eds., *The Molecular Basis of Circadian Rhythms*, Berlin, Dahlem Konferenzen, pp. 193–213.

Joenje, H., Frants, R. R., Arwert, F., and Eriksson, A. 1978. Specific activity of human erythrocyte superoxide dismutase as a function of a donor age: A brief note. *Mech. Ageing Dev.* **8**:265–267.

Johansson, G. 1970. Partition of salts and their effects on partition of proteins in a dextran-poly(ethylene glycol)-water two-phase system. *Biochim. Biophys. Acta* **221**:387–390.

Johnson, O. W. 1961. Reproductive cycle of the mallard duck. *Condor* **63**:351–364.

Johnston, P. G., and Zucker, I. 1980. Photoperiodic regulation of reproductive development in white-footed mice (*Peromyscus leucopus*). *Biol. Reprod.* **22**:983–989.

Joseph, M. M. 1974. Circadian systems in the hormonal regulation of amphibian metamorphosis. *In*: Scheving, L. E., Halberg, F., and Pauly, J. E., eds., *Chronobiology*, Tokyo, Igaku Shoin, pp. 142–146.

Kachi, T. 1979. Demonstration of circadian rhythm in granular vesicle number in pinealocytes of mice and the effect of light. *J. Anat.* **129**:603–614.

Kachi, T., and Ito, T. 1977. Neural control of glycogen content and its diurnal rhythm in mouse pineal cell. *Am. J. Physiol.* **232**:E584–E589.

Kachi, T., Matsushima, S., and Ito, T. 1975. Postnatal observations on the dirunal rhythm and the light-responsiveness in the pineal glycogen content in mice. *Anat. Rec.* **183**:39–46.

Kahan, B. W., and Ephrussi, B. 1970. Developmental potentialities of clonal *in vitro* cultures of mouse testicular teratoma. *J. Natl. Cancer Inst.* **44**:1015–1029.

Kanungo, M. S. 1980. *Biochemistry of Aging*, New York, Academic Press.

Kanungo, M. S., and Singh, S. N. 1965. Effect of age on the isozymes of lactic dehydrogenase of the heart and the brain of rat. *Biochem. Biophys. Res. Commun.* **21**:454–459.

Karran, P., and Ormerod, M. G. 1973. Is the ability to repair damage to DNA related to the proliferative capacity of a cell? The rejoining of X-ray-produced strand breaks. *Biochim. Biophys. Acta* **299**:54–64.

Kasal, C. A., Menaker, M., and Perez-Polo, J. R. 1979. Circadian clock in culture: *N*-acetyltransferase activity of chick pineal gland oscillates *in vitro*. *Science* **203**:656–658.

Kauffman, S. A., and Wille, J. J. 1976. Evidence that the mitotic "clock" in *Physarum polycephalum* is a limit cycle oscillator. *In*: Hastings, J. W., and Schweiger, H. G., eds., *The Molecular Basis of Circadian Rhythms*, Berlin, Dahlem Konferenzen, pp. 421–431.

Kavaliers, M. 1979. The pineal organ and circadian organization of teleost fish. *Rev. Can. Biol.* **38**:281–292.

Kavaliers, M. 1980. Social groupings and circadian activity of the killifish, *Fundulus heteroclitus*. *Biol. Bull.* **158**:69–76.

Kavaliers, M. 1981. Circadian organization in white suckers, *Catostomus commersoni*: The role of the pineal gland. *Comp. Biochem. Physiol.* **68A**:127–129.

Kavaliers, M., and Ralph, C. L. 1980. Circadian organization of an animal lacking a pineal organ; the young American alligator, *Alligator mississippiensis*. *J. Comp. Physiol.* **139**:287–292.

Kavaliers, M., Firth, B. T., and Ralph, C. L. 1980. Pineal control of the circadian rhythms of colour change in the killifish (*Fundulus heteroclitus*). *Can. J. Zool.* **58**:456–460.

Kayser, C. and Petrovic, A. 1958. Rôle du cortex surrénalien dans le méchanisme du sommeil hivernal. *C. R. Soc. Biol.* **152**:519–528.

Kennaway, D. J., Obst, J. M., Dunstan, E. A., and Friesen, H. G. 1981. Ultradian and seasonal rhythms in plasma gonadotropins, prolactin, cortisol, and testosterone in pinealectomized rams. *Endocrinology* **108**:639–646.

Kennes, B., Hubert, C., Brohee, D., and Neve, P. 1981. Early biochemical events associated with lymphocyte activation in ageing. I. Evidence that Ca^{2+} dependent processes induced by PHA are impaired. *Immunology* **42**:119–126.

King, J. R., and Farner, D. S. 1974. Biochronometry and bird migration: General prespective [sic!]. *In*: Scheving, L. E., Halberg, F., and Pauly, J. E., eds., *Chronobiology*, Tokyo, Igaku Shoin, pp. 625–635.

King, R. W. 1974. Photoperiodism and timing mechanisms in the control of flowering. *In*: Scheving, L. E., Halberg, F., and Pauly, J. E., eds., *Chronobiology*, Tokyo, Igaku Shoin, pp. 659–665.

King, T. S., and Dougherty, W. J. 1980. Neonatal development of circadian rhythm in "synaptic" ribbon numbers in the rat pinealocyte. *Am. J. Anat.* **157**:335–343.

Kishimoto, S., Takahama, T., and Mizumachi, H. 1976. *In vitro* immune response to the 2,4,6-trinitrophenyl determinant in aged C57BL/6J mice: Changes in the humoral immune response to avidity for the TNP determinant and responsiveness to LPS effect with aging. *J. Immunol.* **116**:294–300.

Klein, D. C., Namboodiri, M. A. A., and Auerbach, D. A. 1981. The melatonin rhythm generating system: Developmental aspects. *Life Sci.* **28**:1975–1986.

Kolpakov, M. G., Kolaeva, S. G., and Polyak, M. G. 1974. Endogenous mechanisms for the synchronization of corticosteroid production and seasonal rhythms in hibernating mammals. *In*: Scheving, L. E., Halberg, F., and Pauly, J. E., eds., *Chronobiology*, Tokyo, Igaku Shoin, pp. 136–137.

Konopka, R. J., and Benzer, S. 1971. Clock mutants of *Drosophila melanogaster*. *Proc. Natl. Acad. Sci. USA* **68**:2112–2116.

Korf, H. W., Liesner, R., Meissl, H., and Kirk, A. 1981. Pineal complex of the clawed toad, *Xenopus laevis* Daud.: Structure and function. *Cell Tissue Res.* **216**:113–130.

Kripke, D. F. 1974. Ultradian rhythms and sleep: Introduction. *In*: Scheving, L. E., Halberg, F., and Pauly, J. E., eds., *Chronobiology*, Tokyo, Igaku Shoin, pp. 475–477.

Krooth, R. S., Darlington, G. A., and Velazques, I. A. A. 1968. The genetics of cultured mammalian cells. *Annu. Rev. Genet.* **2**:141–164.

Kupila-Ahvenniemi, S., Pihakaski, S., and Pihakaski, K. 1979. Wintertime changes in the ultrastructure and metabolism of the microsporangiate strobili of the Scotch pine. *Planta* **144**:19–29.

Kurtz, D. I., and Sinex, F. M. 1967. Age related differences in the association of brain DNA and nuclear protein. *Biochim. Biophys. Acta* **145**:840–842.

Kurtz, D. I., Russell, A. R., and Sinex, F. M. 1974. Multiple peaks in the derivative melting curve of chromatin from animals of varying age. *Mech. Ageing Dev.* **3**:37–49.

Kurumado, K., and Mori, W. 1977. A morphological study of the circadian cycle of the pineal gland of the rat. *Cell Tissue Res.* **182**:565–568.

Laval-Martin, D. L., Shuch, D. J., and Edmunds, L. N. 1979. Cell cycle-related and endogenously controlled circadian photosynthetic rhythms in *Euglena*. *Plant Physiol.* **63**:495–502.

Lu, K. H., Hopper, B. R., Vargo, T. M., and Yen, S. S. C. 1979. Chronological changes in sex steroid, gonadotropin and prolactin secretion in aging female rats displaying different reproductive states. *Biol. Reprod.* **21**:193–203.

Lues, G. 1971. Die Feinstruktur der Zirbeldrüse normaler, trächtiger, und experimentell beeinflusster Meerschweinchen. *Z. Zellforsch. Mikrosk. Anat.* **114**:38–60.

Lynch, H. J. 1971. Diurnal oscillations in pineal melatonin content. *Life Sci.* **10**:791–795.

McBurney, M. W. 1976. Clonal lines of teratocarcinoma cells *in vitro*: Differentiation and cytogenetic characteristics. *J. Cell. Physiol.* **89**:441–456.

MacGregor, R. 1974. Avian reproductive system: Daily variations in response to hormones. *In*: Scheving, L. E., Halberg, F., and Pauly, J. E., eds., *Chronobiology*, Tokyo, Igaku Shoin, pp. 636–640.

Mackay, I. R. 1972. Ageing and immunological functions in man. *Gerontologia* **18**:285–304.

McMurry, L., and Hastings, J. W. 1972. No desynchronization among four circadian rhythms in the unicellular alga, *Gonyaulax polyedra*. *Science* **175**:1137–1139.

Makinodan, T., and Adler, W. H. 1975. Effects of aging on the differentiation and proliferation potentials of cells of the immune system. *Fed. Proc.* **34**:153–158.

Makinodan, T., Perkins, E. H., and Chen, M. G. 1971. Immunologic activity of the aged. *Adv. Gerontol. Res.* **3**:171–238.

Marshall, A. J., and Williams, M. C. 1959. The pre-nuptial migration of the yellow wagtail (*Motacilla flava*) from latitude 0°04′N. *Proc. Zool. Soc. London* **132**:313–320.

Marshall, M. K., and Donchin, E. 1981. Circadian variation in the latency of brainstem responses and its relation to body temperature. *Science* **212**:356–358.

Martens, C. L., and Sargent, M. C. 1974. Circadian rhythms of nucleic acid metabolism in *Neurospora crassa*. *J. Bacteriol.* **117**:1210–1215.

Martin, D. D. 1974. Hormonal control of orientation in the white-throated sparrow, *Zonotrichia albicollis*. *In*: Scheving, L. E., Halberg, F., and Pauly, J. E., eds., *Chronobiology*, Tokyo, Igaku Shoin, pp. 641–646.

Martin, G. M. 1977. Cellular aging. Part I. Clonal senescence. Part II. Postreplicative cells. *Am. J. Pathol.* **89**:484–530.

Martin, G. M., and Sprague, C. A. 1973. Symposium on *in vitro* studies related to atherogenesis: Life histories of hyperplastoid cell lines from aorta and skin. *Exp. Mol. Pathol.* **18**:125–141.

Matsushima, S., and Reiter, R. J. 1975. Comparative ultrastructural studies on the pineal gland of rodents. *In*: Hess, M., ed., *Ultrastructure of Endocrine and Reproductive Organs*, New York, Wiley, pp. 335–356.

Mattern, M. R., and Cerutti, P. 1975. Age-dependent excision repair of damaged thymidine from irradiated DNA by isolated nuclei from human fibroblasts. *Nature (London)* **254**:450–452.

Matthews, H. R., Hardie, D. G., Inglis, R. J., and Bradbury, E. M. 1976. The molecular basis of control of mitotic cell division. *In*: Hastings, J. W., and Schweiger, H. G., eds., *The Molecular Basis of Circadian Rhythms*, Berlin, Dahlem Konferenzen, pp. 395–408.

Mays, L. L., Lawrence, A. E., Ho, R. W., and Ackley, S. 1979. Age-related changes in function of tRNA of rat livers. *Fed. Proc.* **38**:1984–1988.

Meier, A. H. 1969a. Antigonadal effects of prolactin in the white-throated sparrow, *Zonotrichia albicollis*. *Gen. Comp. Endocrinol.* **13**:222–225.

Meier, A. H. 1969b. Diurnal variations of metabolic responses to prolactin in lower vertebrates. *Gen. Comp. Endocrinol. Suppl.* **2**:55–62.

Meier, A. H., and Davis, K. B. 1967. Diurnal variation of the fattening response to prolactin in the white-throated sparrow, *Zonotrichia albicollis*. *Gen. Comp. Endocrinol.* **8**:110–114.

Meier, A. H., and Dusseau, J. W. 1968. Prolactin and the photoperiodic gonadal response in several avian species. *Physiol. Zool.* **41**:95–103.

Meier, A. H., and Martin, D. D. 1971. Temporal synergism of corticosterone and prolactin controlling fat storage in the white-throated sparrow, *Zonotrichia albicollis*. *Gen. Comp. Endocrinol.* **17**:311–318.

Meier, A. H., Farner, D. S., and King, J. R. 1965. A possible endocrine basis for migratory behavior in the white-crowned sparrow, *Zonotrichia leucophrys gambelii*. *Anim. Behav.* **13**:453–465.

Meier, A. H., Burns, J. T., and Dusseau, J. W. 1969. Seasonal variations in the diurnal rhythm of pituitary prolactin content in the white-throated sparrow, *Zonotrichia albicollis*. *Gen. Comp. Endocrinol.* **12**:282–289.

Meier, A. H., Garcia, L. E., and Joseph, M. M. 1971a. Corticosterone phases a circadian water-drive response to prolactin in the spotted newt, *Diemyctylus viridescens*. *Biol. Bull.* **141**:331–336.

Meier, A. H., Martin, D. D., and MacGregor, R. 1971b. Temporal synergism of corticosterone and prolactin controlling gonadal growth in sparrows. *Science* **173**:1240–1242.

Meier, A. H., Trobec, T. N., Joseph, M. M., and John, T. M. 1971c. Temporal synergism of prolactin and adrenal steroids in the regulation of fat stores. *Proc. Soc. Exp. Biol. Med.* **137**:408–415.

Mergenhagen, D. 1976. Gene expression in its role in rhythms. *In*: Hastings, J. W., and Schweiger, H. G., eds., *The Molecular Basis of Circadian Rhythms*, Berlin, Dahlem Konferenzen, pp. 353–360.

Miller, J. K., Bolla, R., and Denckla, W. D. 1980. Age-associated changes in initiation of RNA synthesis in isolated rat liver nuclei. *Biochem. J.* **188**:55–60.

Milo, G. E., and Hart, R. W. 1976. Age-related alterations in plasma membrane glycoprotein content and scheduled or unscheduled DNA synthesis. *Arch. Biochem. Biophys.* **176**:324–333.

Mogler, R. K. H. 1958. Das Endokrine System des Syrischen Goldhamster unter Berücksichtigung des Natürlichen Winterschaläf. *Z. Morph. Oekol. Tiere* **47**:267–308.

Mohan, C., and Radha, E. 1978. Circadian rhythms in the central cholinergic system in aging animals. *Adv. Exp. Med. Biol.* **108**:275–299.

Moldave, K., Harris, J., Sabo, W., and Sadnik, I. 1979. Protein synthesis and aging: Studies with cell-free mammalian systems. *Fed. Proc.* **38**:1979–1983.

Moore, R. Y., and Smith, R. A. 1971. Postnatal development of a norepinephrine response to light in the rat pineal and salivary glands. *Neuropharmacology* **10**:315–323.

Mugiya, Y., Watabe, N., Yamada, J., Dean, J. M., Dunkelberger, D. G., and Shimizu, M. 1981. Diurnal rhythm in otolith formation in the goldfish, *Carassius auratus*. *Comp. Biochem. Physiol. A* **68**:659–662.

Nakashima, H., Perlman, J., and Feldman, J. F. 1981. Genetic evidence that protein synthesis is required for the circadian clock in *Neurospora*. *Science* **212**:361–362.

Nalbandov, A. V. 1945. A study of the effects of prolactin on broodiness and cock testes. *Endocrinology* **36**:251–258.

Norwood, T. H. 1978. Somatic cell genetics in the analysis of *in vitro* senescence. *In*: Schneider, E. L., ed., *The Genetics of Aging*, New York, Plenum Press, pp. 337–382.

Oksche, A. 1971. Sensory and glandular elements of the pineal organ. *In*: Wolstenholme, G. E. W., and Knight, J., eds., *The Pineal Gland*, Edinburgh, Churchill Livingstone, pp. 127–146.

O'Meara, A., and Herrmann, R. L. 1972. A modified mouse liver chromatin preparation displaying age-related differences in salt dissociation and template ability. *Biochim. Biophys. Acta* **269**:419–427.

Orgel, L. E. 1963. The maintenance of the accuracy of protein synthesis and its relevance to aging. *Proc. Natl. Acad. Sci. USA* **49**:517–521.

Pacifici, M., Fellini, S. A., Holtzer, H., and DeLuca, S. 1981. Changes in the sulfated proteoglycans synthesized by "aging" chondrocytes. I. Dispersed cultured chondrocytes and *in vivo* cartilages. *J. Biol. Chem.* **256**:1029–1037.

Pavlidis, T., and Kauzman, W. 1969. Towards a quantitative biochemical model for circadian oscillators. *Arch. Biochem. Biophys.* **132**:338–348.

Pellegrino de Iraldi, A. 1969. Granulated vesicles in the pineal gland of the mouse, *Z. Zellforsch. Mikrosk. Anat.* **101**:408–418.

Pflugfelder, O. 1956. Physiologie der Epiphyse. *Verh. Dtsch. Zool. Ges.* **50**:53–75.

Philippens, K. M. H. 1974. Circadian variations in rat liver mitochondrial activity. *In*: Scheving, L. E., Halberg, F., and Pauly, J. E., eds., *Chronobiology*, Tokyo, Igaku Shoin, pp. 23–28.

Pieper, D. R., and Gala, R. R. 1979a. The effect of light on the prolactin surges of pseudopregnant and ovariectomized, estrogenized rats. *Biol. Reprod.* **20**:727–732.

Pieper, D. R., and Gala, R. R. 1979b. Lack of an effect of the pineal gland, olfactory bulbectomy and short photoperiod on the afternoon prolactin surge of the ovariectomized, estrogen treated rat. *Biol. Reprod.* **21**:1067–1072.

Pierard, D., Jacqmard, A., Bernier, G., and Salmon, J. 1980. Appearance and disappearance of proteins in the shoot meristem of *Sinapis alba* in transition to flowering. *Planta* **150**:397–405.

Pittendrigh, C. S. 1974. Circadian oscillations in cells and the circadian organization of multicellular systems. *In: The Neurosciences*—Third Study Program, Cambridge, Mass., MIT Press, pp. 437–458.

Pittendrigh, C. S., Bruce, V. G., Rosensweig, N. S., and Rubin, M. L. 1959. Growth patterns in *Neurospora. Nature (London)* **184**:169–170.

Potter, V. R., Baril, E. F., Watanabe, M., and Whittle, E. D. 1968. Systematic oscillations in metabolic functions in liver from rats adapted to controlled feeding schedules. *Fed. Proc.* **27**:1238–1245.

Price, G. B., and Makinodan, T. 1972a. Immunologic deficiencies in senescence. I. Characterization of intrinsic deficiencies. *J. Immunol.* **108**:403–412.

Price, G. B., and Makinodan, T. 1972b. Immunologic deficiencies in senescence. II. Characterization of extrinsic deficiencies. *J. Immunol.* **108**:413–417.

Price, G. B., Modak, S. P., and Makinodan, T. 1971. Age-associated changes in the DNA of mouse tissue. *Science* **171**:917–920.

Pritchett, J. F., Sartin, J. L., Marple, D. N., Harper, W. L., and Till, M. L. 1979. Interaction of aging with *in vitro* adrenocortical responsiveness to ACTH and cyclic AMP. *Horm. Res.* **10**:96–103.

Quay, W. B. 1956. Volumetric and cytologic variation in the pineal body of *Peromyscus leucopus* (Rodentia) with respect to sex, captivity and day-length. *J. Morphol.* **98**:471–495.

Quay, W. B. 1968. Individuation and lack of pineal effect in the rat's circadian locomotor rhythm. *Physiol. Behav.* **3**:109–118.

Quay, W. B. 1970a. Physiological significance of the pineal during adaptation to shifts in photoperiod. *Physiol. Behav.* **5**:353–360.

Quay, W. B. 1970b. Precocious entrainment and associated characteristics of activity patterns following pinealectomy and reversal of photoperiod. *Physiol. Behav.* **5**:1281–1290.

Quay, W. B. 1974. Circadian rhythm and phase-shifting in running activity by feral white-footed mice (*Peromyscus*): Effects of distal pinealectomy. *In*: Scheving, L. E., Halberg, F., and Pauly, J. E., eds., *Chronobiology*,Tokyo, Igaku Shoin, pp. 152–154.

Queiroz, O. 1974. Circadian rhythms and metabolic patterns. *Annu. Rev. Plant Physiol.* **25**115–134.

Ralph, C. L., Hedlund, L., and Murphy, W. A. 1967. Diurnal cycles of melatonin in bird pineal bodies. *Comp. Biochem. Physiol.* **22**:591–599.

Raynal, A. 1979. Evidence for a common cytoplasmic determinant of longevity and senescence in the ascomycete *Podospora anserina. Mol. Gen. Genet.* **175**:281–292.

Reinberg, A. 1974. Aspects of circannual rhythms in man. *In*: Pengelley, E. T., ed., *Circannual Clocks: Annual Biological Rhythms*, New York, Academic Press, pp. 423–505.

Reiss, U., and Gershon, D. 1976. Rat-liver superoxide dismutase: Purification and age-related modifications. *Eur. J. Biochem.* **63**:617–623.

Reiss, U., and Rothstein, M. 1974. Isocitrate lyase from the free-living nematode, *Turbatrix aceti*: Purification and properties. *Biochemistry* **13**:1796–1800.

Reiss, U., and Rothstein, M. 1975. Age-related changes in isocitrate lyase from the free living nematode, *Turbatrix aceti. J. Biol. Chem.* **250**:826–830.

Reiter, R. J. 1971. Influence of the pineal gland and the photoperiod on seasonal reproductive rhythms in golden hamsters. *Anat. Rec.* **169**:410.

Reiter, R. J. 1974. Evidence for a seasonal rhythm in pineal gland function. *In*: Scheving, L. E., Halberg, F., and Pauly, J. E., eds., *Chronobiology*, Tokyo, Igaku Shoin, pp. 155–159.

Reitherman, R., Flanagan, S. D., and Barondes, S. H. 1973. Electromotive phenomena in partition of erythrocytes in aqueous polymer two phase systems. *Biochim. Biophys. Acta* **297**:193–202.

Relkin, R., Adachi, M., and Kahan, S. A. 1972. Effect of pinealectomy and constant light and darkness on prolactin levels in the pituitary and plasma and on pituitary ultrastructure of the rat. *J. Endocrinol.* **54**:263–268.

Reznick, A. Z., and Gershon, D. 1977. Age related alterations in purified fructose-1,6-diphosphate aldolase from the nematode *Turbatrix aceti*. *Mech. Ageing Dev.* **6**:345–353.

Richter, C. P. 1964. Biological clocks and endocrine glands. *Excerpta Med.* **83**:119–123.

Richter, C. P. 1965. *Biological Clocks in Medicine and Psychiatry*, Springfield, Ill., Thomas.

Rizet, G. 1953. Sur l'impossibilité d'obtenir la multiplication végétative ininterrompue et illimitée de l'ascomycete *Podospora anserina*. *C. R. Acad. Sci. Ser. D* **237**:838–840.

Roberts-Thomson, I. C., Whittingham, S., Young-Chaiyud, U., and Mackay, I. R. 1974. Ageing, immune response, and mortality. *Lancet* **1974(2)**:368–370.

Rollag, M. D. Panke, E. S., and Reiter, R. J. 1980. Pineal melatonin content of male hamsters throughout the seasonal reproductive cycle. *Proc. Soc. Exp. Biol. Med.* **165**:330–334.

Romero, J. A. 1978. Biologic rhythms and sympathetic neural control of pineal metabolism. *In*: Samis, H. V., and Capobianco, S., eds., *Aging and Biological Rhythms*, New York, Plenum Press, pp. 235–249.

Romero, J. A., Zatz, M., Kebabian, J. W., and Axelrod, J. A. 1975. Binding of ^{3}H-alprenolol to *beta*-adrenergic receptor sites in rat pineal: Circadian cycles. *Nature (London)* **258**:435–436.

Ronnekleiv, O. K., Krulich, L., and McConn, S. M. 1973. An early morning surge of prolactin in the male rat and its abolition by pinealectomy. *Endocrinology* **92**:1339–1342.

Rothfels, K. H., Kupelwieser, E. B., and Parker, R. C. 1963. Effects of X-irradiated feeder layers on mitotic activity and development of aneuploidy in mouse-embryo cells *in vitro*. *Can. Cancer Conf.* **5**:191–223.

Rowan, W. 1925. Relation of light to bird migration and developmental changes. *Nature (London)* **115**:494–495.

Rowan, W. 1932. Experiments in bird migration. III. The effects of artificial light, castration and certain extracts on the autumn movements of the American crow (*Corvus brachyrhynchos*). *Proc. Natl. Acad. Sci. USA* **18**:659–664.

Rowley, M. J., Buchanan, H., and Mackay, I. R. 1968. Reciprocal change with age in antibody to extrinsic and intrinsic antigens. *Lancet* **1968(2)**:24–26.

Ruby, J. R., Scheving, L. E., Gray, S. B., and White, K. 1973. Circadian rhythm of nuclear DNA in adult rat liver. *Exp. Cell Res.* **76**:136–142.

Ruby, J. R., Scheving, L. E., Gray, S. B., and White, K. 1974. Demonstration of a circadian rhythm of nuclear DNA in liver. *In*: Scheving, L. E., Halberg, F., and Pauly, J. E., eds., *Chronobiology*,Tokyo, Igaku Shoin, pp. 33–37.

Rudeen, P. K., and Reiter, R. J. 1979a. Pineal *N*-acetyltransferase activity in hamsters maintained in shortened light cycles. *J. Endocrinol. Invest.* **2**:19–23.

Rudeen, P. K., and Reiter, R. J. 1979b. Photoperiodic control of rat pineal serotonin *N*-acetyltransferase activity. *Int. J. Chronobiol.* **6**:211–218.

Rudeen, P. K., and Reiter, R. J. 1980. Influence of a skeleton photoperiod on reproductive organ atrophy in the male golden hamster. *J. Reprod. Fertil.* **60**:279–283.

Rutledge, J. T. 1974. Circannual rhythm of reproduction in male European starlings (*Sturnus vulgaris*). *In*: Pengelley, E. T., ed., *Circannual Clocks: Annual Biological Rhythms*, New York, Academic Press, pp. 297–345.

Sacher, G. A. 1978. Longevity and aging in vertebrate evolution. *BioScience* **28**:497–501.

Sachsenmaier, W. 1976. Control of synchronous nuclear mitosis in *Physarum polycephalum*. *In*: Hastings, J. W., and Schweiger, H. G., eds., *The Molecular Basis of Circadian Rhythms*, Berlin, Dahlem Konferenzen, pp. 409–420.

Salisbury, F. B., and Denney, A. 1971. Separate clocks for leaf movements and photoperiodic flowering in *Xanthium strumarium* L. (cocklebur). *In*: Menaker, M., ed., *Biochronometry*, Washington, D.C., National Academy of Sciences, pp. 292–311.

Salisbury, F. B., and Denney, A. 1974. Noncorrelation of leaf movements and photoperiodic clocks in *Xanthium strumarium* L. *In*: Scheving, L. E., Halberg, F., and Pauly, J. E., eds., *Chronobiology*, Tokyo, Igaku Shoin, pp. 679–686.

Samarasinghe, D., and Delahunt, B. 1980. The ependyma of the saccular pineal gland in the non-eutherian mammal *Trichosurus vulpecula*. *Cell Tissue Res.* **213**:417–432.

Samis, H. V., Wulff, V. J., and Falzone, J. A. 1964. The incorporation of [^{3}H]-cytidine into RNA of liver nuclei of young and old rats. *Biochim. Biophys. Acta* **91**:223–232.

Sargent, M. L., and Woodward, D. O. 1969. Genetic determinants of circadian rhythmicity in *Neurospora*. *J. Bacteriol.* **97**:861–866.

Sargent, M. L., Briggs, W. R., and Woodward, D. O. 1966. The circadian nature of a rhythm expressed by an invertaseless strain of *Neurospora crassa*. *Plant Physiol.* **41**:1343–1349.

Satter, R. L., Marinoff, P., and Galston, A. 1970. Phytochrome controlled nyctinasty in *Albizzia julibrissin*. II. Potassium flux as a basis for leaflet movement. *Am. J. Bot.* **57**:916–926.

Sawai, T. 1979. Cyclic changes in the cortical layer of non-nucleated fragments of the newt's egg. *J. Embryol. Exp. Morphol.* **51**:183–193.

Scheving, L. E., and Pauly, J. E. 1973. Cellular mechanisms involving biorhythms with emphasis on those rhythms associated with the S and M stages of the cell cycle. *Int. J. Chronobiol.* **1**:269–286.

Schneider, E. L., ed. 1978. *The Aging Reproductive System,* New York, Raven Press, pp. 193–212.

Schoenmakers, H. J. N. 1977. Steroid synthesis of *Asterias rubens*. *Proc. Int. Union Physiol. Sci.* **13**:673.

Schoenmakers, H. J. N. 1979a. *In vitro* biosynthesis of steroids from cholesterol by the ovaries and pyloric caeca of the starfish *Asterias rubens*. *Comp. Biochem. Physiol.* **63B**:179–184.

Schoenmakers, H. J. N. 1979b. *Steroids and Reproduction of the Female Asterias rubens,* Utrecht, The Netherlands, University of Utrecht, Thesis.

Schoenmakers, H. J. N. 1980a. The possible role of steroids in vitellogenesis in the starfish *Asterias rubens*. *In*: Clark, W. H., and Adams, T. S., eds., *Advances in Invertebrate Reproduction*, Amsterdam, Elsevier/North-Holland, pp. 127–150.

Schoenmakers, H. J. N. 1980b. The variation of 3β-hydroxysteroid dehydrogenase activity of the ovaries and pyloric caeca of the starfish *Asterias rubens* during the annual reproductive cycle. *J. Comp. Physiol.* **138**:27–30.

Schoenmakers, H. J. N., and Dieleman, S. J. 1981. Progesterone and estrone levels in the ovaries, pyloric ceca, and perivisceral fluid during the annual reproductive cycle of starfish, *Asterias rubens*. *Gen. Comp. Endocrinol.* **43**:63–70.

Schoenmakers, H. J. N., and Voogt, P. A. 1980. *In vitro* biosynthesis of steroids from progesterone by the ovaries and pyloric caeca of the starfish, *Asterias rubens*. *Gen. Comp. Endocrinol.* **41**:408–416.

Schulte, B. A., Seal, U. S., Plotka, E. D., Letellier, M. A., Verme, L. J., Ozoga, J. J., and Parsons, J. A. 1981. The effect of pinealectomy on seasonal changes in prolactin secretion in the white-tailed deer (*Odocoileus virginianus borealis*). *Endocrinology* **108**:173–178.

Schweiger, H. G. 1977. Circadian rhythms in unicellular organisms: An endeavor to explain the molecular mechanism. *Int. Rev. Cytol.* **51**:315–342.

Segre, D., and Segre, M. 1976. Humeral immunity in aged mice. II. Increased suppressor T cell activity in immunologically deficient old mice. *J. Immunol.* **116**:735–738.

Seifert, J. 1980. Circadian variations in pyrimidine nucleotide synthesis in rat liver. *Arch. Biochem. Biophys.* **201**:194–198.

Shapiro, B. H., and Leathem, J. H. 1971. Aging and adrenal Δ^5-3β-hydroxysteroid dehydrogenase in female rats. *Proc. Soc. Exp. Biol. Med.* **136**:19–20.

Sharma, H. K., and Rothstein, M. 1978. Age-related changes in properties of enolase from *Turbatrix aceti*. *Biochemistry* **17**:2869–2876.

Sharma, H. K., Gupta, S. K., and Rothstein, M. 1976. Age-related alteration of enolase in the free-living nematode *Turbatrix aceti*. *Arch. Biochem. Biophys.* **174**:324–332.

Sharma, H. K., Prasanna, H. R., and Rothstein, M. 1980. Altered phosphoglycerate kinase in aging rats. *J. Biol. Chem.* **255**:5043–5050.

Shaw, C. R., and Barto, E. 1963. Genetic evidence for the subunit structure of lactate dehydrogenase isozymes. *Proc. Natl. Acad. Sci. USA* **50**:211–214.

Shimo, A. 1980. Aging of hepatocytes. *In*: Oota, K., Makinodan, T., Iriki, M., and Baker, L. S., eds., *Aging Phenomena: Relationships among Different Levels of Organization,* New York, Plenum Press, pp. 59–70.

Simpkins, J. W., Kalra, P. S., and Kalra, S. P. 1981. Alterations in daily rhythms of testosterone and progesterone in old male rats. *Exp. Aging Res.* **7**:25–32.

Singh, S. N., and Kanungo, M. S. 1968. Alterations in lactate dehydrogenase of the brain, heart, skeletal muscle, and liver of rats of various ages. *J. Biol. Chem.* **243**:4526–4529.

Singhal, R. P., Kopper, R. A., Nishimura, S., and Shindo-Okada, N. 1981. Modification of guanine to queuine in transfer RNAs during development and aging. *Biochem. Biophys. Res. Commun.* **99**:120–126.

Smith, S. G., and Stetson, M. H. 1980. Maturation of the clock-timed gonadotropin release mechanism in hamsters: A key event in the pubertal process? *Endocrinology* **107**:1334–1337.

Southam, C. M. 1974. Areas of relationship between immunology and clinical oncology. *Am. J. Clin. Pathol.* **62**:224–242.

Steger, R. W., Huang, H. H., Hodson, C. A., Leung, F. D., Meites, J., and Sacher, G. A. 1980. Effects of advancing age on hypothalamic–hypophysial–testicular functions in the male white-footed mouse (*Peromyscus leucopus*). *Biol. Reprod.* **22**:805–809.

Steinhagen-Thiessen, E., and Hilz, H. 1976. The age-dependent decrease in creatine kinase and aldolase activities in human striated muscle is not caused by an accumulation of faulty proteins. *Mech. Ageing Dev.* **5**:447–457.

Steinhagen-Thiessen, E., and Hilz, H. 1979. Aldolase activity and cross-reacting material in lymphocytes of aged individuals. *Gerontology* **25**:132–135.

Stetson, M. H. 1971. Neuroendocrine control of photoperiodically induced fat deposition in white-crowned sparrows. *J. Exp. Zool.* **176**:409–414.

Stetson, M. H. 1978. Circadian organization and female reproductive cyclicity. *In*: Samis, H. V., and Capobianco, S., eds., *Aging and Biological Rhythms,* New York, Plenum Press, pp. 251–274.

Stetson, M. H., and Erickson, J. E. 1972. Hormonal control of photoperiodically induced fat deposition in white-crowned sparrows. *Gen. Comp. Endocrinol.* **19**:355–362.

Stetson, M. H., and McMillan, J. P. 1974. Some neuroendocrine and endocrine correlates in the timing of bird migration. *In*: Scheving, L. E., Halberg, F., and Pauly, J. E., eds., *Chronobiology,* Tokyo, Igaku Shoin, pp. 630–635.

Stevens, L. C. 1967. The biology of teratomas. *Adv. Morphog.* **6**:1–31.

Stockdale, F. E. 1971. DNA synthesis in differentiating skeletal muscle cells: Initiation by ultraviolet light. *Science* **171**:1145–1147.

Stowe, S. J. 1980. Rapid synthesis of photoreceptor membrane and assembly of new microvilli in a crab at dusk. *Cell Tissue Res.* **211**:419–440.

Straley, S. C., and Bruce, V. G. 1979. Stickiness to glass: Circadian changes in the cell surface of *Chlamydomonas reinhardi. Plant Physiol.* **63**:1175–1181.

Strumwasser, F. 1965. The demonstration and manipulation of a circadian rhythm in a single neuron. *In*: Aschoff, J., ed., *Circadian Clocks,* Amsterdam, North-Holland, pp. 442–462.

Subramanian, M. G., and Gala, R. R. 1976. The influence of cholinergic, adrenergic, and serotonergic drugs on the afternoon surge of plasma prolactin in ovariectomized, estrogen-treated rats. *Endocrinology* **98**:842–848.

Sulzman, F. M., and Edmunds, L. M. 1972. Persisting circadian oscillations in enzyme activity in non-dividing cultures of *Euglena. Biochem. Biophys. Res. Commun.* **47**:1338–1344.

Sweeney, B. M. 1963. Resetting the biological clock in *Gonyaulax* with ultraviolet light. *Plant Physiol.* **38**:704–708.

Sweeney, B. M., and Hastings, J. W. 1958. Rhythmic cell division in populations of *Gonyaulax polyedra. J. Protozool.* **5**:217–224.

Takimoto, A., and Hamner, K. C. 1964. Effect of temperature and preconditioning on photoperiodic responses of *Pharbitis nil. Plant Physiol.* **39**:1024–1030.

Talal, N., and Steinberg, A. D. 1974. *Curr. Top. Microbiol. Immunol.* **61**:79–103.

Tamarkin, L., Reppert, S. M., Klein, D. C., Pratt, B., and Goldman, B. D. 1980. Studies on the daily pattern of pineal melatonin in the Syrian hamster. *Endocrinology* **107**:1525–1529.

Teller, M. N. 1972. Age changes and immune resistance to cancer. *Adv. Gerontol. Res.* **4**:25–43.

Theron, J. J., Biagio, R., Meyer, A. C., and Boekkooi, S. 1979. Microfilaments, the smooth endoplasmic reticulum, and synaptic ribbon fields in the pinealocytes of the baboon (*Papio ursinus*). *Am. J. Anat.* **154**:151–161.

Trobec, T. N. 1974. Daily rhythms in the hormonal control of fat storage in lizards. *In*: Scheving, L. E., Halberg, F., and Pauly, J. E., eds., *Chronobiology*, Tokyo, Igaku Shoin, pp. 147–151.

Truman, J., and Riddiford, L. 1970. Neuroendocrine control of ecdysis in silkmoths. *Science* **167**:1624–1626.

Tudzynski, P., and Esser, K. 1979. Chromosomal and extrachromosomal control of senescence in the ascomycete *Podospora anserina. Mol. Gen. Genet.* **173**:71–84.

Utsumi, K., and Natori, S. 1980. Changes in head proteins of *Sarcophaga peregrina* with age. *FEBS Lett.* **111**:419–422.

Vanden Driessche, T. 1975. Circadian rhythms and molecular biology. *BioSystems* **6**:188–201.

Vollrath, L., and Huss, H. 1973. Synaptic ribbons of the guinea-pig pineal gland under normal and experimental conditions. *Z. Zellforsch. Mikrosk. Anat.* **139**:417–429.

Volm, M. 1964. Die Tagesperiodik der Zellteilung von *Paramecium bursaria. Z. Vgl. Physiol.* **481**:157–180.

von Hahn, H. P., and Fritz, E. C. 1966. Age-related alterations in the structure of DNA. *Gerontologia* **12**:237–250.

Wagner, E. 1976. Endogenous rhythmicity in energy metabolism: Basis for timer–photoreceptor interactions in photoperiodic control. *In*: Hastings, J. W., and Schweiger, H. G., eds., *The Molecular Basis of Circadian Rhythms*, Berlin, Dahlem Konferenzen, pp. 215–238.

Wagner, E., and Frosch, S. 1974. Endogenous rhythmicity and energy transduction. VI. Rhythmicity in reduced and oxidized pyridine nucleotide levels in seedlings of *Chenopodium rubrum. J. Interdiscip. Cycle Res.* **5**:231–239.

Wagner, E., Stroebele, L., and Frosch, S. 1974. Endogenous rhythmicity and energy transduction. V. Rhythmicity in adenine nucleotides and energy charge in seedlings of *Chenopodium rubrum* L. *J. Interdiscip. Cycle Res.* **3**:77–88.

Walker, P. R., and van Potter, R. 1974. Diurnal rhythms of hepatic enzymes from rats adapted to controlled feeding schedules. *In*: Scheving, L. E., Halberg, F., and Pauly, J. E., eds., *Chronobiology*, Tokyo, Igaku Shoin, pp. 17–22.

Walter, H., and Selby, F. W. 1966. Counter-current distribution of red blood cells of slightly different ages. *Biochim. Biophys. Acta* **112**:146–153.

Walter, H., Krob, E. J., Tamblyn, C. H., and Seaman, G. V. F. 1980. Surface alterations of erythrocytes with cell age: Rat red cell is not a model for human red cell. *Biochem. Biophys. Res. Commun.* **97**:107–113.

Walther, W. G., and Edmunds, L. N. 1970. Periodic increase in DNase activity during the cell cycle in synchronized *Euglena. J. Cell Biol.* **46**:613–617.

Watanabe, M., Potter, V. R., and Pitot, H. C. 1968. Systematic oscillations in tyrosine transaminase and other metabolic functions also in liver of normal and adrenalectomized rats on controlled feeding schedules. *J. Nutr.* **95**:207–227.

Weber, A., Szajnert, M. F., and Beck, G. 1980. Age-related changes of liver tyrosine aminotransferase in senescent rats. *Biochim. Biophys. Acta* **631**:412–419.

Weeks, D. P., and Collis, P. S. 1979. Induction and synthesis of tubulin during the cell cycle and life cycle of *Chlamydomonas reinhardi. Dev. Biol.* **69**:400–407.

Weigle, W. O. 1980. Analysis of autoimmunity through experimental models of thyroiditis and allergic encephalomyelitis. *Adv. Imunol.* **30**:159–273.

Weise, C. M. 1967. Castration and spring migration in the white-throated sparrow. *Condor* **69**:49–68.

Weiss, B. 1971. Ontogenetic development of adenyl cyclase and phosphodiesterase in rat brain. *J. Neurochem.* **18**:469–477.

Wever, R. A. 1979. *The Circadian System of Man: Results of Experiments under Temporal Isolation,* Berlin, Springer-Verlag.

Wieland, T., and Pfleiderer, H. 1957. Nachweis der Hetergenität von Milchsäure-dehydrogenasen verschiedenen Ursprungs durch Trägerelektrophorese. *Biochem. Z.* **329**:112–116.

Wille, J. J., and Ehret, C. F. 1968. Light synchronization of an endogenous circadian rhythm of cell division in *Tetrahymena. J. Protozool.* **15**:785–789.

Woolum, J. C., and Strumwasser, F. 1980. The differential effects of ionizing radiation on the circadian oscillator and other functions in the eye of *Aplysia. Proc. Natl. Acad. Sci. USA* **77**:5542–5546.

Wright, W. E., and Hayflick, L. 1975. Contributions of cytoplasmic factors to *in vitro* cellular senescence. *Fed. Proc.* **34**:76–79.

Yamamoto, K. T., and Smith, W. O. 1981. Alkyl and ω-amino alkyl agaroses as probes of light-induced changes in phytochrome from pea seedlings (*Pisum sativum* cv *Alaska*). *Biochim. Biophys. Acta* **668**:27–34.

Zimmermann, J. L. 1966. Effects of extended tropical photoperiod and temperature on the dickcissel. *Condor* **68**:377–387.

Zs-Nagy, I. 1979. The role of membrane structure and function in cellular aging: A review. *Mech. Ageing Dev.* **9**:237–246.

Zweig, M., Snyder, S. H., and Axelrod, J. 1966. Evidence for a nonretinal pathway of light to the pineal gland of newborn rats. *Proc. Natl. Acad. Sci. USA* **56**:515–520.

CHAPTER 7

Aadeen, L., *et al.* 1979. Revised nomenclature for antigen-nonspecific T cell proliferation and helper factors. *J. Immunol.* **123**:2928–2929.

Abney, E. R., and Parkhouse, R. M. E. 1974. Candidate for immunoglobulin D present on murine B lymphocytes. *Nature (London)* **252**:600–602.

Abney, E. R., Cooper, M. D., Kearney, J. F., Lawton, A. R., and Parkhouse, R. M. E. 1978. Sequential expression of immunoglobulin on developing mouse B lymphocytes: A systematic survey suggests a model for the generation of immunoglobulin isotype diversity. *J. Immunol.* **120**:2041–2049.

Abo, T., Kawate, T., Itoh, K., and Kumagai, K. 1981. Studies on bioperiodicity of the immune response. I. Circadian rhythms of human T, B, and K cell traffic in the peripheral blood. *J. Immunol.* **126**:1360–1363.

Al-Adra, A. R., Pilarski, L. M., and McKenzie, I. F. C. 1980. Surface markers on the T-cells that regulate cytotoxic T-cell responses. I. The Ly phenotype of suppressor T-cells changes as a function of time, and is distinct from that of helper or cytotoxic T-cells. *Immunogenetics* **10**:521–533.

Al-Hamdani, M. M., Atkinson, M. E., and Mayhew, T. M. 1981. Ultrastructural morphometry of blastogenesis. II. Stimulated lymphocytes, the progeny of blast cells induced *in vivo* with DNCB. *Cell Tissue Res.* **215**:643–649.

Alt, F. W., Bothwell, A. M. M., Knapp, M., Siden, E., Mather, E., Koshland, M., and Baltimore, D. 1980. Synthesis of secreted and membrane-bound immunoglobulin μ heavy chains is directed by mRNAs that differ at their 3′ ends. *Cell* **20**:293–302.

Anderson, C. L., and Spiegelberg, H. L. 1981. Macrophage receptors for IgE: Binding of IgE to specific IgE Fc receptors in a human macrophage cell line, V937. *J. Immunol.* **126**:2470–2473.

Azuma, T., Steiner, L. A., and Eisen, H. N. 1981. Identification of a third type of λ light chain in mouse immunoglobulins. *Proc. Natl. Acad. Sci. USA* **78**:569–573.

Badenoch-Jones, P., Rouveix, B., and Turk, J. L. 1981. Absorption of macrophage aggregating factor of guinea-pig peritoneal exudate calls. *Immunology* **43**:67–74.

Baglioni, C., Zonta, L. A., Cioli, D., and Carbonara, A. 1966. Allelic antigenic factor Inv(a) of the light chains of human immunoglobulins: Chemical basis. *Science* **152**:1517–1519.

Bargatze, R. F., and Katz, D. H. 1980. "Allergic breakthrough" after antigen sensitization: Height of IgE snythesis is temporally related to diurnal variation of endogeneous steroid production. *J. Immunol.* **125**:2306–2310.

Barnstable, C. J., Jones, E. A., Bodmer, W. T., Bodmer, J. G., Arce-Gomez, B., Snary, D., and Crumpton, J. J. 1977. Genetics and serology of H1-A-linked human Ia antigens. *Cold Spring Harbor Symp. Quant. Biol.* **41**:443–455.

Basch, R. S., and Goldstein, G. 1974. Induction of T cell differentiation *in vitro* by thymin, a purified polypeptide hormone of the thymus. *Proc. Natl. Acad. Sci. USA* **71**:1474–1478.

Benacerraf, B., and Dorf, M. E. 1977. Genetic control of specific immune suppressions by I-region genes. *Cold Spring Harbor Symp. Quant. Biol.* **41**:465–475.

Benner, R., Rijnbeek, A. M., Bernabé, R. R., Martinez-Alonso, C., and Coutinho, A. 1981. Frequencies of background immunoglobulin-secreting cells in mice as a function of organ, age, and immune states. *Immunobiology* **158**:225–238.

Bernard, C. C. A., Bordmann, G., Blomberg, B., and DuPasquier, L. 1981. Genetic control of T-helper cell function in the clawed toad *Xenopus laevis. Eur. J. Immunol.* **11**:151–155.

Bernard, O., and Gough, N. M. 1980. Nucleotide sequence of heavy chain joining segments between translated V^h and μ constant region genes. *Proc. Natl. Acad. Sci. USA* **77**:3630–3634.

Bernard, O., Hozumi, N., and Tonegawa, S. 1978. Sequences of mouse immunoglublin light chain genes before and after somatic changes. *Cell* **15**:1133–1144.

Beverley, P. C. L., Woody, J., Dunkley, M., Feidmann, M., and McKenzie, I. 1976. Separation of suppressor and killer T cells by surface phenotype. *Nature (London)* **262**:495–497.

Bienenstock, J., and Befus, A. D. 1980. Mucosal immunology. *Immunology* **41**:249–270.

Binz, H., and Wigzell, H. 1975. Shared idiotypic determinants on B and T lymphocytes reactive against the same antigenic determinants. II. Determination of frequency and characteristics of idiotype T and B lymphocytes in normal rats using direct visualization. *J. Exp. Med.* **142**:1218–1240.

Bliznakov, E. G. 1980. Suppression of immunological responsiveness in aged mice and its relationship with coenzyme Q deficiency. *In:* Escobar, M. R., and Friedman, H., eds., *Macrophages and Lymphocytes: Nature, Functions, and Interaction*, New York, Plenum Press, Part A, pp. 361–369.

Boime, I., McWilliams, D., Szczesna, E., and Camel, M. 1976. Synthesis of human placental lactogen messenger RNA as a function of gestation. *J. Biol. Chem.* **251**:820–825.

Bolivar, F., Rodrigues, R., Greene, P., Betlach, M., Heynecker, H., and Boyer, H. 1977. Construction and characterization of new cloning vehicles. II. A multipurpose cloning system. *Gene* **2**:95–113.

Boltz-Nitulescu, G., and Spiegelberg, H. L., 1981. Receptors specific for IgE on rat alveolar and peritoneal macrophages. *Cell. Immunol.* **59**:106–114.

Borel, Y., and Young, M. C., 1980. Nucleic acid-specific suppressor T cells. *Proc. Natl. Acad. Sci. USA* **77**:1593–1596.

Boswell, H. S., Ahmed, A., Scher, I., and Singer, A. 1980. Role of accessory cells in B cell activation. II. *J. Immunol.* **125**:1340–1348.

Bothwell, A. L. M., Paskind, M., Reth, M., Imanishi-Kari, T., Rajewsky, K., and Baltimore, D.

1981. Heavy chain variable region contribution to the NP[b] family of antibodies: Somatic mutation evident in a γ2a variable region. *Cell* **24**:625–637.

Braciale, T. J., Andrew, M. E., and Braciale, V. L. 1981. Heterogeneity and specificity of cloned lines of influenza-virus-specific cytotoxic T lymphocytes. *J. Exp. Med.* **153**:910–923.

Bridgen, J., Snary, D., Crumpton, M. J., Barnstable, C., Goodfellow, P., and Bodmer, W. F. 1976. Isolation and N-terminal amino acid sequence of membrane bound human HLA-A and HLA-B antigens. *Nature (London)* **261**:200–205.

Broder, S., Humphrey, R., Durm, M. Blackman, M., Meade, B., Goldman, C., Strober, W., and Waldman, T. 1975. Impaired synthesis of polyclonal (non-paraprotein) immunoglobulins by circulating lymphocytes from patients with multiple myeloma: Role of suppressor cells. *N. Engl. J. Med.* **293**:887–892.

Brunner, K. T., Mauel, J., Cerottini, J. C., and Chapuis, B. 1968. Quantitative assay of the lytic action of immune lymphoid cells on [57]Cr-labeled allogeneic target cells *in vitro*. *Immunology* **14**:181–196.

Burrows, P. D., Beck, G. B., and Wabl, M. R. 1981. Expression of μ and γ immunoglobulin heavy chains in different cells of a cloned mouse lymphoid line. *Proc. Natl. Acad. Sci. USA* **78**:564–568.

Burton, R. C., and Winn, H. J. 1981. Studies on natural killer (NK) cells. I. NK cell specific antibodies in CE anti-CBA serum. *J. Immunol.* **126**:1985–1989.

Calderon, J., Kiely, J. M., Lefko, J., and Unanue, E. R. 1975. The modulation of lymphocyte functions by molecules secreted by macrophages. I. Description and partial biochemical analysis. *J. Exp. Med.* **142**:151–164.

Cantor, H., and Boyse, E. A. 1975. Cooperation between subclasses of Ly bearing cells in the generation of killer activity. *J. Exp. Med.* **141**:1390–1399.

Cantor, H., Shen, F. W., and Boyse, E. A. 1976. Separation of helper T cells from suppressor T cells expressing different Ly components. II. Activation by antigen after immunization: Antigen-specific suppressor and helper activity are mediated by distinct T cell subclasses. *J. Exp. Med.* **143**:1391–1401.

Capra, J. D., and Kehoe, J. M. 1975. Hypervariable regions, idiotypy, and the antibody-combining site. *Adv. Immunol.* **20**:1–40.

Capron, M., Capron, A., Dessaint, J. P., Torpier, G., Johansson, S. G. O., and Prin, L. 1981. Fc receptors for IgE on human and rat eosinophils. *J. Immunol.* **126**:2087–2092.

Cayre, Y., de Sostoa, A., and Silverstone, A. E. 1981. Isolation of a subset of thymocytes inducible for terminal transferase biosynthesis. *J. Immunol.* **126**:553–556.

Cebra, J. J., Gearhart, P. J., Kamat, R., Robertson, S. M., and Tseng, J. 1977. Origin and differentiation of lymphocytes involved in the secretory IgA response. *Cold Spring Harbor Symp. Quant. Biol.* **41**:201–215.

Cerottini, J. C., and Brunner, K. T. 1974. Cell-mediated cytotoxicity, allograft rejection, and tumor immunity. *Adv. Immunol.* **18**:67–132.

Chandrasekaran, E. V., Mendicino, A., Garver, F. A., and Mendicino, J. 1981. Structures of sialylated *O*-glycosidically and *N*-glycosidically linked oligosaccharides in a monoclonal immunoglobulin light chain. *J. Biol. Chem.* **256**:1549–1555.

Charmot, D., Mawas, C., Kristensen, T., and Mercier, P. 1981. The *HLA-D* system: At least two loci and four distinct phenotypic traits per haplotype. *Immunogenetics* **13**:57–84.

Chen, W., Teodorescu, M., McKenzie, I. F. C., and Mayer, E. P. 1981. Functional characterization of mouse lymphocyte subpopulations identified by their natural binding of bacteria. II. *Immunology* **42**:285–295.

Claman, H. N., Chaperon, E. A., and Triplet, R. F. 1966. Thymus–marrow cell combinations: Synergism in antibody production. *Proc. Soc. Exp. Biol. Med.* **122**:1167–1171.

Clark, E. A., and Holly, R. D. 1981. Activation of natural killer (NK) cells *in vivo* with H-2 and non-H-2 alloantigens. *Immunogenetics* **12**:221–235.

Clark, E. A., Russell, P. H., Egghart, M., and Horton, M. A. 1979. Characteristics and genetic control of NK-cell-mediated cytotoxicity activated by naturally acquired infection in the mouse. *Int. J. Cancer* **24**:688–699.

Cobleigh, M. A., Braun, D. P., and Harris, J. E. 1980. Age-dependent changes in human peripheral blood B cells and T-cell subsets: Correlation with mitogen responsiveness. *Clin. Immunol. Immunopathol.* **15**:162–174.

Cohen, F. E., Novotný, J., Sternberg, M. J. E., Campbell, D. G., and Williams, A. F. 1981. Analysis of structural similarities between brain Thy-1 antigen and immunoglobulin domains. *Biochem. J.* **195**:31–40.

Cohn, M., Blomberg, B., Geckler, W., Raschke, W., Riblet, R., and Weigert, M. 1977. First order considerations in analyzing the generator of diversity. *In*: Sercarz, E. E., Herzenberg, L. A., and Fox, C. F., eds., *The Immune System: Genetics and Regulation*, New York, Academic Press, pp. 89–117.

Cooper, M. D., Peterson, R. D. A., South, M. A., and Good, R. A. 1966. The functions of the thymus system and the bursa system in the chicken. *J. Exp. Med.* **123**:75–102.

Coutinho, A., and Forni, L. 1981. The enhancement of antibody response by IgM antibodies is dependent on antigen-specific T helper cells. *Immunobiology* **158**:182–190.

Damacco, F., Michielsen, T. E., and Natvig, J. B. 1972. The hinge region of IgG3, an extended part of the molecule. *FEBS Lett.* **28**:121–124.

Dausset, J. 1981. The major histocompatibility complex in man. *Science* **213**:1469–1474.

Davis, M. M., Calame, K., Early, P. W., Livant, D. L., Joho, R., Weissman, I. L., and Hood, L. 1980. An immunoglobulin heavy-chain gene is formed by at least two recombinational events. *Nature (London)* **283**:733–739.

Delovitch, T. L., and Sohn, U. 1979. *In vitro* analysis of allogeneic lymphocyte interaction. III. Generation of helper allogeneic effect factor (AEF) across an I–J subregion disparity. *J. Immunol.* **122**:1528–1534.

Deslauriers-Boisvert, N., Mercier, G., and Lafleur, L. 1980. Size separation and polyclonal activation to immunoglobulin secretion of early precursors of B lymphocytes. *J. Immunol.* **125**:47–53.

DeWeck, A. L., Kristensen, F., and Landy, M., eds. 1980. *Biochemical Characterization of Lymphokines*, New York, Academic Press.

Dillon, L. S. 1978. *The Genetic Mechanism and the Origin of Life*, New York, Plenum Press.

Dillon, L. S. 1981. *Ultrastructure, Macromolecules, and Evolution*, New York, Plenum Press.

Doll, R., Muir, C., and Waterhouse, J., eds. 1970. *Cancer Incidence in Five Continents*, Berlin, Springer-Verlag.

Draper, L. P., and Süssdorf, D. H. 1957. The serum hemolysin response in intact and splenectomized rabbits following immunization by various routes. *J. Infect. Dis.* **100**:147–161.

Dunlap, D., Bach, F. H., and Bach, M. L. 1978. Cell surface changes in alloantigen activated T. lympocytes. *Nature (London)*. **271**:253–255.

Dutton, R. W., Falkoff, R., Hirst, J., Hoffmann, M. K., Kappler, J., Kettman, J., Lesley, J., and Vann, D. 1971. Is there evidence for a nonantigen specific diffusible chemical mediator from the thymus derived cells in the initiation of the immune response? *In*: Amos, B., ed., *Progress in Immunology*, New York, Academic Press, pp. 355–368.

Early, P. W., Davis, M. M., Kaback, D. B., Davidson, N., and Hood, L. 1979. Immunoglobulin heavy chain gene organization in mice: Analysis of a myeloma genomic clone containing variable and α constant regions. *Proc. Natl. Acad. Sci. USA* **76**:857–861.

Early, P., Huang, H., Davis, M., Calame, K., and Hood, L. 1980. An immunoglobulin heavy chain variable region gene is generated from three segments of DNA: V_H, D and J_H. *Cell* **19**:981–992.

Early P., Rogers, J., Davis, M., Calame, K., Bond, M., Wall, R., and Hood, L. 1981. Two mRNAs can be produced from a single immunoglobulin μ gene by alternative RNA processing pathways. *Cell* **20**:313–319.

Edelman, G. M., Cunningham, B. A., Gall, W. E., Gottlieb, P. D., Rutishauser, U., and Waxdal,

M. J. 1969. The covalent structure of an entire γG immunoglobulin molecule. *Proc. Natl. Acad. Sci. USA* **63**:78–85.

Eichmann, K. 1978. Expression and function of idiotypes on lymphocytes. *Adv. Immunol.* **26**:195–254.

Ellis, E. F. 1969. Immunologic basis of atopic disease. *Adv. Pediatr.* **16**:65–98.

Endres, R. O., and Grey, H. M. 1980. Antigen recognition by T cells. I. Suppressor T cells fail to recognize cross-reactivity between native and denatured ovalbumin. *J. Immunol.* **125**:1515–1520.

Erb, P., and Feldmann, M. 1975. The role of macrophages in the generation of T helper cells. II. The genetic control of the macrophage–T cell interaction for helper cell induction with soluble antigen. *J. Exp. Med.* **142**:460–472.

Everett, N. B., and Tyler, R. W. 1967. Lymphopoiesis in the thymus and other tissues: Functional implications. *Int. Rev. Cytol.* **22**:205–237.

Fahey, J. L., and Solomon, A. 1963. Two types of γ-myeloma proteins, β_{2A} myeloma-proteins, γ1-macroglobulins, and Bence–Jones proteins identified by two groups of common antigenic determinants. *J. Clin. Invest.* **42**:811–822.

Fanger, M. W., and Smyth, D. G. 1972. The oligosaccharide units of rabbit immunoglobulin G: Multiple carbohydrate attachment sites. *Biochem. J.* **127**:757–765.

Farrar, J. J., Simon, P. L., Farrar, W. L., Koopman, J., and Fuller-Bonar, J. 1980. Role of mitogenic factor, lymphocyte activating factor, and immune interferon in the induction of humoral and cell-mediated immunity. *Ann. N.Y. Acad. Sci.* **332**:303–315.

Farrar, W. L., Mizel, S. B., and Farrar, J. J. 1980. Participation of lymphocyte activating factor (interleukin 1) in the production of cytotoxic T cell responses. *J. Immunol.* **124**:1371–1377.

Farrar, W. L., Johnson, H. M., and Farrar, J. J. 1981. Regulation of the production of immune interferon and cytotoxic T lymphocytes by interleukin 2. *J. Immunol.* **126**:1120–1125.

Feldmann, M., and Kotiainen, S. 1976. Suppressor cell induction *in vitro*. II. Cellular requirements of suppressor cell induction. *Eur. J. Immunol.* **6**:302–305.

Finke, J. H., Orosz, C. G., and Battisto, J. R. 1977. Splenic T-killer cells can be generated by allogeneic thymic cells in conjunction with assisting factor. *Nature (London)* **267**:353–354.

Fishelson, Z., and Berke, G. 1981. Tumor cell destruction by cytotoxic T lymphocytes: The basis of reduced antitumor cell activity in syngeneic hosts. *J. Immunol.* **126**:2048–2052.

Forni, L., Coutinho, A., Köhler, G., and Jerne, N. K. 1980. IgM antibodies induce the production of antibodies of the same specificity. *Proc. Natl. Acad. Sci. USA* **77**:1125–1128.

Fournier, C., and Charreire, J. 1981. Autologous mixed lymphocytic reaction in man. I. Relation with age and sex. *Cell. Immunol.* **60**:212–219.

Frangione, B., and Milstein, C. 1968. Variations in the S–S bridges of immunoglobulins G: Interchain disulphide bridges of γG3 myeloma proteins. *J. Mol. Biol.* **33**:893–906.

Frangione, B., Milstein, C., and Franklin, E. C. 1969. Chemical typing of immunoglobulins. *Nature (London)* **221**:149–151.

Franklin, E. C. 1962. Two types of γ_{1A}-globulin in sera from normals and patients with multiple myeloma. *Nature (London)* **195**:393–394.

Franklin, E. C., and Frangione, B. 1969. Immunoglobulins. *Annu. Rev. Med.* **20**:155–174.

Friedman, S. M., Hunter, S. B., Irigoyen, O. H., Kung, P. C., Goldstein, G., and Chess, L. 1981. Functional analysis of human T cell subsets defined by monoclonal antibodies. II. Collaborative T–T interactions in the generation of TNP-altered-self-reactive cytotoxic T lymphocytes. *J. Immunol.* **126**:1702–1705.

Fu, S. M., Winchester, R. J., and Kunkel, H. G. 1975. Similar idiotypic specificity for the membrane IgD and IgM of human B lymphocytes. *J. Immunol.* **114**:250–254.

Fulton, A. M., and Levy, J. G., 1981. The induction of nonspecific T suppressor lymphocytes by prostaglandin E. *Cell. Immunol.* **59**:54–60.

Gadd, K. J., and Reid, K. B. M. 1981. Importance of the integrity of the inter-heavy-chain disulphide bond of rabbit IgG in the activation of the alternative pathway of human complement by the F(ab')$_2$ region of rabbit IgG antibody in immune aggregates. *Immunology* **42**:75–82.

Gahrton, G., Robèrt, K. H., Friberg, K., Zech, L., and Bird, A. G. 1980. Nonrandom chromosomal aberrations in chronic lymphocytic leukemia revealed by polyclonal B-cell-mitogen stimulation. *Blood* **56**:640–647.

Galili, N., Devens, B., Naor, D., Becker, S., and Klein, E. 1978. Immune reponses to weakly immunogenic virally induced tumors. *Eur. J. Immunol.* **8**:17–22.

Gally, J. A., and Edelman, G. M. 1972. The genetic control of immunoglobulin synthesis. *Annu. Rev. Genet.* **6**:1–46.

Garver, F. A., Chang, L. S., Kiefer, C. R., Mendicino, J., Chandrasekaran, E. V., Isobe, T., and Osserman, E. F. 1981. Localization of the carbohydrate units in a human immunoglobulin light chain, protein Smλ. *Eur. J. Biochem.* **115**:643–652.

Gately, M. K., and Martz, E. 1981. T11: A new protein marker on activated murine T lymphocytes. *J. Immunol.* **126**:709–714.

Gathings, W. E., Cooper, M. D., Lawton, A. R., and Alford, C. A. 1976. B cell ontogeny in humans. *Fed. Proc.* **35**:276.

Gathings, W. E., Lawton, A. R., and Cooper, M. D. 1977. Immunofluorescent studies of the development of pre-B cells, B lymphocytes and immunoglobulin isotype diversity in humans. *Eur. J. Immunol.* **7**:804–810.

Gearhart, P. J., Johnson, N. D., Douglas, R., and Hood, L. 1981. IgG antibodies to phosphorylcholine exhibit more diversity than their IgM counterparts. *Nature (London)* **291**:29–34.

Gery, I., and Waksman, B. H. 1972. Potentiation of the T-lymphocyte response to mitogens. II. The cellular source of potentiating factors. *J. Exp. Med.* **136**:143–155.

Gilbert, W. 1979. Introns and exons: Playgrounds of evolution. *ICN–UCLA Symp. Mol. Cell. Biol.* **14**:1–10.

Glimcher, L., Shen, F. W., and Cantor, H. 1977. Identification of a cell surface antigen selectively expressed on the natural killer cell. *J. Exp. Med.* **145**:1–9.

Goding, J. W., and Layton, J. E. 1976. Antigen-induced co-capping of IgM and IgD-like receptors on murine B cells. *J. Exp. Med.* **144**:852–857.

Goding, J. W., Scott, D. W., and Layton, J. E. 1977. Genetics, cellular expression and function of IgD and IgM receptors. *Immunol. Rev.* **37**:152–186.

Goldstein, G., Scheid, M. P., Hämmerling, U., Boyse, E. A., Schlesinger, D. H., and Niall, H. D. 1975. Isolation of a polypeptide that has lymphocyte differentiation properties and is probably present universally in living cells. *Proc. Natl. Acad. Sci. USA* **72**:11–15.

Golub, E. S. 1977. *The Cellular Basis of the Immune Response*, Sunderland, Mass., Sinauer.

Golub, E. S. 1981. Suppressor T cells and their possible role in the regulation of autoreactivity. *Cell* **24**:595–596.

Goodman, J. W. 1963. Antigenic determinants in fragments of gamma globulin from rabbit serum. *Science* **139**:1292–1293.

Gormus, B. J., Crandall, R. B., and Shands, J. W. 1974. Endotoxin-stimulated spleen cells: Mitogenesis, the occurrence of the C3 receptor, and the production of immunoglobulin. *J. Immunol.* **112**:770–775.

Gormus, B. J., Basara, M. L., Cossman, J., Arneson, M. A., and Kaplan, M. E. 1980. The bacteria (B)–antibody (A)–complement (C) (BAC) rosette method for detecting C3 receptors (R): Binding specificity and capping of human peripheral blood lymphocyte C3R. *Cell. Immunol.* **55**:94–105.

Götze, D. 1977. *The Major Histocompatibility System in Man and Animals*, Berlin, Springer-Verlag.

Gough, N. M., and Bernard, O. 1981. Sequences of the joining region genes for immunoglobulin heavy chains and their role in generation of antibody diversity. *Proc. Natl. Acad. Sci. USA* **78**:509–513.

Greenstein, J. L., Lord, E. M., Horan, P., Kappler, J. W., and Marrack, P. 1981. Functional aspects of B cells defined by quantitative differences in surface I-A. *J. Immunol.* **126**:2419–2423.

Grey, H. M., and Kunkel, H. G. 1964. H chain subgroups of myeloma proteins and normal 7S λ-globulins. *J. Exp. Med.* **120**:253–266.

Grossi, C. E., Webb, S. R., Zicia, A., Lydyard, P. M., Moretta, L., Mingari, M. C., and Cooper, M. D. 1978. Morphological and histochemical analyses of two human T-cell subpopulations bearing receptors for IgM or IgG. *J. Exp. Med.* **147**:1408–1417.

Haas, M. 1974. Continuous production of radiation leukemia virus in C57BL thymoma tissue culture lines: Purification of the leukemogenic virus. *Cell* **1**:79–89.

Hafeman, D. G., and Lucas, Z. J. 1979. Polymorphonuclear leukocyte-mediated, antibody-dependent, cellular cytotoxicity against tumor cells: Dependent on oxygen and respiratory burst. *J. Immunol.* **123**:55–62.

Hansson, M., Kiessling, R., Andersson, B., Kärre, K., and Roder, J. 1979a. NK cell-sensitive T-cell subpopulation in thymus: Inverse correlation to host NK activity. *Nature (London)* **278**:174–176.

Hansson, M., Kärre, K., Kiessling, R., Roder, J., Andersson, B., and Häyry, P. 1979b. Natural NK-cell targets in the mouse thymus: Characteristics of the sensitive cell population. *J. Immunol.* **123**:765–771.

Hansson, M., Kiessling, R., and Andersson, B. 1981. Human fetal thymus and bone marrow contain target cells for natural killer cells. *Eur. J. Immunol.* **11**:8–12.

Haynes, B. F., and Fauci, A. S. 1977. Activation of human B lymphocytes. III. Concanavalin A-induced generation of suppressor cells of the plaque-forming cell response of normal human B lymphocytes. *J. Immunol.* **118**:2281–2287.

Hayward, A. R., Simons, M. A., Lawton, A. R., Mage, R. G., and Cooper, M. D. 1977. Pre-B and B cells in rabbits: Ontogeny and allelic exclusion of kappa light chain genes. *J. Exp. Med.* **148**:1367–1377.

Hellström, K. E., and Hellström, I. 1974. Lymphocyte-mediated cytotoxicity and blocking serum activities to tumor antigens. *Adv. Immunol.* **18**:209–277.

Henney, C. S. 1973. On the mechanism of T-cell mediated cytolysis. *Transplant. Rev.* **17**:37–56.

Henson, P. M. 1971. Release of biologically active constituents from blood cells and its role in antibody-mediated tissue injury. *In*: Amos, B., ed., *Progress in Immunology*, New York, Academic Press, Vol. I, pp. 155–171.

Herberman, R. B., and Ortaldo, J. R. 1981. Natural killer cells: Their role in defenses against disease. *Science* **214**:24–30.

Herberman, R. B., Nunn, M. E., and Lavrin, D. H. 1975. Natural cytotoxic reactivity of mouse lymphoid cells against syngeneic and allogeneic tumors. *Int. J. Cancer* **16**:216–229.

Herberman, R. B., Holden, H. T., Varesio, L., Taniyama, T., Puccetti, P., Kirchner, H., Gerson, J., White, S., and Keisari, Y. 1980. Immunologic reactivity of lymphoid cells in tumors. *Contemp. Top. Immunobiol.* **10**:61–78.

Hildemann, W. H., and Jokiel, P. L. 1979. Immunocompetence in the lowest metazoan phylum: Transplantation immunity in sponges. *Science* **204**:420–422.

Hildemann, W. H., and Thoenes, G. H. 1969. Immunological responses of Pacific hagfish. I. Skin transplantation immunity. *Transplantation* **7**:506–521.

Hilschmann, N. 1967. Die chemische Struktur von zwei Bence-Jones-Proteinen (Roy and Cum.) von κ-Typ. *Hoppe-Seyler's Z. Physiol. Chem.* **348**:1077–1080.

Hoessli, D. C., and Vassalli, P. 1980. High molecular weight surface glycoproteins of murine lymphocytes. *J. Immunol.* **125**:1758–1763.

Hoffmann, M. K. 1980. Macrophages and T cells control distinct phases of B cell differentiation in the humoral immune response *in vitro*. *J. Immunol.* **125**:2076–2081.

Hoffmann, M. K., and Dutton, R. W. 1971. Immune response restoration with macrophage culture supernatants. *Science* **172**:1047–1048.

Hoffmann, M. K., and Watson, J. 1979. Helper T cell replacing factors secreted by thymus-derived cells and by macrophages: Cellular requirements for B cell activation and synergistic properties. *J. Immunol.* **122**:1371–1375.

Hoffmann, M. K., Hämmerling, U., Simon, M., and Oettgen, H. F. 1976. Macrophage requirements of CR⁻ and CR⁺ B lymphocytes for antibody production *in vitro*. *J. Immunol.* **116**:1447–1451.

Honjo, T., and Kataoka, T. 1978. Organization of immunoglobulin heavy chain genes and allelic deletion model. *Proc. Natl. Acad. Sci. USA* **75**:2140–2144.

Horwitz, D. A., Kight, N., Temple, A., and Allison, A. C. 1979. Spontaneous and induced cytotoxic properties of human adherent mononuclear cells. *Immunology* **36**:221–228.

Huber, B., Devinsky, O., Gershon, R. K., and Cantor, H. 1976. Cell-mediated immunity: Delayed type hypersensitivity and cytotoxic responses are mediated by different T-cell subclasses. *J. Exp. Med.* **143**:1534–1539.

Humphrey, J. H., and Dourmashkin, R. R. 1969. The lesions in cell membrane caused by complement. *Adv. Immunol.* **11**:75–115.

Humphrey, J. H., and Grennan, D. 1981. Different macrophage populations distinguished by means of fluorescent polysaccharides: Recognition and properties of marginal-zone macrophages. *Eur. J. Immunol.* **11**:221–228.

Ishizaka, K., and Adachi, T. 1976. Generation of specific helper cells and suppressor cells *in vitro* for the IgE and IgG antibody responses. *J. Immunol.* **117**:40–47.

Jaffe, B. M., Behrman, H. R., and Parker, C. W. 1973. Radioimmunoassay measurement of prostaglandins E, A, and F in human plasma. *J. Clin. Invest.* **52**:398–405.

Johanson, R. A., Shaw, A. R., and Schlamowitz, M. 1981. Evidence that the C_H2 domain of IgG contains the recognition unit for binding by the fetal rabbit yolk sac membrane receptor. *J. Immunol.* **126**:194–199.

Johnson, B. J. 1977. Complement: A host defense mechanism ready for pharmacological manipulation. *J. Pharmacol. Sci.* **66**:1367–1376.

Jones, P. P., Murphy, D. B., and McDevitt, H. O. 1978. Two-gene control of the expression of a murine Ia antigen. *J. Exp. Med.* **148**:925–939.

Kabat, E. A., Wu, T. T., and Bilofsky, H. 1979. *Sequences of Immunoglobulin Chains*, Bethesda, National Institutes of Health.

Kanellopoulos, J. M., Liu, T. Y., Poy, G., and Metzger, H. 1980. Composition and subunit structure of the cell receptor for immunoglobulin E. *J. Biol. Chem.* **255**:9060–9066.

Kano, S., Oshimi, K., Sumiya, M., and Gonda, N. 1980. Activation of secondary cytotoxic lymphocytes by cell-free factors from I-region-primed and D-region-primed lymphocytes. *Immunology* **41**:653–662.

Katz, D. H. 1977. *Lymphocyte Differentiation, Recognition, and Regulation*, New York, Academic Press.

Katz, D. H. 1980a. Recent studies on the regulation of IgE antibody synthesis in experimental animals and man. *Immunology* **41**:1–24.

Katz, D. H. 1980b. Adaptive differentiation of lymphocytes: Theoretical implications for mechanisms of cell–cell recognition and regulation of immune responses. *Adv. Immunol.* **29**:137–207.

Katz, D. H., Hamaoka, T., and Benacerraf, B. 1973. Cell interactions between histoincompatible T and B lymphocytes. II. Failure of physiological cooperative interactions between T and B lymphocytes from allogeneic donor strains in humoral response to hapten–protein conjugates. *J. Exp. Med.* **137**:1405–1418.

Katz, D. H., Chiorazzi, N., McDonald, J., and Katz, L. R. 1976. Cell interactions between histoincompatible T and B lymphocytes. IX. The failure of histocompatible cells is not due to suppression and cannot be circumvented by carrier-priming T cells with allogeneic macrophages. *J. Immunol.* **117**:1853–1859.

Kawate, T., Abo, T., Hinuman, S., and Kumagai, K. 1981. Studies on the bioperiodicity of the immune response. II. Co-variations of murine T and B cells in the role of a corticosteroid. *J. Immunol.* **126**:1364–1367.

Keller, R. 1976. Cytostatic and cytocidal effects of activated macrophages. *In*: Nelson, D. S., ed., *Immunobiology of the Macrophage*, New York, Academic Press, pp. 487–508.

Kempner, D. H., Liebold, W., and Gatti, R. A. 1980. T-cell regulation of B-lymphoblastoid cell line function. *Cell. Immunol.* **55**:32–41.

Keystone, E. C., Gladman, D. D., and Cane, D. 1980. Antigen-specific suppressor cell activity in man. 1. Temporal, antigenic, and proliferative requirements. *Cell. Immunol.* **55**:136–144.

Kiessling, R. W., and Welsh, R. M. 1980. Killing of normal cells by activated mouse natural killer cells: Evidence for two patterns of genetic regulation of lysis. *Int. J. Cancer* **25**:611–615.

Kinoshita, T., Hong, K., Kondo, K., and Inoue, K. 1981. Fifth component of guinea pig complement: Purification and characterization. *J. Immunol.* **126**:2414–2418.

Kishimoto, T., Hirano, T., Kuritani, T., Yamamura, Y., Ralph, P., and Good, R. A. 1978. Induction of IgG production in human B lymphoblastoid cell lines with normal human T cells. *Nature (London)* **271**:756–758.

Kisielow, P., Hirst, J. A., Shiku, H., Beverley, P. C. L., Hoffmann, M. K., Boyse, E. A., and Oettgen, H. F. 1975. Ly antigens as markers for functionally distinct subpopulations of thymus-derived lymphocytes of the mouse. *Nature (London)* **253**:219–220.

Kitamura, Y., Shimada, M., Hatanaka, K., and Miyano, Y. 1977. Development of mast cells from grafted bone marrow cells in irradiated mice. *Nature (London)* **268**:442–443.

Kitamura, Y., Shimada, M., and Go, S. 1979a. Presence of mast cell precursors in fetal liver of mice. *Dev. Biol.* **70**:510–514.

Kitamura, Y., Hatanaka, K., Murakami, M., and Shibata, H. 1979b. Decrease of mast cells in W/W^v mice and their increase by bone marrow transplantation. *Blood* **52**:447–452.

Kitamura, Y., Yokoyama, M., Matsuda, H., Ohno, T., and Mori, K. J. 1981. Spleen colony-forming cell as common precursor for tissue mast cells and granulocytes. *Nature (London)* **291**:159–160.

Klassen, D. K., and Sagone, A. L. 1980. Evidence for both oxygen and non-oxygen dependent mechanisms of antibody sensitized target cell lysis by human monocytes. *Blood* **56**:985–992.

Klaus, G. G. B., Halpern, M. S., Koshland, M. E., and Goodman, J. W. 1971. A polypeptide chain from leopard shark 19S immunoglobulin analogous to mammalian J chain. *J. Immunol.* **107**:1785–1787.

Klein, B. Y, and Naor, D. 1979. Anti-YAC cell mediated cytotoxicity induced by immunization of syngeneic mice with YAC cellular fractions. *Isr. J. Med. Sci.* **15**:884.

Klein, B. Y., Frenkel, S., Ahituv, A., and Naor, D. 1980. Immunogenicity of subcellular fractions and molecular species of MuLV-induced tumors. *J. Immunol. Methods* **38**:325–341.

Klein, B. Y., Caraux, J., Thierry, C., Gauci, L., Causse, A., and Serrou, B. 1981a. Human T-lymphocyte colonies: Generation of colonies in different lymphocyte subpopulations. *Immunology* **43**:39–45.

Klein, B. Y., Devens, B., Deutsch, O., Ahituv, A., Frenkel, S., Kobrin, B. J., and Naor, D. 1981b. Isolation of immunogenic and suppressorgenic determinants of the nonimmunogenic YAC tumor and the change in immunogenic repertoire after *in vitro* cultivation. *Transplant. Proc.* **13**:790–797.

Knapp, W., Bolhuis, R. L. H., Radl, J., and Hijmans, W. 1973. Independent movement of IgD and IgM molecules on the surface of individual lymphocytes. *J. Immunol.* **111**:1295–1298.

Knox, R. B., and Clarke, A. E. 1980. Discrimination of self and non-self in plants. *Contemp. Top. Immunobiol.* **9**:1–36.

Kobayashi, K., Vaerman, J. P., Bazin, H., Lebacq-Verheden, A. M., and Heremans, J. F. 1973. Identification of J chain in polymeric immunoglobulins from a variety of species by cross-reaction with rabbit antisera to human J chain. *J. Immunol.* **111**:1590–1594.

Parker, C. D., Fothergill, J. J., and Wadsworth, D. C. 1979. B lymphocyte activation by insoluble immunoglobulin: Induction of immunoglobulin secretion by a T cell-dependent soluble factor. *J. Immunol.* **123**:931–941.

Parkhouse, R. M. E., Abney, E. R., Bourgois, A., and Willcox, H. N. A. 1977. Functional and structural characterization of immunoglobulin on murine B lymphocytes. *Cold Spring Harbor Symp. Quant. Biol.* **41**:193–200.

Passwell, J. H., Colten, H. R., Schneeberger, E. L., Marom, Z., and Merler, E. 1980. Modulation of human monocyte functions by Fc fragments of IgG. *Immunology* **41**:217–226.

Paul, W. E., and Benacerraf, B. 1977. Functional specificity of thymus-dependent lymphocytes. *Science* **195**:1293–1300.

Pernis, B., Forni, L., and Amante, L. 1971. Immunoglobulins as cell receptors. *Ann. N.Y. Acad. Sci.* **190**:420–431.

Pernis, B., Brouet, J. C., and Seligmann, M. 1974. IgD and IgM on the membrane of lymphoid cells in macroglobulinemia. *Eur. J. Immunol.* **4**:776–778.

Pernis, B., Forni, L., and Knight, K. L. 1975. The problem of an IgD equivalent in non-primates. *In:* Seligmann, M., Preud'homme, J. L., and Kourilsky, F. M., eds., *Membrane Receptors of Lymphocytes,* Amsterdam, North-Holland, pp. 57–64.

Pernis, B., Forni, L., and Luzzati, A. C. 1976. Synthesis of multiple immunoglobulin classes by single lymphocytes. *Cold Spring Harbor Symp. Quant. Biol.* **41**:175–183.

Perry, R. P., and Kelley, D. E. 1979. Immunoglobulin RNAs in murine cell lines that have characteristics of immature B lymphocytes. *Cell* **18**:1333–1339.

Pierres, M., and Germain, R. N. 1978. Antigen-specific T cell-mediated suppression. IV. Role of macrophages in generation of L-glutamic acid[60]-L-alanine[30]-L-tyrosine[10] (GAT)-specific suppressor T cells in responder mouse strains. *J. Immunol.* **121**:1306–1314.

Pilarski, L. M. 1977. A requirement for antigen-specific helper T cells in the generation of cytotoxic T cells from thymocyte precursors. *J. Exp. Med.* **145**:709–725.

Pillai, P. S., and Scott, D. W. 1981. Hapten-specific murine colony-forming B cells: *In vitro* response of colonies to fluoresceinated thymus independent antigens. *J. Immunol.* **126**:1883–1886.

Plate, J. M. D. 1976. Soluble factors substitute for T–T cell collaboration in generation of T killer cells. *Nature (London)* **260**:329–331.

Plate, J. M. D. 1980. Genetic mapping of an H-2-associated antigen expressed on regulatory T cells. *J. Immunol.* **125**:1102–1112.

Plate, J. M. D. 1981. Major histocompatibility complex restriction of soluble helper molecules in T cell response to altered self. *J. Exp. Med.* **153**:1102–1112.

Plater, C., Debré, P., and Leclerc, J. C. 1981. T cell-mediated immunity to oncornavirus-induced tumors. III. Specific and nonspecific suppression in tumor-bearing mice. *Eur. J. Immunol.* **11**:39–44.

Plaut, M., Lichtenstein, L. M., Gillespie, E., and Henney, C. S. 1973. Studies on the mechanism of lymphocyte-mediated cytolysis. IV. Specificity of the histamine receptor on effector T cells. *J. Immunol.* **111**:389–394.

Plaut, M., Lichtenstein, L. M., and Henney, C. S. 1975. Properties of a subpopulation of T cells bearing histamine receptors. *J. Clin. Invest.* **55**:856–874.

Poulsen, P. B., and Claësson, M. H. 1980. B lymphocyte colony formation *in vitro:* Ultrastructural development of individual colonies. *Differentiation* **17**:77–84.

Prager, M. D., and Baechtel, F. S. 1973. Methods for modification of cancer cells to enhance their antigenicity. *Methods Cancer Res.* **9**:339–400.

Press, E. M., and Hogg, N. M. 1970. The amino acid sequences of the Fd fragments of two human γ1 heavy chains. *Biochem. J.* **117**:641–660.

Primi, D., Lewis, G. K., and Goodman, J. W. 1980. The role of immunoglobulin receptors and T cell mediators in B lymphocyte activation. *J. Immunol.* **125**:1286–1292.

Pross, H. F., and Baines, M. G. 1977. Spontaneous human lymphocyte-mediated cytotoxicity against tumor target cells. VI. A brief review. *Cancer Immunol. Immunother.* **3**:75–94.

Putnam, D., Storb, U., and Clagett, J. 1977. Synthesis of kappa chains from thymus RNA by cell free translation. *ICN–UCLA Symp. Mol. Cell. Biol.* **6**:71–77.

Putnam, F. W., Florent, G., Paul, C., Shinoda, T., and Shinizu, A. 1973. Complete amino acid sequence of the mu heavy chain of a human IgM immunoglobulin. *Science* **182**:287–291.

Quinnan, G. V., and Manischewitz, J. E. 1979. The role of natural killer cells and antibody-dependent cell-mediated cytotoxicity during murine cytomegalovirus infection. *J. Exp. Med.* **150**:1549–1554.

Raff, M. C. 1977. Development and modulation of B lymphocytes: Studies on newly formed B cells and their putative precursors in the hemopoietic tissue of mice. *Cold Spring Harbor Symp. Quant. Biol.* **41**:159–162.

Raff, M C., Owen, J. J. T., Cooper, M. D., Lawton, A. R., Megson, M., and Gathings, W. E. 1975. Differences in susceptibility of mature and immature mouse B lymphocytes to anti-immunoglobulin induced immunoglobulin suppression *in vitro*. *J. Exp. Med.* **142**:1052–1064.

Raff, M. C., Megson, M., Owen, J. J. T., and Cooper, M. D. 1976. Early production of intracellular IgM by B lymphocyte precursors in mouse. *Nature (London)* **259**:224–226.

Ralph, P., Nakoinz, I., Diamond, B., and Yelton, D. 1980. All classes of murine IgG antibody mediate macrophage phagocytosis and lysis of erythrocytes. *J. Immunol.* **125**:1885–1888.

Randazzo, B., Hirschberg, T., and Hirschberg, H. 1979. Cytotoxic effect of activated human monocytes and lymphocytes to anti-D-treated human erythrocytes *in vitro*. *Scand. J. Immunol.* **9**:351–358.

Reinherz, E. L., and Schlossman, S. F. 1979. Con A-inducible suppression of MLC: Evidence for mediation by the TH$_2^+$ T cell subset in man. *J. Immunol.* **122**:1335–1341.

Reinherz, E. L., Kung, P. C., Goldstein, G., and Schlossman, S. F. 1979a. Separation of functional subsets of human T cells by a monoclonal antibody. *Proc. Natl. Acad. Sci. USA* **76**:4061–4065.

Reinherz, E. L., Kung, P. C., Goldstein, G., and Schlossman, S. F. 1979b. Further characterization of the human inducer T cell subsets defined by monoclonal antibody. *J. Immunol.* **123**:2894–2896.

Reinherz, E. L., King, P. C., Goldstein, G., Levey, R. H., and Schlossman, S. F. 1980. Discrete stages in human intrathymic differentiation: Analysis of normal thymocytes and leukemic lymphoblasts of T lineage. *Proc. Natl. Acad. Sci. USA* **77**:1588–1592.

Reyes, F., Lejonc, J. L., Gourdin, M. F., Mannoni, P., and Dreyfus, B. 1975. The surface morphology of human B lymphocytes as revealed by immunoelectron microscopy. *J. Exp. Med.* **141**:392–410.

Ricardo, M. J. 1980. Heterogeneity of Fc-receptors on guinea pig T lymphocytes. *J. Immunol.* **125**:2009–2016.

Riccardi, C., Santoni, A., Barlozzari, T., and Herberman, R. B. 1981. *In vivo* reactivity of mouse natural killer (NK) cells against normal bone marrow cells. *Cell. Immunol.* **60**:136–143.

Rice, L., Laughter, A. H., and Twomey, J. J. 1979. Three suppressor systems in human blood that modulate lymphoproliferation. *J. Immunol.* **122**:991–996.

Rivat-Peran, L., Tischendorf, F. W., Dumitresco, S. M., Rivat, C., Tischendorf, M. M., Haas, H., and Deutsch, H. F. 1980. The variable region of human immunoglobulins. I. Serologic and structural correlations of antigenic markers common to VλI and VλIV proteins (isotypic cross-reactivities). *J. Immunol.* **125**:270–277.

Rocklin, R. E. 1976. Modulation of cellular-immune responses *in vivo* and *in vitro* by histamine receptor-bearing lymphocytes. *J. Clin. Invest.* **57**:1051–1058.

Rocklin, R. E. 1977. Histamine-induced suppressor factor (HSF): Effect on migration inhibitory factor (MIF) production and proliferation. *J. Immunol.* **118**:1734–1738.

Rocklin, R. E., Entremeder, D., Littman, B. M., and Melmon, K. L. 1978. Modulation of cellular immune function *in vitro* by histamine receptor-bearing lymphocytes: Mechanism of action. *Cell. Immunol.* **37**:162–173.

Rocklin, R. E., Bendtzen, K., and Greineder, D. 1980. Mediators of immunity: Lymphokines and monokines. *Adv. Immunol.* **29**:55–136.

Roder, J. C., Argov, S., Klein, M., Petersson, C., Kiessling, R., Anderson, K., and Hansson, M. 1980. Target–effect or cell interaction in the natural killer cell system. V. Energy requirements, membrane integrity and the possible involvement of lysosomal enzymes. *Immunology* **40**:107–116.

Rogers, J., Early, P., Carter, C., Calame, K., Bond, M., Hood, L., and Wall, R. 1980. Two mRNAs with different 3′ ends encode membrane-bound and secreted forms of immunoglobulin μ chain. *Cell.* **20**:303–312.

Roitt, I. M. 1974. *Essential Immunology,* 2nd ed., Oxford, Blackwell.

Ron, Y., De Baetselier, P., and Segal, S. 1981. Involvement of the spleen in murine B cell differentiation. *Eur. J. Immunol.* **11**:94–96.

Rosenthal, A. S. 1978. Determinant selection and macrophage function in genetic control of the immune response. *Immunol. Rev.* **40**:136–152.

Rosenthal, A. S., and Shevach, E. M. 1973. The function of macrophages in antigen recognition by guinea pig T lymphocytes. I. Requirement for histocompatible macrophages and lymphocytes. *J. Exp. Med.* **138**:1194–1212.

Rosenthal, A. S., Blake, J. T., Ellner, J. J., Greineder, D. K., and Lipsky, P. E. 1976. Macrophage function in antigen recognition by T lymphocytes. *In:* Nelson, D. S., ed., *Immunobiology of the Macrophage,* New York, Academic Press, pp. 131–160.

Rosenwasser, L. J., and Rosenthal, A. S. 1978. Adherent cell function in murine T lymphocyte antigen recognition. II. Definition of genetically restricted and nonrestricted macrophage functions in T cell proliferation. *J. Immunol.* **121**:2497–2501.

Roth, R. A., and Koshland, M. E. 1981. Identification of a lymphocyte enzyme that catalyzes pentamer immunoglobulin M assembly. *J. Biol. Chem.* **256**:4633–4639.

Rowe, D. A., Hug, K., Forni, L., and Pernis, B. 1973. Immunoglobulin D as a lymphocyte receptor. *J. Exp. Med.* **138**:965–972.

Rowley, D. A. 1950a. The effect of splenectomy on the formation of circulating antibody in the adult male albino rat. *J. Immunol.* **64**:289–295.

Rowley, D. A. 1950b. The formation of circulating antibody of the splenectomized human being following intravenous injection of heterologous erythrocytes. *J. Immunol.* **65**:515–521.

Rubin, B., Hertel-Wulff, B., and Kimura, A. 1979. Alloantigen-specific idiotype-bearing receptors on mouse thymocytes. *J. Exp. Med.* **150**:307–321.

Rups, E. C., Giroir, B. P., and Borel, Y. 1981. The fine specificity of immune suppression to individual nucleosides. *J. Immunmol* **126**:1542–1546.

Ruscetti, F. W., Morgan, D. A., and Gallo, R. C. 1977. Functional and morphologic characterization of human T-cells continuously grown *in vitro*. *J. Immunol.* **119**:131–138.

Russell, M. W., Brown, T. A., and Mestecky, J. 1981. Role of serum IgA. Hepatobiliary transport of circulating antigen. *J. Exp. Med.* **153**:968–976.

Sakano, H., Huppi, K., Heinrich, G., and Tonegawa, S. 1979. Sequences at the somatic recombination sites of immunoglobulin light chains. *Nature (London)* **280**:288–294.

Sakano, H., Maki, R., Kurosawa, Y., Roeder, W., and Tonegawa, S. 1980. Two types of somatic recombination are necessary for the generation of complete immunoglobulin heavy-chain genes. *Nature (London)* **286**:676–683.

Sakano, H., Kurosawa, Y., Weigert, M., and Tonegawa, S. 1981. Identification and nucleotide sequence of a diversity DNA segment (D) of immunoglobulin heavy-chain genes. *Nature (London)* **290**:562–565.

Saluk, P. H., and Clem, L. W. 1971. The unique molecular weight of the heavy chain from human IgG3. *J. Immunol.* **107**:298–301.

Scher, I., Berning, A. K., Kessler, S., and Finkelman, F. D. 1980. Development of B lymphocytes in the mouse: Studies of the frequency and distribution of surface IgM and IgD in normal and immune-defective CBA/N F$_1$ mice. *J. Immunol.* **125**:1686–1693.

Schimpl, A., and Wecker, E. 1972. Replacement of T-cell function by a T-cell product. *Nature New Biol.* **237**:15–17.

Schrohenloher, R. E., Mestecky, J., and Acton, R. T. 1973. Molecular weight of a human J chain. *Biochim. Biophys. Acta* **295**:576–581.

Schwartz, R. C., Sonenschein, G. E., Bothwell, A., and Gefter, M. L. 1981. Multiple expression of Ig λ-chain encoding RNA species in murine plasmacytoma cells. *J. Immunol.* **126**:2104–2108.

Segal, A. W., Garcia, R., Goldstone, A. H., Cross, A. R., and Jones, O. T. G. 1981. Cytochrome b_{245} of neutrophils is also present in human monocytes, macrophages and eosinophils. *Biochem. J.* **196**:363–367.

Sell, S. 1980. *Immunology, Immunopathology, and Immunity*, 3rd ed., New York, Harper & Row.

Sell, S., and Gell, P. G., H. 1965. Studies on rabbit lymphocytes *in vitro*. *J. Exp. Med.* **122**:423–441.

Senik, A., Maury, C., and Gressor, I. 1979. Interferon enhancement of NK cell activity. *Transplant. Proc.* **11**:993–996.

Shaw, G. M., Levy, P. C., and LoBuglio, A. F. 1978. Human monocyte antibody dependent cell-mediated cytotoxicity to tumor cells. *J. Clin. Invest.* **62**:1172–1180.

Shen, L., and Fanger, M. W. 1981. Secretory IgA antibodies synergize with IgG in promoting ADCC by human polymorphonuclear cells, monocytes, and lymphocytes. *Cell. Immunol.* **59**:75–81.

Sherr, D. H., Francus, T., Szewczuk, R., Kim, Y. T., Sogan, D., and Siskind, G. W. 1981. Ontogeny of B lymphocyte function. X. Strain differences in maturation of capacity of the B lymphocyte population to produce a high-affinity antibody response. *Eur. J. Immunol.* **11**:32–38.

Shiku, H., Kisielow, P., Bean, M. A., Takahashi, T., Boyse, E. A., Oettgen, H. F., and Old, L. J. 1975. Expression of T-cell differentiation antigens on effector cells in cell-mediator cytotoxicity *in vitro*. *J. Exp. Med.* **141**:227–241.

Shinoda, T., Takahashi, N., Takayasu, T., Okuyama, T., and Shimizu, A. 1981. Complete amino-acid sequence of the Fc region of a human δ chain. *Proc. Natl. Acad. Sci. USA* **78**:785–789.

Shiozawa, C., Singh, B., Rubinstein, S., and Diener, E. 1977. Molecular control of B cell triggering by antigen-specific T cell-derived helper factor. *J. Immunol.* **118**:2199–2205.

Shiozawa, C., Sonik, S., Singh, B., and Diener, E. 1979. Purification and B cell triggering properties of antigen-specific T cell derived helper factor. *ICN–UCLA Symp. Mol. Cell. Biol.* **16**:391–400.

Shiozawa, C., Longenecker, M. B., and Diener, E. 1980. *In vitro* cooperation of antigen-specific T cell-derived helper factor, B cells, and adherent cells or their secretory-product in primary IgM response to chicken MHC antigens. *J. Immunol.* **125**:68–73.

Shortman, K., Layton, J. E., and Baker, J. 1981. Cell surface markers and surface immunoglobulin status of a class of intermediate (pre-progenitor) B cells. *Dev. Immunol.* **15**:121–132.

Shou, L., Schwartz, S. A., and Good, R. A. 1976. Suppressor cell activity after concanavalan A treatment of lymphocytes from normal donors. *J. Exp. Med.* **143**:1100–1110.

Shou, L., Schwartz, S. A., Good, R. A., Peng, R., and Chen, C. L. 1980. A human soluble suppressor factor affecting lymphocyte responses *in vitro*. *Proc. Natl. Acad. Sci. USA* **77**:6096–6100.

Sidman, C. I. 1981. B lymphocyte differentiation and the control of IgM μ chain expression. *Cell* **23**:379–389.

Sidman, C. I., and Unanue, E. R. 1975. Receptor mediated inactivation of early B lymphocytes. *Nature (London)* **257**:149–151.

Silver, D. M., and Lane, D. P. 1979. A heirarchy of responsiveness and the production of non-precipitating antibodies to F-antigen. *Immunogenetics* **8**:65–70.

Silver, D. M., and Lane, D. P. 1981. Polygenic control of the immune response to F antigen. *Immunogenetics* **12**:237–251.

Silverstone, A. E., Rosenberg, N., Baltimore, D., Sato, V. L., Scheid, M. P., and Boyse, E. A. 1978. Correlating terminal deoxynucleotidyl transferase and cell-surface markers in the pathway of lymphocyte ontogeny. *Cold Spring Harbor Conf. Immunol. Cell Prolif.* **5**:433–453.

Simon, M. M., and Abenhardt, B. 1980. Generation of effector cells from T cell subsets. II. Lyt-123 T cells contain the precursors for all primary cytotoxic effector cells and for cells involved in the regulation of cytotoxic responses. *Eur. J. Immunol.* **10**:334–341.

Simon, M. M., and Eichmann, K. 1980. T cell subsets participating in the generation of cytotoxic T cells. *Springer Semin. Immunopathol.* **3**:39–62.

Simon, M. M., Edwards, A. J., Hämmerling, U., McKenzie, I. F. C., Eichmann, K., and Simpson, E. 1981. Generation of effector cells from T cell subsets. III. Synergy between Lyt-1 and Lyt-123/23 lymphocytes in the generation of H-2-restricted and alloreactive cytotoxic T cells. *Eur. J. Immunol.* **11**:246–250.

Simon, P. L., Farrar, J. J., and Kind, P. D. 1979. Biochemical relationship between murine immune interferon and killer cell helper factor. *J. Immunol.* **122**:127–132.

Singer, P. A., Singer, H. H., and Williamson, A. R. 1980. Different species of messenger RNA encode receptor and secretory IgM μ chains differing at their carboxyl termini. *Nature (London)* **285**:294–301.

Slomski, R., and Cohen, E. P. 1980. Isolation and cell-free translation of mRNA specifying thymus-leukemia antigens. *Biochemistry* **19**:5659–5664.

Smith, F. I., and Miller, J. F. A. P. 1978. Delayed type hypersensitivity to allogeneic cells in mice. II. Cell transfer studies. *Int. Arch. Allergy Appl. Immunol.* **58**:295–301.

Smith, F. I., and Miller, J. F. A. P. 1979. Delayed type hypersensitivity to allogeneic cells in mice. III. Sensitivity to cell surface antigens coded by the MHC and other genes. *J. Exp. Med.* **150**:965–976.

Smith, W. G., Usinger, W. R., and Splitter, G. A. 1981. Bovine Con A-induced suppressor cells: Generation, macrophage requirements and possible mechanisms of regulatory action. *Immunology* **43**:91–100.

Snary, D., Barnstable, C., Bodmer, W. F., Goodfellow, P., and Crumpton, M. L. J. 1977. Human Ia antigens—Purification and molecular structure. *Cold Spring Harbor Symp. Quant. Biol.* **41**:379–386.

South, M. A., Cooper, M. D., Wollheim, F. A., Hong, R., and Good, R. A. 1966. The IgA system. I. Studies of the transport and immunochemistry of IgA in the saliva. *J. Exp. Med.* **123**:615–627.

Sprent, J. 1978. Role of the *H-2* complex in induction of T helper cells *in vivo*. I. Antigen-specific selection of donor T cells to sheep erythrocytes in irradiated mice dependent upon sharing of *H-2* determinants between donor and host. *J. Exp. Med.* **148**:478–489.

Sprent, J., and Alpert, B. 1981. Role of the *H-2* complex in induction of T helper cells *in vivo*. II. Negative selection of discrete subgroups of T cells restricted by I-A and I-A/E determinants. *J. Exp. Med.* **153**:823–831.

Springer, T. A., Kaufman, J. F., Siddoway, L. A., Giphart, M., Mann, D. L., Terhorst, C., and Strominger, J. L. 1977. Chemical and immunological characterization of HL-A-linked B-lymphocyte alloantigens. *Cold Spring Harbor Symp. Quant. Biol.* **41**:387–396.

Stafford, H. A., and Fanger, M. W. 1980. Receptors for IgA on rabbit lymphocytes. I. Distribution, specificity, and modulation. *J. Immunol.* **125**:2461–2466.

Stanwick, T. L., Campbell, D. E., and Nahmias, A. J. 1981. Cells infected with herpes simplex virus induce human monocyte-macrophages to produce interferon. *Immunobiology* **158**:207–212.

Stashenko, P., Nadler, L. M., Hardy, R., and Schlossman, S. F. 1980. Characterization of a human B lymphocyte specific antigen. *J. Immunol.* **125**:1678–1685.

Stevenson, F. K., Morris, D., and Stevenson, G. T. 1980. Immunoglobulin produced by guinea-pig leukaemic B lymphocytes: Its source and use as a monitor of tumour load. *Immunology* **41**:313–322.

Storb, U., Hager, L., Wilson, R., and Putnam, D. 1977. Expression of immunoglobulin and globin genes in B and T lymphocytes and other cells. *Biochemistry* **16**:5432–5438.

Strausser, H. R., and Rosenstein, M. M. 1980. Immunosuppression as a homeostatic mechanism in disease and aging. *In*: Escobar, M. R., and Friedman, H., eds., *Macrophages and Lymphocytes: Nature, Functions, and Interaction*, New York, Plenum Press, Part B, pp. 277–281.

Stuart, A. E. 1970. *The Reticuloendothelial System*, Edinburgh, Livingstone.

Sunday, M. E., Benacerraf, B., and Dorf, M. E. 1981. Hapten-specific T cell responses to 4-hydroxy-3-nitrophenyl acetyl. *J. Exp. Med.* **153**:811–822.

Sunderland, C. A., McMaster, W. R., and Williams, A. F. 1979. Purification with monoclonal antibody of a predominant leucocyte-common antigen and glycoprotein from rat thymocytes. *Eur. J. Immunol.* **9**:155–159.

Svedmyr, E. A., Deinhardt, F., and Klein, G. 1974. Sensitivity of different target cells to the killing action of peripheral lymphocytes stimulated by autologous lymphoblastoid cell lines. *Int. J. Cancer* **13**:891–903.

Svedmyr, E. A., Jondal, M., and Leibold, W. 1975. Stimulation of normal lymphocytes with autologous lymphoid cell lines: Properties of derived killer cells. *Scand. J. Immunol.* **4**:721–734.

Tada, T., Taniguchi, M., and David, C. S. 1976. Suppressive and enhancing T cell factors as I-region gene products: Properties and the subregion assignment. *Cold Spring Harbor Symp. Quant. Biol.* **41**:119–127.

Tanaka, Y., Sugamura, K., Hinuma, Y., Sato, H., and Okochi, K. 1980. Memory of Epstein–Barr virus-specific cytotoxic T cells in normal seropositive adults as revealed by an *in vitro* restimulation method. *J. Immunol.* **125**:1426–1431.

Taramelli, D., Holden, H. T., and Varesio, L. 1981. *In vitro* induction of tumoricidal and suppressor macrophages by lymphokines: Possible feedback regulation. *J. Immunol.* **126**:2123–2128.

Taussig, M. J. 1980. Antigen-specific T-cell factors. *Immunology* **41**:759–787.

Teale, J. M., Liu, F. T., and Katz, D. H. 1981a. A clonal analysis of the IgE response and its implications with regard to isotope commitment. *J. Exp. Med.* **153**:783–792.

Teale, J. M., Lafrenz, D., Klinman, N. R., and Strober, S. 1981b. Immunoglobulin class commitment exhibited by B lymphocytes separated according to surface isotype. *J. Immunol.* **126**:1952–1957.

Terhorst, C., Parham, P., Mann, D. L., and Strominger, J. L. 1976. Structure of HLA antigens: Amino acid and carbohydrate compositions and N-terminal sequences as four antigen preparations. *Proc. Natl. Acad. Sci. USA* **73**:910–914.

Terry, W. D., and Fahey, J. L. 1964. Subclasses of human γ_2-globulin based on differences in the heavy polypeptide chains. *Science* **146**:400–401.

Thoenes, G. H., and Hildemann, W. H. 1970. *In*: Sternback, R. A., and Riha, I., eds., *Developmental Aspects of Antibody Formation and Structure*, New York, Academic Press, Vol. II.

Thomas, Y., Huchet, R., and Granjon, D. 1981. Histamine-induced suppressor cells of lymphocyte mitogenic response. *Cell. Immunol.* **59**:268–275.

Tischendorf, F. W., Tischendorf, M. M., and Osserman, E. F. 1970. Subgroup-specific antigenic marker of immunoglobulin λ-chains: Identification of three subtypes of the variable region. *J. Immunol.* **105**:1033–1035.

Tokuyama, H., and Tanigaki, N. 1981. Separation and comparison of human TL-like antigens and HLA(A,B,C) antigens expressed on cultured T cells. *Immunogenetics* **13**:147–165.

Tomasi, T. B., and Bienenstock, J. 1968. Secretory immunoglobulins. *Adv. Immunol.* **9**:1–96.

Tomasi, T. B., Tam, E. M., Solomon, A., and Prendergast, R. A. 1965. Characteristics of an immune system common to certain external secretions. *J. Exp. Med.* **121**:101–124.

Tourville, D., Adler, R., Bienenstock, J., and Tomasi, T. B. 1969. The human secretory immunoglobulin system: Immunohistological localization of γA, secretory "piece" and lactoferrin in normal human tissues. *J. Exp. Med.* **129**:411–429.

Treves, A. J. 1978. *In vitro* induction of cell-mediated immunity against tumor cells by antigen-fed macrophages. *Immunol. Rev.* **40**:205–226.

Triebel, F., Robinson, W. A., Hayward, A. R., and de LaForest, P. G. 1981. Characterization of the T lymphocyte colony-forming cells and evidence for the acquisition of T cell markers in the absence of the thymic microenvironment in man. *J. Immunol.* **126**:2020–2023.

Trotter, J. A. 1981. The organization of action in spreading macrophages. *Exp. Cell Res.* **132**:235–248.

Trowbridge, I. S., Ralph P., and Bevan, M. J. 1975. Differences in the surface proteins of mouse B and T cells. *Proc. Natl. Acad. Sci. USA* **72**:157–161.

Tse, H. Y., Mond, J. J., and Paul, W. E. 1981. T lymphocyte-dependent B lymphocyte proliferative response to antigen. I. Genetic restriction of the stimulation of B lymphocyte proliferation. *J. Exp. Med.* **153**:871–882.

Tsoukas, C. D., Fox, R. I., Slovin, S. F., Carson, D. A., Pellegrino, M., Fong, S., Pasquali, J. L., Ferrone, S., Kung, P., and Vaughan, J. H. 1981. T lymphocyte-mediated cytotoxicity against autologous EBV-genome-bearing B cells. *J. Immunol.* **126**:1742–1746.

Tsukuda, K., Tsukuda, Y., and Klein, G. 1981. Suppressor T cells activated by lymphoblastoid cell lines inhibit pokeweed mitogen-induced immunoglobulin synthesis. *Cell. Immunol.* **60**:191–202.

Tzehoval, E., De Baetselier, P., Feldman, M., and Segal, S. 1981. The peritoneal antigen-presenting macrophage: Control and immunogenic properties of distinct subpopulations. *Eur. J. Immunol.* **11**:323–328.

Uhr, J. W., Capra, J. D., Vitetta, E. S., and Cook, R. G. 1979. Organization of the immune response genes. *Science* **206**:292–297.

Utsumi, S., and Karush, F. 1965. Peptic fragmentation of rabbit γG-immunoglobulin. *Biochemistry* **4**:1766–1779.

Van Halbeek, H., Dorland, L., and Vliegenthart, J. F. G. 1981. Primary structure of the asparagine-563-linked carbohydrate chain of an immunoglobulin M from a patient with Waldenstrom's macroglobulinemia. *Biochem. Biophys. Res. Commun.* **99**:886–892.

Van Wauwe, J., and Goossens, J. 1981. Monoclonal anti-human T-lymphocyte antibodies: Enumeration and characterization of T-cell subsets. *Immunology* **42**:157–164.

Veit, B. C. 1981. Variable occurrence of splenic suppressor macrophages in normal and tumor-inoculated rats. *Cell. Immunol.* **59**:367–377.

Viallat, J., Svedmyr, E., Steinctz, M., and Klein, G. 1978. Stimulation of peripheral human lymphocytes by autologous EBV genome-carrying lymphoblastoid cell lines. *Cell. Immunol.* **38**:68–75.

Vitetta, E. S., and Uhr, J. W. 1975. Immunoglobulin-receptors revisited. *Science* **189**:964–969.

Vitetta, E. S., Cambier, J., Forman, J., Kettman, J. R., Yuan, D., and Uhr, J. W. 1977. Immunoglobulin receptors on murine B lymphocytes. *Cold Spring Harbor Symp. Quant. Biol.* **41**:185–191.

Vogler, L. B., Preud'homme, J. L., Seligmann, M., Gathings, W. E., Crist, W. M., Cooper, M. D., and Bollun, F. J. 1981. Diversity of immunoglobulin-expression on leukemic cells resembling B-lymphocyte precursors. *Nature (London)* **290**:339–341.

Vos, J. G., Roholl, P. J. M., and Leene, W. 1980. Ultrastructural studies of peripheral blood lymphocytes in T cell-depleted rabbits. *Cell Tissue Res.* **213**:221–235.

Vranian, G., Conrad, D. H., and Ruddy, S. 1981. Specificity of C3 receptors that mediate phagocytosis by rat peritoneal mast cells. *J. Immunol.* **126**:2302–2306.

Wabl, M. R., Johnson, J. P., Haas, I. G., Tenkhoff, I. G., Meo, T., and Inan, R. 1980. Simultaneous expression of mouse immunoglobulins M and D is determined by the same homology of chromosome 12. *Proc. Natl. Acad. Sci. USA* **77**:6793–6796.

Walfield, A. M., Storb, U., Selsing, E., and Zentgraf, H. 1980. Comparison of different rearranged immunoglobulin kappa genes of a myeloma by electronmicroscopy and restriction mapping of cloned DNA: Implications for "allelic exclusion." *Nucleic Acids Res.* **8**:4689–4707.

Walfield, A. M., Selsing, E., Arp, B., and Storb, U. 1981. Misalignment of V and J gene segments resulting in a nonfunctional immunoglobulin gene. *Nucleic Acids Res.* **9**:1101–1109.

Wang, A. C., Gergely, J., and Fudenberg, H. H. 1973. Amino acid sequences at constant and variable regions of heavy chains of monotypic immunoglobulins G and M of a single patient. *Biochemistry* **12**:528–534.

Warner, N. L. 1974. Membrane immunoglobulins and antigen receptors on B and T lymphocytes. *Adv. Immunol.* **19**:67–216.

Weinberger, O., Herrmann, S., Mescher, M. F., Benacerraf, B., and Burakoff, S. J. 1981. Antigen-presenting cell function in induction of helper T cells for cytotoxic T-lymphocyte responses: Evidence for antigen processing. *Proc. Natl. Acad. Sci. USA* **78**:1796–1799.

Weinheimer, P. F., Mestecky, J., and Acton, R. T. 1971. Species distribution of J chain. *J. Immunol.* **107**:1211–1212.

Weiss, S., and Dennert, G. 1981. T cell lines active in the delayed-type hypersensitivity reaction (DTH). *J. Immunol.* **126**:2031–2035.

Weissman, I. L., Baird, S., Gardner, R. L., Papaioannou, E., and Raschke, W. 1976. Normal and neoplastic maturation of T-lineage lymphocytes. *Cold Spring Harbor Symp. Quant. Biol.* **41A**:9–21.

Welsh, R. M., Zinkernagel, R. M., and Hallenbeck, L. A. 1979. Cytotoxic cells induced during lymphocytic choriomeningitis virus infection of mice. II. "Specificities" of the NK cells. *J. Immunol.* **122**:475–481.

Wetzel, G. D., and Kettman, J. R. 1981. Activation of murine B lymphocytes. III. Stimulation of B lymphocyte clonal growth with lipopolysaccharide and dextran sulfate. *J. Immunol.* **126**:723–728.

Wicker, L. S., and Hildemann, W. H. 1981. Two distinct high immune response phenotypes are both controlled: *H-2* genes mapping in *K* or *I-A*. *Immunogenetics* **12**:253–265.

Wikler, M., and Putnam, F. W. 1970. Amino acid sequence of human λ chains. III. Tryptic peptides, chymotryptic peptides, and sequence of protein Bo. *J. Biol. Chem.* **245**:4488–4507.

Williams, R. C., and Korsmeyer, S. J. 1978. Studies of human lymphocyte interactions with emphasis on soluble suppressor activity. *Clin. Immunol. Immunopathol.* **9**:335–349.

Wood, D. D., Cameron, P. M., Poe, M. T., and Morris, C. A. 1976. Resolution of a factor that enhances the antibody response of T cell-depleted murine splenocytes from several other monocyte products. *Cell. Immunol.* **21**:88–96.

Yamashita, U., and Shevach, E. M. 1977. The expression of Ia antigens on immunocompetent cells in the guinea pig. II. Ia antigens on macrophages. *J. Immunol.* **119**:1584–1588.

Yonemasu, K., and Sasaki, T. 1981. Purification and characterization of subcomponent Clq of the first component of mouse complement. *Biochem. J.* **193**:621–629.

Yowell, R. L., Araneo, B. A., Miller A., and Sercarz, E. E. 1979. Amputation of a suppressor determinant on lysozyme reveals underlying T cell reactivity to other determinants. *Nature (London)* **279**:70–71.

Zettergren, L. D., Lydyard, P. M., and Parkhouse, R. M. E. 1977. Liver as a site of B cell generation in *Xenopus laevis*. *Fed. Proc.* **36**:1239.

CHAPTER 8

Aufderheide, K. J., Frankel, J., and Williams, N. E. 1980. Formation and positioning of surface-related structures in protozoa. *Microbiol. Rev.* **44**:252–302.

Baltimore, D. 1981. Somatic mutation gains its place among the generators of diversity. *Cell* **26**:295–296.

Baralle, F. E., Shoulders, C. C., and Proudfoot, N. J. 1980. The primary structure of the human ε-globin gene. *Cell* **21**:621–626.

Barrell, B. G., Seidman, J. G., Guthrie, C. and McClain, W. H. 1974. The nucleotide sequence of a precursor to serine and proline tRNA's. *Proc. Natl. Acad. Sci. USA* **71**:413–416.

Bechmann, H., Haid, A., Schweyen, R. J., Mathews, S., and Kaudewitz, F. 1981. Expression of the "split gene" COB in yeast mtDNA. *J. Biol. Chem.* **256**:3525–3531.

Bernard, O., Hozumi, N., and Tonegawa, S. 1978. Sequences of mouse immunoglobulin light chain genes before and after somatic changes. *Cell* **15**:1133–1144.

Bibb, M. J., Van Etten, R. A., Wright, C. T., Walberg, M. W., and Clayton, D. A. 1981. Sequence and gene organization of mouse mitochondrial DNA. *Cell* **26**:167–180.

Bigelow, S., Hough, R., and Rechsteiner, M. 1981. The selective degradation of injected proteins occurs principally in the cytosol rather than in lysosomes. *Cell* **25**:83–93.

Bohnert, H. J., Priesel, A. J., Crouse, E. J., Gordon, K., Herrmann, R. G., Steinmetz, A., Mubumbila, M., Keller, M., Burkard, G., and Weil, J. H. 1979. Presence of a tRNA gene in the spacer sequence between the 16S and 23S rRNA genes of spinach chloroplast genes. *FEBS Lett.* **103**:52–56.

Boissel, J. P., Wajcman, H., and Labie, D. 1980. Hemoglobins of an amphibia, the neotenous *Ambystoma mexicanum*. *Eur. J. Biochem.* **103**:613–621.

Bothwell, A. L. M., Paskind, M., Raph M., Imanishi-Kari, T., Rajewsky, K., and Baltimore, D. 1981. Heavy chain variable region contribution to the NP[b] family of antibodies: Somatic mutation evident in a γ2a variable region. *Cell* **24**:625–637.

Brack, C., Hirama, M., Lenhard-Schuller, R., and Tonegawa, S. 1978. A complete immunoglobulin gene is created by somatic recombination. *Cell* **15**:1–14.

Breathnach, R., Benoist, C., O'Hare, K., Gannon, F., and Chambon, P. 1978. Ovalbumin gene: Evidence for a leader sequence in mRNA and DNA sequence at the exon–intron boundaries. *Proc. Natl. Acad. Sci. USA* **75**:4853–4857.

Calvin, M. 1956. Chemical evolution and the origin of life. *Am. Sci.* **44**:248–263.

Calvin, M. 1969. *Chemical Evolution: Molecular Evolution towards the Origin of Living Systems on the Earth and Elsewhere,* London, Oxford University Press.

Calvin, M. 1975. Chemical evolution. *Am. Sci.* **63**:1969–1977.

Catterall, J. F., O'Malley, B. W., Robertson, M. A., Staden, R., Tanaka, Y., and Brownlee, G. G. 1978. Nucleotide sequence homology at 12 intron–exon junctions in the chick ovalbumin gene. *Nature (London)* **275**:510–513.

Chapman, B. S., Tobin, A. J., and Hood, L. E. 1981. Complete amino acid sequence of the major early embryonic β-like globin in chickens. *J. Biol. Chem.* **256**:5524–5531.

Chauvet, J. P., and Acher, R. 1972. Phylogeny of hemoglobins: β chain of frog (*Rana esculenta*) hemoglobin. *Biochemistry* **11**:916–927.

Clarkson, S. G., Birnstiel, M. L., and Serra, V. 1973. Reiterated tRNA genes of *Xenopus laevis*. *J. Mol. Biol.* **79**:391–410.

Cleary, M. L., Schon, E. A., and Lingrel, J. B. 1981. Two related pseudogenes are the result of a gene duplication in the goat β-globin locus. *Cell* **26**:181–190.

Clegg, J. B., and Gagnon, J. 1981. Structure of the ζ chain of human embryonic hemoglobin. *Proc. Natl. Acad. Sci. USA* **78**:6076–6080.

Colby, D., Leboy, P. S., and Guthrie, C. 1981. Yeast tRNA precursor mutated at a splice junction is correctly processed *in vivo*. *Proc. Natl. Acad. Sci. USA* **78**:415–419.

Cory, S., and Adams, J. M. 1980. Deletions are associated with somatic rearrangement of immunoglobulin heavy chain genes. *Cell* **19**:37–51.

Cory, S., Adams, J. M., and Kemp, D. J. 1980. Somatic rearrangements forming active immunoglobulin μ-genes in B and T lymphoid cell lines. *Proc. Natl. Acad. Sci. USA* **77**:4943–4947.

Crews, S., Griffin, J., Huang, H., Calame, K., and Hood, L. 1981. A single V$_H$ gene segment encodes the immune response to phosphorylcholine: Somatic mutation is correlated with the class of the antibody. *Cell* **25**:59–66.

DeFranco, D., Schmidt, O., and Söll, D. 1980. Two control regions for eukaryotic tRNA gene transcription. *Proc. Natl. Acad. Sci. USA* **77**:3365–3368.

Delaney, A., Dunn, R., Grigliatti, T. A., Tener, G. M., Kaufman, T. C., and Suzuki, D. T. 1976. Quantitation and localization of tRNA genes of *Drosophila melanogaster*. *Fed. Proc.* **35**:1676.

Dickinson, D. G., and Baker, R. F. 1978. Evidence for translocation of DNA sequences during sea urchin embryogenesis. *Proc. Natl. Acad. Sci. USA* **75**:5627–5630.

Diesseroth, A., Nienhuis, A., Turner, P., Velez, R., Anderson, W. F., Ruddle, F., Lawrence, J., Creagan, R., and Kucherlapati, R. 1977. Localization of the human α-globin structural gene to chromosome 16 in somatic cell hybrids by molecular hybridization assay. *Cell* **12**:205–218.

Dillon, L. S. 1962. Comparative cytology and the evolution of life. *Evolution* **16**:102–117.

Dillon, L. S. 1963. A reclassification of the major groups of organisms based upon comparative cytology. *Syst. Zool.* **12**:71–82.

Dillon, L. S. 1966. The life cycle of the species: An extension of current concepts. *Syst. Zool.* **15**:112–126.

Dillon, L. S. 1970. Speciation and changing environments. *Am. Zool.* **10**:27–39.

Dillon, L. S. 1973. Origins of the genetic code. *Bot. Rev.* **39**:301–345.

Dillon, L. S. 1978a. *The Genetic Mechanism and the Origin of Life,* New York, Plenum Press.

Dillon, L. S. 1978b. *Evolution: Concepts and Consequences,* St. Louis, Mosby.

Dillon, L. S. 1981. *Ultrastructure, Macromolecules, and Evolution,* New York, Plenum Press.

Dolan, M., Sugarman, B. J., Dodgson, J. B., and Engel, J. D. 1981. Chromosomal arrangement of the chicken β-type globin genes. *Cell* **24**:669–677.

Duester, G., Campen, R. K., and Holmes, W. M. 1981. Nucleotide sequence of an *Escherichia coli* tRNA (Leu 1) operon and identification of the transcription promoter signal. *Nucleic Acids Res.* **9**:2121–2129.

Early, P., and Hood, L. 1981. Allelic exclusion and nonproductive immunoglobulin gene rearrangements. *Cell* **24**:1–3.

Efstratiadis, A., Posakony, J. W., Maniatis, T., Lawn, R. M., O'Connell, C., Spritz, R. A., DeRiel, J. K., Slightom, J. L., Blechl, A. E., Smithies, O., Baralle, F. E., Shoulders, C. C., and Proudfoot, N. J. 1980. The structure and evolution of the human β-globin gene family. *Cell* **21**:653–668.

Etcheverry, T., Colby, D., and Guthrie, C. 1979. A precursor to a minor species of yeast tRNA[Ser] contains an intervening sequence. *Cell* **18**:11–26.

Flavell, R. A., Kooter, J. M., DeBoer, E., Little, P. F. R., and Williamson, R. 1978. Analysis of the β-δ-globin gene loci in normal and Hb Lepore DNA: Direct determination of gene linkage and intergene distance. *Cell* **15**:25–41.

Földi, J., Cohen-Sola, M., Valentin, C., Blouquit, Y., Hollán, S. R., and Rosa, J. 1980. The human α-globin gene: The protein products of the duplicated genes are identical. *Eur. J. Biochem.* **109**:463–470.

Fox, S. W. 1980. Metabolic microspheres: Origins and evolution. *Naturwissenschaften* **67**:378–383.

Fox, S. W., and Nakashima, T. 1980. The assembly and properties of protobiological structures: The beginnings of cellular peptide synthesis. *BioSystems* **12**:155–166.

Fox, T. D., and Leaver, C. J. 1981. The *Zea mays* mitochondrial gene coding cytochrome oxidase subunit II has an intervening sequence and does not contain TGA codons. *Cell* **26**:315–323.

Fritsch, E. F., Lawn, R. M., and Maniatis, T. 1980. Molecular cloning and characterization of the human β-like globin gene cluster. *Cell* **19**:959–972.

Gallwitz, D., and Sures, I. 1980. Structure of a split gene: Complete nucleotide sequence of the actin gene in *Saccharomyces cerevisiae*. *Proc. Natl. Acad. Sci. USA* **77**:2546–2550.

Gearhart, P. J., Johnson, N. D., Douglas, R., and Hood, L. 1981. IgG antibodies to phosphoryl-choline exhibit more diversity than their IgM counterparts. *Nature (London)* **291**:29–34.

Gershenfeld, H. K., Tsukamoto, A., Weissman, I. L., and Joho, R. 1981. Somatic diversification is required to generate the V_κ genes of MOPC 511 and MOPC 167 myeloma proteins. *Proc. Natl. Acad. Sci. USA* **78**:7674–7678.

Ghysen, A., and Celis, J. E. 1974. Joint transcription of two $tRNA_1^{Tyr}$ genes from *E. coli*. *Nature (London)* **249**:418–421.

Gilbert, W. 1981. DNA sequencing and gene structure. *Science* **214**:1305–1312.

Gō, M. 1981. Correlations of DNA exonic regions with protein structural units in hemoglobin. *Nature (London)* **291**:90–92.

Gorini, L. 1970. Informational suppression. *Annu. Rev. Genet.* **4**:107–134.

Gough, N. M., and Bernard, O. 1981. Sequences of the joining region genes for immunoglobulin heavy chains and their role in generation of antibody diversity. *Proc. Natl. Acad. Sci. USA* **78**:509–513.

Gould, S. J. 1980. *Ontogeny and Phylogeny*, Cambridge, Mass., Belknap Press.

Gray, M. W., and Spencer, D. F. 1981. Is wheat mitochondrial 5S ribosomal RNA prokaryotic in nature? *Nucleic Acids Res.* **9**:3523–3529.

Grigliatti, T. A., White, B. N., Tener, G. M., Kaufman, T. C., and Suzuki, D. T. 1974. The localization of transfer RNA_5^{Lys} genes from *Drosophila melanogaster*. *Proc. Natl. Acad. Sci. USA* **71**:3527–3531.

Grosveld, G. C., Shewmaker, C. K., Jat, P., and Flavell, R. A. 1981. Localization of DNA sequences necessary for transcription of the rabbit β-globin gene *in vitro*. *Cell* **25**:215–226.

Gruss, P., Efstratiadis, A., Karathanasis, S., König, M., and Khoury, G. 1981. Synthesis of stable unspliced mRNA from an intronless simian virus 40-rat preproinsulin gene recombinant. *Proc. Natl. Acad. Sci. USA* **78**:6091–6095.

Hardison, R. C., Butler, E. T., Lacy, E., Maniatis, T., Rosenthal, N., and Efstratiadis, A. 1979. The structure and transcription of four linked rabbit β-like globin genes. *Cell* **18**:1285–1297.

Heckman, J. E., Sarnoff, J., Alzner-DeWeerd, B., Yin, S., and RajBhandary, U.L. 1980. Novel features in the genetic code and codon reading patterns in *Neurospora crassa* mitochondria based on sequences of six mitochondrial tRNA's. *Proc. Natl. Acad. Sci. USA* **77**:3159–3163.

Heintz, N., Zernik, M., and Roeder, R. G. 1981. The structure of the human histone genes: Clustered but not tandemly repeated. *Cell* **24**:661–668.

Henseon, P. 1978. The presence of single stranded regions in mammalian DNA. *J. Mol. Biol.* **119**:487–506.

Hodgson, G. W., and Ponnamperuma, C. A. 1968. Prebiological porphyrin synthesis: Porphyrins from electric discharge in methane, ammonia, and water vapor. *Proc. Natl. Acad. Sci. USA* **59**:22–28.

Hurrell, J. G. R., and Leach, S. J. 1977. The amino acid sequence of soybean leghaemoglobin c_2. *FEBS Lett.* **80**:23–26.

Inoué, S. 1953. Polarization optical studies of the mitotic spindle. *Chromosoma* **5**:487–500.

Jahn, C. L., Hutchison, C. A., Phillips, S. J., Weaver, S., Haigwood, N. L., Voliva, C. F., and Edgell, M. H. 1980. DNA sequence organization of the β-globin complex in the BALB/c mouse. *Cell* **21**:159–168.

Jensen, E. Ø., Paludan, K., Hyldig-Nielsen, J. J., Jørgensen, P., and Marcker, K. A. 1981. The structure of a chromosomal leghemoglobin gene from soybean. *Nature (London)* **291**:677–679.

Johnson, J. D., Ogden, R., Johnson, P., Abelson, J., Dembeck, P., and Itakura, K. 1980. Transcription and processing of a yeast tRNA gene containing a modified intervening sequence. *Proc. Natl. Acad. Sci. USA* **77**:2561–2568.

Knapp, G., Beckmann, J. S., Johnson, P. F., Fuhrman, S. A., and Abelson, J. 1978. Transcription and processing of intervening sequences in yeast tRNA genes. *Cell* **14**:221–236.

Knapp, G., Ogden, R. C., Peebles, C. L., and Abelson, J. 1979. Splicing of yeast tRNA precursors: Structure of the reaction intermediates. *Cell* **18**:37–45.

Koch, W., Edwards, K., and Kossel, H. 1981. Sequencing of the 16 S–23 S spacer in a ribosomal RNA operon of the *Zea mays* chloroplast DNA reveals two split tRNA genes. *Cell* **25**:205–213.

Konkel, D. A., Tilghman, S. M., and Leder, P. 1978. The sequence of the mouse β-globin major gene: Homologies in capping, splicing and poly(A) sites. *Cell* **15**:1125–1132.

Konkel, D. A., Maizel, J. V., and Leder, P. 1979. The evolution and sequence comparison of two recently diverged mouse chromosomal β-globin genes. *Cell* **18**:865–873.

Lacy, E., and Maniatis, T. 1980. The nucleotide sequence of a rabbit β-globin pseudogene. *Cell* **21**:545–553.

Lacy, E., Hardison, R. C., Quon, D., and Maniatis, T. 1979. The linkage arrangement of four rabbit β-like globin genes. *Cell* **18**:1273–1283.

Lalanne, J. L., Bregegere, F., Delarbre, C., Gachelin, G., and Kourilsky, P. 1982. Comparison of nucleotide sequences of mRNAs belonging to the mouse H-2 multigene family. *Nucl. Acids Res.* **10**:1039–1049.

Landy, A., Foeller, C., and Ross, W. 1974. DNA fragments carrying genes for tRNA$_1^{Tyr}$. *Nature (London)* **249**:738–742.

Lauer, J., Shen, C. K. J., and Maniatis, T. 1980. The chromosomal arrangement of human α-like globin genes: Sequence homology and α-globin gene deletions. *Cell* **20**:119–130.

Leder, P., Hanse, J. N., Konkel, D., Leder, A., Nishioka, Y., and Talkington, C. 1980. Mouse globin system: A functional and evolutionary analysis. *Science* **209**:1336–1342.

Lewin, B. 1980. Alternatives for splicing an intron-coded protein. *Cell* **22**:645–646.

Lewin, R. 1981a. Biggest challenge since the double helix. *Science* **212**:28–32.

Lewin, R. 1981b. How conversational are genes? *Science* **212**:313–315.

Lewin, R. 1981c. Evolutionary history written in globin genes. *Science* **214**:426–429.

Liebhaber, S. A., Goossens, M., and Kan, Y. W. 1981. Homology and concerted evolution at the α1 and α2 loci of human α-globin. *Nature (London)* **290**:26–29.

Lohmann, K., and Schubert, L. 1980. Qualitative changes in DNA indicating differential DNA replication during early embryogenesis of the newt *Triturus vulgaris*. *J. Embryol. Exp. Morphol.* **57**:61–70.

Maki, R., Kearney, J., Paige, C., and Tonegawa, S. 1980. Immunoglobulin gene rearrangement in immature B cells. *Science* **209**:1366–1369.

Masters, C. J., and Winzor, D. J. 1981. Physiochemical evidence against the concept of an interaction between aldolase and glyceraldehyde-3-phosphate dehydrogenase. *Arch. Biochem. Biophys.* **209**:185–190.

Mazzara, G. P., Plunkett, G., and McClain, W. H. 1981. DNA sequence of the transfer RNA region of bacteriophage T4: Implications for transfer RNA synthesis. *Proc. Natl. Acad. Sci. USA* **78**:889–892.

Michelson, A. M., and Orkin, S. M. 1980. The 3' untranslated regions of the duplicated human α-globin genes are unexpectedly divergent. *Cell* **22**:371–377.

Miller, S. L. 1953. A production of amino acids under possible primitive earth conditions. *Science* **117**:528–529.

Morgan, E. A., Ikemura, T., and Nomura, M. 1977. Identification of spacer tRNA genes in individual ribosomal RNA transcription units of *Escherichia coli*. *Proc. Natl. Acad. Sci. USA* **74**:2710–2714.

Naveh-Many, T., and Cedar, H. 1981. Active gene sequences are undermethylated. *Proc. Natl. Acad. Sci. USA* **78**:4246–4250.

Nishioka, Y., and Leder, P. 1979. The complete sequence of a chromosomal mouse α-globin gene reveals elements conserved throughout vertebrate evolution. *Cell* **18**:875–882.

Nishioka, Y., Leder, A., and Leder, P. 1980. Unusual α-globin-like gene that has lost both globin intervening sequences. *Proc. Natl. Acad. Sci. USA* **77**:2806–2809.

Nute, P. E. 1974. Multiple hemoglobin α-chain loci in monkeys, apes, and man. *Ann. N.Y. Acad. Sci.* **241**:39–60.

Nute, P. E. 1981. Hemoglobin α-gene duplication in macaques: Individual *Macaca nemestrina* with three structurally different α chains. *Arch. Biochem. Biophys.* **206**:346–352.

O'Farrell, P. Z., Cordell, B., Valenzuela, P., Rutter, W. J., and Goodman, H. M. 1978. Structure and processing of yeast precursor tRNAs containing intervening sequences. *Nature (London)* **274**:438–445.

Ohno, S. 1980. Origin of intervening sequences within mammalian genes and the universal signal for their removal. *Differentiation* **17**:1–15.

Olson, M. V., Montgomery, D. L., Hopper, A. K., Page, G. S., Horodyski, F., and Hall, B. D. 1977. Molecular characterisation of the tyrosine tRNA genes of yeast. *Nature (London)* **267**:639–641.

Orkin, S. H., and Goff, S. C. 1981. The duplicated human α-globin genes: Their relative expression as measured by RNA analysis. *Cell* **24**:345–351.

Peebles, C. L., Ogden, R. C., Knapp, G., and Abelson, J. 1979. Splicing of yeast tRNA precursors: A two stage reaction. *Cell* **18**:27–35.

Peffley, D. M., and Sogin, M. L. 1981. A putative tRNA^{Trp} gene cloned from *Dictyostelium discoideum:* Its nucleotide sequence and association with repetitive DNA. *Biochemistry* **20**:4015–4021.

Pribnow, D. 1975. Nucleotide sequence of an RNA polymerase binding site at an early T_7 promoter. *Proc. Natl. Acad. Sci. USA* **72**:784–788.

Proudfoot, N. J., and Maniatis, T. 1980. The structure of a human α-globin pseudogene and its relationship to α-globin gene duplication. *Cell* **21**:537–554.

Proudfoot, N. J., Shander, M. H. M., Manley, J. L., Gefter, M. L., and Maniatis, T. 1980. Structure and *in vitro* transcription of human globin genes. *Science* **209**:1329–1336.

Quincey, R. V., and Wilson, S. H. 1969. The utilization of genes for rRNA, 5S RNA, and tRNA in liver cells of adult rats. *Proc. Natl. Acad. Sci. USA* **64**:981–988.

Rogers, J., and Wall, R. 1980. A mechanism for RNA splicing. *Proc. Natl. Acad. Sci. USA* **77**:1877–1879.

Ross, J., and Knecht, D. A. 1978. Precursors of α and β globin messenger RNAs. *J. Mol. Biol.* **119**:1–20.

Sanderson, K. E. 1967. Revised linkage map of *Salmonella typhimurium. Bacteriol. Rev.* **31**:354–372.

Sassone-Corsi, P., Corden, J., Kédinger, C., and Chambon, P. 1981. Promotion of specific *in vitro* transcription by excised "TATA" box sequences inserted in a foreign nucleotide environment. *Nucleic Acids Res.* **9**:3941–3958.

Schmelzer, C., Haid, A., Grosch, G., Schweyen, R. J., and Kaudewitz, F. 1981. Pathways of transcript splicing in yeast mitochondria. *J. Biol. Chem.* **256**:7610–7619.

Schwarz, Z., Kössel, H., Schwarz, E., and Bogorad, L. 1981. A gene coding for tRNA^{Val} is located near 5' terminus of 16S rRNA gene in *Zea mays* chloroplast genome. *Proc. Natl. Acad. Sci. USA* **78**:4748–4752.

Schweizer, E., MacKechnie, C., and Halvorson, H. O. 1969. The redundancy of the ribosomal and transfer RNA genes in *Saccharomyces cerevisiae. J. Mol. Biol.* **40**:261–277.

Sekiya, T., and Nishimura, S. 1979. Sequence of the gene for isoleucine tRNA$_1$ at the surrounding region in a ribosomal RNA operon of *E. coli. Nucleic Acids Res.* **6**:575–592.

Sekiya, T., Gait, M. J., Noris, K., Rammamoorthy, B., and Khorana, H. G. 1976. The nucleotide sequence in the promoter region for the gene for an *Escherichia coli* tyrosine transfer RNA. *J. Biol. Chem.* **251**:4481–4489.

Sekiya, T., Mori, M., Takahashi, N., and Nishimura, S. 1980. Sequence of the distal tRNA$_1^{\text{Asp}}$ gene and the transcription termination signal in the *E. coli* ribosomal RNA operon rrn F (or G). *Nucleic Acids Res.* **8**:3809–3827.

Sekiya, T., Kuchino, Y., and Nishimura, S. 1981. Mammalian tRNA genes: Nucleotide sequence of rat genes for tRNA^{Asp}, tRNA^{Gly}, and tRNA^{Glu}. *Nucleic Acids Res.* **9**:2239–2250.

Sharp, S., DeFranco, D., Dingermann, T., Farrell, P., and Söll, D. 1981. Internal control regions for transcription of eukaryotic tRNA genes. *Proc. Natl. Acad. Sci. USA* **78**:6657–6661.

Shen, C. K. J., and Maniatis, T. 1980. Tissue-specific DNA methylation in a cluster of rabbit β-like globin genes. *Proc. Natl. Acad. Sci. USA* **77**:6634–6638.

Slightom, J. L., Blechl, A. E., and Smithies, O. 1980. Human fetal $^Gγ$- and $^Aγ$-globin genes: Complete nucleotide sequences suggest that DNA can be exchanged between these duplicated genes. *Cell* **21**:627–638.

Smith, G. H., and Vonderhaar, B. K. 1981. Functional differentiation in mouse mammary gland epithelium is attained through DNA synthesis, inconsequent of mitosis. *Dev. Biol.* **88**:167–179.

Snyder, M., Hirsh, J., and Davidson, N. 1981. The cuticle genes of *Drosophila:* A developmentally regulated gene cluster. *Cell* **25**:165–177.

Spencer, D. F., Bonen, L., and Gray, M. W. 1981. Primary sequence of wheat mitochondrial 5S ribosomal RNA: Functional and evolutionary implications. *Biochemistry* **20**:4022–4029.

Spohr, G., Reith, W., and Sures, I. 1981. Organization and sequence analysis of a cluster of repetitive DNA elements from *Xenopus laevis. J. Mol. Biol.* **151**:573–592.

Spritz, R. A., deRiel, J. K., Forget, B. G., and Weissman, S. M. 1980. Complete nucleotide sequence of the human δ-globin gene. *Cell* **21**:639–646.

Squires, C., Konrad, B., Kirschbaum, J., and Carbon, J. 1973. Three adjacent tRNA genes in *E. coli. Proc. Natl. Acad. Sci. USA* **70**:438–441.

Steinmetz, M., and Zachau, H. G. 1980. Two rearranged immunoglobulin kappa light chain genes in one mouse myeloma. *Nucleic Acids Res.* **8**:1693–1707.

Stephenson, E. C., Erba, H. P., and Gall, J. G. 1981. Histone gene clusters of the newt *Notophthalmus* are separated by long tracts of satellite DNA. *Cell* **24**:639–647.

Tanksley, S. D., Zamir, D., and Rick, C. M. 1981. Evidence for extensive overlap of sporophytic and gametophytic gene expression in *Lycopersicum esculentum. Science* **213**:453–455.

Valbuena, O., Marcu, K. B., Weigert, M., and Perry, R. P. 1978. Multiplicity of germline genes specifying a group of related mouse κ chains with implications for the generation of immunoglobulin diversity. *Nature (London)* **276**:780–784.

Valenzuela, P., Venegas, A., Weinberg, F., Bishop, R., and Rutter, W. J. 1978. Structure of yeast phenylalanine-tRNA genes: An intervening DNA segment within the region coding for the tRNA. *Proc. Natl. Acad. Sci. USA* **75**:190–194.

Van Arsdell, S. W., Denison, R. A., Bernstein, L. B., Weiner, A. M., Manser, T., and Gesteland, R. F. 1981. Direct repeats flank three small nuclear RNA pseudogenes in the human genome. *Cell* **26**:11–17.

van Ooyen, A, van den Berg, J., Mantei, N., and Weissman, C. 1979. Comparisons of total sequence of a cloned rabbit β-globin gene and its flanking regions with a homologous mouse sequence. *Science* **206**:337–344.

Villeponteau, B., and Martinson, H. 1981. Isolation and characterization of the complete chicken β-globin gene region: Frequent deletion of adult β-globin genes in λ. *Nucleic Acids Res.* **9**:3731–3746.

Weber, A. L., and Miller, S. L. 1981. Reasons for the occurrence of the twenty coded protein amino acids. *J. Mol. Evol.* **17**:273–284.

Weigert, M. G., and Riblet, R. 1976. Genetic control of antibody variable regions. *Cold Spring Harbor Symp. Quant. Biol.* **41**:837–846.

Weigert, M. G., Cesari, H. M., Yonkovich, S. J., and Cohn, M. 1970. Variability in the lambda light chain sequences of mouse antibody. *Nature (London)* **228**:1045–1047.

Weigert, M. G., Gatmaitan, L., Loh, E., Schilling, J., and Hood, L. 1978. Rearrangement of genetic information may produce immunoglobulin diversity. *Nature (London)* **276**:785–790.

Wilson, J. T., deRiel, J. K., Forget, B. G., Marotta, C. A., and Weissman, S. M. 1977. Nucleotide sequence of 3′ untranslated portion of human alpha globin mRNA. *Nucleic Acids Res.* **4**:2353–2368.

Wilson, J. T., Wilson, L. B., Reddy, V. B., Cavallesco, C., Ghosh, P. K., deRiel, J. K., Forget, B. G., and Weissman, S. M. 1980. Nucleotide sequence of the coding portion of a human α globin mRNA. *J. Biol. Chem.* **255**:2807–2815.

Wortzman, M. S., and Baker, R. F. 1980. Specific sequences within single-stranded regions in the sea urchin embryo genome. *Biochim. Biophys. Acta* **609**:84–96.

Wortzman, M. S., and Baker, R. F. 1981. Two classes of single-stranded regions in DNA from sea urchin embryos. *Science* **211**:588–590.

Yao, M. C., and Yao, C. H. 1981. Repeated hexanucleotide C—C—C—C—A—A is present near free ends of macronuclear DNA of *Tetrahymena*. *Proc. Natl. Acad. Sci. USA* **78**:7436–7439.

Yao, M. C., Blackburn, E., and Gall, J. 1981. Tandemly repeated C—C—C—C—A—A hexanucleotide of *Tetrahymena* rDNA is present elsewhere in the genome and may be related to the alteration of the somatic genome. *J. Cell Biol.* **90**:515–520.

Yao, M. C. 1982. Elimination of specific DNA sequences from the somatic nucleus of the ciliate *Tetrahymena*. *J. Cell Biol.* **92**:783–789.

Young, J. R., Donelson, J. E., Majiwa, P. A. O., Shapiro, S. Z., and Williams, R. O. 1982. Analysis of genomic rearrangements associated with two variable antigen genes of *Trypanosoma*. *Nucl. Acids Res.* **10**:803–809.

Zimmer, E. H., Martin, S., Beverly, S. M., Kan, Y. W., and Wilson, A. C. 1980. Rapid duplication and loss of genes coding for the α chains of hemoglobin. *Proc. Natl. Acad. Sci. USA* **77**:2158–2162.

Index

Page numbers in **bold** type refer to illustrations.